Pathogenicity Islands
and Other Mobile Virulence Elements

Pathogenicity Islands and Other Mobile Virulence Elements

EDITED BY

James B. Kaper

Center for Vaccine Development
and Department of Microbiology and Immunology
University of Maryland School of Medicine
Baltimore, Maryland

AND

Jörg Hacker

Institut für Molekulare Infektionsbiologie
Universität Würzburg
Würzburg, Germany

ASM PRESS

WASHINGTON, D.C.

Library of Congress Cataloging-in-Publication Data

Pathogenicity islands and other mobile virulence elements / edited by
    James B. Kaper and Jörg Hacker.
            p.   cm.
    Includes bibliographical references and index.
    ISBN 1-55581-161-2 (hardcover)
    1. Virulence (Microbiology)—Molecular aspects.   2. Bacterial
genetics.   3. Mobile genetic elements.   4. Plasmids.   I. Kaper,
James B.   II. Hacker, Jörg (Jörg Hinrich).
QR175.P375   1999
616'.014—dc21   99-24324
                                                       CIP

Cover photo: Enteropathogenic *Escherichia coli* (EPEC) inducing pedestal formation on cultured epithelial cells. This phenotype, which is seen as an ''attaching and effacing'' histopathology in intestinal specimens from patients infected with EPEC, is encoded by the locus of enterocyte efface-ment (LEE) pathogenicity island. The long filaments radiating from the bacterial cell are the type III secretion system translocon, encoded on the LEE, which is believed to serve as the conduit for effector proteins to be translocated from the bacterial cell to the eukaryotic cell. Courtesy of Stuart Knutton, University of Birmingham.

CONTENTS

CONTRIBUTORS

Reiko Akakura • Section of Microbiology, Cornell University, Ithaca, New York 14853

Anne-Béatrice Blanc-Potard • Department of Molecular Microbiology, Howard Hughes Medical Institute, Washington University School of Medicine, St. Louis, Missouri 63110

Gabriele Blum-Oehler • Institut für Molekulare Infektionsbiologie, Universität Würzburg, Röntgenring 11, D-97070 Würzburg, Germany

George Bonheyo • Department of Microbiology, University of Illinois, Urbana, Illinois 61801

Veit Braun • Institut für Medizinische Mikrobiologie und Hygiene, Johannes-Gutenberg-Universität Mainz, D-55101 Mainz, Germany

Daniela Brem • Max von Pettenkofer-Institut für Hygiene und Mikrobiologie, Ludwig-Maximilians-Universität München, Pettenkoferstrasse 9a, D-80336 Munich, Germany

Brian F. Cheetham • Division of Molecular and Cellular Biology, School of Biological Sciences, University of New England, Armidale, New South Wales 2351, Australia

Guy R. Cornelis • Microbial Pathogenesis Unit, Christian de Duve Institute of Cellular Pathology and Faculty of Medicine, Catholic University of Louvain, B-1200 Brussels, Belgium

Antonello Covacci • Department of Molecular Biology, Immunobiological Research Institute of Siena, Chiron Vaccines, Via Fiorentina 1, 53100 Siena, Italy

Jorge Frias • Department of Microbiology, University of Illinois, Urbana, Illinois 61801

Werner Goebel • Lehrstuhl für Mikrobiologie, Biozentrum Universität Würzburg, D-97074 Würzburg, Germany

Friedrich Götz • Mikrobielle Genetik, Universität Tübingen, Auf der Morgenstelle 28, D-72076 Tübingen, Germany

Eduardo A. Groisman • Department of Molecular Microbiology, Howard Hughes Medical Institute, Washington University School of Medicine, St. Louis, Missouri 63110

Jörg Hacker • Institut für Molekulare Infektionsbiologie, Universität Würzburg, Röntgenring 11, D-97070 Würzburg, Germany

Jürgen Heesemann • Max von Pettenkofer-Institut für Hygiene und Mikrobiologie, Ludwig-Maximilians-Universität München, Pettenkoferstrasse 9a, D-80336 Munich, Germany

Steven W. Hutcheson • Department of Cell Biology and Molecular Genetics, Microbiology Building, University of Maryland, College Park, Maryland 20742

Maite Iriarte   •   Microbial Pathogenesis Unit, Christian de Duve Institute of Cellular Pathology and Faculty of Medicine, Catholic University of Louvain, B-1200 Brussels, Belgium

Samina Jafri   •   Section of Microbiology, Cornell University, Ithaca, New York 14853

Britta Janke   •   Institut für Molekulare Infektionsbiologie, Universität Würzburg, Röntgenring 11, D-97070 Würzburg, Germany

Virginia Kalogeraki   •   Section of Microbiology, Cornell University, Ithaca, New York 14853

James B. Kaper   •   Center for Vaccine Development and Department of Microbiology and Immunology, University of Maryland School of Medicine, 685 West Baltimore Street, Baltimore, Maryland 21201

David K. R. Karaolis   •   Division of Hospital Epidemiology, University of Maryland School of Medicine, Baltimore, Maryland 21201

Margaret E. Katz   •   Division of Molecular and Cellular Biology, School of Biological Sciences, University of New England, Armidale, New South Wales 2351, Australia

Jürgen Kreft   •   Lehrstuhl für Mikrobiologie, Biozentrum Universität Würzburg, D-97074 Würzburg, Germany

Jay L. Mellies   •   Center for Vaccine Development and Department of Microbiology and Immunology, University of Maryland School of Medicine, 685 West Baltimore Street, Baltimore, Maryland 21201

Gabor Nagy   •   Institut für Molekulare Infektionsbiologie, Universität Würzburg, Röntgenring 11, D-97070 Würzburg, Germany

James P. Nataro   •   Center for Vaccine Development and Department of Pediatrics, University of Maryland School of Medicine, Baltimore, Maryland 21201

Eva Ng   •   Lehrstuhl für Mikrobiologie, Biozentrum Universität Würzburg, D-97074 Würzburg, Germany

Knut Ohlsen   •   Institut für Molekulare Infektionsbiologie, Universität Würzburg, Röntgenring 11, D-97070 Würzburg, Germany

Claude Parsot   •   Unité de Pathogénie Microbienne Moléculaire, Unité INSERM U389, Institut Pasteur, 25 rue du Dr Roux, 75724 Paris Cedex 15, France

Cosima Pelludat   •   Max von Pettenkofer-Institut für Hygiene und Mikrobiologie, Ludwig-Maximilians-Universität München, Pettenkoferstrasse 9a, D-80336 Munich, Germany

Alexander Rakin   •   Max von Pettenkofer-Institut für Hygiene und Mikrobiologie, Ludwig-Maximilians-Universität München, Pettenkoferstrasse 9a, D-80336 Munich, Germany

Rino Rappuoli   •   Department of Molecular Biology, Immunobiological Research Institute of Siena, Chiron Vaccines, Via Fiorentina 1, 53100 Siena, Italy

Werner Reichardt   •   Institut für Experimentelle Mikrobiologie, Friedrich-Schiller-Universität Jena, Winzerlaer Strasse 10, 07745 Jena, Germany

Joachim Reidl   •   Zentrum für Infektionsforschung, Universität Würzburg, Röntgenring 11, D-97070 Würzburg, Germany

Abigail Salyers   •   Department of Microbiology, University of Illinois, Urbana, Illinois 61801

Philippe J. Sansonetti   •   Unité de Pathogénie Microbienne Moléculaire, Unité INSERM U389, Institut Pasteur, 25 rue du Dr Roux, 75724 Paris Cedex 15, France

Sören Schubert   •   Max von Pettenkofer-Institut für Hygiene und Mikrobiologie, Ludwig-Maximilians-Universität München, Pettenkoferstrasse 9a, D-80336 Munich, Germany

Nadja Shoemaker   •   Department of Microbiology, University of Illinois, Urbana, Illinois 61801

Keiichi Uchiya   •   Department of Molecular Microbiology, Howard Hughes Medical Institute, Washington University School of Medicine, St. Louis, Missouri 63110

José-Antonio Vázquez-Boland   •   Grupo de Patogénesis Molecular Bacteriana, Microbiología e Inmunología, Facultad de Veterinaria, Universidad Complutense de Madrid, E-28040 Madrid, Spain

Christoph von Eichel-Streiber   •   Institut für Medizinische Mikrobiologie und Hygiene, Johannes-Gutenberg-Universität Mainz, D-55101 Mainz, Germany

Gabrielle Whittle   •   Division of Molecular and Cellular Biology, School of Biological Sciences, University of New England, Armidale, New South Wales 2351, Australia

Stephen C. Winans   •   Section of Microbiology, Cornell University, Ithaca, New York 14853

Wolfgang Witte   •   Robert-Koch-Institut, Bereich Wernigerode, Burgstrasse 37, 38855 Wernigerode, Germany

Qi Xia   •   Section of Microbiology, Cornell University, Ithaca, New York 14853

Wilma Ziebuhr   •   Institut für Molekulare Infektionsbiologie, Universität Würzburg, Röntgenring 11, D-97070 Würzburg, Germany

FOREWORD

Pathogenicity Islands and Other Mobile Virulence Elements contains a collection of chapters by some of the very best students of pathogenic microbes. The broadly termed concept of pathogenicity islands was clearly enunciated less than 10 years ago and has provided us with an intellectual springboard to understand the professional bacterial pathogen more clearly than ever before. The idea of pathogenicity islands arrives along with the new age of microbial genomics, in which the complete genetic blueprint of virtually all bacterial pathogens will be solved (at least once, anyway) in the next 5 years. The development of new molecular methods to identify genes and the marriage of cell biology and cellular immunology to study host-parasite interactions from the earliest moments of contact to the agonal phase of disease bring us to the brink of being able to describe microbial infection in fairly complete biological terms.

A given bacterial pathogen appears to be a clone or cell line, and disease outbreaks and increases in infection frequency can be traced to distinct bacterial subclones that typically possess unique combinations of virulence genes. Multilocus electrophoretic studies and now DNA sequencing data support the idea that many pathogenic bacteria actually manifest a relatively limited set of additional genes compared to commensal species of the same taxonomic group. This observation suggests that pathogens probably arose by descent from a single progenitor, rather than by convergence from a number of different progenitors arising by constant gene flow. By no means does this suggest that genetic variation is stultified in bacterial pathogens; rather, temporal variation in disease frequency and severity is often associated with clonal replacement, much as influenza epidemics are driven by antigenic shifts. The basic platform of virulence genes, however, remains generally intact, and the disease remains a reflection of a relatively few fundamental effector molecules. These effectors are usually proteins with some enzymatic capacity to alter a host defense system or a surface molecule designed to thwart the same or other host defenses. On one hand, bacteria are rather cautious about bestowing their unique constellation of virulence attributes on other microbes, even those closely related to them. On the other hand, when faced with the fact that bacterial pathogens usually possess distinct constellations of genes absent from commensal species, we have had to ask, "Where do the pathogenicity sequences come from?"

We have known for some time that bacterial plasmids play a key role as carriers of essential components of pathogenicity in the haploid world of bacteria. Some virulence genes are even part of mobile transposons, which span the worlds of the extrachromosomal element and the chromosomal mass. However, I do not think we expected to find that pathogens—at least gram-negative ones—almost universally carry large inserts of DNA called pathogenicity islands, which are totally absent from nonpathogenic members of the same and closely related genera. The chapters in this volume document the extraordinary flowering of thought and definitive information that has arisen since the concept of the pathogenicity island was first suggested by Jörg Hacker and his colleagues. The initial observations made with uropathogenic *Escherichia coli* were promptly extended to other pathogenic *E. coli* strains and then to salmonellae. As documented in this volume, the number of pathogenic species shown to possess pathogenicity islands has grown to encompass a significant number of pathogenic microorganisms of humans, plants, and animals.

A pathogenicity island is a large insert of DNA that contains a number of essential virulence genes. Usually there is a precise junction between the ends of the unique genes found in a pathogenicity island and chromosomal genes common to both commensal and pathogenic species of the same genus or even family of bacteria. Often, but not always, the pathogenicity island DNA inserts are adjacent to a tRNA locus that encodes an uncommon amino acid or an uncommon codon used by the species. Almost without exception, the DNA composition of the pathogenicity island differs markedly from the overall DNA composition pattern of the rest of the chromosome, which suggests that pathogenicity island DNA is "alien" to the host chromosome. Remarkably, significant homologs of the effector-encoding genes on plasmids found in pathogenic yersiniae and shigellae are found in the chromosomal pathogenicity islands in enteropathogenic *E. coli*, *Salmonella typhimurium*, and *Salmonella typhi*.

What has emerged from the availability of DNA sequence information is the realization that pathogenicity islands and DNA inserts into virulence plasmids encode a defined secretory pathway (type III and type IV secretory systems), often complete with regulatory elements and molecular ushers to bring about the transport of a set of effector genes to a location on the bacterial surface juxtaposed with a specific receptor on the host cell. In several cases, the secretory system is known to be keyed to specific environmental cues and cellular contact so that the pathogenicity island is mobilized in the most efficient and, in one sense, most deadly way. The most conserved regions of the chromosomal pathogenicity islands and their plasmid counterparts are the secretory pathways, while the effector molecules show more in the way of individuality consonant with the characteristics and specificity of each pathogenic species. It is almost as if there were a common secretory platform into which was inserted a cassette of different effector (specialized) genes that provided the microorganism with a selective advantage. After all, pathogenicity is a selective advantage in the sense that the pathogen, unlike its commensal relative, has the advantage of occupying a niche within a host that is usually devoid of most other microbial competitors and is rich in nutrients. The pathogen gains this niche by virtue of the genes it employs to breach the host cellular and anatomic barriers, as well as avoiding, circumventing, or subverting host defense mechanisms.

Not only has the examination of pathogenicity islands helped us to appreciate a common theme in bacterial pathogenicity, but it provides us with a glimpse into what might have been the evolution of pathogenicity as a molecular specialization. For example, the examination of the evolution of *Escherichia*, *Salmonella*, and *Shigella* from a common ancestor puts an interesting new light on how pathogens "got that way." From the examination of DNA sequences and the measurement of divergence, it appears that some 130 million years ago an ancestral facultative microorganism, which had learned to colonize the gastrointestinal tract, split off into two distinct clones, one to become the escherichiae and the other to become the modern-day salmonellae. This split appears to coincide with the acquisition of a pathogenicity island, now termed SPI-1, which provided this microbe, now called *Salmonella bongori*, with the ability to breach the epithelial barrier of the small bowel, possibly the Peyer's patch equivalent of birds and cold-blooded animals. The next evolutionary step for the salmonellae followed the acquisition of yet another distinct pathogenicity island, now termed SPI-2, which permitted the organism to survive and replicate within resident phagocytic cells just beyond the epithelial barrier. It is from this ancestral line that the second clonal *Salmonella* emerged to become modern-day *Salmonella enterica*. The story does not end here; it is still in the process of being written in the pages that follow and in years to come. Some salmonellae that inhabited warm-blooded animals also inherited a plasmid that contributes to systemic spread and survival in the host animal. More to the point, the examination of the *Salmonella* chromosome goes on to reveal the presence of other DNA insertions acquired at different times in the course of evolution that seem to contribute to both the unique attributes of particular salmonellae and, in the more general sense, the capacity of these bacteria to become specialists in intracellular life, survival, and long-term colonization of the host. The clone we call *Shigella* broke off from the escherichiae with the acquisition of a virulence plasmid some 90 million years ago. It is remarkable that the plasmid virulence genes are closely homologous to the SPI-1 pathogenicity island, both in the order of genes and in the function of their effector molecules. Pathogenicity islands seem likely to have been mobile in their own right at some time in evolution. As we trace the homology pathway of virulence genes, we come away with the idea that some parts of the secretory pathway common in many gram-negative bacteria must have derived from flagellar genes. Perhaps of more interest, many plant pathogens contain pathogenicity islands that are clearly related to those found in the pathogens of humans. What new wonders will unfold in the next 10 years of study of these islands?

The concept of the pathogenicity island swiftly has brought a new chapter to the study of the biology of parasitism. Pathogenicity islands, despite their large size, probably do not contain sufficient information to convert a commensal into a pathogen in one genetic event. Determinants on extrachromosomal elements and other blocks of DNA somehow come together in a particular clone, leading to the emergence of a cell line that can occupy a new, unique niche in a host animal. Yet the pathogenicity island represents a large piece of the puzzle, the piece that sometimes turns a maze of indistinct shapes into a recognizable picture. It is not likely a coincidence that the discovery of pathogenicity islands and pathogenicity islets occurred as one of the initial findings of the genomic era. The concept of the pathogenicity island also influences our thinking as the study of bacteria inexorably wends its way from studies in the confines of the laboratory container to the real world, including the tissues of infected animal hosts. This volume represents one of the first serious compendia of scientific research concerned with the discovery and characterization of pathogenicity islands from a variety of microbial species. I recommend that you read this book in the spirit of discovery suggested by Thomas Huxley: "Sit down before fact as a little child, be prepared to give up every preconceived notion, follow humbly wherever and to whatever abysses nature leads, or you shall learn nothing."

Stanley Falkow
Department of Microbiology and Immunology
Stanford University School of Medicine

Pathogenicity Islands and Other Mobile Virulence Elements
Edited by J. B. Kaper and J. Hacker
© 1999 American Society for Microbiology, Washington, D.C.

Chapter 1

The Concept of Pathogenicity Islands

Jörg Hacker and James B. Kaper

FROM TAXONOMY TO PATHOGENICITY

In traditional microbiology, a pathogen is defined as a member of a certain species with the capacity to cause infectious disease. This taxonomic approach was developed by Robert Koch (1843–1910) and his mentor, Ferdinand Cohn (1828–1898), at the end of the nineteenth century for so-called obligate pathogens and was based on the taxonomic status of infectious agents such as anthrax bacilli, mycobacteria, and cholera bacteria (20). It soon became obvious that especially in species whose members belong to the group of so-called facultative pathogens, e.g., *Escherichia coli,* staphylococci, and *Pseudomonas,* there were differences in the pathogenic potential between isolates and variants of the same species. These differences included important pathogenic functions such as host cell adherence, invasion capacity, and toxin production (10). Several observations led to the conclusion that specific genes which encode the corresponding pathogenicity factors, e.g., adhesins, invasins, and toxins, should be present in the genome of pathogenic members of a particular genus or species but absent in nonpathogenic variants (39). Since the discovery of virulence plasmids and toxin-converting phages in the 1950s and 1960s, it was accepted that "virulence-associated genes" can be members of extrachromosomal elements and are horizontally transferable (31, 38). In the early 1980s it was discovered that chromosomal regions may carry blocks of virulence-associated genes and may differ between related members of certain species or genera (14, 24). These regions were termed pathogenicity islands (PAIs) (15).

WHAT IS A PATHOGENICITY ISLAND?

The basic observation leading to the concept of PAIs was the finding that particular genomic regions of pathogens carry virulence-associated genes together with loci whose presence strongly indicates horizontal gene transfer of these regions between different species or even genera. The concept of PAIs was developed on the basis of data on genome structure and pathogenicity of pathogenic enterobacteria, especially pathogenic *E. coli* (3,

Jörg Hacker • Institut für Molekulare Infektionsbiologie, Universität Würzburg, Röntgenring 11, D-97070 Würzburg, Germany. *James B. Kaper* • Center for Vaccine Development and Department of Microbiology and Immunology, University of Maryland School of Medicine, 685 W. Baltimore St., Baltimore, MD 21201.

4, 26) (see chapters 3 and 4). However, it also seems to be valid for other gram-negative and gram-positive pathogens. From our point of view, PAIs represent distinct pieces of DNA, which have most if not all of the following features in common (16).

- PAIs carry genes encoding one or more virulence factors. As indicated in Table 1, different types of virulence factors, i.e., adhesins, invasins, iron uptake systems, toxins, and type III and IV protein secretion systems, are encoded by PAIs. It is likely that additional types of PAI-encoded virulence factors will be discovered.
- PAIs are present in the genome of pathogenic bacteria but absent from the genome of nonpathogenic members of the same or a closely related species. PAIs were first found as chromosomal regions, but the increasing amount of sequence data also available for virulence plasmids seems to support the view that parts of virulence plasmids may also be considered PAIs. This is true for the invasion region of *Shigella* plasmids, the Yop-encoding DNA of *Yersinia* plasmids, and the T-DNA of Ti plasmids of *Agrobacterium* (see chapters 6, 8, and 15).
- PAIs occupy relatively large genomic regions. The majority of PAIs cover DNA regions of 10 to 20 kb to 200 kb or more, which may reflect the introduction of large DNA pieces via horizontal gene transfer into new hosts. Strains of certain bacterial species with different pathogenic potency, however, may also carry insertions of small pieces of DNA, 1 to 10 kb, which may encode virulence factors. These small pieces of DNA, in contrast to the larger islands, have been termed islets (13, 29). From a heuristic point of view, it seems to be useful to distinguish between the islands and islets. Thus, the 1.6-kb *sifA* region or fimbrial gene clusters of *Salmonella typhimurium* (2, 40) or the 6.0-kb element carrying the fragilysin gene of *Bacteroides fragilis* (29) should be considered islets rather than islands.
- PAIs very often consist of DNA sequences which differ from the rest of the genome by differences in the G+C content and by different codon usage. This property reflects the generation of PAIs by horizontal gene transfer. During evolution, however, the G+C content and

Table 1. Virulence features encoded by PAIs

Virulence feature	Examples
Adherence factor	Diarrheagenic *E. coli*, UPEC, *V. cholerae*, *Listeria* spp.
Toxin	UPEC, *S. aureus*
Iron uptake system	UPEC, *S. flexneri*, *Yersinia* spp.
Invasion	Diarrheagenic *E. coli*, *Salmonella* spp., *Shigella* spp., *Listeria* spp.
Type II secretion system	Enterohemorrhagic *E. coli*
Type III secretion system	Diarrheagenic *E. coli*, *P. syringae*, *Erwinia* spp., *Yersinia* spp., *Salmonella* spp., *Shigella* spp.
Type IV secretion system	*H. pylori*

the codon usage of newly acquired DNA have the tendency to assume properties similar to the rest of the host genome. It is trivial but necessary to mention here that differences in G+C content between PAIs and the core genome will not be seen if the DNAs of the donors and recipients have similar or identical G+C consensus. It is also possible that a codon usage pattern for virulence genes that differs from codon usage in housekeeping genes will offer an advantage in virulence gene expression during the course of infection (8, 35).

- PAIs represent distinct genetic elements often flanked by small directly repeated (DR) DNA sequences. These sequences may be generated following integration of PAI-specific DNA regions into the host genome via recombination.

- PAIs are often associated with tRNA genes. In many prokaryotic and some eukaryotic organisms, tRNA genes often act as target sites for the integration of foreign DNA. This also seems to be true for processes leading to PAI formation. In addition, the 3′ regions of tRNA loci are often identical to attachment sites for bacteriophages (7, 36). The association of PAIs and tRNA genes and the occurrence of even cryptic phage integrase genes next to the tRNA loci may indicate that many PAIs or parts of PAIs represent bacteriophage-derived elements.

- PAIs often carry cryptic or functional genes encoding mobility factors such as integrases, transposases, or parts of insertion elements (IS elements). PAIs often do not represent homogeneous pieces of DNA but, rather, are made up of mosaic-like structures which have been generated by multistep processes including DNA rearrangements via IS elements. While the presence of phage integrase genes on PAIs illustrates that PAIs may represent former phages, the occurrence of (often cryptic) plasmid origins as well as transfer genes argues for the existence of plasmid-derived PAIs.

- PAIs often represent unstable DNA regions. Deletions of PAIs may occur via the DR sequences at their ends or via IS elements and other homologous sequences located in PAIs. In *Yersinia pseudotuberculosis,* PAIs can move from one tRNA target site to another within a matter of days (5) (see chapter 5). PAIs of staphylococci and *V. cholerae* can be mobilized and transmitted by bacteriophages (see chapters 9 and 14). Whenever PAIs are able to replicate or even spread autonomously between strains, they seem to represent integrated plasmids, conjugative transposons, or bacteriophages.

WHERE ARE PATHOGENICITY ISLANDS FOUND?

PAIs occur in the genomes of various pathogens with the capacity to cause infections not only in humans but also in animals and even in plants. The list of PAIs described up to now (Table 2) includes those in bacteria for which frequent gene transfer via plasmids, bacteriophages, and conjugative transposons has been described. It seems that PAIs do not frequently occur in species with natural competence which take up DNA via transfor-

Table 2. PAIs and PAI-associated genes of various pathogens

Organism[a]	Description	Functions	Size (kb)	Junction	Associated sequence(s)
E. coli 536 (UPEC)	PAI I$_{536}$	Hemolysin	70	DR 16 bp	*selC*
E. coli 536 (UPEC)	PAI II$_{536}$	Hemolysin, P fimbriae	190	DR 18 bp	*leuX*
E. coli 536 (UPEC)	PAI III$_{536}$	S fimbriae	25		*thrW*
E. coli 536 (UPEC)	PAI IV$_{536}$	Yersiniabactin synthesis, uptake	45		*asnT*
E. coli J96 (UPEC)	PAI I$_{J96}$	Hemolysin, P fimbriae	170		*pheV*
E. coli J96 (UPEC)	PAI II$_{J96}$	Hemolysin, P fimbriae, cytotoxic necrotizing factor 1	110	DR 135 bp	*pheR*
E. coli CFT073 (UPEC)	PAI I$_{CFT073}$	Hemolysin, P fimbriae	58	DR 9 bp	*metV*
E. coli K1	*kps* PAI	Capsule	ND[b]		*pheV*
E. coli E2348/69 (EPEC)	LEE	Type III secretion, invasion	35		*selC*
E. coli O157:H7 (EHEC)	LEE	Type III secretion, invasion	43		*selC*
E. coli EPEC2	LEE	Type III secretion, invasion	>35		*pheU*
E. coli ETEC	Tia-PAI	Invasion	46		*selC*
Y. enterocolitica	HPI	Yersiniabactin synthesis, transport	43		*asnT*
Y. pseudotuberculosis	HPI	Yersiniabactin synthesis, transport	36	DR 16 bp	*asnTUW*
Y. pestis	HPI (*pgm* locus)	Yersiniabactin synthesis, transport; hemin uptake	102	IS*100*, DR 16 bp	*asnT*
Yersinia spp.	Yop virulon	Type III secretion, effectors (YOPs)	47	IS elements	Plasmid
S. flexneri 2a	SHI I	Enterotoxin, immunoglobulin A protease	51	IS elements	
S. flexneri	SHI II	Aerobactin synthesis, transport	ND		*selC*

Table 2. *Continued*

Organism[a]	Description	Functions	Size (kb)	Junction	Associated sequence(s)
Shigella spp.	Entry region	Type III secretion, invasion	37		Plasmids
S. enterica	SPI-1	Type III secretion, invasion into epithelial cells, apoptosis	40		
S. enterica	SPI-2	Type III secretion, invasion into monocytes	40		*valV*
S. enterica	SPI-3	Invasion, survival in monocytes	17		*selC*
S. enterica	SPI-4	Invasion, survival in monocytes	25		Putative tRNA gene
V. cholerae	VPI	Tcp adhesin, regulator	40	DR 136 bp	*ssrA*
H. pylori	*cag* PAI	Type IV secretion, *cag* antigen	40	DR 31 bp	*glr*
C. difficile	PaLoc	Large clostridal cytotoxins	20		
D. nodosus	*vap* region	Vap antigens	12	DR 19 bp	*serV*
D. nodosus	*vrl* region	Vrl antigens	27		
P. syringae	*hrp* cluster	Type III secretion, effectors	35		
Erwinia spp.	*hrp* cluster	Type III secretion, effectors			
A. tumefaciens	T-DNA	Crown gall tumor induction, opine production	20	DR 25 bp	Plasmid
L. ivanovii	*vis* gene cluster	Internalins, sphinomyelinase	23		
S. aureus	SaPI1	Toxic shock syndrome toxin 1, putative superantigen	15.2	DR 17 bp	

[a] EPEC, enteropathogenic *E. coli*; EHEC, enterohemorrhagic *E. coli*; ETEC, enterotoxigenic *E. coli*.
[b] ND, not determined.

mation, such as *Streptococcus pneumoniae, Haemophilus influenzae, Neisseria gonorrhoeae,* and *N. meningitis.* In these organisms, small pieces of DNA seem to be continually introduced into their genomes by homologous recombination, leading to new variants of genes such as new pilin genes of *N. gonorrhoeae* (28) and novel variants of penicillin-binding protein genes of *S. pneumoniae* (30). It is obvious from Table 2 that PAIs occur in a wide spectrum of species, most of which are gram negative. Recent observations, however, indicate that PAIs exhibiting the ''classical'' features mentioned above are also present in a number of gram-positive species such as *Listeria ivanovii* and *Staphylococcus aureus* (see chapters 12 and 14).

As shown for uropathogenic *E. coli* (UPEC), bacterial PAIs may even carry gene clusters specific for eukaryotic organisms, such as intron sequences (see chapter 4). However, it is not known whether genomic regions comparable to PAIs also exist in genomes of eukaryotic pathogens such as parasites or pathogenic fungi. The existence of PAIs in eukaryotic pathogens can be predicted, because gene transfer also exists in eukaryotic organisms, transposable elements frequently occur, and retroviruses have a tendency to integrate into tRNA genes (25). All these processes lead to a plasticity of the genomes of eukaryotes which, in general, is a prerequisite for the development of PAIs in various organisms.

PRE-, POST-, AND REAL PATHOGENICITY ISLANDS: WHAT MAKES THE DIFFERENCE?

The various PAIs of different microorganisms (Table 2) have a number of common features. On the one hand, they represent a rather heterogeneous group of DNA elements which can vary in size, composition, encoded functions, and boundary sequences. While some PAIs, such as those of *Salmonella enterica* or the locus of enterocyte effacement (LEE) element of diarrheagenic *E. coli* (9, 17, 32), represent compact genetic elements carrying functionally related clusters of genes (see chapters 3 and 7), other PAIs, such as those from UPEC, carry many cryptic genes, open reading frames of unrelated and even unknown functions, pseudogenes, and junk DNA sequences (see chapter 4). PAIs of *Salmonella* and intestinal *E. coli* seem to be stably inherited, whereas other PAIs, such as those of *Helicobacter pylori, Yersinia* spp., and UPEC, show a high tendency for deletion, and staphylococcal and *V. cholerae* PAIs can even be mobilized by bacteriophages (3, 4, 6, 19) (see chapters 4, 5, 9, 10, and 14).

From our point of view, PAIs represent a group of genetic elements whose different structures strongly reflect different stages in microbial evolution. Some of the PAIs are, from an evolutionary view point, rather old, while others represent recently acquired DNA segments. Thus, *Salmonella* PAI 1 (SPI-1) is present in strains of *S. enterica* as well as of *S. bongori* (17). The two species diverged more than 100 million years ago, a very long period for the evolution of PAIs. However, considering that microorganisms appeared on Earth 2,400 million years ago, this is a recent event, which means that PAIs, including SPI-1, still represent ''novel'' genetic elements.

Some processes presumably involved in the evolution of PAIs are indicated in Fig. 1. It is now accepted that the generation of PAIs often starts with the integration of plasmids, phages, conjugative transposons, or cointegrates of these into specific target genes, preferentially on the chromosomes. These targets are very often tRNA genes. An integrated

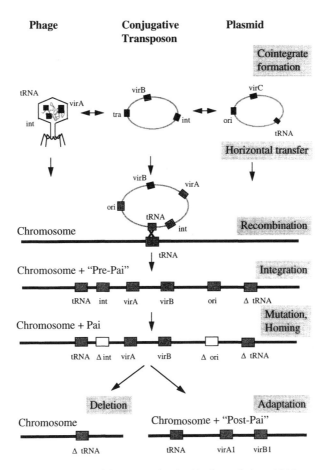

Figure 1. Potential processes involved in the evolution of PAIs.

element has been termed pre-PAI by Lee (23) because it has the potential to develop into a PAI over time. Under specific selective pressures, successful combinations of ancient genes located in the core genome and newly acquired sequences may be genetically optimized by recombination. This event physically combines unlinked genes with common functions (nearest-neighbor hypothesis), thereby leading to the development of large gene clusters, e.g., those coding for secretion or transport processes. In addition, pre-PAIs optimally integrated into a certain host genome may be frozen by deletions of genes not further used and/or by inactivation of such genes by point mutations. This is particularly true for certain mobility genes, such as those encoding integrases and excisases, to immobilize and stabilize the newly acquired elements in the genome. These processes can also be termed homing. The homing status is usually the evolutionary stage for the majority of PAIs indicated in Table 2. Some PAIs still have the tendency to be deleted, while other PAIs are already completely immobilized in the host genome. Such PAIs have been developed by further mutations leading to adaptation and now exhibit features similar to the rest of the chromosomes, including a similar G+C content and a comparable codon usage. Such structures can be termed post-PAIs. *Salmonella* PAIs and the *prf* virulence gene cluster of *Listeria monocytogenes* may now be considered post-PAIs (see chapters 7 and 12).

The so-called high pathogenicity island (HPI) found in the three pathogenic *Yersinia* species and in other enterobacteria may reflect different stages in the evolution of PAIs. In *Y. pseudotuberculosis,* but not in certain *Y. enterocolitica* strains, the integrase gene located in the PAI is still active (5). Therefore, only in *Y. pseudotuberculosis* has the HPI element retained the capacity to move from one target Asn-specific tRNA locus to another. In *E. coli* HPIs, the integrase is still active but one of the DR sequences on one end of the PAIs is deleted, leading to an immobilization of the HPI element (see chapter 5). Together, the HPI elements of *Y. pseudotuberculosis* still have the capacity to move whereas the elements in *Y. enterocolitica* and *E. coli,* for different reasons, are immobilized in the genome. These PAIs are on the track to post-PAI status.

PATHOGENICITY ISLANDS IN NONPATHOGENIC MICROBES?

The concept of PAIs became popular at the same time as the first complete genome sequences of pathogenic as well as nonpathogenic organisms were published (12, 27, 41). From these sequence data, it became obvious that a microbial genome consists of core sequences with rather homogeneous G+C content and codon usage and additional DNA sequences which have been recently acquired via horizontal transmission. The overall amount of horizontally transferred DNA in *E. coli* K-12 has been calculated to be about 17% (22). Single structural genes (islets), IS elements, transposases, prophages, and, as shown for *Streptomyces* and other organisms, integrated plasmids may belong to the bulk of newly acquired DNA (34). As demonstrated for PAIs of pathogenic bacteria, nonpathogenic species also carry large fragments of foreign DNA integrated into their genomes, which, by analogy to PAIs, have been termed genomic islands.

Recently, integrated plasmids carrying genes whose products are involved in nitrogen fixation as well as in chlorocatechol degradation have been described in *Mesorhizobium loti* and *Pseudomonas putida* (33, 42). The integrated plasmids of mesorhizobia were termed symbiosis islands, and indeed they exhibit similarities to PAIs in various aspects: they are integrated into phenylalanine-tRNA genes like PAIs of pathogenic *E. coli,* and they encode additional functions relative to the core genome. DNA sequence analysis of a similar symbiosis plasmid of a different organism (11) showed a number of motifs, such as mobility genes, which are also found on large PAIs.

Furthermore, in staphylococci, the *mecA* regions represent such genomic islands (1). In addition, other DNA regions carrying resistance genes, such as many conjugative and nontransferable transposons (nonreplicative *Bacteroides* units), genetic elements encoding secretion proteins of pathogenic and nonpathogenic bacteria, and genetic units of certain *Salmonella senftenberg* strains, may be considered genomic islands (18, 37). The units of *S. senftenberg* are parts of conjugative transposons and encode important metabolic functions such as sucrose uptake. In conclusion, it is our opinion that while these islands were initially discovered in pathogenic bacteria, the underlying genetic mechanisms are not restricted to pathogens. Rather, the initial discovery was just the tip of the iceberg. It has now become apparent that these genetic mechanisms are much more widespread and that they encompass different functions in phylogenetically diverse organisms. The concept of genomic islands is also demonstrated in Fig. 2.

In most cases, it is not clear which driving forces lead to the evolution of pathogenic strains from nonpathogenic ancestors. Many of the islands which in specific cases increase the pathogenic capacity of strains may also contribute to adaptation of these strains in other environments. Thus, the *Yersinia* HPI, which carries genes encoding an iron uptake system, is also present in the genome of about 30% of nonpathogenic *E. coli* strains isolated from the human intestinal tract (see chapter 5). The function of the HPI in nonpathogens is to increase the capacity of the respective strains to compete with other microbes and even with the eukaryotic host organism to acquire a suitable amount of iron. The HPI in nonpathogens may function as a fitness island rather than a pathogenicity island. A similar situation may be true for an island of *Shigella flexneri,* carrying the aerobactin gene cluster, for SPI-1 in nonpathogenic *Salmonella bongori* strains, and for PAIs coding for P fimbriae of UPEC, which are also present in normal, nonpathogenic *E. coli* strains from birds (17, 21, 43). Evolutionary pressure to incorporate the respective genetic units into the genomes of the microbes was presumably not caused by increasing their pathogenic potency but, rather, by providing advantages in replication and survival in particular ecological niches.

Thus, from an evolutionary point of view, the distinction between the genetic units which are described as genomic islands, fitness islands, or PAIs often becomes unclear. From our point of view, we consider all genetic elements which contain the typical genetic structures described above to be genomic islands. If the presence of an island confers an advantage to the survival of the respective bacteria in an ecological niche, the islands should be termed fitness islands. If, however, the niche is a given host (human, animal, or plant) and the result is an infection that damages the host and whose functions can be linked to the island, it should be called a pathogenicity island. In addition to the strict grammatical definitions, one should consider the answer a famous taxonomist gave to the question, ''What is a species?'' His response, ''A species is what a good microbiologist terms a species,'' can, by analogy, be applied to our question, ''What is a pathogenicity

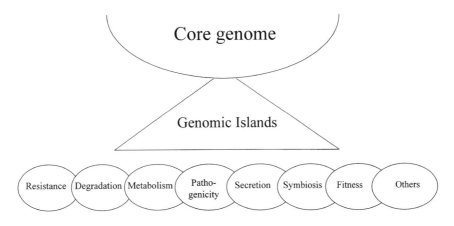

Figure 2. Genomic islands encode a variety of functions.

island?'' The statement ''A pathogenicity island is what a good microbiologist terms a pathogenicity island'' rests finally in the eyes of the beholder and therefore in our understanding and interpretation of the processes contributing to microbial pathogenesis.

Acknowledgments. We thank Ute Hentschel (Universität Würzburg) for comments and Claudia Borde (Universität Würzburg) for editorial assistance.

REFERENCES

1. **Archer, G. L., and D. M. Niemeyer.** 1994. Origin and evolution of DNA associated with resistance to methicillin in staphylococci. *Trends Microbiol.* **2:**343–347.
2. **Bäumler, A. J., A. J. Gilde, R. M. Tsolis, A. W. M. van der Velden, B. M. M. Ahmer, and F. Heffron.** 1997. Contribution of horizontal gene transfer and deletion events to development of distinctive patterns of fimbrial operons during evolution of *Salmonella* serotypes. *J. Bacteriol.* **179:**317–322.
3. **Blum, G., M. Ott, A. Lischewski, A. Ritter, H. Imrich, H. Tschäpe, and J. Hacker.** 1994. Excision of large DNA regions termed pathogenicity islands from tRNA-specific loci in the chromosome of an *Escherichia coli* wild-type pathogen. *Infect. Immun.* **62:**606–614.
4. **Blum, G., V. Falbo, A. Caprioli, and J. Hacker.** 1995. Gene clusters encoding the cytotoxic necrotizing factor type 1, Prs-fimbriae and α-hemolysin form the pathogenicity island II of the uropathogenic *Escherichia coli* strain J96. *FEMS Microbiol. Lett.* **126:**189–196.
5. **Buchrieser, C., R. Brosch, S. Bach, A. Guiyoule, and E. Carniel.** 1998. The high pathogenicity island of *Yersinia tuberculosis* can be inserted into any of the three chromosomal *asn* tRNA genes. *Mol. Microbiol.* **30:**965–978.
6. **Censini, S., C. Lange, Z. Xiang, J. E. Crabtree, P. Ghiara, M. Borodovsky, R. Rappuoli, and A. Covacci.** 1996. *cag,* a pathogenicity island of *Helicobacter pylori,* encodes type I-specific and disease-associated virulence factors. *Proc. Natl. Acad. Sci. USA* **93:**14648–14653.
7. **Cheetham, B. F., and M. E. Katz.** 1995. A role for bacteriophages in the evolution and transfer of bacterial virulence determinants. *Mol. Microbiol.* **18:**201–208.
8. **Dobrindt, U., P. S. Cohen, M. Utley, I. Mühldorfer, and J. Hacker.** 1998. The *leuX*-encoded tRNA$_5^{Leu}$ but not the pathogenicity islands I and II influence the survival of the uropathogenic *Escherichia coli* strain 536 in CD-1 mouse bladder mucus in the stationary phase. *FEMS Microbiol. Lett.* **162:**135–141.
9. **Elliott, S. J., L. A. Wainwright, T. K. McDaniel, K. G. Jarvis, Y. K. Deng, L. C. Lai, B. P. McNamara, M. S. Donnenberg, and J. B. Kaper.** 1998. The complete sequence of the locus of enterocyte effacement (LEE) from enteropathogenic *Escherichia coli* E2348/69. *Mol. Microbiol.* **28:**1–4.
10. **Finlay, B. B., and S. Falkow.** 1997. Common themes in microbial pathogenicity revised. *Microbiol. Mol. Biol. Rev.* **61:**136–169.
11. **Freiberg, C., R. Fellay, A. Bairoch, W. J. Broughton, A. Rosenthal, and X. Perret.** 1997. Molecular basis of symbiosis between *Rhizobium* and legumes. *Nature* **387:**394–401.
12. **Groisman, E. A., and H. Ochman.** 1996. Pathogenicity islands: bacterial evolution in quantum leaps. *Cell* **87:**791–794.
13. **Groisman, E. A., and H. Ochman.** 1997. How *Salmonella* became a pathogen. *Trends Microbiol.* **5:** 343–349.
14. **Hacker, J., S. Knapp, and W. Goebel.** 1983. Spontaneous deletions and flanking regions of the chromosomal inherited hemolysin determinant of an *Escherichia coli* O6 strain. *J. Bacteriol.* **154:**1145–1152.
15. **Hacker, J., L. Bender, M. Ott, J. Wingender, B. Lund, R. Marre, and W. Goebel.** 1990. Deletions of chromosomal regions coding for fimbriae and hemolysins occur *in vivo* and *in vitro* in various extraintestinal *Escherichia coli* isolates. *Microb. Pathog.* **8:**213–225.
16. **Hacker, J., G. Blum-Oehler, I. Mühldorfer, and H. Tschäpe.** 1997. Pathogenicity islands of virulent bacteria: structure, function and impact on microbial evolution. *Mol. Microbiol.* **23:**1089–1097.
17. **Hensel, M., J. E. Shea, A. J. Bäumler, C. Gleeson, F. Blattner, and D. W. Holden.** 1997. Analysis of the boundaries of *Salmonella* pathogenicity island 2 and the corresponding chromosomal region of *Escherichia coli* K-12. *J. Bacteriol.* **179:**1105–1111.
18. **Hochhut, B., K. Jahreis, J. W. Lengeler, and K. Schmid.** 1997. CT*nscr94,* a conjugative transposon found in enterobacteria. *J. Bacteriol.* **179:**2097–2101.
19. **Karaolis, D. K. R., J. A. Johnson, C. C. Bailey, E. C. Boedeker, J. B. Kaper, and P. R. Reeves.** 1998.

A *Vibrio cholerae* pathogenicity island associated with epidemic and pandemic strains. *Proc. Natl. Acad. Sci. USA* **95**:3134–3139.

20. **Koch, R.** 1876. Untersuchungen über Bakterien. V. Die Aetiologie der Milzbrandkrankheit, begründet auf der Entwicklungsgeschichte des *Bacillus anthracis. Beitr. Biol. Pflanz.* **2**:277–310.

21. **Kusters, G., and W. Gaastra.** 1994. Fimbrial operons and evolution, p. 179–196. *In* P. Klemm (ed.), *Fimbriae, Adhesion, Genetics, Biogenesis, and Vaccines.* CRC Press, Inc., Boca Raton, Fla.

22. **Lawrence, J. G., and H. Ochman.** 1998. Molecular archaeology of the *Escherichia coli* genome. *Proc. Natl. Acad. Sci. USA* **95**:9413–9417.

23. **Lee, C. A.** 1996. Pathogenicity islands and the evolution of bacterial pathogens. *Infect. Agents Dis.* **5**:1–7.

24. **Low, D., V. David, D. Lark, G. Schoolnik, and S. Falkow.** 1984. Gene clusters governing the production of hemolysin and mannose-resistant hemagglutination are closely linked in *Escherichia coli* serotype O4 and O6 isolates from urinary tract infections. *Infect. Immun.* **43**:353–358.

25. **Marschalek, R., T. Brechner, E. Amon-Böhm, and T. Dingermann.** 1989. Transfer RNA genes: landmarks for integration of mobile genetic elements in *Dictyostelium discoideum. Science* **244**:1493–1496.

26. **McDaniel, T. K., K. G. Jarvis, M. S. Donnersberg, and J. B. Kaper.** 1995. A genetic locus of enterocyte effacement conserved among diverse enterobacterial pathogens. *Proc. Natl. Acad. Sci. USA* **92**:1664–1668.

27. **Mecsas, J., and E. J. Strauss.** 1996. Molecular mechanisms of bacterial virulence: type III secretion and pathogenicity islands. *Emerging Infect. Dis.* **2**:271–288.

28. **Meyer, T.** 1991. Evasion mechanisms of pathogenic neisseriae. *Behring Inst. Mitt.* **88**:194–199.

29. **Moncrief, J. S., A. J. Duncan, R. L. Wright, L. A. Barroso, and T. D. Wilkins.** 1998. Molecular characterization of the fragilysin pathogenicity islet of enterotoxigenic *Bacteroides fragilis. Infect. Immun.* **66**: 1735–1739.

30. **Munoz, R., C. G. Dowson, M. Daniels, T. J. Coffey, C. Martin, R. Hakenbeck, and B. G. Spratt.** 1992. Genetics of resistance to third-generation cephalosporins in clinical isolates of *Streptococcus pneumoniae. Mol. Microbiol.* **6**:2461–2465.

31. **Pappenheimer, A. M.** 1993. The story of a toxic protein, 1988–1992. *Protein Sci.* **2**:292–298.

32. **Perna, N. T., G. F. Mayhew, G. Posfai, S. Elliott, M. S. Donnenberg, J. B. Kaper, and F. R. Blattner.** 1998. Molecular evolution of a pathogenicity island from enterohemorrhagic *Escherichia coli* O157:H7. *Infect. Immun.* **66**:3810–3817.

33. **Ravatn, R., S. Studer, D. Springael, A. J. B. Zehnder, and J. R. van der Meer.** 1998. Chromosomal integration, tandem amplification, and deamplification in *Pseudomonas putida* F1 of a 105-kilobase genetic element containing the chlorocatechol degradative genes from *Pseudomonas* sp. strain B13. *J. Bacteriol.* **180**:4360–4369.

34. **Raynal, A., K. Tuphile, C. Gerbaud, T. Luther, M. Guerlineau, and J. L. Pernodet.** 1998. Structure of the chromosomal insertion site for pSAM2: functional analysis in *Escherichia coli. Mol. Microbiol.* **28**: 333–342.

35. **Ritter, A., D. Gally, P. B. Olsen, U. Dobrindt, A. Friedrich, P. Klemm, and J. Hacker.** 1997. The Pai-associated *leuX* specific tRNA$_5$^{Leu} affects type 1 fimbriation in pathogenic *Escherichia coli* by control of FimB recombinase expression. *Mol. Microbiol.* **25**:871–882.

36. **Schmidt, H., J. Scheef, C. Janetzki-Mittermann, M. Datz, and H. Karch.** 1997. An *ileX* tRNA gene is located close to the Shiga toxin II operon in enterohemorrhagic *Escherichia coli* O157 and non-O157 strains. *FEMS Microbiol. Lett.* **149**:39–44.

37. **Shoemaker, N. B., G. R. Wang, and A. A. Salyers.** 1996. The *Bacteroides* mobilizable insertion NBU1 integrates into the 3′ end of a Leu-tRNA gene and has an integrase that is a member of the lambda integrase family. *J. Bacteriol.* **178**:3594–3600.

38. **Smith, H. W.** 1968. The transmissible nature of the genetic factor in *Escherichia coli* that controls enterotoxin production. *J. Gen. Microbiol.* **52**:319–334.

39. **So, M., H. W. Boyer, M. Betlach, and S. Falkow.** 1976. Molecular cloning of an *Escherichia coli* plasmid determinant that encodes for the production of heat-stable enterotoxin. *J. Bacteriol.* **128**:463–472.

40. **Stein, M. A., K. Y. Leung, M. Zwick, F. G. del Portillo, and B. B. Finlay.** 1996. Identification of a *Salmonella* virulence gene required for formation of filamentous structures containing lysosomal membrane glycoproteins within epithelial cells. *Mol. Microbiol.* **20**:151–164.

41. **Strauss, E. J., and S. Falkow.** 1997. Microbial pathogenesis: genomics and beyond. *Science* **276**:707–712.

42. **Sullivan, J. T., and C. W. Ronson.** 1998. Evolution of rhizobia by acquisition of a 500-kb symbiosis island that integrates into a phe-tRNA gene. *Proc. Natl. Acad. Sci. USA* **95**:5145–5149.

43. **Volkes, S. A., A. G. Torres, S. A. Reeves, and S. M. Payne.** The aerobactin iron transport system genes in *Shigella flexneri* are present within a pathogenicity island. *Mol. Microbiol.*, in press.

Chapter 2

Methods and Strategies for the Detection of Bacterial Virulence Factors Associated with Pathogenicity Islands, Plasmids, and Bacteriophages

Joachim Reidl

During this decade some elegant molecular biological techniques have been developed which represent valuable tools for the detection and characterization of virulence gene clusters. Many examples involving large regions of chromosomal DNA called pathogenicity islands (PAIs) (21, 24, 36) are described in this book. For almost all of the PAIs, no common origin has been identified and the process of how they became a physical part of the host chromosome remains obscure, although they are assumed to belong to or constitute parts of former mobile elements such as phages or plasmids (36). Homologs of recombinases, transposases, or phage integrases have been identified near inverted repeats which flank such PAIs (24). Other common features of phages and PAIs are the location of their insertion or attachment sites, which are often associated with tRNA genes (see chapter 1) (12, 14), and repeats in the flanking DNA regions (24). PAIs encode single and clusters of virulence genes, and some examples in which different PAIs are present in a single bacterial isolate have been reported (24).

In addition, many bacterial pathogens harbor plasmids, phages, and other mobile elements which code for important virulence factors (see chapters 5 and 7) (12, 13, 15). Quite often, specific combinations of plasmid-encoded virulence factors occur, which argues for coevolution of specific properties, such as adhesins and toxins in enterotoxigenic *Escherichia coli* or invasins and type III secretion proteins in, e.g., *Shigella flexneri* and *Yersinia* spp. Also, a large number of toxins are encoded by temperate phages (5) that specifically express these molecules during the lysogenic phase of their life cycle. Of course, most of these elements are self-transmissible or can spread by mobilization and horizontal transfer. The loss of such vehicles, including PAI structures, spontaneously converts such pathogens into nonpathogenic strains (7, 23, 56).

Recent technical developments (e.g., complete genome sequencing and various genetic techniques) may help to detect further mobile elements or PAI structures as a common

Joachim Reidl • Zentrum für Infektionsforschung, Universität Würzburg, Röntgenring 11, 97070 Würzburg, Germany.

Table 1. Methods developed to detect virulence genes by differential analysis

Method	Aim	Function	Reference(s)
Promoter-trapping systems	To identify host-specific in vivo-expressed and responding genes, to be further characterized as virulence factors	Plasmid-borne systems, used to generate libraries containing short DNA fragments which potentially encode promoter regions, controlling a suitable reporter gene(s)	
IVET	To identify promoter fragments which respond to in vivo expression signals and induce in vivo relevant virulence factors; especially valuable tool for intracellular bacterial pathogens	Synthetic operon uses positive selection marker, e.g., *purA* or antibiotic marker and reporter gene *lacZ*, to determine on/off situation of *ivi*-controlled promoter	41
DFI	To identify promoter fragments which respond to in vivo expression signals, which can be detected in single cells	A highly active form of the green fluorescent protein-encoding gene (*gfp*) is used as a reporter gene to monitor expression of in vivo-controlled promoters; in combination with FACS, the isolation of in vivo-induced *gfp* and ex vivo uninduced *gfp* fusions can be achieved	67
Differential or subtractive display methods	To expose differences in genome structure (additional genes or polymorphism) or to identify differential gene expression (DD and DD-PCR are essentially like IVET and DFI)	Differential expression of genes in one organism under different growth conditions (DD, DD-PCR) and differential analysis between the genotypes of two organisms (RDA)	
DD	To identify a differentially expressed mRNA signal by the generation and amplification of cDNA	Utilizes reverse mRNA transcriptase to generate cDNA; after cDNA subtractive hybridization by physical separation methods and subsequent amplification, an enrichment of specific cDNA is obtained, resulting in the identification of differential expressed genes	51
DD-PCR	To identify a differentially expressed mRNA signal by generation and amplification of cDNA	Essentially like DD, cDNA is amplified in PCR and radioactively labeled; however, no subtractive hybridization is performed and isolation of different generated DNA fragments is performed by comparable separation on a sequencing urea gel	33, 37
RDA	To seek genomic differences between two related organisms	RDA uses the DNA of two comparable organisms (tester and driver), and by an applied PCR and subtractive amplification procedure a representational difference analysis allows the identification of tester-specific DNA, not contained in the driver strain	38

Table 1. *Continued*

Method	Aim	Function	Reference(s)
Transposons	To characterize knockout mutations and phenotypes	Used to generate random insertions by the action of the transposase	
STM	To identify specific gene products, necessary to survive in the bacterial host environment	Utilizes individually tagged transposons, which are suitable as identifiers of generated knockout mutations, leading to an essential gene	27
In vivo transposition	To expose virulence genes by their secretory pathways or their gene regulation pattern associated with other virulence genes	Utilizes designed and specialized transposon systems suitable to produce randomized mutagenesis and to screen for translational or transcriptional fusions, further identified as virulence factors by specific location or transcriptional control	53, 60, 61
In vitro transposition	To mutagenize isolated genome in the test tube and to assign essential function to gene products	Specially designed transposition systems, which can transpose without the cell context (in a test tube); after the generation of insertions, one can test whether defined insertions can be accommodated by the living cell, indicating essential gene function	2, 3
Physical genome-mapping techniques	To assemble complete genome maps, allowing a comparison of genomes or large DNA fragments by restriction analysis	Construction of physical DNA fragments derived from one genome and assembly as restriction maps and ordered contig maps	
PFGE	To determine macrorestriction analysis with rare restriction enzymes (8-bp cutters) to compare and resolve genomes or large DNA fragments (up to 10 Mbp can be separated by agarose gel electrophoresis)	Separation of large DNA fragments in an alternating electric field, causing separation by the orientation phase of the large DNA fragments toward the force line of the changing electric field	59
Gene maps	To dissect a chromosome or genome to an ordered gene library in which cloned DNA fragments are ordered according to the gene order of the respective chromosome	Construction of gene libraries or long contig encoding vector-based libraries; ordered library generation by restriction and hybridization analysis	30
Island probing	To investigate the potential of introducing deletions into PAI regions or to delete PAIs	Suspected PAI structure(s) tagged by Tn10, and subsequent deletions in or around such PAI(s) are provoked by applying the fusaric acid positive selection (Bochner method)	52
Genomics-proteomics	To preselect for possible PAI targets and deduced information source	Comprehensive database information and access to suspected and putative PAI region by sequence analysis	24
DAP[a] labeling	To expose bacterium-specific protein synthesis in host environments	DAP labeling allows the specific labeling of bacterial protein synthesis in the human host environment, since DAP is a nonmetabolizable substrate in mammalian cells	10

[a] DAP, diaminopimelic acid.

feature of pathogenic variants of otherwise harmless or commensal bacteria. As many techniques to study individual genes (e.g., by knockout mutations, such as insertion, in-frame, point, and deletion mutations) become available, more complex genetic structures like plasmids, phage genomes, and PAIs can also be addressed. For example, depending on the structural and functional properties of a specific PAI, the PAI might be recognized by DNA structural features, indicated by deductive and comparable analysis (e.g., genome sequence analysis, G+C content, heteroduplex formation, and tRNA integration sites) or by genetic approaches (e.g., identification of essential virulence or host survival genes, their differential expression responses, and identification by genome subtractive techniques and island probing).

Specific PAIs are reviewed in great detail in the other chapters of this volume. This chapter provides a summary and overview of recently developed strategies to detect virulence genes in PAIs and other genetic elements (summarized in Table 1).

PROMOTER-TRAPPING SYSTEMS TO STUDY IN VIVO EXPRESSION

The complex context of host-specific environments is sensed by the microorganisms, enabling them to respond in a specific and appropriate way to adapt best to the host ecology. The term which addresses this kind of gene expression regulation is ''in vivo induction.'' ''In vivo'' describes the special environmental situations where the bacterium occurs in nature normally; these can range from a hot spring environment (*Archaea*) to endosymbionts (nitrogen-fixing bacteria) to a lysosome compartment of a human macrophage (intracellular bacterial pathogens). These induced genes include ones that encode virulence-associated gene products (cytotoxins, adhesins, invasins, regulators, antibiotic resistance, etc.), as well as those involved in general and specialized biosynthetic pathways (nutrition acquisition, nucleotide biosynthesis, stress response) (26). Some of these expressed systems make essential contributions to colonization and persistence in the host system. To identify these classes of in vivo-induced genes, several techniques including promoter-trapping systems have been invented (for recent reviews, see references 26 and 68).

In Vivo Expression Technology

In vivo expression technology (IVET) is a positive selection scheme for bacterial genes which are specifically induced when bacteria are committed to infection or passage through the host (41). As illustrated in Fig. 1, a suicide plasmid system (pIVET1 [41]) harboring a synthetic operon containing the promoterless *purA* gene (adenylosuccinate synthetase for purine synthesis) of *Salmonella typhimurium* and the promoterless *lacZY* genes of *E. coli* (for β-galactosidase and the lactose uptake system) was constructed. pIVET1 was used to generate a plasmid-based DNA library containing small fragments of ligated *S. typhimurium* DNA in the region upstream of *purA*. If such fragments containing promoter structures were oriented toward the *purA lacZY* operon transcriptional direction, transcription was initiated and PurA and LacZ activities were observed. *purA* served as a positive selection marker, which could be replaced by antibiotic selection markers (42), and *lacZ* represented the reporter gene. Conjugation of pIVET-based *S. typhimurium* fragment libraries into an *S. typhimurium purA* strain, which by itself would not survive within the

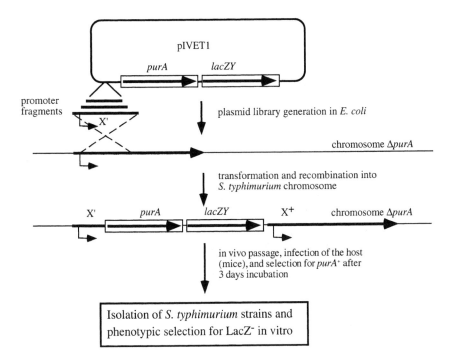

Figure 1. IVET (41). A plasmid library containing putative promoter fragments cloned in front of *purA lacZY* on pIVET1 was constructed. These plasmids were then conjugated to *S. typhimurium purA* and integrated into the chromosome, generating a merodiploid state (*X::purAlacZY* and *X⁺*). Pooled transconjugants were then used to infect mice. After incubation for 3 days, *S. typhimurium* cells were recovered from the spleens and plated onto MacConkey lactose plates. In vivo LacZ⁺ colonies were then recognized under ex vivo conditions as LacZ⁻ colonies and further identified as containing *ivi* genes.

mouse, and subsequent infection into mice would select for in vivo survivors, provided that *purA* was expressed (Fig. 1). After a 3-day incubation period, *S. typhimurium* cells were then extracted from the mouse spleen and screened for the LacZ⁻ phenotype. Isolates which had lost the ability to express *lacZ* represented candidates which encode in vivo-induced (*ivi*) specific promoters.

Using this method, Heithoff et al. (25) performed a comprehensive study in which more than 100 *ivi* genes in *S. typhimurium* that were specifically expressed during infection in mice or cultured macrophages were identified. They identified genes that corresponded to adhesins and invasins of prokaryotic and eukaryotic pathogens. They also found these genes clustered in several regions with low G+C content, indicating PAI structures. Further analysis revealed that some regions can be found in only some *S. typhimurium* isolates, distinguishing broad-host-range from host-adapted serovars (17).

Differential Fluorescence Induction

Another newly developed promoter-based selection method, differential fluorescence induction (DFI), was used to identify bacterial genes that are preferentially expressed under in vivo conditions. This method (67) relies on the differential fluorescence activity caused by the highly active form of the reporter gene *gfp* (18), encoding the green fluorescent protein, and was combined with fluorescence-activated cell sorting (FACS). Via flow cytometry (66), it was possible to detect bacterium-specific gene expression within the infection model (e.g., macrophages and animal tissues), and no limitation to other tractable genetic systems or strain manipulations was necessary.

DFI also requires construction of a plasmid DNA library, consisting of short promoter-containing DNA fragments subcloned in front of a promoterless *gfp* gene. Transformation of such libraries into *S. typhimurium* strains resulted in *gfp*-expressing isolates. With these constructs, it was possible to screen for and identify in vivo-induced *S. typhimurium* genes during macrophage infection (67). For these experiments, *S. typhimurium* cells containing *gfp*-fused libraries were used to infect macrophages and differentially activated *gfp* fusions were then sorted by FACS. The isolated macrophages were lysed, and *S. typhimurium* cells were recovered and grown under ex vivo conditions. Gfp-specific isolates of the grown culture were obtained again by the FACS mechanism on the basis of low or no fluorescent activity, indicating a down-regulated promoter under ex vivo conditions (see above for a discussion of the LacZ⁻ phenotype of IVET). By using this procedure, 14 in vivo-induced promoters, belonging to genes associated with virulence factors (67) and characterized as under the control of four independent regulatory systems, were identified. Also, the expression of a type III secretion system, encoded on a PAI (SPI II [67]), was found to be induced under in vivo conditions in BALB/c mice, and active fusions of macrophage-inducible genes (*mig*) in *S. typhimurium* were identified in infected splenocytes and hepatocytes.

DIFFERENTIAL DISPLAY AND SUBTRACTIVE TECHNIQUES

Identification of the differences between two complex genomes or between the expression patterns of the same organism under different environmental conditions (see above) is also the subject of differential display (DD) and subtractive hybridization techniques. Starting in 1984, applied subtractive hybridization techniques led to the isolation and cloning of the Y chromosome (32), the Duchenne muscular dystrophy locus (34), and the choroidermia locus (50). The following sections specifically address the techniques of DD and representational difference analysis (RDA) applicable to prokaryotes.

Differential Display and Differential Display-PCR

DD techniques were initially developed for eukaryotic cell systems and only recently introduced as methods for use in the prokaryotic field. Investigating the induction of *Mycobacterium avium* gene expression following phagocytosis in human macrophages, Plum and Clark-Curtiss (51) developed a DD scheme applicable to bacteria and based on the genomic subtraction technique of Straus and Ausubel (62). The basic scheme is illustrated in Fig. 2, which shows that broth- or macrophage-cultured bacterial cells were used for mRNA extraction and that cDNA was produced by the action of the reverse transcriptase. cDNA was then ligated with primer/adapter oligonucleotides (Fig. 2A), and further ligation resulted in the generation of cosmid-based clones. Subsequent PCR amplification and biotin labeling were performed only with the broth culture-derived cDNA, and

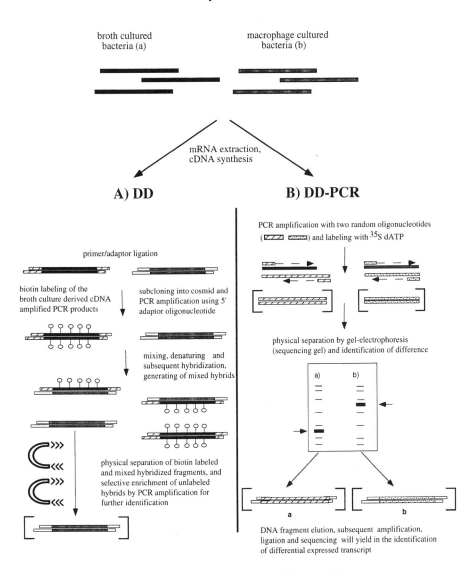

Figure 2. DD (51) and DD-PCR (33, 37) techniques. Different mRNA expression patterns of one species will be compared; e.g., mRNA extracted from broth-cultured bacteria is compared to mRNA extracted from bacteria cultured in macrophages. In a first step, cDNA is synthesized from mRNA. (A) After primer-adapter ligation, these cDNA fragments were subcloned and cDNA derived from step a was amplified and biotin labeled. cDNA derived from steps a and b was denatured, mixed, and hybridized. By magnetic separation, the biotin-labeled and mixed hybridized fragments were removed. By using macrophage-derived adapter-specific oligonucleotides in PCR amplification, the remaining fragments were amplified, isolated, and further characterized as macrophage-induced genes. (B) For DD-PCR, after production of cDNA as a template, two sets of random primers were used to amplify and simultaneously label the cDNA-derived DNA fragments with ^{35}S-dATP. Subsequent separation by gel electrophoresis allowed the identification of differently positioned DNA fragments, which were eluted and amplified for further subcloning and identification.

denaturation of both pools and subsequent mixed hybridization produced double-stranded products between broth- and macrophage-expressed cDNAs. Use of streptavidin-coated paramagnetic particles for magnetic separation and removal of the biotin-labeled fragments resulted in the relative enrichment of the macrophage-cultured *M. avium*-derived cDNA pool. PCR-amplified DNA was then identified as "macrophage-only" expressed genes. One identified open reading frame was found to be unique in *M. avium,* and the reverse transcriptase PCR technique, confirmed that its expression is induced during macrophage phagocytosis (51). Another application of this technique resulted in the identification of unique sequences of *E. coli* chromosomal DNA of a virulent strain of avian pathogenic *E. coli* (APEC) (9). Brown and Curtiss (9) performed a genomic subtraction procedure, described by Straus and Ausubel (62), between APEC (strain χ7122) and K-12. Their analysis revealed that 12 unique regions were found in that APEC isolate, including 5 previously identified clusters such as the group II capsule, *rfb* gene cluster, and inserted DNA segments in regions which were otherwise occupied by other PAIs (PAI I, locus of enterocyte effacement, or PAI II). They also assessed the role of each segment by replacing such regions with K-12 DNA in the APEC strain. They subsequently identified impaired colonization phenotypes for some of the replaced regions, e.g., for the *rfb* gene cluster or a cluster located near *thr* and *carA* operon.

Another technique involves the PCR-DD approach (37), which was originally also developed for eukaryotic cells. This technique (Fig. 2B) is also based on the isolation of mRNA from two differently cultured cell populations at a given time point. Subsequent synthesis of cDNA was produced by the action of the reverse transcriptase. The cDNA products were then amplified and labeled (with ^{35}S-dATP) by PCR, using polyadenyl-based oligonucleotides and randomly generated oligonucleotide primers. After amplification, the two samples were separated by urea gel electrophoresis. PCR-DD products at different locations in the comparable sample footprinting were referred to as differentially produced transcripts and were eluted out of the polyacrylamide gel. Such isolated material was used as templates in PCR, and the same oligonucleotides were used for reamplification. Subsequent cloning and sequencing led to the identification of the products. Recently, this system was adapted to be applicable for prokaryotic organisms and was used to investigate differential gene expression in *Legionella pneumophila* (33). Using two randomly designed oligonucleotides in the amplification and labeling steps, the authors were able to compare gene expression between in vitro-cultured (BCYE medium) and intracellularly (macrophage-like U937) cultured *L. pneumophila* cells. As a result, the identification of a region called early-stage macrophage-induced locus (*eml*) was performed with a 700-bp transcript, also found exclusively in *L. pneumophila*. This transcript was observed in the first few hours postinfection but was then down-regulated by 12 h postinfection. Further analysis revealed that on a 3.7-kb region encoding this early 700-bp transcript, minitransposon insertions caused a lowered cytopathicity compared with the wild type, indicating that this gene was necessary for intracellular survival.

Representative Difference Analysis

RDA addresses the differential analysis of genomes by a reduced complexity ("representations") in combining subtractive and kinetic enrichment methods and using PCR and DNA hybridization only. This technique was introduced in 1993 by Lisitsyn et al. (38)

and has since been used on several biological systems (for recent reviews, see references 39 and 40). In principle, this system does not depend on mRNA expression and cDNA synthesis and does not involve any physical separation techniques. It starts with the generation of so-called tester and driver amplicons generated by restriction fragments derived from two genomes which are being compared. First, the tester and driver DNA samples are digested with a restriction endonuclease that cuts relatively infrequently. Subsequently, driver- and tester-specific oligonucleotides (adapters) are annealed and ligated onto the restriction fragments. Then the driver and tester are amplified by PCR to generate the so-called driver and tester amplicons. The oligonucleotides (adapters) which were used for amplicon generation are then cut away by a restriction enzyme which recognizes a site in the adapter and are removed. Next, the hybridization-amplification step is performed (Fig. 3). Only the fragments of the tester amplicons are ligated to new adapters; then the tester and driver amplicons are mixed, denatured, and hybridized to form hybrids. At the end of the hybridization, *Taq* polymerase is added to fill in the cohesive ends, and finally the tester-specific primers are used to specifically amplify (exponentially by PCR) the remaining tester-tester combination to an extent where it could be used for ligation and further characterization.

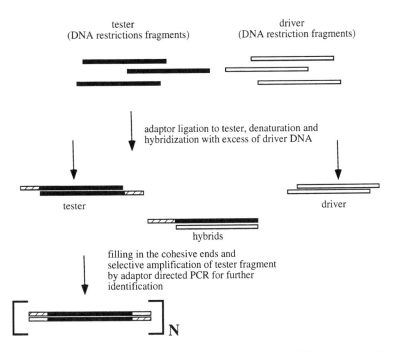

Figure 3. RDA (38). This analysis allows the detection of genomic differences of related species. Starting material was genomic DNA of organism 1 (tester) and organism 2 (driver). After the generation of restriction fragments, ligation of adapters (consisting of long oligonucleotide adapters and nonligated short oligonucleotide) to tester DNA led to tester-specific amplicons. Tester and driver fragments were then denatured, mixed, and hybridized to form tester-tester, tester-driver, and driver-driver fragments. Subsequent exponential amplification of tester-specific fragments led to organism (tester)-specific DNA.

This method was successfully used in a modified form to analyze differences between the closely related pathogenic *Neisseria* species *N. meningitidis* and *N. gonorrhoeae* (65). The result of the RDA analysis yielded the identification of three distinct chromosomal regions (regions 1, 2, and 3) which were found only in *N. meningitidis*. Region 1 was referred to as a PAI and contained the capsule A gene cluster, whereas region 3 contained parts of a defective prophage. Furthermore, the authors were able to identify further meningococcus-specific genes without any known homology to other neisserial sequences. In addition, modified RDA analysis has been used to identify DNA specific for *N. meningitidis* compared to *N. lactamica*. This study resulted in the identification of an *N. meningitidis*-specific restriction-modification system (20a). RDA was also used to verify the presence of the cagA PAI(s) called cagI and cagII in type I *Helicobacter pylori* strains (see chapter 10) (13). These studies were conducted to elucidate the evolutionary development of type I *H. pylori* strains that are associated with severe forms of gastroduodenal disease (see chapter 10). Another recent application of RDA in a modified form was reported for *Vibrio cholerae* (11). The authors used RDA to examine genomic differences between *V. cholerae* O1 and O139 serogroups and between the O1 classical and O1 El-Tor biotypes. The results of this study revealed a greater genetic difference between the two O1 biotypes than between the O1 and O139 biotypes. Also, RDA analysis has been used for *Bordetella* species. When *B. pertussis* was compared with *B. bronchiseptica,* species-specific DNA fragments containing genes encoding a transcriptional factor, transport systems, DNA modification systems, and metabolic enzymes were found (21a).

TRANSPOSON INSERTION MUTAGENESIS

With the introduction of selectable transposon mutagenesis systems in the 1980s (for a comprehensive overview, see reference 61), valuable tools became available to study the phenotypes of knockout mutations. Numerous virulence genes have been discovered by using transposon mutagenesis, and highly sophisticated transposon constructions and mutagenesis schemes have been established to address the detection and regulation of biosynthetic pathways of secreted or membrane-associated virulence genes. Some examples of recently developed transposon techniques which address the identification of virulence factors encoded on PAIs are described here.

Signature-Tagged Mutagenesis

The signature-tagged mutagenesis (STM) method (Fig. 4) was developed by Hensel et al. (27) and is based on an insertional mutagenesis system involving transposons which carry unique DNA sequence tags. With the aim of identifying bacterial genes which are responsible for survival within a given host system, STM has been used so far to detect potential virulence genes in *S. typhimurium* (27), *Staphylococcus aureus* (47), *V. cholerae* (16), and *Haemophilus influenzae* (28a), some of which were characterized and found to be located within newly discovered PAIs (28).

The details of the method devised by Hensel et al. involve a Tn5-based minitransposon, which on one end contains a double-stranded DNA tag comprising a different sequence of 40 bp ($[NK]_{20}$; N = A, C, G, or T; K = G or T) flanked by invariant 20-bp sequences which are common to all of the tags (Fig. 4A). The variable sequence is designed so that

A) Signature tag composition

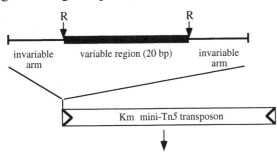

mutagenesis and generation of tagged transposon insertions

B) In vivo screen for attenuated mutations (signature-tagged mutants)

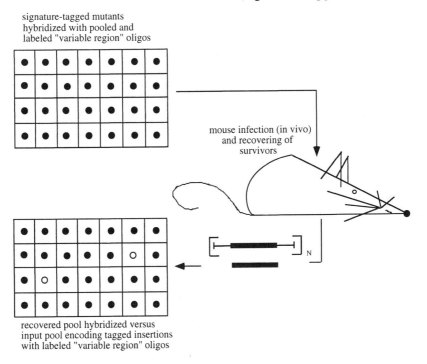

Figure 4. STM (27). (A) The design of a tagged transposon system is shown by the Km mini-Tn5 transposon containing the kanamycin resistance gene and the tag region. This region contained a restriction site (R), which could be used to isolate the variable region, which was used as hybridization probe DNA. (B) An input pool of tagged insertion mutants was generated in *S. typhimurium* and used to infect mice, after which the spleens were removed and bacterial cells were isolated. Probe DNA of the variable regions of the recovered pool was produced and hybridized with the input pool. Nonhybridizing representatives were observed, and such clones were further identified to contain transposon insertions in genes essential for surviving in the in vivo model.

the same sequence should occur only once in 2×10^{17} molecules. The invariant regions contain two amplification primer sequences, which allow the amplification and labeling of the central region by PCR with radiolabeled dCTP. The transposon system (mini-Tn5Km2) was contained on a suicide plasmid (R6K based [49]), and after conjugation into *S. typhimurium,* stable chromosomal insertions of the transposon were obtained. About 1,510 individual mutants were generated and were separated and cultured in 96-well microtiter dishes. These isolates represented the "input pool." As indicated in Fig. 4B, these mutants were then pooled and used to infect mice (mouse model of typhoid); after 3 days, the spleens were removed and the remaining *S. typhimurium* cells were recovered under ex vivo conditions. The isolates were combined (recovered pool), their DNA was prepared, and the tags were PCR amplified by using primers for the invariant region. These labeled PCR products were then hybridized against the input pool. Isolates from the input pool that failed to hybridize with the recovered pool represented mutants which had failed to survive the infection, persistence, and replication state in the mice (in vivo). Hence, these specific transposon tags were inserted into genes which were essential for survival or persistence (virulence genes). By using this method, Hensel et al. recovered 28 mutations which contribute to an attenuation of *S. typhimurium* in the mouse model (27). Some of these genes were located within a newly defined PAI structure (see chapter 7) encoding a type III secretion system (28, 60).

In Vivo Transposon Mutagenesis

In vivo transposon mutagenesis refers to the ability to use a transposon system directly in a given bacterial species under either laboratory or environmental conditions. One specific application is in the detection of secreted or membrane-associated gene products which were the target of so-called translational gene fusion systems. To detect such secreted gene products, suitable transposon systems and reporter genes such as *phoA* (alkaline phosphatase [43]) or *blaM* (β-lactamase [53, 63]) have been used. These reporter genes were aligned with the flanking insertion elements (IS elements) so as to contain only the mature form of the encoding reporter genes (i.e., without a signal sequence). The reporter gene and the IS elements were cloned so that they were linked in a single open reading frame. Therefore, detectable levels of PhoA or β-lactamase activity are produced only by cells that carry an insertion in the correct reading frame of a targeted gene encoding a membrane or exported gene product. Tn*phoA* has been particularly useful in detecting genes encoding virulence determinants which were identified by their typical extracellular or cell surface localization (44). By using Tn*phoA* mutagenesis, it was possible to detect phage-located potential virulence factors (*bor* and *lom*), which then were found to be associated with phenotypes of increased serum resistance and suspected invasiveness. Both genes were located on the genome of phage λ (4). Another example of the use of Tn*phoA* resulted in the identification of the toxin-coregulated pilus biogenesis gene cluster in *V. cholerae* (64), which was found to be structured as a PAI (see chapter 9) (29, 31).

Recently, a specialized transposon mutagenesis scheme suitable for detecting phage-derived secreted gene products was developed and utilized small, phage-linked gene fusions encoding chimeric β-lactamase hybrid proteins in lysogenic bacteria (Fig. 5). The element (53), termed Tn*10d-bla,* used in this scheme is a mere 861 bp in total length and can be efficiently complemented in *trans* for transposition. Tn*10d-bla* is composed of

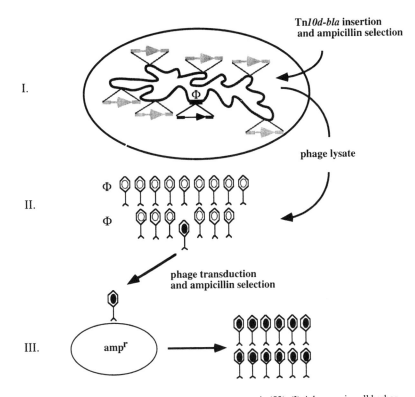

Figure 5. Example of an in vivo transposon mutagenesis (53). (I) A lysogenic cell harboring an integrated bacteriophage (represented by a black bar, Φ) was mutagenized with Tn*10d-bla*, and randomized insertion was selected by ampicillin resistance. (II) Phage lysate production was induced to obtain a heterogeneous lysate, containing the Tn*10d-bla* insertion on the phage genome. (III) The phage lysate was then used to infect a reference strain, and ampicillin-resistant transductants were selected. Subsequent isolation of such colonies and further phage purification steps resulted in the isolation of lysogenic expressed and phage-encoded β-lactamase hybrid proteins, indicating secreted or membrane-derived phage products to be further identified as potential virulence factors.

DNA encoding the mature portion of β-lactamase flanked by two 29-bp oligonucleotides corresponding to the minimal functional ends of insertion sequence IS*10*. This system has been used to characterize the O1 *V. cholerae* phage K139 (53) and to tag the Shiga-toxin-encoding gene *stxA* to study in vivo transduction behavior (1).

In Vitro Transposition

In contrast to the in vivo approaches described above, an in vitro transposon mutagenesis technique allows a direct manipulation of isolated chromosomal DNA or amplified fragments derived by long-distance PCR techniques in the test tube. This technique requires purified components, such as transposase, target DNA (chromosome or PCR fragments), and transposon DNA. It is especially valuable if the organisms under study show a high specificity and effectiveness for the uptake of homospecific DNA, as, for example, *Bacil-*

lus, Campylobacter, Haemophilus, Helicobacter, Neisseria, and *Streptococcus* spp. Recently, two methods have been introduced; one uses the defined in vitro activity of the transposon system Tn7 (3), and the other uses the widespread and diverse family of animal transposons called mariner (Himar1) (35). Only the latter is explained in more detail, as follows.

Genomic analysis and mapping by in vitro transposition (GAMBIT) was developed by Akerley et al. (2) to specifically detect essential gene products contained on genomic segments that are necessary for bacterial growth and viability. GAMBIT involves long-distance PCR, in vitro transposition (mariner system), recombination of the targeted insertions onto the chromosome, and subsequent footprinting to determine the location of permissive and nonpermissive insertion targets. However, by the GAMBIT approach, it was possible to target "essential" genes and identify them by their inability to acquire such in vitro-tagged insertions. By using this approach, Akerley et al. have identified numerous conserved hypothetical genes of *H. influenzae* and *S. pneumoniae* that encode essential products (2).

PHYSICAL GENOME-MAPPING TECHNIQUES

Physical genome mapping was made possible by the introduction of pulsed-field gel electrophoresis (PFGE)-based methods and the establishment of gene maps (for a recent review, see reference 20).

Pulsed-Field Gel Electrophoresis

PFGE (59) is based on the separation of long DNA fragments in agarose gels with low-ionic-strength buffers and involves alternately pulsed, perpendicularly oriented electrical fields. The duration of the applied pulses can vary from 1 to 90 s to separate DNAs with sizes from 30 to 2,000 kb. Separation is caused by relapsing reorientation phases of the large DNA molecules to the force line of the electric field (59). By using rare-cutting restriction enzymes (8-base cutter), this technique was subsequently extended for fingerprint analysis of macrorestriction fragments. PFGE was used to characterize two PAIs (PAI I and PAI II) of uropathogenic *E. coli* 536 (7). These PAIs were mapped at chromosome positions 82 and 97 min, respectively, on the *E. coli* K-12 linkage map, and mutants with deletions of these regions were investigated by a combination of PFGE and hybridization analysis.

PFGE was also extensively used for genome analysis in *Pseudomonas aeruginosa* for strain typing (22). A higher resolution of complex restriction patterns and restriction mapping of chromosomes was demonstrated by Schmidt et al. (58). They differentiated *P. aeruginosa* clone C isolates from cystic fibrosis patients, isolates from aquatic habitats, and a wound isolate (*P. aeruginosa* PAO) and detected significant restriction length polymorphism. The clone C variant was also detected in aquatic habitats and differs from type PAO in having a larger genome extended by large DNA insertions. Furthermore, differences among *P. aeruginosa* C strains were found, again by high-resolution PFGE, indicating large inversions (1×10^6 to 5×10^6 bp) among such isolates (54). A combination of genomic subtraction, PFGE, and Southern hybridization techniques was used to compare two *P. aeruginosa* C strains, one isolate from a cystic fibrosis patient and one aquatic isolate; this study revealed that the overall gene order remained relatively constant although insertions and deletions of large blocks of DNA in defined regions of the chromosome were observed (57). Whether such DNA segments represent PAIs will be elucidated after their sequences are determined. However, among bacteria, genome conservation within species covers a broad range from species with an almost absolute gene order to species in which no long-range conservation of the genetic map can be detected (20).

Genetic Maps

Genetic maps, also called gene encyclopedias, refer to gene libraries in which cloned DNA fragments are ordered according to the gene order of the chromosome. In 1987, Kohara et al. (30) introduced a completely ordered gene library encoded on 3,400 λ phages. By deducing from these clones, they assembled a 4,700-kb restriction map for eight restriction enzymes (Kohara map). In general, the establishment of genetic maps is very time-consuming and depends on one isolate. In the first step, a library must be constructed by using vectors with a high capacity for insert length (e.g., yeast artificial chromosomes, or phage λ-, P1-, and OriF-based vectors). In the second step, the ordered library has to be assembled, which is done by analyzing for overlapping regions by hybridization or restriction analysis and subsequent computer analysis. The last step includes the ordered generation and compilation of a restriction map and the generation of defined insertions of selectable markers (Tn) for mapping studies (20).

Island Probing

By using the well-established method of Bochner et al (8) for selection of loss of tetracycline resistance, a positive selection procedure to generate deletions of Tn*10*-tagged PAIs was developed and was termed island probing. Rajakumar et al. (52) applied the Bochner method to identify an S. flexneri PAI called *she*. They generated Tn*10* insertions in the *she* locus to investigate whether this region was deletable. Selecting on a fusaric acid medium (which counterselects for the active tetracycline pump activity), they showed that tetracycline-sensitive revertants occurred with a frequency of about 10^{-5} to 10^{-6}. Subsequent molecular analysis confirmed the loss of the *she*::Tn*10* insertions in the chromosome. Within these deleted regions, a 25-kbp sequenced fragment encoded insertion sequence-like elements and proteins with homology to immunoglobulin A protease.

Target Screening

Blanc-Potard and Groisman (6) identified suspected PAI structures by using the predilection of PAIs to insert at tRNA genes (6). Since the *selC* tRNA gene in uropathogenic or enteropathogenic *E. coli* strains is targeted as the integration locus for PAI I and the locus of enterocyte effacement island, respectively (7, 46), these investigators examined the possibility of a PAI integration in the *selC* locus in *S. typhimurium*. In a PCR analysis with primers surrounding the *selC* region, they identified an insertion and subsequently characterized it as a 17-kb DNA segment. Within this DNA segment, they identified an Mg^{2+}-uptake system (*mgtCB*), which is regulated by the two-component system PhoP-PhoQ (48) and is required for survival inside macrophages and growth in low-Mg^{2+} media

(6) (chapter 7). By DNA hybridization they showed that this region was also present in *Y. enterocolitica.*

GENOMICS AND PROTEOMICS

In addition to the above-described techniques, the use of complete genome sequencing and the application of proteomics are future sources of important biological information. Knowledge of the complete genome sequence of a given pathogen, in combination with the above-described techniques, will represent the most powerful approach to the identification of PAI structures and associated virulence factors. Since the complete sequencing of the genome of *H. influenzae* Rd in 1995 (19), the genomes of some 30 additional pathogenic bacteria have been or are currently being sequenced (overview provided by The Institute of Genomic Research; Web site http://www.tigr.org/tdb/mdb/hidb/hidb.html) and many PAI structures were suspected or found to be located on the genomes of *M. tuberculosis, V. cholerae, H. pylori,* and other organisms described in this book. Identification of potential PAIs is confirmed mainly by the finding of certain characteristics, as described by Hacker et al. (24), such as different G+C content, insertion site into tRNA genes, flanking DNA repeats, and colocalized integrase structural genes.

Another recent approach which served to identify protein expression profiles of whole organisms (proteomics) was introduced and allowed the monitoring of bacterial protein expression of intracellular *S. typhimurium* (10). This method is based on the detection or profiling of proteins by the technique of protein labeling and two-dimensional gel electrophoresis. To differentiate bacterial from host protein synthesis and to specifically label bacterial proteins, a labeled lysine precursor, diaminopimelic acid, was used, which cannot be utilized by mammalian cells. By this technique, Burns-Keliher et al. (10) could detect about 57 proteins synthesized by *S. typhimurium* growing in a human intestinal epithelial cell line. They further found that 34 of the 57 proteins were specifically expressed due to the intracellular environment. Future protein identification of these spots will reveal whether such identified proteins are encoded by genes located on some of the SP⁻ PAIs in *S. typhimurium.*

CONCLUSIONS

As we proceed further into the so-called "postgenomic era," enormous amounts of DNA sequencing and deduced data will become available. This type of biological information reveals chromosomal features and will tell us more about evolution and the formation of pathogenic variants and species. The methods reviewed in this chapter only begin to describe the large battery of highly developed molecular tools that can be applied to the identification and characterization of PAIs. Furthermore, new developments of powerful integrative methods such as DNA chip technology (for an overview, see reference 45), which allows screening for differential gene expression on microfabricated chips as published recently for *E. coli* (15), *H. influenzae* (55), and *S. pneumoniae* (55), and fast and reliable detection techniques like strand displacement amplification (69) are just two examples. These techniques will also be helpful in the future to detect virulence factors encoded by PAIs and will be used as diagnostic tools to identify pathogens containing PAIs.

In the future, sophisticated genetic approaches in combination with genomics- and proteomics-derived information and methods will allow us to efficiently investigate aspects of bacterial pathogenesis, addressing the evolution of pathogenic bacteria and their molecular analysis, diagnosis, prevention, and therapy.

Acknowledgments. For critical reading of the manuscript, suggestions, and comments, I thank Jörg Hacker, Mark Herbert, Inge Mühldorfer, and Stefan Schlör. The portions of this work that are from my laboratory were funded by BMBF grant 01KI8906.

REFERENCES

1. **Acheson, D. W. K., J. Reidl, X. Zhang, G. T. Keusch, J. J. Mekalanos, and M. K. Waldor.** 1998. In vivo transduction with Shiga toxin 1-encoding phage. *Infect. Immun.* **66:**4496–4498.
2. **Akerley, B. J., E. J. Rubin, A. Camilli, D. J. Lampe, H. M. Robertson, and J. J. Mekalanos.** 1998. Systematic identification of essential genes by *in vitro* mariner mutagenesis. *Proc. Natl. Acad. Sci. USA* **95:**8927–8932.
3. **Bainton, R. J., K. M. Kubo, J. N. Feng, and N. L. Craig.** 1993. Tn7 transposition: target DNA recognition is mediated by multiple Tn7-encoded proteins in a purified *in vitro* system. *Cell* **72:**931–943.
4. **Barondess, J., and J. Beckwith.** 1990. A bacterial virulence determinant encoded by lysogenic coliphage lambda. *Nature* **346:**871–874.
5. **Bishai, W. R., and J. R. Murphy.** 1988. Bacteriophage gene products that cause human disease, p. 683–724. *In* R. Calendar (ed.), *The Bacteriophages.* Plenum Press, New York, N.Y.
6. **Blanc-Potard, A. B., and E. A. Groisman.** 1997. The *Salmonella selC* locus contains a pathogenicity island mediating intramacrophage survival. *EMBO J.* **16:**5376–5385.
7. **Blum, G., M. Ott, A. Lischewski, A. Ritter, H. Imrich, H. Tschäpe, and J. Hacker.** 1994. Excision of large DNA regions termed pathogenicity islands from tRNA-specific loci in the chromosome of an *Escherichia coli* wild-type pathogen. *Infect. Immun.* **62:**606–614.
8. **Bochner, B. R., H. C. Huang, G. L. Schieven, and B. N. Ames.** 1980. Positive selection for loss of tetracycline resistance. *J. Bacteriol.* **143:**926–933.
9. **Brown, P. K., and R. Curtiss III.** 1996. Unique chromosomal regions associated with virulence of an avian pathogenic *Escherichia coli* strain. *Proc. Natl. Acad. Sci. USA* **93:**11149–11154.
10. **Burns-Keliher, L. L., A. Portteus, and R. Curtiss III.** 1997. Specific detection of *Salmonella typhimurium* proteins synthesized intracellularly. *J. Bacteriol.* **179:**3604–3612.
11. **Calia, K. E., M. K. Waldor, and S. B. Calderwood.** 1998. Use of representational difference analysis to identify genomic differences between pathogenic strains of *Vibrio cholerae. Infect. Immun.* **66:**849–852.
12. **Campbell, A. M.** 1992. Chromosomal insertion sites for phages and plasmids. *J. Bacteriol.* **174:**7495–7499.
13. **Censini, S., C. Lange, Z. Xiang, J. E. Crabtree, P. Ghiara, M. Borodovsky, R. Rappuoli, and A. Covacci.** 1996. cag, a pathogenicity island of *Helicobacter pylori,* encodes type I-specific and disease-associated virulence factors. *Proc. Natl. Acad. Sci. USA* **93:**14648–14653.
14. **Cheetham, B. F., and M. E. Katz.** 1995. A role for bacteriophages in the evolution and transfer of bacterial virulence determinants. *Mol. Microbiol.* **18:**201–208.
15. **Cheng, J., E. L. Sheldon, L. Wu, A. Uribe, L. O. Gerrue, J. Carrino, M. J. Heller, and J. P. O'Connell.** 1998. Preparation and hybridization analysis of DNA/RNA from *E. coli* on microfabricated bioelectronic chips. *Nat. Biotechnol.* **16:**541–546.
16. **Chiang, S. L., and J. J. Mekalanos.** 1998. Use of signature-tagged transposon mutagenesis to identify *Vibrio cholerae* genes critical for colonization. *Mol. Microbiol.* **27:**797–805.
17. **Conner, C. P., D. M. Heithoff, S. M. Julio, R. L. Sinsheimer, and M. J. Mahan.** 1998. Differential patterns of acquired virulence genes distinguish *Salmonella* strains. *Proc. Natl. Acad. Sci. USA* **95:**4641–4645.
18. **Cormack, B., R. H. Valdivia, and S. Falkow.** 1996. FACS-optimized mutants of the green fluorescent protein (GFP). *Gene* **173:**33–38.
19. **Fleischmann, R. D., M. D. Adams, O. White, R. A. Clayton, E. F. Kirkness, A. R. Kerlavage, C. J. Bult, J. F. Tomb, B. A. Dougherty, J. M. Merrick, K. McKenney, G. Sutton, W. FitzHugh, C. Fields, J. D. Gocayne, J. Scott, R. Shirley, L. I. Liu, A. Glodek, J. M. Kelley, J. F. Weidman, C. A. Phillips,**

T. Spriggs, E. Hedblom, M. D. Cotton, T. R. Utterback, M. C. Hanna, D. T. Nguyen, D. M. Saudek, R. C. Brandon, L. D. Fine, J. L. Frichman, J. L. Fuhrmann, N. S. M. Geoghagen, C. L. Gnehm, L. A. McDonald, K. V. Small, C. M. Fraser, H. O. Smith, and J. C. Venter. 1995. Whole-genome random sequencing and assembly of *Haemophilus influenzae* Rd. *Science* **269**:496–512.

20. Fonstein, M., and R. Haselkorn. 1995. Physical mapping of bacterial genomes. *J. Bacteriol.* **177**: 3361–3369.

20a. Frosch, M., and U. Vogel. Personal communication.

21. Groisman, E. A., and H. Ochman. 1996. Pathogenicity islands: bacterial evolution in quantum leaps. *Cell* **87**:791–794.

21a. Gross, R., and B. Middendorf. Personal communication.

22. Grothues, D., and B. Tuemmler. 1987. Genome analysis of *Pseudomonas aeruginosa* by field inversion gel electrophoresis. *FEMS Microbiol. Lett.* **48**:419–422.

23. Hacker, J., L. Bender, M. Ott, J. Wingender, B. Lund, R. Marre, and W. Goebel. 1990. Deletions of chromosomal regions coding for fimbriae and hemolysins occur *in vivo* and *in vitro* in various extraintestinal *Escherichia coli* isolates. *Microb. Pathog.* **8**:213–225.

24. Hacker, J., G. Blum-Oehler, I. Mühldorfer, and H. Tschäpe. 1997. Pathogenicity island of virulent bacteria: structure, function and impact on microbial evolution. *Mol. Microbiol.* **23**:1089–1097.

25. Heithoff, D. M., C. P. Conner, P. C. Hanna, S. M. Julio, U. Hentschel, and M. J. Mahan. 1997. Bacterial infection as assessed by *in vivo* gene expression. *Proc. Natl. Acad. Sci. USA* **94**:934–939.

26. Heithoff, D. M., C. P. Conner, and M. J. Mahan. 1997. Dissecting the biology of a pathogen during infection. *Trends Microbiol.* **5**:509–513.

27. Hensel, M., J. E. Shea, C. Gleeson, M. D. Jones, E. Dalton, and D. W. Holden. 1995. Simultaneous identification of bacterial virulence genes by negative selection. *Science* **269**:400–403.

28. Hensel, M., J. E. Shea, B. Raupach, D. Monack, S. Falkow, C. Gleeson, T. Kubo, and D. W. Holden. 1997. Functional analysis of *ssaJ* and the *ssaK/U* operon, 13 genes encoding components of the type III secretion apparatus of *Salmonella* pathogenicity island 2. *Mol. Microbiol.* **24**:155–167.

28a. Herbert, M., and R. Moxom. Personal communication.

29. Karaolis, D. K., J. A. Johnson, C. C. Bailey, E. C. Boedeker, J. B. Kaper, and P. R. Reeves. 1998. A *Vibrio cholerae* pathogenicity island associated with epidemic and pandemic strains. *Proc. Natl. Acad. Sci. USA* **95**:3134–3139.

30. Kohara, Y., K. Akiyama, and K. Isono. 1987. The physical map of the whole *E. coli* chromosome: application of a new strategy for rapid analysis and sorting of a large genomic library. *Cell* **50**:495–508.

31. Kovach, M. E., M. D. Shaffer, and K. M. Peterson. 1996. A putative integrase gene defines the distal end of a large cluster of ToxR-regulated colonization genes in *Vibrio cholerae. Microbiology* **142**:2165–2174.

32. Kunkel, L. M., A. P. Monaco, W. Middlesworth, D. Ochs, and S. A. Latt. 1985. Specific cloning of DNA fragments absent from the DNA of a male patient with an X chromosome deletion. *Proc. Natl. Acad. Sci. USA* **82**:4778–4782.

33. Kwaik, Y. A., and L. L. Pederson. 1996. The use of differential display-PCR to isolate and characterize a *Legionella pneumophila* locus induced during the intracellular infection of macrophages. *Mol. Microbiol.* **21**:543–556.

34. Lamar, E. E., and E. Palmer. 1984. Y-encoded, species-specific DNA in mice: evidence that the Y chromosome exists in two polymorphic forms in inbred strains. *Cell* **37**:171–177.

35. Lampe, D. J., M. E. Churchill, and H. M. Robertson. 1996. A purified mariner transposase is sufficient to mediate transposition *in vitro. EMBO J.* **15**:5470–5479.

36. Lee, C. A. 1996. Pathogenicity islands and the evolution of bacterial pathogens. *Infect. Agents Dis.* **5**:1–7.

37. Liang, P., and A. B. Pardee. 1992. Differential display of eukaryotic messenger RNA by means of the polymerase chain reaction. *Science* **257**:967–971.

38. Lisitsyn, N., N. Lisitsyn, and M. Wigler. 1993. Cloning the difference between two complex genomes. *Science* **259**:946–951.

39. Lisitsyn, N., and M. Wigler. 1995. Representational difference analysis in detection of genetic lesions in cancer. *Methods Enzymol.* **254**:291–304.

40. Lisitsyn, N. A. 1995. Representational difference analysis: finding the differences between genomes. *Trends Genet.* **11**:303–307.

41. Mahan, M. J., J. M. Slauch, and J. J. Mekalanos. 1993. Selection of bacterial virulence genes that are specifically induced in host tissues. *Science* **259**:686–688.

42. **Mahan, M. J., J. W. Tobias, J. M. Slauch, P. C. Hanna, R. J. Collier, and J. J. Mekalanos.** 1995. Antibiotic-based IVET selection for bacterial virulence genes that are specifically induced during infection of a host. *Proc. Natl. Acad. Sci. USA* **92:**669–673.

43. **Manoil, C., and J. Beckwith.** 1985. Tn*phoA*: a transposon probe for protein export signals. *Proc. Natl. Acad. Sci. USA* **82:**8129–8133.

44. **Manoil, C., J. J. Mekalanos, and J. Beckwith.** 1990. Alkaline phosphatase fusions: sensors of subcellular location. *J. Bacteriol.* **172:**515–518.

45. **Marshall, A., and J. Hodgson.** 1998. DNA chips: an array of possibilities. *Nat. Biotechnol.* **16:**27–31.

46. **McDaniel, T. K., K. G. Jarvis, M. S. Donnenberg, and J. B. Kaper.** 1995. A genetic locus of enterocyte effacement conserved among diverse enterobacterial pathogens. *Proc. Natl. Acad. Sci. USA* **92:**1664–1668.

47. **Mei, J. M., F. Nourbakhsh, C. W. Ford, and D. W. Holden.** 1997. Identification of *Staphylococcus aureus* virulence genes in a murine model of bacteraemia using signature-tagged mutagenesis. *Mol. Microbiol.* **26:** 399–407.

48. **Miller, S. I., A. M. Kukral, and J. J. Mekalanos.** 1989. A two-component regulatory system (*phoP phoQ*) controls *Salmonella typhimurium* virulence. *Proc. Natl. Acad. Sci. USA* **86:**5054–5058.

49. **Miller, V. L., and J. J. Mekalanos.** 1988. A novel suicide vector and its use in construction of insertion mutations: osmoregulation of outer membrane proteins and virulence determinants in *Vibrio cholerae* requires *toxR. J. Bacteriol.* **170:**2575–2583.

50. **Nussbaum, R. L., J. G. Lesko, R. A. Lewis, S. Ledbetter, and D. H. Ledbetter.** 1987. Isolation of anonymous DNA sequences from within a submicroscopic X chromosomal deletion in a patient with choroideremia, deafness, and mental retardation. *Proc. Natl. Acad. Sci. USA* **84:**6521–6525.

51. **Plum, G., and J. E. Clark-Curtiss.** 1994. Induction of *Mycobacterium avium* gene expression following phagocytosis by human macrophages. *Infect. Immun.* **62:**476–483.

52. **Rajakumar, K., C. Sasakawa, and B. Adler.** 1997. Use of a novel approach, termed island probing, identifies the *Shigella flexneri she* pathogenicity island which encodes a homolog of the immunoglobulin A protease-like family of proteins. *Infect. Immun.* **65:**4606–4614.

53. **Reidl, J., and J. J. Mekalanos.** 1995. Characterization of *Vibrio cholerae* bacteriophage K139 and use of a novel mini-transposon to identify a phage-encoded virulence factor. *Mol. Microbiol.* **18:**685–701.

54. **Roemling, U., K. D. Schmidt, and B. Tuemmler.** 1997. Large chromsomal inversions occur in *Pseudomonas aeruginosa* clone C strains isolated from cystic fibrosis patients. *FEMS Microbiol. Lett.* **150:**149–156.

55. **Saizieu, A., U. Certa, J. Warrington, C. Gray, W. Keck, and J. Mous.** 1998. Bacterial transcript imaging by hybridization of total RNA to oligonucleotide arrays. *Nat. Biotechnol.* **16:**45–48.

56. **Salyers, A. A., and D. D. Whitt.** 1994. *Bacterial Pathogenesis: a Molecular Approach.* ASM Press, Washington, D.C.

57. **Schmidt, K. D., T. Schmidt-Rose, U. Roemling, and B. Tuemmler.** 1998. Differential genome analysis of bacteria by genomic subtractive hybridization and pulsed field gel electrophoresis. *Electrophoresis* **19:** 509–514.

58. **Schmidt, K. D., B. Tuemmler, and U. Roemling.** 1996. Comparative genome mapping of *Pseudomonas aeruginosa* PAO with *P. aeruginosa* C, which belongs to a major clone in cystic fibrosis patients and aquatic habitats. *J. Bacteriol.* **178:**85–93.

59. **Schwartz, D. C., and C. R. Cantor.** 1984. Separation of yeast chromosome-sized DNAs by pulsed field gradient gel electrophoresis. *Cell* **37:**67–75.

60. **Shea, J. E., M. Hensel, C. Gleeson, and D. W. Holden.** 1996. Identification of a virulence locus encoding a second type III secretion system in *Salmonella typhimurium. Proc. Natl. Acad. Sci. USA* **93:**2593–2597.

61. **Slauch, J. M., and T. J. Silhavy.** 1991. Genetic fusion as experimental tools. *Methods Enzymol.* **204:** 13–48.

62. **Straus, D., and F. M. Ausubel.** 1990. Genomic subtraction for cloning DNA corresponding to deletion mutations. *Proc. Natl. Acad. Sci. USA* **87:**1889–1893.

63. **Tadayyon, M., and J. K. Broome-Smith.** 1993. Tn*blaM:* a transposon for directly tagging bacterial genes encoding cell envelope and secreted proteins. *Gene* **111:**21–26.

64. **Taylor, R. K., V. L. Miller, D. B. Furlong, and J. J. Mekalanos.** 1987. Use of *phoA* gene fusions to identify a pilus colonization factor coordinately regulated with cholera toxin. *Proc. Natl. Acad. Sci. USA* **84:**2833–2837.

65. **Tinsley, C. R., and X. Nassif.** 1996. Analysis of the genetic difference between *Neisseria meningitidis* and

Neisseria gonorrhoeae: two closely related bacteria expressing two different pathogenicities. *Proc. Natl. Acad. Sci. USA* **93:**11109–11114.

66. **Valdivia, R. H., and S. Falkow.** 1996. Bacterial genetics by flow cytometry: rapid isolation of *Salmonella typhimurium* acid-inducible promoters by differential fluorescence induction. *Mol. Microbiol.* **22:**367–378.

67. **Valdivia, R. H., and S. Falkow.** 1997. Fluorescence-based isolation of bacterial genes expressed within host cells. *Science* **277:**2007–2011.

68. **Valdivia, R. H., and S. Falkow.** 1997. Probing bacterial gene expression within host cells. *Trends Microbiol.* **5:**360–363.

69. **Walker, G. T., C. P. Linn, and J. G. Nadeau.** 1996. DNA detection by strand displacement amplification (SDA) and fluorescence polarization with signal enhancement using a DNA binding protein. *Nucleic Acids Res.* **24:**348–353.

Chapter 3

Pathogenicity Islands and Other Mobile Genetic Elements of Diarrheagenic *Escherichia coli*

James B. Kaper, Jay L. Mellies, and James P. Nataro

Escherichia coli is the prototypic "normal-flora" species of humans, since it is the predominant facultative anaerobe of the human colonic flora. However, some strains can cause a variety of intestinal and extraintestinal infections in normal hosts due to the presence of specific genes encoding virulence factors that are largely absent from normal-flora *E. coli* strains. These virulence genes are usually encoded on a variety of pathogenicity islands (PAIs), bacteriophages, plasmids, and transposons (Table 1). Three general clinical syndromes result from infection with inherently pathogenic *E. coli* strains: (i) urinary tract infection, (ii) sepsis and meningitis, and (iii) enteric and diarrheal disease (with a subset of these infections leading to systemic toxin-mediated disease including hemolytic-uremic syndrome [HUS]) (78). The PAIs of uropathogenic *E. coli* were the first PAIs to be described, and they are reviewed in detail in chapter 4. PAIs in *E. coli* strains associated with newborn sepsis and meningitis are not as well characterized, but a recent study shows that large blocks of DNA containing virulence genes in this pathogen are inserted at the same chromosomal sites as PAIs for uropathogenic *E. coli* J96 (92). This chapter focuses on diarrheagenic *E. coli* strains and the various PAIs and other mobile genetic elements that differentiate these pathogens from normal-flora *E. coli*.

At least six categories of diarrheagenic *E. coli* strains have been defined. Five of these categories, enteropathogenic *E. coli* (EPEC), enterohemorrhagic *E. coli* (EHEC), enteroaggregative *E. coli* (EAEC), enterotoxigenic *E. coli* (ETEC), and enteroinvasive *E. coli* (EIEC), are reviewed here. A sixth category, diffusely adherent *E. coli* (DAEC), is a heterogeneous group of organisms, and epidemiological studies have given conflicting results about the true clinical significance of these strains. No clear picture of pathogenesis has emerged for DAEC, and no PAIs or other mobile virulence elements have yet been reported. The pathogenesis, epidemiology, diagnosis, and clinical considerations of disease due to all six categories of diarrheagenic *E. coli* have recently been reviewed (78).

James B. Kaper and Jay L. Mellies • Department of Microbiology and Immunology and Center for Vaccine Development, University of Maryland School of Medicine, Baltimore, MD 21201. ***James P. Nataro*** • Center for Vaccine Development and Department of Pediatrics, University of Maryland School of Medicine, Baltimore, MD 21201.

Table 1. Mobile genetic elements encoding virulence factors in human diarrheagenic *E. coli*

Element	Present in:	Phenotype
Pathogenicity islands		
LEE	EPEC, EHEC	A/E histopathology
HPI (*Yersinia*)	EAEC	Iron utilization
Tia-PAI	ETEC	Invasion
EspC islet	EPEC	EspC enterotoxin
Virulence plasmids		
EAF plasmid	EPEC	Type IV pili, regulator
pO157	EHEC	Hemolysin, protease, toxin
ENT plasmids	ETEC	LT and ST enterotoxins, CFA and CS colonization factors
pAA	EAEC	Pet and EAST1 enterotoxins, fimbriae, mucosal-cell exfoliation
INV plasmids	EIEC	Invasion
Bacteriophage		
Stxφ	EHEC	Stx1 and Stx2
Transposons/IS elements		
Tn*1681*	ETEC	ST
EAST1 IS	EAEC, EHEC, EPEC, normal-flora *E. coli*	ST-like enterotoxin

ENTEROPATHOGENIC *E. COLI*

EPEC strains are a major cause of infant diarrhea in the developing world. EPEC can also cause outbreaks of infant diarrhea in day care centers and pediatric wards in developed countries, and atypical EPEC strains have been linked to outbreaks of diarrheal disease in adults in the United States and Finland (reviewed in reference 78). EPEC strains cause a characteristic intestinal histopathology known as "attaching and effacing" (A/E), which is characterized by effacement of intestinal epithelial-cell microvilli and intimate adherence between the bacterium and the epithelial-cell membrane. Directly beneath the adherent bacterium, marked cytoskeletal changes are seen in the epithelial cell, including the accumulation of polymerized actin. Related *E. coli* strains that produce A/E intestinal histopathologic changes can cause diarrhea in rabbits, dogs, pigs, and other animals. These strains are collectively known as A/E *E. coli* strains.

The LEE PAI

Structure

The locus of enterocyte effacement (LEE) PAI is responsible for the A/E intestinal histopathologic changes exhibited by EPEC, EHEC, and related animal pathogens. The first gene described for this PAI was the *eae* gene, which was discovered by Jerse et al. (52), who screened a collection of Tn*phoA* mutants of EPEC E2348/69 for mutants which abolished the A/E phenotype. A second mutation which abolished this phenotype was located 5 kb downstream of the *eae* gene and was initially named *eaeB* and later named *espB* by Donnenberg et al. (24). McDaniel et al. (70) characterized additional mutations which abolished the A/E phenotype and discovered that the genes disrupted by the transposon mutations along with the *eae* and *espB* genes were located in a 35-kb region that was present in EPEC and EHEC O157:H7 and A/E pathogens of animals but absent from *E. coli* K-12 strains, normal-flora *E. coli* strains, and ETEC strains. Characterization of the junction between unique EPEC E2348/69 DNA and K-12 DNA revealed that this 35-kb region was inserted next to the *selC* locus which encodes the tRNA for selenocysteine. The insertion site is exactly the same insertion site for PAI I of uropathogenic *E. coli* (see chapter 4). (Other EPEC strains may have a different insertion site for this region, as described below.) This region was named the LEE PAI.

The complete DNA sequence of the LEE has been determined for the prototypical EPEC strain E2348/69 (O127:H6) (27). The G+C content of the EPEC LEE is 38.3%, which is significantly lower than the 50.8% G+C content of the total *E. coli* genome. The 35,624-bp LEE contains 41 open reading frames (ORFs) that encode predicted proteins larger than 50 amino acid residues (Fig. 1; Table 2). The genes contained on the LEE are sufficient to confer the A/E phenotype on an *E. coli* K-12 strain when cloned on a plasmid (71). The LEE is organized into three regions with known functions.

The middle part of the LEE contains the *eae* and *tir* genes. The *eae* gene encodes intimin, a 94- to 97-kDa outer membrane protein that is an intestinal adherence factor. The importance of intimin in intestinal adherence has been demonstrated in studies of volunteers experimentally infected with *eae* mutants of EPEC (23) and in studies of gnotobiotic piglets infected with *eae* mutants of EHEC O157:H7 (reviewed in references 56 and 78). The Tir protein was initially identified as a 90-kDa eukaryotic cytoskeletal protein (Hp90) that became phosphorylated on a tyrosine residue in response to EPEC infection. It was subsequently shown that Tir is a bacterial protein encoded in the LEE that is translocated into the host cell via a type III secretion system (60). Upon entry into the host cell, it serves as a receptor for the intimin protein. In EPEC E2348/69 (93) and EHEC O26:H− (20), the Tir protein (also called EspE) is tyrosine phosphorylated, but in O157:H7, it is not (49). Tir may also serve to nucleate host cell actin following intimin binding and to transmit signals to the host cell once Tir-intimin binding occurs (60). Between the *tir* and *eae* genes is the *cesT* (previously called *orfU*) gene, which encodes

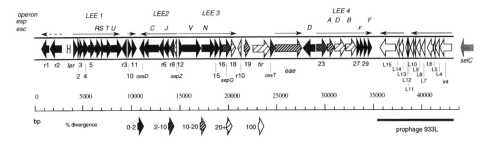

Figure 1. Diagram of the LEE PAIs of EPEC E2348/69 (O127:H6) (27) and EHEC EDL933 (O157:H7) (88). The different patterns of the large arrows indicate the nucleotide divergence between the EPEC and EHEC genes. Small arrows indicate operons within the LEE; the four polycistronic operons demonstrated for the LEE are designated LEE1 through LEE4. The 933L prophage on the right side of the LEE is present in EHEC O157:H7 but not in EPEC O127:H6.

Table 2. Major gene products of the EPEC LEE[a]

Gene product	Similar protein in other gram-negative pathogens:			Similar protein in E. coli K-12	Specific function in EPEC
	Yersinia	Salmonella	Shigella		
Type III secretion apparatus components					
EscR	YscR	SsaR	Spa24		
EscS	YscS	SsaS	Spa9		
EscT	YscT	SsaT	Spa29		
EscU	YscU	SsaU	Spa40		
EscC	YscC	SpiA	MxiD		
EscJ	YscJ	SsaJ	MxiJ		
EscV	YscV	SsaV	MxiA		
EscN	YscN	SsaN	Spa47		
EscD	YscD	SpiB			
EscF	YscF				
SepZ					
SepQ		SsaQ			
Attachment					
Intimin	InvA			02383	Outer membrane adhesin
Secreted proteins					
Tir					Translocated intimin receptor
EspA[b]					Translocation filament subunit
EspD	YopB	SipB	IpaB		
EspB[b]	YopB				Pore formation
EspF					
Chaperones					
CesD	SycD	SicA	Ippl		Chaperone for EspD
CesT	SycH				Chaperone for Tir
Regulation					
Ler		StpA		StpA	Positive regulator of LEE operons

[a] Not all LEE products are shown, only those with functions established experimentally or with compelling homology to other gene products.
[b] Also part of the type III secretion apparatus.

a chaperone for the Tir protein (28). Although the evidence showing that Tir serves as a receptor for intimin is quite convincing, recent data suggest that intimin can also bind to a carbohydrate moiety (37), thus suggesting that intimin may bind to a carbohydrate-containing receptor before the Tir protein is translocated into the host cell.

On the left side of the LEE, as shown in Fig. 1, is a set of genes encoding a type III secretion system. These genes were originally called *sep* (51), but a subset with homologs in other type III secretion systems were renamed *esc* (27) to follow the *Yersinia* nomenclature for type III secretion genes (see chapter 6). Two *esc* genes, *escD* and *escF,* are located downstream of *eae* on the right side of the LEE. Additional genes located in polycistronic operons containing *esc* genes, *sepZ* and *sepQ,* are involved in type III secretion but have no homology to other type III systems. The *cesD* gene, located downstream of *escC,* encodes a chaperone essential for secretion of EspD and EspB (115).

On the right side of the LEE are the *espA, espB, espD,* and *espF* genes, which encode proteins secreted via the type III system. Mutation of any of the first three genes abolishes the A/E phenotype (36, 61, 63), while mutation of *espF* results in no obvious change in phenotype (72). The EspA protein was recently shown by Knutton et al. (62) to form a filamentous structure on the surface of EPEC that is presumed to be the conduit by which Tir and other EPEC proteins are translocated into the host cell. The EspB protein is translocated into the host cell membrane and cytoplasm (109, 121), and recent evidence suggests that it forms a pore in the host cell membrane that serves as the distal end of the EspA filament (37), although a role for EspB in signal transduction events in the host cell has also been proposed (109). The function of the secreted EspD protein is unknown. EspA and EspB are clearly produced during the course of disease, since volunteers experimentally infected with EPEC develop strong antibody responses to these proteins (51).

In contrast to many other PAIs, the LEE of EPEC E2348/69 lacks direct repeats at each end and also lacks obvious phage sequences. (The LEE of EHEC O157:H7 contains a lysogenic phage at one end, but it probably integrated into the LEE after the chromosomal insertion of the LEE [see below].) However, at the right side of the LEE is a 440-bp region with 89 and 77% identity to IS*600* and IS*660,* respectively (22). Despite repeated attempts, we have never observed mobilization or deletion of the LEE, as has been observed with some other PAIs.

Regulation

Recent studies have provided insights into how genes on the LEE are regulated. Expression of many LEE genes is controlled by a regulatory element called Per, which is encoded on the EAF plasmid present in most EPEC strains (see below). Per was initially discovered because of its ability to activate the transcription of the *eae* gene. Recently, Mellies et al. (73) have shown that Per also activates transcription of the four polycistronic operons of the LEE which encode the type III secretion system and secreted EspABD proteins (Fig. 1). However, Per acts directly only on the first operon (*LEE1*) and acts indirectly on the other operons. Within the first operon is an ORF (previously called *orf1*) that encodes a regulator which we have called Ler (for LEE-encoded regulator). This 14-kDa protein has amino acid homology to the H-NS family of transcriptional regulators (24% identity and 44% similarity to H-NS of *Salmonella*). Expression of the Ler protein activates transcription of the *LEE2, LEE3,* and *LEE4* operons in a K-12 background. The presence of a regulator controlling type III secretion systems in a PAI is reminiscent of the situation in other enteric pathogens such as *Salmonella* and *Shigella.* These recent studies show that a regulatory cascade controls the expression of virulence factors in EPEC: Per activates Ler, which in turn activates other genes of the type III secretion system. PerA is an AraC homolog (see below), and many members of this family of regulators act in concert with DNA bending, which is in turn affected by the presence of H-NS-type proteins (such as Ler). Although Ler also controls expression of these genes in the LEE of EHEC O157:H7, *per* genes are not found in EHEC.

Another level of control of the genes encoding the type III secretion system was recently reported by Sperandio et al. (105), who showed that the *LEE1* and *LEE2* operons are regulated by quorum sensing. The existence of a quorum-sensing system in *E. coli* K-12 and O157:H7 was recently shown by Surette and Bassler (107), but no target *E. coli* genes that are regulated by this mechanism were identified. Regulation of *LEE1* by quorum sensing in turn increases the expression of the *LEE3* and *LEE4* operons via the Ler protein encoded in *LEE1*. The mechanistic details of these multiple regulatory systems are currently being elucidated, and it is likely that additional positive or negative regulatory elements are yet to be discovered for this system.

Epithelial-Cell Response

The host cell exhibits a variety of responses to EPEC infection, most of which are absolutely dependent upon proteins encoded by the LEE (reviewed in references 37, 54, 55, and 78). The cell cytoskeleton is altered, and localized actin filament depolymerization within microvilli results in retraction of microvilli and effacement. Tir protein is translocated and serves as a nucleator of actin repolymerization beneath adherent bacteria. Other cytoskeletal components such as α-actinin, ezrin, and talin are recruited to join actin in forming pedestals characteristic of the A/E lesion. Protein kinase C is rapidly activated and then deactivated and phospholipase C is activated by tyrosine phosphorylation. Myosin light-chain kinase is activated, leading to phosphorylation of myosin and loosening of tight junctions. NF-κB is translocated to the nucleus, leading to increased transcription of the interleukin-8 gene. Interleukin-8 induces an inflammatory response including migration of polymorphonuclear leukocytes (PMNs) through the paracellular space and into the lumen.

The mechanism(s) of diarrhea due to EPEC infection is not definitely known, but these cellular responses could provide numerous mechanisms by which LEE-containing pathogens could induce diarrhea. Activation of protein kinase C can lead to phosphorylation and activation of the cystic fibrosis transmembrane regulator, the same chloride channel that is activated by cholera toxin. Transepithelial migration of PMNs can induce chloride secretion, since luminal PMNs release AMP which is converted to adenosine, a potent mediator of intestinal secretion. Attachment of EPEC to Caco-2 cells has recently been reported to stimulate chloride secretion (15), although the mechanisms responsible for this secretion are not known. Loosening of tight junctions via myosin light-chain phosphorylation would increase intestinal permeability, which could contribute to diarrhea. Finally, the loss of the absorptive surface provided by the brush border could lead to malabsorption, which would also contribute to diarrhea. It is likely that multiple mechanisms operate simultaneously, although *espB* (108) or *eae* (23) mutants are greatly reduced in diarrheagenicity in volunteers, thereby underscoring the importance of the LEE PAI in EPEC pathogenesis.

EPEC Adherence Factor Plasmid

Prior to the discovery of the LEE, a ca. 60-MDa plasmid called the EPEC adherence factor (EAF) plasmid had been associated with the pathogenesis of disease due to this organism. The majority of EPEC strains associated with diarrhea possess the EAF plasmid and are referred to as typical EPEC strains, while EPEC strains that do not possess EAF plasmids are referred to as atypical EPEC strains (78). Atypical EPEC strains can be isolated from cases of diarrhea, but they are usually not significantly associated with disease in case-control epidemiological studies (78). Although the EAF plasmid was found in 1983 to be essential for the in vitro adherence of EPEC to HEp-2 cells and in 1985 to be essential for full virulence in volunteer studies, it was not until 1991 that a specific virulence factor encoded by this plasmid was described (reviewed in reference 78). This factor is the bundle-forming pilus (BFP) (40), which is a member of the type IV family of pili and which was initially thought to mediate the initial adherence of EPEC to epithelial cells. However, a recent study with intestinal epithelial cells freshly harvested from children undergoing biopsy or surgery suggests that BFP is involved primarily in mediating bacterium-to-bacterium rather than bacterium-to-epithelial-cell adherence (46). The BFP is encoded by a set of 14 genes (*bfpA* to *bfpL, bfpP,* and *bfpU*) contained on the EAF plasmid (reviewed in reference 22). Strains mutated in the *bfpA* or *bfpF* gene were tested in volunteers and found to be significantly attenuated (8). The *bfp* genes are highly conserved between the two strains from which the gene cluster has been sequenced, but some O128ab:H2 and O119:H2 EPEC strains that contain part of the *bfpA* gene encoding the major pilin subunit have the rest of the *bfp* gene cluster deleted (11). Adjacent to the deleted region is an IS66 element, which is proposed to play a role in the deletion of the *bfp* operon in these strains.

A second set of genes located on the EAF plasmid regulates most, if not all, of the EPEC virulence genes described so far. The Per regulator is encoded by a set of three genes called *perABC* that are located 5 kb downstream of the *bfp* operon. As noted above, the product of the first gene, *perA,* is a member of the AraC family of bacterial regulators, but all three ORFs are required for full activation of the regulated genes (41). The Per regulator was initially discovered by the ability of the cloned *per* genes to increase the transcription of the chromosomal *eae* gene (41). Subsequently, it was shown that these genes also regulate expression of the *bfpA* gene (110); the genes previously named *perABC* were confusingly named *bfpTVW* in the later study. Recent studies have shown that the Per regulator also activates genes encoding the type III secretion system in the LEE through the Ler regulator in a cascade fashion (see above).

The EAF plasmid has apparently been introduced at multiple times into EPEC strains (see below). EAF plasmids isolated from different strains of EPEC range in size from ca. 50 to 70 MDa, and hybridization studies show extensive homology among plasmids isolated from different strains (79). The *bfp* and *perABC* gene clusters contain 38.4 and 29.6% G+C, respectively. Just downstream of the last genes in the operons, *bfpL* and *perC,* are genes with much higher G+C contents (*bfpM,* 48.9% G+C, and *perD* or *orfx,* 48.8% G+C), which are highly homologous to transposons. This pattern suggests possible mobility of the *bfp* and *per* genes at one time in the past, although they are now apparently incapable of mobilization. Interestingly, although the EAF plasmid is highly stable in vitro (<1% spontaneous plasmid cure rate), 67% of the challenge strain isolates recovered from volunteer stool specimens had lost this plasmid (65). The potential for loss of the plasmid has implications for the classification of atypical and typical EPEC strains (78).

EspC Pathogenicity Islet

The *espC* gene (106) encodes a 110-kDa protein that has homology to members of the autotransporter protein family, which includes immunoglobulin A proteases of *Neisseria gonorrhoeae* and *Haemophilus influenzae,* Tsh protein produced by avian pathogenic *E. coli,* and SepA of *Shigella flexneri* (45). Two other members of this family are EspP of EHEC and Pet of EAEC (see below). Stein et al. (106) showed that mutation of the *espC* gene did not disrupt the ability of EPEC to form A/E lesions in tissue culture or in animal

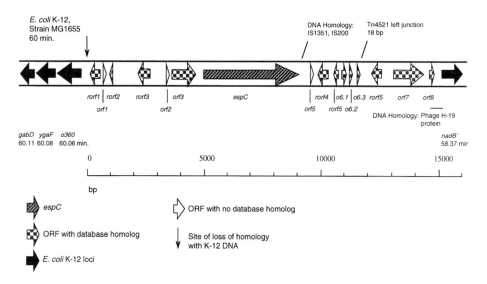

Figure 2. EspC pathogenicity islet from EPEC E2348/69.

models. We have recently shown that the EspC protein has enterotoxic activity and can increase the short-circuit current in rat jejunum mounted in Ussing chambers (74).

The *espC* gene of EPEC E2348/69 is located outside the LEE in a 15-kb region that is absent from *E. coli* K-12 (74). The majority of genes within this region have homology to transposons and insertion elements (IS elements), although these elements are apparently incomplete and nonfunctional (Fig. 2). The *espC* gene is the only obvious gene that encodes a virulence factor, although another ORF upstream of *espC* encodes a predicted protein with 19% identity and 37% similarity to VirA of *Shigella*. We would therefore call this region a pathogenicity islet rather than a PAI. The sequences on the "left" side of the region as presented in Fig. 2 are K-12 sequences located at 60 min. However, the junction with K-12 sequences on the "right" side is not as clear, and preliminary characterization of this region reveals a *nadB′* gene which is located at 58.37 min in K-12. The G+C content of this region is 41.2%. Further sequence analysis may reveal additional non-K-12 sequences before the true junction with the K-12 chromosome is established. Such a pattern would be reminiscent of uropathogenic *E. coli* PAIs that are interrupted by stretches of K-12 DNA (see chapter 4) and would suggest that major deletions and rearrangements of this region of the *E. coli* chromosome have occurred. Examination of other EPEC and EHEC strains shows that the *espC* islet is present only in a minority of EPEC strains of the DEC1 and DEC2 clonal groups (see below) and is absent from any EHEC strains examined to date.

ENTEROHEMORRHAGIC *E. COLI*

EHEC strains are responsible for numerous food- and water-borne outbreaks of bloody diarrhea (hemorrhagic colitis), nonbloody diarrhea, and HUS. The most notorious EHEC serotype is O157:H7, which has caused large outbreaks involving up to 8,000 individuals in Japan, as well as in the United States, United Kingdom, and other industrialized countries. Nomenclature for this pathogen can be confusing, with the terms EHEC, Shiga toxin (Stx)-producing *E. coli* (STEC), and verocytotoxin-producing *E. coli* (VTEC) being used in different reports. EHEC strains represent a subset of *E. coli* which produce Stx (STEC) and are usually considered to contain the LEE PAI and the pO157 virulence plasmid (see below). EHEC O157:H7, the most common human EHEC serotype, expresses a variety of virulence factors which are encoded on PAIs, virulence plasmids, and toxin-encoding bacteriophages. The genome of O157:H7 contains an extra 1 Mb of DNA compared to K-12, and these mobile genetic elements make up at least part of this extra DNA in this pathogen (10).

The LEE PAI

Like EPEC, EHEC O157:H7 and other EHEC serotypes produce the LEE-encoded A/E lesion in tissue culture and animal models. The sequence of the LEE PAI from EHEC O157:H7 strain EDL933 has been determined and compared to that of EPEC E2348/69 (88). A major difference between the two LEEs is that the O157:H7 LEE is larger, containing 43,359 bp compared with 35,624 bp from E2348/69. Most of the size difference is explained by a 7.5-kb putative prophage with homology to the P4 family of prophages. This prophage, designated 933L, is inserted at the end of the LEE closest to the *selC* locus (Fig. 1). The prophage is not present in E2348/69 but is present in an O55:H7 EPEC strain, the EPEC serotype that is most closely related to O157:H7 (see below). The position of the prophage suggests that it was involved in mobilization of the LEE; however, the placement of the putative *att* sites suggests that this scenario is unlikely (88) and that the prophage inserted after chromosomal integration of the LEE. The remaining 41 genes are present in both LEEs in exactly the same order and number. Similar to the low G+C content of the E2348/69 LEE, the 41 genes of the O157:H7 LEE contain 39.59% G+C; the G+C content of the 933L prophage is 51.72%.

The average nucleotide identity for the 41 shared genes is 93.9%, although the rate of divergence is heterogeneous along the LEE. The *esc* genes encoding components of the type III secretion system are highly conserved, with 98 to 100% nucleotide identity. However, genes encoding proteins known to interact directly with the host are much more divergent. The *eae* genes encoding intimin are 87.23% identical, with the majority of the divergence occurring in the 3' end, which encodes the putative receptor-binding portion. The genes encoding the secreted Esp proteins are quite divergent: *espB* (74% identity), *espA* (84.6% identity), and *espD* (80.4% identity). Most divergent of all is the *tir* gene, with 66.5% identity. The variability between the EPEC and O157:H7 LEEs suggests that the variable proteins may be subject to natural selection for adaptation to either host specificity or evasion of the host immune system. Additional genes of unknown function, *sepZ, orf19, rorf10,* and *orf18,* also show striking divergence between the two LEEs. Two genes, *eae* (2, 3, 56) and *tir* (87), have been sequenced from a number of EPEC and EHEC strains. Considerable sequence variation was seen in these loci, with four major families of sequences being found for each gene. Little information is available to correlate functional phenotypic differences with sequence divergence, but it is notable that while the Tir protein of EPEC is tyrosine phosphorylated in host cells, the quite divergent Tir protein of O157:H7 is not tyrosine phosphorylated. Furthermore, although the cloned EPEC LEE from E2348/69 confers the A/E phenotype when cloned into *E. coli* K-12, the cloned LEE from O157:H7 does not confer this phenotype on K-12 when tested on HEp-2 cells (29).

The LEE is present in all O157:H7 strains and is also present in the majority of non-O157:H7 STEC strains implicated in human disease (reviewed in references 55 and 78). In contrast, the majority of STEC strains isolated from animals do not contain the LEE. Although numerous LEE-negative non-O157:H7 strains have been isolated from sporadic human infections as well as from two small outbreaks, possession of the LEE is associated with the most virulent clones of STEC.

Bacteriophages

Stx, the most important virulence factor of EHEC, is encoded on lysogenic bacteriophages. Stx is an A-B subunit toxin which inhibits protein synthesis by depurinating a critical residue in the 28S rRNA of eukaryotic ribosomes. In the intestine, Stx can kill epithelial cells and cause severe inflammation and extensive histological damage, resulting in bloody or nonbloody diarrhea. Stx produced in the intestine is assumed to translocate to the bloodstream (although toxin has never been detected in the blood of patients), thereby leading to HUS. The pathogenesis of HUS is believed to involve direct damage of the glomerular endothelial cells of the kidney by Stx, leading to decreased glomerular filtration rates, thrombocytopenia, microangiopathic hemolytic anemia, and, ultimately, kidney failure.

There is an Stx family composed of two major immunologically non-cross-reactive groups called Stx1 and Stx2, which have 55 and 57% sequence identity in the A and B subunits, respectively. While Stx1 is highly conserved, sequence variation exists within Stx2, and the different variants are designated Stx2c, Stx2v, Stx2vhb, Stxt2e, etc. Stx1 is essentially identical to the Stx produced by *Shigella dysenteriae* 1, but the toxin in *Shigella* is chromosomally encoded rather than phage encoded. EHEC isolated from human disease may express either Stx1 or Stx2 or both; the Stx2e variant is classically associated with pig edema disease rather than human disease and, unlike other *E. coli* members of the Stx family, is chromosomally encoded. *E. coli* strains belonging to over 200 serotypes (i.e., O:H antigen combinations, not just O serogroups) can express Stx, but within most serotypes, both Stx-positive and Stx-negative strains can be found (53). The *stx2* gene has also been found in some strains of *Citrobacter freundii* and *Enterobacter* spp. (99). The genetics, mechanism of action, and role in pathogenesis of Stx toxins have been extensively reviewed (78, 84, 101).

The lambdoid-like bacteriophages encoding Stx1 or Stx2 from O157 strains are similar in genomic size (62 to 73 kb) and have extensive DNA homology, although Stx phages from non-O157 strains may show greater variability (91). The larger phage genome size compared to lambda phage (48.5 kb) suggests that other virulence factors may be encoded on these phages besides the Stx. These phages are responsible for considerable genomic variation within *E. coli* O157:H7 and non-O157 EHEC strains. In vitro transduction of Stx between *E. coli* strains has been known for many years, and in vivo transduction in a mouse model has recently been demonstrated (1). Stx phage can be lost upon in vitro subculture, and some non-O157:H7 serotypes are particularly prone to phage loss (57). In vivo phage loss in humans has also been reported. In one study of seven patients who shed O157 in their stools for over 32 days, two of the patients eventually shed O157 variants which had lost an *stx* gene (58). The chromosomal insertion site of the 933W prophage encoding Stx2 in O157:H7 strain EDL933 is the *wrbA* gene (9), but the full range of phage insertion sites in different strains is not known. Restriction fragment length polymorphism (RFLP) patterns based on Stx phage sequences have been used as an epidemiological tool for discriminating among O157 strains. By using λ DNA as a hybridization probe, Paros et al. (86) found 23 different RFLP patterns among 72 human and bovine O157:H7 isolates. How much of the RFLP variability is due to differences in phage insertion sites rather than differences within phage sequences is not known.

Plasmids

A 92-kb plasmid is highly conserved among EHEC strains of the O157:H7 serotype and is also common in EHEC strains of other serotypes associated with human disease (66). The DNA sequence of this plasmid, called pO157, has been determined from two different strains, the well-studied EDL 933 strain isolated in 1982 from an outbreak in Michigan (14) and a recently isolated strain from the massive 1996 outbreak in Japan (68). The sequence analysis reveals a composite structure with two possible replication origins (of IncFI and IncFII plasmids) and up to 18 partial or complete IS elements scattered around the plasmid (Fig. 3). A third replication region is interrupted by an IS*629* insertion. Several potential virulence factors are encoded on this plasmid. A hemolysin belonging to the RTX family of toxins is encoded by the *hlyABCD* genes, whose predicted protein products have ca. 60 to 70% identity to the *hlyABCD* gene products of uropathogenic *E. coli* (6, 98). A 104-kDa serine protease encoded by the *espP* gene belongs to the autotransporter protein family and has striking homology to the chromosomally encoded EspC protein of EPEC (64% similarity in the N-terminal region and 89% similarity in the C-terminal region) (13). This protease has also been found in an O26:H− EHEC strain,

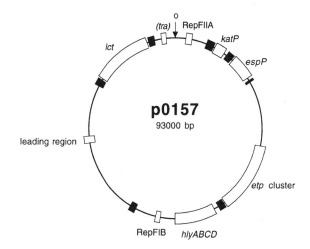

Figure 3. Map of the pO157 plasmid based on the complete sequence determination by Makino et al. (68) and Burland et al. (14). Solid boxes indicate locations of major IS elements.

where it was called PssA (21). Adjacent to the *espP* gene (separated by an IS*629* element) is the *katP* gene encoding a bifunctional catalase peroxidase (12, 14). A type II secretion system with similarity to the pullulanase secretion pathway of *Klebsiella* is encoded by the *etp* genes on this plasmid, but the specific proteins that are actually secreted by this system are unknown (97). An unusually large ORF on this plasmid, encoding 3,169 amino acids, shows strong sequence similarity in the first 700 residues to the toxin family known as the large clostridial toxins that includes ToxA and ToxB from *Clostridium difficile* (14, 68).

No definitive evidence exists to link any of the pO157-encoded factors to disease caused by EHEC, but this lack of evidence is probably due to the lack of an appropriate animal model that reproduces all aspects of EHEC disease. Numerous studies have drawn variable conclusions showing either substantial or insignificant contributions of the plasmid (reviewed in reference 78). There is a strong correlation, however, between the presence of this plasmid and human disease (78). Essentially all O157:H7 isolates possess this plasmid, and some 95% of non-O157 Stx-producing *E. coli* strains isolated from patients possess it. In contrast, only a minority of non-O157 STEC strains from cattle possess it. There is also a strong correlation between the presence of the pO157 plasmid and the LEE PAI. In one study of human and animal STEC strains, 44 of 45 non-O157 isolates were either positive for both probes or negative for both probes (4). Interestingly, there is some heterogeneity among pO157 plasmids isolated from different strains. Karch et al. (59) found that 100% of O157 strains hybridized with an *hly* gene probe (which corresponds to the CVD419 probe of Levine et al. [66]) and with an *etp* probe while only 66% of strains hybridized with the *katP* or *espP* probe. Among non-O157 STEC strains, 95% hybridized with the *hly* genes, 52% hybridized with the *etp* genes, and 36% hybridized with the *espP* genes. No doubt the numerous IS elements present on this plasmid contribute to the deletions and variability seen among different plasmid isolates.

A 6.7-kb plasmid called pColD157 has been isolated from many O157 strains. This plasmid encodes colicinogenic activity, and it has been suggested that this activity could inhibit the normal gut flora, thereby giving O157 strains a selective advantage in the intestine (47). Interestingly, 16 of 46 O157 strains isolated in Germany between 1987 and 1991 harbored this plasmid whereas only 1 of 50 strains isolated during 1996 carried it, thus suggesting continuing evolution of the O157 pathogen (47). Finally, a 3.3-kb plasmid named p4821 was found in 8% of the O157:H7 strains isolated in Germany in 1996 (43). This plasmid is >98% identical to the core region of the antibiotic resistance plasmid NTP16 of *Salmonella typhimurium* but apparently does not encode any virulence factors or antibiotic resistance.

Clonal Evolution of A/E *E. coli*

A considerable body of work has described the evolution of *E. coli* strains based on multilocus enzyme electrophoresis (MLEE) patterns of housekeeping proteins. Whittam and colleagues (116–119) have made important contributions to this field and have described at least 23 distinct clones of *E. coli* strains associated with enteric disease which are referred to as DEC (diarrheagenic *E. coli*) clones. Based on MLEE analysis, two clusters of EPEC strains and two clusters of EHEC strains have been defined: EPEC1 (containing DEC groups 1 and 2 and serotypes such as O127:H6 and O55:H6), EPEC2

(DEC groups 11 and 12 and serotypes such as O128:H2, O111:H2, O111:NM, and O45:H2), EHEC1 (DEC groups 3 and 4 and O157:H7 and O157:H− serotypes), and EHEC2 (DEC groups 8 and 9 and serotypes such as O111:H8, O111:H11, O26:H11, and O26:NM). In addition, Stx-producing *E. coli* strains that do not contain the LEE are grouped into two other clusters called STEC1 and STEC2. The MLEE patterns plus variations in the LEE insertion site and sequence variation in *stx, eae,* and other genes allow the construction of a possible model for the evolution of EPEC and EHEC and other A/E *E. coli* strains (Fig. 4).

The LEE is found in one of at least three different chromosomal insertion sites, and the specific insertion site differs according to the clonal phylogeny of the strains (104, 120). From an ancestral strain lacking the LEE, one branch of the A/E pathogens acquired the LEE at the *selC* locus and further evolved along two paths. One path acquired the EAF plasmid and became the cluster known as EPEC1; a subgroup of the EPEC1 strains acquired the *espC* islet. A second fork of the *selC* lineage contained O55:H7 strains, which further evolved along two different lines. One line became the present-day O55:H7 EPEC strains, which comprise DEC5. These strains are EAF negative and *espC* negative and presumably never acquired these elements. A second line of the O55:H7 lineage acquired the Stx2 phage and subsequently acquired an *rfb* gene cluster encoding the O157 lipopolysaccharide (33, 117). Further evolution of this cluster included the acquisition of the pO157 plasmid and the Stx1 phage to become the present-day O157:H7 EHEC.

A second branch of A/E pathogens acquired the LEE at the *pheU* locus and evolved along two paths. One path became the EPEC2 cluster, which includes both EAF-positive and EAF-negative strains. Another path acquired Stx phages and the pO157 plasmid to

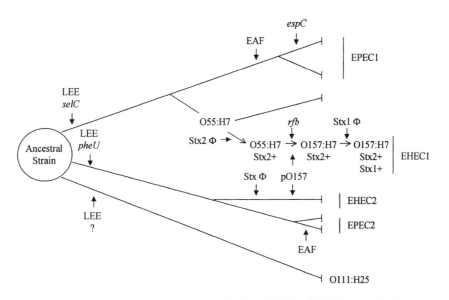

Figure 4. Proposed model for the clonal evolution of EPEC and EHEC strains showing the hypothesized insertion of the LEE PAI, the EAF and pO157 plasmids, the Stx phage, the *espC* islet, and the *rfb* genes encoding the O157 lipopolysaccharide.

become the EHEC2 cluster. The LEE PAIs in this second branch of the A/E pathogens have acquired additional DNA, including IS elements, so that the LEEs in this branch are larger than those in the *selC* branch (104). Finally, a third group, containing O111ab:H25 strains, acquired the LEE at a site other than *selC* or *pheU,* the identity of which is currently unknown (104). These strains lack the EAF plasmid.

It is likely that multiple acquisitions and losses of the Stx bacteriophages and EAF and pO157 plasmids occurred during this evolution. While the sequence variation of genes within the LEE PAIs is consistent with the evolution along phylogenetic lines, the high conservation of plasmid sequences in strains with considerable chromosomal variation argues for lateral transfer of the plasmids among EPEC and EHEC strains. Conversely, even within the highly clonal O157:H7 serotype, differences among the pO157 plasmid are found (see above). The evolutionary model described is obviously very simplified but is consistent with the available data. Additional information on the evolution of EHEC O157:H7 and other EPEC, EHEC, and STEC strains can be found in the papers by Whittam and colleagues (33, 116–119).

ENTEROAGGREGATIVE *E. COLI*

EAEC is defined by aggregative adherence (AA) to HEp-2 cells in culture. EAEC has been associated characteristically with persistent diarrhea among infants, particularly in the developing world (reviewed in references 78 and 80). However, recent outbreaks and volunteer studies suggest that EAEC strains are virulent in adults (50, 81) and have a global distribution (48).

The virulence factors of EAEC are not as well understood as those of other *E. coli* pathotypes. However, several putative virulence factors have been described, and there is evidence supporting the roles of some of these in pathogenesis (Table 3). Although the full pathogenetic paradigm has not been formulated for EAEC, available evidence supports

Table 3. Putative virulence genes in EAEC

Factor	Product	Genomic location	Evidence for role in virulence
AAF/I	Fimbria	Plasmid	Adherence to human epithelial cell lines in vitro (76)
AAF/II	Fimbria	Plasmid	Adherence to human colonic explants (16); associated with diarrhea in epidemiologic study (85)
EAST	Enterotoxin	Plasmid	Rises in Isc in rabbit tissue (94)
Pet	Cytoskeleton-altering enterotoxin	Plasmid	Elicits damage to human colonic explants (44)
Pic	Protease	Chromosome	Associated with disease in epidemiologic study[a] (112); associated with colonization of mouse gastrointestinal tract (44)
ShET1	Enterotoxin	Chromosome	Associated with disease in epidemiologic study (112)
Yersiniabactin	Siderophore	Chromosome	None
Tia	Invasin	Chromosome	Invasion of epithelial cells in culture (35)

[a] Cannot be differentiated from ShET1 due to overlapping configuration of the *pic/set* genes.

a model comprising mucosal colonization followed by enterotoxin and probably cytotoxin production.

Plasmid-Borne Virulence Genes

The large majority of EAEC strains harbor a 60- to 65-MDa plasmid (designated pAA) that confers the defining AA phenotype (5, 111). In the best-studied examples, this phenotype is mediated by the plasmid-borne fimbrial antigen AAF/I or AAF/II (16, 76); these antigens are both related to the Dr class of *E. coli* adhesins (83). Interestingly, although mutants with null mutations in these fimbrial genes are deficient in AA, many strains that do not express AAF/I or AAF/II are nonetheless capable of adhering to HEp-2 cells in the AA pattern. Several investigators have therefore proposed that various fimbrial and nonfimbrial surface factors may also contribute to expression of the AA phenotype (19, 114).

The 65-MDa pAA plasmid (designated pAA2) from the pathogenic EAEC strain 042 has been studied in some detail (Fig. 5). pAA2 encodes the AAF/II fimbria as well as the enterotoxins Pet and EAST, all within a cluster of approximately 25 kb (Fig. 5) (see below). pAA2 is considered prototypical of the pAA family, since most EAEC strains share at least one gene with pAA2. This observation was first suggested by Baudry et al. (5), who described a ca. 800-bp fragment that is present on pAA2 and that serves as a

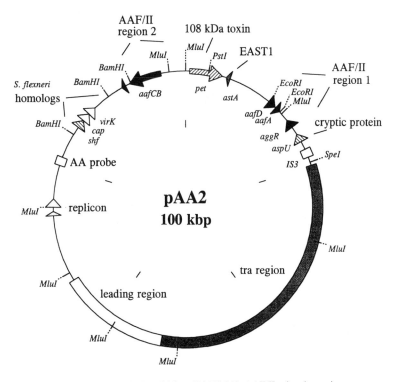

Figure 5. Map of the pAA2 plasmid from EAEC 042. AAF/II-related proteins are represented by solid black arrows. Secreted proteins are designated by hatching.

useful marker for pAA plasmids. Thus, EAEC is like EPEC, EHEC, and *Shigella,* in that virulent strains apparently harbor a partially conserved pathotype-specific virulence plasmid.

Approximately 18% of EAEC strains carry the gene encoding Pet, a 108-kDa protein with enterotoxic and cytoskeleton-altering effects (31). Pet has 55% amino acid identity to the EspP protein of EHEC. When applied to HEp-2 cells, purified Pet induces rounding and detachment of cells, accompanied by early loss of microfilaments (82); the cells remain viable until after they have detached from the substratum. In support of a pathogenetic role for this toxin, Nataro et al. (77) have shown that EAEC strains induce exfoliation of mucosal cells and widening of crypt openings in human colonic tissue maintained in organ culture. Null mutations of *pet* induce significantly less toxic effect in this model, whereas the effect is restored when the *pet* mutation is complemented in *trans* (44).

The Pet protein is a member of the autotransporter class of proteins secreted from gram-negative organisms. This class is named for a distinctive secretion mechanism, first described for the immunoglobulin A (IgA) protease of *Neisseria gonorrhoeae* (45). Auto-transporter proteins possess a signal sequence that is presumed (but not proven) to mediate inner membrane secretion via the Sec apparatus. Once in the periplasm, a ca. 30-kDa C-terminal domain forms a beta-barrel structure, which inserts into the outer membrane and serves as a pore for the passage of the mature (or passenger) domain of the protein. Upon translocation, the passenger protein is cleaved and is released into the extracellular milieu. Flanking the *pet* gene and indeed the genes of the close homologs of this secreted protein lie remnants of insertion sequences, generally IS*629* and IS*911*. The presence of these remnants provides a potential mechanism to explain the presence of autotransporters in only some members of a particular pathotype and upon the plasmid (EHEC and EAEC) or the chromosome (EPEC).

The *pet* gene of strain 042 lies between two gene clusters, each of which is required for biogenesis of the AAF/II fimbrial antigen (26) (Fig. 5). The AAF/II genes feature a unique organization in which a P-fimbria-like chaperone (called here *aafD*), the fimbrial subunit (*aafA*), and a *trans*-acting transcriptional regulator (*aggR*) are present in a cluster designated region 1. A second gene cluster (region 2) (26), encoding the *aafC* fimbrial usher and the product of a smaller gene with homology to the Dr-family putative invasin genes (38), lies 13 kb away from region 1. Upstream from *aafC* lies a pseudogene with significant nucleotide homology to the chaperone family. Notably, the genes of region 1 have closest homology to those encoding the AAF/I fimbrial antigen (95) and exhibit a similarly low G+C content whereas the genes of region 2 are more closely related to those encoding the afimbrial Dr adhesins and have a similarly high G+C content (26). Both region 1 and region 2 genes are flanked by IS elements. Taken together, these observations suggest that the AAF/II biogenesis genes arose by a novel mechanism. The region 1 cluster was probably the original AAF/II biogenesis cluster, at some point comprising an AAF/I-like cluster of chaperone-usher-invasin-pilin genes (95). However, it appears that the pAA2 ancestral plasmid underwent insertion of a complete Dr-like gene cluster by virtue of the flanking IS elements of the Dr-like gene cluster. In support of this conjecture, Garcia et al. (39) have demonstrated transposition of a Dr-family cluster as a complete transposon. Following the insertion of the new fimbrial antigen, genes from each AAF/II cluster were lost by deletion or point mutation, giving rise to the current novel organization.

The AAF/I and AAF/II fimbriae are each present in only a minority of EAEC strains (16). However, the activator of transcription for each of these fimbriae (*aggR*) is present in a much higher proportion of EAEC isolates (ca. 60 to 80%) (17, 85). These data suggest that other, as yet undescribed AAFs may exist and that these may also be under the control of the AggR regulator.

Also encoded within the 25-kb pAA2 virulence gene cluster is the EAST1 gene (*astA*). This gene encodes a low-molecular-weight ST-like toxin that elicits increases in short-circuit current in rabbit tissue mounted in the Ussing chamber (94). The *astA* gene resides within an IS-like element (26), explaining the observation that it is found on either the chromosome or a plasmid of many *E. coli* pathotypes as well as in a large number of commensal *E. coli* strains (96). A role for EAST1 in enteric pathogenesis has yet to be demonstrated.

Also located on many pAA plasmids is a cluster of three genes that have close (93% identical) homologs in *Shigella flexneri* (89). The third gene of this cluster is *virK*, which has been described as a posttranslational regulator of VirG expression (75). Upstream from *virK* lie a gene (termed *shf*) whose predicted product is a cryptic 30-kDa protein and a gene designated *cap*, which has homology to the superfamily of hexosyltransferase genes (44). The *cap* gene product may serve to modify the O antigen expressed by strain 042. No role for these genes in EAEC virulence has yet been described.

Further analysis of pAA2 reveals an IncFVII-like replicon, as well as other genes required for replication and maintenance of IncF plasmids (Fig. 5) (25). In addition, an apparently complete *tra* region has been identified and conjugal transfer of pAA2 has been demonstrated (85). This observation presumably explains the presence of close pAA2 homologs widely dispersed throughout the phylogenetic map of EAEC (17).

Chromosomal Virulence Genes

Although no well-defined PAIs have been described for EAEC strains, three chromosomal loci that may play roles in virulence have been identified. Czeczulin et al. (17) have shown that 57% of the EAEC strains that they examined carried genes homologous to the *S. flexneri* chromosomal gene *she*, which encodes a 116-kDa mucinase. This gene is notable in that *Shigella* enterotoxin 1 (ShET1) is encoded on the *she* antisense strand in an overlapping configuration (32). Moreover, a null mutation in the *she* allele (designated *pic*) in EAEC 042 confers a 2-log-unit-lower colonization of the mouse gastrointestinal tract than does the wild-type parent (44). Thus, these overlapping genes are likely to represent virulence factors.

The complete sequence of the *she/pic* island has not been determined in any strain, but Rajakumar et al. (90) have suggested that another high-molecular-weight secreted protein (SigA) is linked to the *she* gene in *S. flexneri*. However, we have found that the *sigA* gene is not present in *she*-positive EAEC strains, suggesting that the *she* chromosomal locus differs between *Shigella* and EAEC.

Schubert et al. (100) have reported that most EAEC strains harbor the 45-kb high pathogenicity island (HPI) of *Yersinia enterocolitica* (see chapter 5). This island encodes the siderophore yersiniabactin and its uptake protein, FyuA. Nucleotide sequence analysis reveals that the island in EAEC 17-2 is complete, highly homologous to that of *Y. enterocol-*

itica, and also inserted into the chromosomal *asnT* locus (100). Notably, the *hms* genes, part of the HPI of *Y. pestis,* are not present in EAEC strains.

Fleckenstein et al. (35) have described a chromosomal gene designated *tia* that encodes a 25-kDa putative invasin protein in ETEC. The *tia* gene is located in a 46-kb PAI in ETEC, which is described below. Although the distribution of the entire PAI has not yet been described, the *tia* gene has been found in prototype EAEC 042 but as yet in no other EAEC strains. Further investigation of this locus is under way.

ENTEROTOXIGENIC *E. COLI*

ETEC strains are major causes of weanling diarrhea in children in the developing world and of traveler's diarrhea in adults from industrialized countries traveling to developing countries. ETEC strains elaborate at least one member of two defined groups of enterotoxins: LT (heat-labile enterotoxin) and ST (heat-stable enterotoxin) (reviewed in references 78 and 101). LT is related to cholera toxin and acts primarily by increasing intracellular cyclic AMP (cAMP) levels, which ultimately leads to altered epithelial-cell ion transport and diarrhea. STa is a small peptide that acts by binding to the extracellular portion of the membrane-spanning guanylate cyclase protein, leading to increased intracellular cGMP levels and ultimately to altered ion transport. A second class of heat-stable enterotoxins, STb, is associated primarily with ETEC strains isolated from pigs. The mechanism by which STb causes diarrhea is not known, but it does not increase intracellular cAMP or cGMP levels.

ETEC strains colonize the human intestine via surface structures that are called colonization factor antigens (CFAs) or CS antigens. These colonization factors can be divided into groups based on morphology: rigid, bundle forming, fibrillar, or nonfimbrial (78). At least 19 different colonization factors have been reported for ETEC strains isolated from humans, and additional colonization factors have been found in animal ETEC isolates.

Mobile Genetic Elements

Most ETEC enterotoxins and colonization factors are encoded on plasmids. In fact, ETEC virulence factors were the first bacterial virulence factors shown to be plasmid encoded (102). The ETEC plasmids generally belong to the IncFI and IncFII incompatibility classes, but some plasmids belong to other classes such as I, P, and X (67). Molecular analysis of enterotoxin plasmids shows that strains with the same O serotype and toxigenicity carry closely related plasmids (18). Interestingly, enterotoxin plasmids from serotypes frequently associated with *E. coli* diarrhea are generally nonconjugative, whereas toxin plasmids from serotypes rarely associated with diarrhea are usually conjugative (18). Both enterotoxins and colonization factors may be encoded on the same plasmid, or they may be encoded on separate plasmids within the same strain. Duplicate copies of enterotoxin genes may be encoded on separate plasmids within the same strain, and many enterotoxin plasmids contain genes encoding resistance to a variety of antibiotics. In some cases, regulatory elements essential for expression of colonization factors may be present on one plasmid while the structural genes are present on a second plasmid or even on the chromosome. Enterotoxin-encoding plasmids can also encode antibiotic resistance, and transmission of these plasmids has been observed under the selective pressure of increased antibiotic use (42). Another factor in the evolution of ETEC is the fact that the gene encoding STa can be present on a functional transposon in some strains (103).

Unlike the *Yersinia* and *Shigella* virulence plasmids, the enterotoxin-encoding plasmids of ETEC have not been reported to contain 10- to 30-kb blocks of DNA which encode multiple virulence factors involved in pathogenesis. The lack of such reports may not reflect the true situation but may instead reflect the fact that the great majority of research in ETEC pathogenesis has concentrated on LT and ST and the colonization factors and relatively little attention has been paid to other potential virulence factors. No enterotoxin plasmids have been sequenced as of this writing, but such future studies will provide insights into the evolution of these plasmids.

A potential chromosomal PAI has recently been described in a prototypical ETEC strain, H10407, by Fleckenstein et al. (35). Discovery of this PAI arose from investigations of the *tia* locus, which was shown to mediate in vitro invasion into cultured intestinal epithelial cells (34). (A second gene associated with ETEC invasion in vitro, *tib*, is unlinked to the *tia* locus and is found only in CFAI-containing ETEC strains [30].) The *tia* gene is located in a ca. 46-kb region that is inserted at *selC*, the same site of insertion as that for the LEE of E2348/69 and O157:H7 and for PAI I from uropathogenic *E. coli* 536. Preliminary sequence information for a 37-kb portion of this region revealed a G+C content of 43.7% compared to the 50.8% G+C content of *E. coli* K-12. Within this region are genes encoding proteins with homology to P4 integrase, retronphage R73 integrase, and IS2. The first ORF within this island (next to the *selC* gene) is nearly identical to the gene encoding integrase from the 933L prophage from the EHEC O157:H7 LEE. At the opposite end of this island are four ORFs with high homology to the L7 to L10 ORFs of the 933L prophage. Thus, all available information indicates that this region is indeed a PAI, but the relevance of this PAI to disease caused by ETEC has yet to be established.

ENTEROINVASIVE *E. COLI*

EIEC strains are biochemically and genetically closely related to *Shigella* species and closely resemble *Shigella* species in possessing a virulence plasmid encoding the ability to penetrate epithelial cells. The plasmid virulence genes and other aspects of pathogenesis of EIEC are virtually identical to those of *Shigella* species, which are reviewed in chapter 8.

EIEC and *Shigella* species produce aerobactin, an iron-binding protein which is associated with enhanced virulence. The *iuc* genes, encoding aerobactin, together with the *iutA* gene, encoding an aerobactin receptor, were recently found by Vokes et al. (113) to be located within a PAI in *S. flexneri*. This island, called Shi II for *Shigella* aerobactin island, is inserted into the *selC* locus in this species and is at least 26 kb. This island contains the *int* gene encoding the prophage integrase gene found in the O157:H7 LEE, and the region sequenced to date has a G+C content of 43%, not counting the numerous partial and complete IS element genes which may have transposed into this region after acquisition of the island. The *iuc* genes are also present in EIEC, but many other genes of Shi II are missing from *E. coli*. The insertion site of the *iuc* and *iutA* genes in EIEC is unknown, but these genes are inserted at a chromosomal site other than *selC*. In many *E. coli* strains associated with septicemia, the aerobactin genes are inserted in a plasmid, whose prototype is pColV (reviewed by Vokes et al. [113]). The mobility of the *uic* genes, which are found in at least three different locations in the *E. coli-Shigella* group (two chromosomal locations and one plasmid), may be explained by the presence of the integrase gene and the IS elements on Shi II.

A concept that is the opposite of PAIs was recently proposed for EIEC and *Shigella* species. It has long been known that EIEC and *Shigella* species are lysine decarboxylase (LDC) negative, in contrast to the great majority of *E. coli* strains, which are LDC positive. Maurelli et al. (69) introduced the gene for LDC, *cadA,* into *S. flexneri* 2a and observed that virulence became attenuated and enterotoxin activity was greatly inhibited. The product of the reaction catalyzed by LDC, cadaverine, was identified as the inhibitor of enterotoxin activity. The *cadA* gene was shown to be in a region of up to 90 kb that is present around 90 min in the *E. coli* K-12 chromosome but deleted from EIEC and *Shigella* species. The authors propose that as EIEC and *Shigella* evolved from commensal *E. coli* to become pathogens, they not only acquired virulence genes on a plasmid but also shed genes via deletions. They named these blocks of deleted genes ''black holes'' and proposed that deletion of such genes, which are detrimental to a pathogenic lifestyle, can provide an evolutionary mechanism that enables a pathogen to enhance virulence.

CONCLUSIONS

The genome size of natural isolates of *E. coli* can vary by as much as 1 Mb, from 4.5 to 5.5 Mb (7). Much of the extra DNA in pathogenic strains can be accounted for by PAIs, virulence plasmids, and toxin-encoding bacteriophages, as reviewed here. However, some DNA that is present in K-12 strains is missing from pathogenic strains, and there is evidence to suggest that the deletion of certain K-12 sequences, the so-called black holes, actually enhances virulence (69). A comprehensive picture of one of these pathogens, EHEC O157:H7, is emerging from the genomic sequencing project being completed in the Blattner laboratory. The O157:H7 genome contains ca. 1 Mb of unique DNA that is absent from K-12, while ca. 0.54 Mb of K-12 DNA is absent from O157:H7 (9). The unique DNA insertions and deletions are not concentrated in only one or two sites but are scattered throughout the chromosome.

The best-characterized PAI of *E. coli* O157:H7 and EPEC, and of diarrheagenic *E. coli* in general, is the LEE. The LEE (35,624 bp for strain E2348/69) is considerably smaller than most PAIs of uropathogenic *E. coli,* which can be as large as 190 kb (see chapter 4). The prototypical LEE PAI of EPEC E2348/69 is relatively ''lean,'' with nearly all of the 41 ORFs being required for formation of the A/E phenotype, and less than 2% of the LEE contains the IS-like sequences that are so prominent in many other PAIs. It is striking that so many PAIs in diarrheagenic *E. coli* and other enteric pathogens are inserted at the *selC* locus, including the LEE of EPEC O127:H6 and EHEC O157:H7, the *tia*-associated PAI of ETEC, Shi II of *S. flexneri,* SPI-3 of *Salmonella enteritidis* (see chapter 7), and PAI I of uropathogenic *E. coli* (see chapter 4). While this insertion site is the most prominent so far described, the LEE is present in at least two other chromosomal sites. Additional PAIs of diarrheagenic *E. coli* that are inserted at other tRNA genes will no doubt be described.

In *E. coli* K-12, an estimated 755 of the 4,288 ORFs have been introduced into the *E. coli* genome in at least 234 lateral transfer events since this species diverged from *Salmo-*

nella some 100 million years ago (64). Many of these horizontally transferred regions, which constitute ca. 18% of the K-12 genome, are inserted at 1 of up to 19 different tRNA genes (64). The great variety of mobile genetic elements present in diarrheagenic *E. coli,* including plasmids, bacteriophages, transposons, and PAIs, on a K-12 backbone with so many horizontally transferred regions indicates an enormous genomic plasticity that complicates both our efforts to categorize the existing subgroups into sharply delineated pathotypes and our attempts to predict what novel combination of virulence factors may emerge in the future.

Acknowledgments. Work in our laboratories was supported by Public Health Service grants AI-21657 and AI-41325 to J.B.K. and AI-33096 to J.P.N. We thank Mohamed Karmali, Vanessa Sperandio, and Jane Michalski for assistance in preparation of this chapter.

REFERENCES

1. **Acheson, D. W. K., J. Reidl, X. Zhang, G. T. Keusch, J. J. Mekalanos, and M. K. Waldor.** 1998. In vivo transduction with Shiga toxin 1-encoding phage. *Infect. Immun.* **66:**4496–4498.
2. **Adu-Bobie, J., G. Frankel, C. Bain, A. G. Goncalves, L. R. Trabulsi, G. Douce, S. Knutton, and G. Dougan.** 1998. Detection of intimins α, β, γ, and δ. Four intimin derivatives expressed by attaching and effacing microbial pathogens. *J. Clin. Microbiol.* **36:**662–668.
3. **Agin, T. S., and M. K. Wolf.** 1997. Identification of a family of intimins common to *Escherichia coli* causing attaching-effacing lesions in rabbits, humans, and swine. *Infect. Immun.* **65:**320–326.
4. **Barrett, T. J., J. B. Kaper, A. E. Jerse, and I. K. Wachsmuth.** 1992. Virulence factors in Shiga-like toxin-producing *Escherichia coli* isolated from humans and cattle. *J. Infect. Dis.* **165:**979–980.
5. **Baudry, B., S. J. Savarino, P. Vial, J. B. Kaper, and M. M. Levine.** 1990. A sensitive and specific DNA probe to identify enteroaggregative *Escherichia coli,* a recently discovered diarrheal pathogen. *J. Infect. Dis.* **161:**1249–1251.
6. **Bauer, M. E., and R. A. Welch.** 1996. Characterization of an RTX toxin from enterohemorrhagic *Escherichia coli* O157:H7. *Infect. Immun.* **64:**167–175.
7. **Bergthorsson, U., and H. Ochman.** 1998. Distribution of chromosome length variation in natural isolates of *Escherichia coli. Mol. Biol. Evol.* **15:**6–16.
8. **Bieber, D., S. W. Ramer, C. Wu, W. J. Murray, T. Tobe, R. Fernandez, and G. K. Schoolnik.** 1998. Type IV pili, transient bacterial aggregates, and virulence of enteropathogenic *Escherichia coli. Science* **280:**2114–2118.
9. **Blattner, F. R.** 1999. Personal communication.
10. **Blattner, F. R., G. I. Plunkett, N. T. Perna, Y. Shao, J. Gregor, G. F. Mayhew, B. Mau, N. W. Davis, H. A. Kirkpatrick, D. Rose, and M. Goeden.** 1997. Comparative genome sequencing of *E. coli* O157:H7 versus *E. coli* K-12. *Microb. Comp. Genomics* **2:**174. (Abstract.)
11. **Bortolini, M. R., L. R. Trabulsi, R. Keller, G. Frankel, and V. Sperandio.** Virulence properties and characterization of a conserved deletion in the *bfp* operon in enteropathogenic *Escherichia coli* (EPEC) strains from O128ab:H2 and O119:H2 serotypes. Submitted for publication.
12. **Brunder, W., H. Schmidt, and H. Karch.** 1996. KatP, a novel catalase-peroxidase encoded by the large plasmid of enterohaemorrhagic *Escherichia coli* O157:H7. *Microbiology* **142:**3305–3315.
13. **Brunder, W., H. Schmidt, and H. Karch.** 1997. EspP, a novel extracellular serine protease of enterohaemorrhagic *Escherichia coli* O157:H7 cleaves human coagulation factor V. *Mol. Microbiol.* **24:**767–778.
14. **Burland, V., Y. Shao, N. T. Perna, G. Plunkett, H. J. Sofia, and F. R. Blattner.** 1998. The complete DNA sequence and analysis of the large virulence plasmid of *Escherichia coli* O157:H7. *Nucleic Acids Res.* **26:**4196–4204.
15. **Collington, G. K., I. W. Booth, and S. Knutton.** 1998. Rapid modulation of electrolyte transport in Caco-2 cell monolayers by enteropathogenic *Escherichia coli* (EPEC) infection. *Gut* **42:**200–207.
16. **Czeczulin, J. R., S. Balepur, S. Hicks, A. Phillips, R. Hall, M. H. Kothary, F. Navarro-Garcia, and J. P. Nataro.** 1997. Aggregative adherence fimbria II, a second fimbrial antigen mediating aggregative adherence in enteroaggregative *Escherichia coli. Infect. Immun.* **65:**4135–4145.

17. **Czeczulin, J. R., T. S. Whittam, I. R. Henderson, and J. P. Nataro.** 1999. Phylogenetic analysis of enteroaggregative and diffusely adherent *Escherichia coli*. *Infect. Immun.* **67**:2692–2699.

18. **Danbara, H., K. Komase, H. Arita, H. Abe, and M. Yoshikawa.** 1988. Molecular analysis of enterotoxin plasmids of enterotoxigenic *Escherichia coli* of 14 different O serotypes. *Infect. Immun.* **56**:1513–1517.

19. **Debroy, C., J. Yealy, R. A. Wilson, M. K. Bhan, and R. Kumar.** 1995. Antibodies raised against the outer membrane protein interrupt adherence of enteroaggregative *Escherichia coli*. *Infect. Immun.* **63**: 2873–2879.

20. **Deibel, C., S. Krämer, T. Chakraborty, and F. Ebel.** 1998. EspE, a novel secreted protein of attaching and effacing bacteria, is directly translocated into infected host cells where it appears as a tyrosine-phosphorylated 90 kDa protein. *Mol. Microbiol.* **28**:463–474.

21. **Djafari, S., F. Ebel, C. Deibel, S. Krämer, M. Hudel, and T. Chakraborty.** 1997. Characterization of an exported protease from Shiga toxin-producing *Escherichia coli*. *Mol. Microbiol.* **25**:771–784.

22. **Donnenberg, M. S., L. Lai, and K. A. Taylor.** 1997. The locus of enterocyte effacement pathogenicity island of enteropathogenic *Escherichia coli* encodes secretion functions and remnants of transposons at its extreme right end. *Gene* **184**:107–114.

23. **Donnenberg, M. S., C. O. Tacket, S. P. James, G. Losonsky, J. P. Nataro, S. S. Wasserman, J. B. Kaper, and M. M. Levine.** 1993. Role of the *eaeA* gene in experimental enteropathogenic *Escherichia coli* infection. *J. Clin. Investig.* **92**:1412–1417.

24. **Donnenberg, M. S., J. Yu, and J. B. Kaper.** 1993. A second chromosomal gene necessary for intimate attachment of enteropathogenic *Escherichia coli* to epithelial cells. *J. Bacteriol.* **175**:4670–4680.

25. **Dubovsky, F., and J. P. Nataro.** 1999. Unpublished observations.

26. **Elias, W. P., Jr., J. R. Czeczulin, I. R. Henderson, L. R. Trabulsi, and J. P. Nataro.** 1999. Organization of biogenesis genes for aggregative adherence fimbria II defines a virulence gene cluster in enteroaggregative *Escherichia coli*. *J. Bacteriol.* **181**:1779–1785.

27. **Elliott, S., L. A. Wainwright, T. McDaniel, B. MacNamara, M. Donnenberg, and J. B. Kaper.** 1998. The complete sequence of the locus of enterocyte effacement (LEE) from enteropathogenic *Escherichia coli* E2348/69. *Mol. Microbiol.* **28**:1–4.

28. **Elliott, S. J., M. S. Dubois, S. W. Hutcheson, L. A. Wainwright, M. Batchelor, G. Frankel, S. Knutton, and J. B. Kaper.** Identification of CesT, a chaperone for the type III secretion of Tir in enteropathogenic *Escherichia coli*. Submitted for publication.

29. **Elliott, S. J., J. Yu, and J. B. Kaper.** The cloned locus of enterocyte effacement (LEE) from enterohemorrhagic *Escherichia coli* O157:H7 is unable to confer the attaching-effacing phenotype on *E. coli* K-12. Submitted for publication.

30. **Elsinghorst, E. A., and J. A. Weitz.** 1994. Epithelial cell invasion and adherence directed by the enterotoxigenic *Escherichia coli tib* locus is associated with a 104-kilodalton outer membrane protein. *Infect. Immun.* **62**:3463–3471.

31. **Eslava, C. E., F. Navarro-Garcia, J. R. Czeczulin, I. R. Henderson, A. Cravioto, and J. P. Nataro.** 1998. Pet, an autotransporter enterotoxin from enteroaggregative *Escherichia coli*. *Infect. Immun.* **66**: 3155–3163.

32. **Fasano, A., F. Noriega, J. Liao, W. Wang, and M. M. Levine.** 1997. Effect of *Shigella* enterotoxin 1 (ShET1) on rabbit intestine in vitro and in vivo. *Gut* **40**:505–511.

33. **Feng, P., K. A. Lampel, H. Karch, and T. S. Whittam.** 1998. Genotypic and phenotypic changes in the emergence of *Escherichia coli* O157:H7. *J. Infect. Dis.* **177**:1750–1753.

34. **Fleckenstein, J. M., D. J. Kopecko, R. L. Warren, and E. A. Elsinghorst.** 1996. Molecular characterization of the *tia* invasion locus from enterotoxigenic *Escherichia coli*. *Infect. Immun.* **64**:2256–2265.

35. **Fleckenstein, J. M., N. J. Snellings, E. A. Elsinghorst, and L. E. Lindler.** 1997. The *tia* gene of the prototypical ETEC strain H10407 is encoded on a large chromosomal element inserted within the *selC* tRNA gene, p. 37. *In Abstracts of the Meeting on Microbial Pathogenesis and Host Response*. Cold Spring Harbor Laboratory Press, Cold Spring Harbor, N.Y.

36. **Foubister, V., I. Rosenshine, M. S. Donnenberg, and B. B. Finlay.** 1994. The *eaeB* gene of enteropathogenic *Escherichia coli* (EPEC) is necessary for signal transduction in epithelial cells. *Infect. Immun.* **62**: 3038–3040.

37. **Frankel, G., A. D. Phillips, I. Rosenshine, G. Dougan, J. B. Kaper, and S. Knutton.** 1998. Enteropathogenic and enterohaemorrhagic *Escherichia coli*: more subversive elements. *Mol. Microbiol.* **30**:911–921.

38. **Garcia, M. I., P. Gounon, P. Courcoux, A. Labigne, and C. Le Bouguénec.** 1996. The afimbrial adhesive

sheath encoded by the *afa-3* gene cluster of pathogenic *Escherichia coli* is composed of two adhesins. *Mol. Microbiol.* **19:**683–693.

39. **Garcia, M. L., A. Labigue, and C. Le Bouguénec.** 1994. Nucleotide sequence of the afimbrial adhesin-encoding *afa-3* gene cluster and its translocation via flanking IS*1* sequences. *J. Bacteriol.* **176:**7601–7613.

40. **Girón, J. A., A. S. Y. Ho, and G. K. Schoolnik.** 1991. An inducible bundle-forming pilus of enteropathogenic *Escherichia coli. Science* **254:**710–713.

41. **Gómez-Duarte, O. G., and J. B. Kaper.** 1995. A plasmid-encoded regulatory region activates chromosomal *eaeA* expression in enteropathogenic *Escherichia coli. Infect. Immun.* **63:**1767–1776.

42. **Gyles, C. L., S. Palchaudhuri, and W. K. Mass.** 1977. Naturally occurring plasmid carrying genes for enterotoxin production and drug resistance. *Science* **198:**198–199.

43. **Haarmann, C., H. Karch, M. Frosch, and H. Schmidt.** 1998. A 3.3-kb plasmid of enterohemorrhagic *Escherichia coli* O157:H7 is closely related to the core region of the *Salmonella typhimurium* antibiotic resistance plasmid NTP16. *Plasmid* **39:**134–140.

44. **Henderson, I. R., S. Hicks, A. Phillips, and J. P. Nataro.** 1999. Unpublished observations.

45. **Henderson, I. R., F. Navarro-Garcia, and J. P. Nataro.** 1998. The great escape: structure and function of the autotransporter proteins. *Trends Microbiol.* **6:**370–378.

46. **Hicks, S., G. Frankel, J. B. Kaper, G. Dougan, and A. D. Phillips.** 1998. Role of intimin and bundle-forming pili in enteropathogenic *Escherichia coli* adhesion to pediatric intestine in vitro. *Infect. Immun.* **66:**1570–1578.

47. **Hofinger, C., H. Karch, and H. Schmidt.** 1998. Structure and function of plasmid pColD157 of enterohemorrhagic *Escherichia coli* O157 and its distribution among strains from patients with diarrhea and hemolytic-uremic syndrome. *J. Clin. Microbiol.* **36:**24–29.

48. **Huppertz, H. I., S. Rutkowski, S. Aleksic, and H. Karch.** 1997. Acute and chronic diarrhoea and abdominal colic associated with enteroaggregative *Escherichia coli* in young children living in western Europe. *Lancet* **349:**1660–1662.

49. **Ismaili, A., D. J. Philpott, M. T. Dytoc, and P. M. Sherman.** 1995. Signal transduction responses following adhesion of verocytotoxin-producing *Escherichia coli. Infect. Immun.* **63:**3316–3326.

50. **Itoh, Y., I. Nagano, M. Kunishima, and T. Ezaki.** 1997. Laboratory investigation of enteroaggregative *Escherichia coli* O untypeable:H10 associated with a massive outbreak of gastrointestinal illness. *J. Clin. Microbiol.* **35:**2546–2550.

51. **Jarvis, K. G., J. A. Girón, A. E. Jerse, T. K. McDaniel, M. S. Donnenberg, and J. B. Kaper.** 1995. Enteropathogenic *Escherichia coli* contains a specialized secretion system necessary for the export of proteins involved in attaching and effacing lesion formation. *Proc. Natl. Acad. Sci. USA* **92:**7996–8000.

52. **Jerse, A. E., J. Yu, B. D. Tall, and J. B. Kaper.** 1990. A genetic locus of enteropathogenic *Escherichia coli* necessary for the production of attaching and effacing lesions on tissue culture cells. *Proc. Natl. Acad. Sci. USA* **87:**7839–7843.

53. **Johnson, R. P., R. C. Clarke, J. B. Wilson, S. C. Read, K. Rahn, S. A. Renwick, K. A. Sandhu, D. Alves, M. A. Karmali, H. Lior, S. A. McEwen, J. S. Spika, and C. L. Gyles.** 1996. Growing concerns and recent outbreaks involving non-O157:H7 serotypes of verotoxigenic *Escherichia coli. J. Food Prot.* **59:**1112–1122.

54. **Kaper, J. B.** 1998. EPEC delivers the goods. *Trends Microbiol.* **6:**169–172.

55. **Kaper, J. B., S. Elliott, V. Sperandio, N. T. Perna, G. F. Mayhew, and F. R. Blattner.** 1998. Attaching and effacing intestinal histopathology and the locus of enterocyte effacement, p. 163–182. *In* J. B. Kaper and A. D. O'Brien (ed.), Escherichia coli *O157:H7 and Other Shiga Toxin-Producing* E. coli *Strains.* American Society for Microbiology, Washington, D.C.

56. **Kaper, J. B., L. J. Gansheroff, W. R. Wachtel, and A. D. O'Brien.** 1998. Intimin-mediated adherence of Shiga toxin-producing *Escherichia coli* and attaching-and-effacing pathogens, p. 148–156. *In* J. B. Kaper and A. D. O'Brien (ed.), Escherichia coli *O157:H7 and Other Shiga Toxin-Producing* E. coli *Strains.* American Society for Microbiology, Washington, D.C.

57. **Karch, H., T. Meyer, H. Rüssmann, and J. Heesemann.** 1992. Frequent loss of Shiga-like toxin genes in clinical isolates of *Escherichia coli* upon subcultivation. *Infect. Immun.* **60:**3464–3467.

58. **Karch, H., H. Rüssmann, H. Schmidt, A. Schwarzkopf, and J. Heesemann.** 1995. Long-term shedding and clonal turnover of enterohemorrhagic *Escherichia coli* O157 in diarrheal disease. *J. Clin. Microbiol.* **33:**1602–1605.

59. **Karch, H., H. Schmidt, and W. Brunder.** 1998. Plasmid-encoded determinants of *Escherichia coli*

O157:H7, p. 183–194. *In* J. B. Kaper and A. D. O'Brien (ed.), Escherichia coli *O157:H7 and Other Shiga Toxin-Producing* E. coli *Strains.* American Society for Microbiology, Washington, D.C.

60. **Kenny, B., R. DeVinney, M. Stein, D. J. Reinscheid, E. A. Frey, and B. B. Finlay.** 1997. Enteropathogenic *E. coli* (EPEC) transfers its receptor for intimate adherence into mammalian cells. *Cell* **91**:511–520.

61. **Kenny, B., L. Lai, B. B. Finlay, and M. S. Donnenberg.** 1996. EspA, a protein secreted by enteropathogenic *Escherichia coli,* is required to induce signals in epithelial cells. *Mol. Microbiol.* **20**:313–324.

62. **Knutton, S., I. Rosenshine, M. J. Pallen, L. Nisan, B. C. Neves, C. Bain, C. Wolff, G. Dougan, and G. Frankel.** 1998. A novel EspA-associated surface organelle of enteropathogenic *Escherichia coli* involved in protein translocation into epithelial cells. *EMBO J.* **17**:2166–2176.

63. **Lai, L.-C., L. A. Wainwright, K. D. Stone, and M. S. Donnenberg.** 1997. A third secreted protein that is encoded by the enteropathogenic *Escherichia coli* pathogenicity island is required for transduction of signals and for attaching and effacing activities in host cells. *Infect. Immun.* **65**:2211–2217.

64. **Lawrence, J. G., and H. Ochman.** 1998. Molecular archaeology of the *Escherichia coli* genome. *Proc. Natl. Acad. Sci. USA* **95**:9413–9417.

65. **Levine, M. M., J. P. Nataro, H. Karch, M. M. Baldini, J. B. Kaper, R. E. Black, M. L. Clements, and A. D. O'Brien.** 1985. The diarrheal response of humans to some classic serotypes of enteropathogenic *Escherichia coli* is dependent on a plasmid encoding an enteroadhesiveness factor. *J. Infect. Dis.* **152**:550–559.

66. **Levine, M. M., J. Xu, J. B. Kaper, H. Lior, V. Prado, B. Tall, J. Nataro, H. Karch, and K. Wachsmuth.** 1987. A DNA probe to identify enterohemorrhagic *Escherichia coli* of O157:H7 and other serotypes that cause hemorrhagic colitis and hemolytic uremic syndrome. *J. Infect. Dis.* **156**:175–182.

67. **Mainil, J. G., F. Bex, P. Dreze, A. Kaeckenbeeck, and M. Couturier.** 1992. Replicon typing of virulence plasmids of enterotoxigenic *Escherichia coli* isolates from cattle. *Infect. Immun.* **60**:3376–3380.

68. **Makino, K., K. Ishii, T. Yasunaga, M. Hattori, K. Yokoyama, C. H. Yutsudo, Y. Kubota, Y. Yamaichi, T. Iida, K. Yamamoto, T. Honda, C. Han, E. Ohtsubo, M. Kasamatsu, T. Hayashi, S. Kuhara, and H. Shinagawa.** 1998. Complete nucleotide sequences of 93-kb and 3.3-kb plasmids of an enterohemorrhagic *Escherichia coli* O157:H7 derived from Sakai outbreak. *DNA Res.* **5**:1–9.

69. **Maurelli, A. T., R. E. Fernández, C. A. Bloch, C. K. Rode, and A. Fasano.** 1998. "Black holes" and bacterial pathogenicity: a large genomic deletion that enhances the virulence of *Shigella* spp. and enteroinvasive *Escherichia coli. Proc. Natl. Acad. Sci. USA* **95**:3943–3948.

70. **McDaniel, T. K., K. G. Jarvis, M. S. Donnenberg, and J. B. Kaper.** 1995. A genetic locus of enterocyte effacement conserved among diverse enterobacterial pathogens. *Proc. Natl. Acad. Sci. USA* **92**:1664–1668.

71. **McDaniel, T. K., and J. B. Kaper.** 1997. A cloned pathogenicity island from enteropathogenic *Escherichia coli* confers the attaching and effacing phenotype on *E. coli* K-12. *Mol. Microbiol.* **23**:399–407.

72. **McNamara, B. P., and M. S. Donnenberg.** 1998. A novel proline-rich protein, EspF, is secreted from enteropathogenic *Escherichia coli* via the type III export pathway. *FEMS Microbiol. Lett.* **166**:71–78.

73. **Mellies, J., S. J. Elliott, V. Sperandio, M. S. Donnenberg, and J. B. Kaper.** A regulatory cascade controlling expression of genes encoding type III secretion components and secreted molecules in the locus of enterocyte effacement in enteropathogenic *E. coli. Mol. Microbiol.,* in press.

74. **Mellies, J. L., F. Navarro-Garcia, J. P. Nataro, and J. B. Kaper.** 1999. The EspC pathogenicity islet encodes an enterotoxin of enteropathogenic *Escherichia coli.* Submitted for publication.

75. **Nakata, N., C. Sasakawa, N. Okada, T. Tobe, I. Fukuda, T. Suzuki, K. Komatsu, and M. Yoshikawa.** 1992. Identification and characterization of *virK,* a virulence-associated large plasmid gene essential for intercellular spreading of *Shigella flexneri. Mol. Microbiol.* **6**:2387–2395.

76. **Nataro, J. P., Y. Deng, D. R. Maneval, A. L. German, W. C. Martin, and M. M. Levine.** 1992. Aggregative adherence fimbriae I of enteroaggregative *Escherichia coli* mediate adherence to HEp-2 cells and hemagglutination of human erythrocytes. *Infect. Immun.* **60**:2297–2304.

77. **Nataro, J. P., S. Hicks, A. D. Phillips, P. A. Vial, and C. L. Sears.** 1996. T84 cells in culture as a model for enteroaggregative *Escherichia coli* pathogenesis. *Infect. Immun.* **64**:4761–4768.

78. **Nataro, J. P., and J. B. Kaper.** 1998. Diarrheagenic *Escherichia coli. Clin. Microbiol. Rev.* **11**:142–201.

79. **Nataro, J. P., K. O. Maher, P. Mackie, and J. B. Kaper.** 1987. Characterization of plasmids encoding the adherence factor of enteropathogenic *Escherichia coli. Infect. Immun.* **55**:2370–2377.

80. **Nataro, J. P., T. S. Steiner, and R. L. Guerrant.** 1998. Enteroaggregative *Escherichia coli. Emerging Infect. Dis.* **4**:251–261.

81. **Nataro, J. P., D. Yikang, S. Cookson, A. Cravioto, S. J. Savarino, L. D. Guers, M. M. Levine,**

and C. O. Tacket. 1995. Heterogeneity of enteroaggregative *Escherichia coli* virulence demonstrated in volunteers. *J. Infect. Dis.* **171**:465–468.

82. Navarro-Garcia, F., C. Sears, C. Eslava, A. Cravioto, and J. P. Nataro. 1999. Cytoskeletal effects induced by Pet, the serine protease enterotoxin of enteroaggregative *Escherichia coli*. *Infect. Immun.* **67**: 2184–2192.

83. Nowicki, B., A. Labigne, S. L. Moseley, R. Hull, S. Hull, and J. Moulds. 1990. The Dr hemagglutinin, afimbrial adhesins AFA-I and AGA-III, and F1845 fimbriae of uropathogenic and diarrhea-associated *Escherichia coli* belong to a family of hemagglutinins with Dr receptor recognition. *Infect. Immun.* **58**: 279–281.

84. O'Brien, A. D., V. L. Tesh, A. Donohue-Rolfe, M. P. Jackson, S. Olsnes, K. Sandvig, A. A. Lindberg, and G. T. Keusch. 1992. Shiga toxin: biochemistry, genetics, mode of action, and role in pathogenesis. *Curr. Top. Microbiol. Immunol.* **180**:65–94.

85. Okeke, I. N., A. Lamikanra, J. R. Czeczulin, J. B. Kaper, and J. P. Nataro. 1999. Unpublished observations.

86. Paros, M., P. I. Tarr, H. Kim, T. E. Besser, and D. D. Hancock. 1993. A comparison of human and bovine *Escherichia coli* O157:H7 isolates by toxin genotype, plasmid profile, and bacteriophage lambda-restriction fragment length polymorphism profile. *J. Infect. Dis.* **168**:1300–1303.

87. Paton, A. W., P. A. Manning, M. C. Woodrow, and J. C. Paton. 1998. Translocated intimin receptors (Tir) of Shiga-toxigenic *Escherichia coli* isolates belonging to serogroups O26, O111, and O157 react with sera from patients with hemolytic-uremic syndrome and exhibit marked sequence heterogeneity. *Infect. Immun.* **66**:5580–5586.

88. Perna, N. T., G. F. Mayhew, G. Pósfal, S. Elliott, M. S. Donnenberg, J. B. Kaper, and F. R. Blattner. 1998. Molecular evolution of a pathogenicity island from enterohemorrhagic *Escherichia coli* O157:H7. *Infect. Immun.* **66**:3810–3817.

89. Rajakumar, K., F. Luo, C. Sasakawa, and B. Adler. 1996. Evolutionary perspective on a composite *Shigella flexneri* 2a virulence plasmid borne locus comprising three distinct genetic elements. *FEMS Microbiol. Lett.* **144**:13–20.

90. Rajakumar, K., C. Sasakawa, and B. Adler. 1997. Use of a novel approach, termed island probing, identifies the *Shigella flexneri she* pathogenicity island which encodes a homolog of the immunoglobulin A protease-like family of proteins. *Infect. Immun.* **65**:4606–4614.

91. Rietra, P. J., G. A. Willshaw, H. R. Smith, A. M. Field, S. M. Scotland, and B. Rowe. 1989. Comparison of Vero-cytotoxin-encoding phages from *Escherichia coli* of human and bovine origin. *J. Gen. Microbiol.* **135**:2307–2318.

92. Rode, C. K., L. J. Melkerson-Watson, A. T. Johnson, and C. A. Bloch. 1999. Type-specific contributions to chromosome size differences in *Escherichia coli*. *Infect. Immun.* **67**:230–236.

93. Rosenshine, I., M. S. Donnenberg, J. B. Kaper, and B. B. Finlay. 1992. Signal transduction between enteropathogenic *Escherichia coli* (EPEC) and epithelial cells: EPEC induces tyrosine phosphorylation of host cell proteins to initiate cytoskeletal rearrangement and bacterial uptake. *EMBO J.* **11**:3551–3560.

94. Savarino, S. J., A. Fasano, D. C. Robertson, and M. M. Levine. 1991. Enteroaggregative *Escherichia coli* elaborate a heat-stable enterotoxin demonstrable in an in vitro rabbit intestinal model. *J. Clin. Investig.* **87**:1450–1455.

95. Savarino, S. J., P. Fox, Y. K. Deng, and J. P. Nataro. 1994. Identification and characterization of a gene cluster mediating enteroaggregative *Escherichia coli* aggregative adherence fimbria I biogenesis. *J. Bacteriol.* **176**:4949–4957.

96. Savarino, S. J., A. McVeigh, J. Watson, A. Cravioto, J. Molina, P. Echeverria, M. K. Bhan, M. M. Levine, and A. Fasano. 1996. Enteroaggregative *Escherichia coli* heat-stable enterotoxin is not restricted to enteroaggregative *E. coli*. *J. Infect. Dis.* **173**:1019–1022.

97. Schmidt, H., B. Henkel, and H. Karch. 1997. A gene cluster closely related to type II secretion pathway operons of gram-negative bacteria is located on a large plasmid of enterohemorrhagic *Escherichia coli* O157 strains. *FEMS Microbiol. Lett.* **148**:265–272.

98. Schmidt, H., C. Kernbach, and H. Karch. 1996. Analysis of the EHEC *hly* operon and its location in the physical map of the large plasmid of enterohaemorrhagic *Escherichia coli* O157:H7. *Microbiology* **142**:907–914.

99. Schmidt, H., M. Montag, J. Bockemühl, J. Heesemann, and H. Karch. 1993. Shiga-like toxin II-related cytotoxins in *Citrobacter freundii* strains from humans and beef samples. *Infect. Immun.* **61**:534–543.

100. **Schubert, S., A. Rakin, H. Karch, E. Carniel, and J. Heeseman.** 1998. Prevalence of the "high pathogenicity island" of *Yersinia* species among *Escherichia coli* strains that are pathogenic to humans. *Infect. Immun.* **66:**480–485.

101. **Sears, C. L., and J. B. Kaper.** 1996. Enteric bacterial toxins: mechanisms of action and linkage to intestinal secretion. *Microbiol. Rev.* **60:**167–215.

102. **Smith, H. W., and M. A. Linggood.** 1971. The transmissible nature of enterotoxin production in a human enteropathogenic strain of *Escherichia coli. J. Med. Microbiol.* **4:**301–305.

103. **So, M., F. Heffron, and B. J. McCarthy.** 1979. The *E. coli* gene encoding heat stable toxin is a bacterial transposon flanked by inverted repeats of IS1. *Nature* **277:**453–456.

104. **Sperandio, V., J. B. Kaper, M. R. Bortolini, B. C. Neves, R. Keller, and L. R. Trabulsi.** 1998. Characterization of the locus of enterocyte effacement (LEE) in different enteropathogenic *Escherichia coli* (EPEC) and Shiga-toxin producing *Escherichia coli* (STEC) serotypes. *FEMS Microbiol. Lett.* **164:**133–139.

105. **Sperandio, V., J. Mellies, W. Nguyen, and J. B. Kaper.** Regulation by quorum sensing of genes encoding the type III secretion system in enterohemorrhagic *Escherichia coli* O157:H7. Submitted for publication.

106. **Stein, M., B. Kenny, M. A. Stein, and B. B. Finlay.** 1996. Characterization of EspC, a 110-kilodalton protein secreted by enteropathogenic *Escherichia coli* which is homologous to members of the immunoglobulin A protease-like family of secreted proteins. *J. Bacteriol.* **178:**6546–6554.

107. **Surette, M. G., and B. L. Bassler.** 1998. Quorum sensing in *Escherichia coli* and *Salmonella typhimurium. Proc. Natl. Acad. Sci. USA* **95:**7046–7050.

108. **Tacket, C. O., G. Losonsky, M. B. Sztein, A. Abe, B. B. Finlay, G. T. Fantry, S. P. James, J. P. Nataro, J. B. Kaper, M. M. Levine, and M. S. Donnenberg.** The role of EspB in experimental human enteropathogenic *Escherichia coli* (EPEC) infection. Submitted for publication.

109. **Taylor, K. A., P. W. Luther, and M. S. Donnenberg.** 1999. Expression of the EspB protein of enteropathogenic *Escherichia coli* within HeLa cells affects stress fibers and cellular morphology. *Infect. Immun.* **67:** 120–125.

110. **Tobe, T., G. K. Schoolnik, I. Sohel, V. H. Bustamante, and J. L. Puente.** 1996. Cloning and characterization of *bfpTVW*, genes required for the transcriptional activation of *bfpA* in enteropathogenic *Escherichia coli. Mol. Microbiol.* **21:**963–975.

111. **Vial, P. A., R. Robins Browne, H. Lior, V. Prado, J. B. Kaper, J. P. Nataro, D. Maneval, A. Elsayed, and M. M. Levine.** 1988. Characterization of enteroadherent-aggregative *Escherichia coli,* a putative agent of diarrheal disease. *J. Infect. Dis.* **158:**70–79.

112. **Vila, J., and J. P. Nataro.** 1999. Unpublished observations.

113. **Vokes, S. A., A. G. Torres, S. A. Reeves, and S. M. Payne.** The aerobactin iron transport system genes in *Shigella flexneri* are present within a pathogenicity island. *Mol. Microbiol.,* in press.

114. **Wai, S. N., A. Takade, and K. Amako.** 1996. The hydrophobic surface protein layer of enteroaggregative *Escherichia coli* strains. *FEMS Microbiol. Lett.* **135:**17–22.

115. **Wainwright, L. A., and J. B. Kaper.** 1998. EspB and EspD require a specific chaperone for proper secretion from enteropathogenic *E. coli. Mol. Microbiol.* **27:**1247–1260.

116. **Whittam, T. S.** 1966. Genetic variation and evolutionary processes in natural populations of *Escherichia coli,* p. 2708–2720. *In* F. C. Neidhardt, R. Curtiss III, J. L. Ingraham, E. C. C. Lin, K. B. Low, B. Magasanik, W. S. Reznikoff, M. Riley, M. Schaechter, and H. E. Umbarger (ed.), Escherichia coli *and* Salmonella*: Cellular and Molecular Biology,* 2nd ed. American Society for Microbiology, Washington, D.C.

117. **Whittam, T. S.** 1998. The evolution of *Escherichia coli* O157:H7 and other Shiga toxin-producing *E. coli* strains, p. 195–209. *In* J. B. Kaper and A. D. O'Brien (ed.), Escherichia coli *O157:H7 and Other Shiga Toxin-Producing* E. coli *Strains.* American Society for Microbiology, Washington, D.C.

118. **Whittam, T. S., and E. A. McGraw.** 1996. Clonal analysis of EPEC serogroups. *Rev. Microbiol. Sao Paulo* **27**(Suppl. 1)**:**7–16.

119. **Whittam, T. S., M. L. Wolfe, I. K. Wachsmuth, F. Orskov, I. Orskov, and R. A. Wilson.** 1993. Clonal relationships among *Escherichia coli* strains that cause hemorrhagic colitis and infantile diarrhea. *Infect. Immun.* **61:**1619–1629.

120. **Wieler, L. H., T. K. McDaniel, T. S. Whittam, and J. B. Kaper.** 1997. Insertion site of the locus of enterocyte effacement in enteropathogenic and enterohemorrhagic *Escherichia coli* differs in relation to the clonal phylogeny of the strains. *FEMS Microbiol. Lett.* **156:**49–53.

121. **Wolff, C., I. Nisan, E. Hanski, G. Frankel, and I. Rosenshine.** 1998. Protein translocation into host epithelial cells by infecting enteropathogenic *Escherichia coli. Mol. Microbiol.* **28:**143–155.

Chapter 4

Pathogenicity Islands of Extraintestinal
Escherichia coli

*Jörg Hacker, Gabriele Blum-Oehler, Britta Janke, Gabor Nagy, and
Werner Goebel*

EXTRAINTESTINAL *ESCHERICHIA COLI*

Escherichia coli Pathotypes and Their Diseases

Strains of *Escherichia coli* have their principal habitat in the bowels of humans and animals. For a long time *E. coli* was considered a harmless commensal. However, the identification and characterization of a wide range of specific virulence factors changed this view. Nowadays, particular variants of *E. coli* are known to be pathogens because of their potential to cause disease in the gastrointestinal tract as well as extraintestinal infections (61, 77). While intestinal *E. coli* strains can be grouped into at least six different pathotypes, extraintestinal *E. coli* strains fall into three groups: MENEC (meningitis *E. coli*) strains, which cause newborn meningitis (NBM), SEPEC (septicemia *E. coli*) strains, which cause meningitis and septicemia, and UPEC (uropathogenic *E. coli*) strains, which are by far the most common cause of uncomplicated cases of urinary tract infections (UTIs). This review focuses mainly on UPEC because urinary tract infections represent, by number, the most important bacterial infectious disease in highly industralized countries. Furthermore, UPEC strains are considered a model system for analysis of the genome structure and the composition of pathogenicity islands (PAIs) of pathogenic bacteria in general.

Uropathogenic *Escherichia coli*

About 80% of the UTIs in outpatients and 40% in hospital patients are due to *E. coli* (81). Most UTIs are ascending infections, where the infectious agents originate from the patient's own fecal flora. The pathogens can migrate through the urethra to the bladder and, in more severe cases, may proceed through the ureters to the kidneys. Occasionally the infecting bacteria invade the bloodstream and cause septicemia. Less common infections occur via hematogenous spread of an organism to the kidneys. Moreover, *E. coli* bacteria colonizing the urinary tracts of pregnant women represent a source of strains that

Jörg Hacker, Gabriele Blum-Oehler, Britta Janke, and Gabor Nagy • Institut für Molekulare Infektionsbiologie, Universität Würzburg, Röntgenring 11, D-97070 Würzburg, Germany. *Werner Goebel* • Lehrstuhl für Mikrobiologie, Biozentrum Universität Würzburg, D-97074 Würzburg, Germany.

cause NBM (10, 57). UTIs are more common in women than in men and manifest themselves as cystitis (95% of all cases in women), pyelonephritis, and, in men, prostatitis. Uncomplicated UTIs are mostly due to *E. coli*, but other species such as *Proteus mirabilis, Klebsiella pneumoniae,* and, in young women, *Staphylococcus saprophyticus* may also contribute to this type of infection (81). Complicated UTIs generally occur in patients with complicated urinary tracts, i.e., with anatomical and functional abnormalities. While the former UTIs are generally responsive to antibiotic treatment, the latter ones are more resistant, and persistent infections may occur.

   E. coli strains causing UTIs possess traits that distinguish them from commensal *E. coli* isolates and other pathotypes causing diarrhea. One important trait is the presence of adherence factors which enable them to adhere to uroepithelial cells (20). These include type 1 fimbrial adhesins binding to mannose oligosaccharides, P fimbrial adhesins binding to Galα(1–4)Gal moieties of glycolipids, S fimbrial adhesins binding to α-sialyl-2,3-β-galactose receptors and F1C fimbriae binding to Galβ(1–3)GalNAc and Gal(31–4)GlcNAc receptors (35, 45, 73). Whereas type 1 fimbriae are common among pathogenic and nonpathogenic *E. coli* strains, P fimbriae are the most prevalent fimbrial type in UPEC strains. In addition, most UPEC strains produce a pore-forming toxin which belongs to the group of Rtx toxins, alpha-hemolysin, and cytotoxic necrotizing factor 1 (CNF1), which causes necrosis of eukaryotic cells (29, 54, 71). They also produce the enterobactin system, as well as additional iron uptake systems such as aerobactin and yersiniabactin (21, 74). Furthermore, most UPEC strains belong to a select group of O types (e.g., O1, O4, O6, O18, and O75), produce a capsule antigen (preferentially K1 or K5), and have the capacity to overcome the human complement system by a complex mechanism termed serum resistance (43). Particular UPEC isolates and strains causing NBM have the capacity to invade epithelial and endothelial cells. Specific gene products encoded by *ibe* are involved in the invasive processes (40).

PATHOGENICITY ISLANDS OF UROPATHOGENIC *E. COLI*

General Features

   PAIs were initially discovered in UPEC strains, and UPEC PAIs are now among the best-understood examples of PAIs (8). In the early 1980s, UPEC strains were shown to contain distinct blocks of DNA carrying closely linked virulence genes (33, 38, 53). The first PAIs were identified in the UPEC strains 536 and J96 (9, 34, 78). Recently, another PAI has been identified in *E. coli* CFT073 (44).

   With a few exceptions, the PAIs of all three strains meet the following criteria typical of PAIs: (i) they occupy large genomic DNA regions (>20 kb), (ii) they carry at least one virulence gene, (iii) they are inserted within or near tRNA genes, (iv) they contain direct repeats and mobility sequences, and (v) they have a G+C content different from that of the respective host bacteria (36). With the recent findings of multiple PAIs in UPEC strains, a uniform nomenclature has become necessary. We therefore propose the following. In agreement with current usage, the PAIs will be numbered chronologically in roman numerals. To acknowledge the bacterial strain in which the PAI was detected, the roman numerals will be followed by the strain designation in subscript letters. Accordingly, PAI I_{536} is the first PAI detected in strain 536.

Composition

UPEC 536 (O6:K15:H31) was isolated from a patient with acute pyelonephritis and is well characterized (4). This strain produces several virulence factors including two alpha-hemolysins (*hly*), three different fimbrial adhesin types (P-related, S, and type 1 fimbriae [*prf, sfa,* and *fim,* respectively]), and the siderophores enterobactin (*ent*) and yersiniabactin (*ybt*), and it exhibits serum resistance (11). Goebel and coworkers initially analyzed the *hly*-flanking sequences of this strain and observed that they are located on large, unstable chromosomal regions, which were termed "hemolysin islands" (33, 47). Further studies revealed the presence of additional virulence genes, namely, the *prf* gene cluster, on one of these regions, which were therefore renamed "pathogenicity islands (PAIs)" (34). It was demonstrated that these virulence genes are closely linked on the chromosome of strain 536 and that codeletion of hemolysin and fimbrial gene clusters can occur.

At least four PAIs are present in the genome of UPEC 536 (Fig. 1). The sizes of the PAIs vary significantly being between ~25 and 190 kb. While PAIs I$_{536}$ and II$_{536}$ carry *hly* and *prf* genes, PAI III$_{536}$ encodes the S fimbrial adhesin (8, 12). PAI IV$_{536}$ is characterized by the presence of the *fyuA* (ferric yersiniabactin uptake) and *irp1* through *irp5* (iron-repressible protein) genes, which encode the yersiniabactin iron uptake (*ybt*) system originally found in the genome of different *Yersinia* species on the so-called "high-patho-

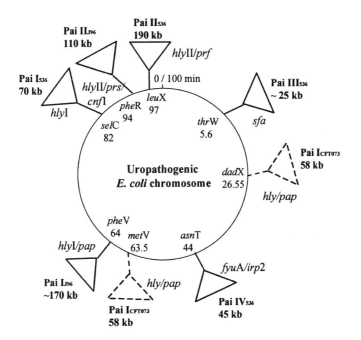

Figure 1. Distribution of PAIs in the UPEC genome. The indicated map positions refer to the *E. coli* K-12 chromosome. The position of PAI I$_{CFT073}$ remains unclear and is shown in dotted lines because the left junction of this PAI maps at 26.55, downstream of the *dadX* gene (alanine racemase), and the right junction maps at 63.5, downstream of the *metV* tRNA gene (44).

genicity island'' (HPI) (15, 27) (for further details, see chapter 5). It could be demonstrated that the HPI is also a part of the genome of other pathogenic *E. coli* strains, especially enteroaggregative (EAEC) and fecal isolates (74). All four PAIs have common features, i.e., the association with tRNA genes at their boundaries and the presence of (often cryptic) integrase genes (Table 1). PAIs I_{536} and II_{536} are flanked by direct repeats of 16 bp (PAI I_{536}) or 18 bp (PAI II_{536}), and one copy each of the direct repeats forms part of the 3' end of tRNA genes. PAI I_{536} is flanked by the *selC* gene (map position 82), a selenocysteine-tRNA, while PAI II_{536} is associated with the leucine-specific tRNA gene *leuX* (map position 97), which is involved in the modulation of virulence gene expression in strain 536 (see below) (8, 69). Whereas PAIs I_{536} and II_{536} can be deleted from the chromosome, possibly by the involvement of the direct repeats in homologous recombination, deletion of PAIs III_{536} and IV_{536} has not been detected yet. In the flanking region of PAI III_{536}, a *thrW* tRNA gene followed by a putative integrase gene (*intD*) of prophage DLP 12 of *E. coli* K-12 could be identified. According to the map position of *thrW* and the flanking genes *proA and proB*, the insertion site of PAI III_{536} could be mapped to 5.6 min (5, 12). Linkage to a tRNA gene, *asnT,* was also shown for PAI IV_{536}, which is inserted at map position 44. Interestingly, a cluster of three additional *asn* tRNA genes is present around map location 44, and these genes can independently serve as integration sites for the HPI in *Y. pseudotuberculosis* (13). Whether integration in different copies of *asn* tRNA genes can also occur in *E. coli* has yet to be determined. In *Yersinia* strains, the HPI regions are flanked by 17-bp direct repeats. In contrast, in *E. coli* strains, only one repeat sequence is intact, while the other repeat is deleted (13, 75).

UPEC J96 (O4 : K6) was isolated from a patient with acute pyelonephritis. It is characterized by the presence of several virulence gene clusters, including those for two alphahemolysins (*hlyI* and *hlyII*), the CNF1 gene (*cnf1*), and genes for two types of P fimbriae (*pap* and P-related sequence [*prs*]), F1C fimbriae (*foc*), and type 1 fimbriae (*fim*); it exhibits serum resistance; and it is colicin V and *ybt* positive (9, 41). Previous work had shown that the *hly, pap,* and *prs* sequences are linked, arguing for the presence of putative PAIs (53, 83). Further investigations showed that there are at least two PAIs on the chromosome of this strain, which are now called PAIs I_{J96} and II_{J96} (Table 1). PAI I_{J96} spans a DNA stretch of at least 170 kb and carries the virulence determinants *hlyI* and *pap*, and PAI II_{J96} is 110 kb in size and contains the *hlyII, prs,* and *cnf1* genes closely linked to each other. The PAIs of J96 are associated with tRNA genes (PAI I_{J96} with *pheV* at 64 min and PAI II_{J96} with *pheR* at 94 min on the K-12 chromosome), a feature which is consistent with the current definition of PAIs. PAI II_{J96} is flanked by 135-bp imperfect direct repeats and can spontaneously remove itself from the chromosome.

E. coli CFT073 was isolated from the blood and urine of a woman with acute pyelonephritis and carries the virulence gene clusters for *hly,* two *pap* operons, *sfa* and *fim* (58). Based on studies with strains 536 and J96, the PAI was identified by the characterization of a *pap*-positive cosmid clone and three further overlapping cosmid clones (78). A region of about 50 kb was present in strain CFT073 but absent from *E. coli* K-12 (44). Sequence analysis of the first identified PAI of this strain showed that it is 57,988 bp, includes an alpha-hemolysin operon and the genes encoding the Pap fimbrial adhesins, and has a G+C content of 42.9% (excluding K-12-specific sequences within the PAI) compared to 50.8% in *E. coli* K-12 (Table 1) (32). According to our new nomenclature, this PAI would be

Table 1. Main features of PAIs of UPEC strains

Strain	Designation of PAI	Insertion site (min)	Target tRNA	Size (kb)	Virulence factors encoded	Integrase	Boundary
536	PAI I$_{536}$	82	*selC*	70	Alpha-hemolysin	ΦR73[a]	16-bp DR[b]
536	PAI II$_{536}$	97	*leuX*	190	Alpha-hemolysin, P fimbriae (Prf)	P4[a]	18-bp DR
536	PAI III$_{536}$	5.6	*thrW*	~25	S fimbriae	DLP12[a]	?
536	PAI IV$_{536}$	44	*asnT*	~40	Yersiniabactin, iron-repressible proteins	P4	?
J96	PAI I$_{J96}$	64	*pheV*	170	Alpha-hemolysin, P fimbriae (Pap)	?	?
J96	PAI II$_{J96}$	94	*pheR*	110	Alpha-hemolysin, P fimbriae (Prs), cytotoxic necrotizing factor 1	?	135-bp IR[b]
CFT073	PAI I$_{CFT073}$	63.5?	Near *metV*	58	Alpha-hemolysin, P fimbriae (Pap)	?	9-bp DR

[a] Cryptic integrase genes.
[b] DR, direct repeats; IR, imperfect repeats.

called PAI I$_{CFT073}$. The insertion site of PAI I$_{CFT073}$ remains unclear because the left junction shows a site of insertion at 26.55 min, 7 bp downstream of the *dadX* gene in the *E. coli* K-12 chromosome, whereas the right junction is localized at 63.5 min, 75 bp downstream of the *metV* tRNA gene. This observation strongly argues for a chromosomal rearrangement, possibly due to the presence of two *pap* operons which could have served as crossover points (44). No deletion could be detected for PAI I$_{CFT073}$, which may be due to the presence of only short (9-bp) direct repeats.

GENES ENCODED ON PATHOGENICITY ISLANDS
OF UROPATHOGENIC *E. COLI*

Virulence-Associated Loci and Novel Genes

Hemolysin and P fimbrial genes are the best-studied virulence factors in UPEC since their proteins can be easily used as phenotypic markers. The best-known examples of PAIs in UPEC 536, J96, and CFT073 were initially identified by localization of the virulence genes on the genome and, for 536 and J96, by the presence of nonhemolytic and/or nonfimbriated PAI deletion mutants (34, 44, 78).

However, more recently, the development of new sequencing techniques made it possible to determine the entire sequences of PAIs. Sample sequencing analysis of PAI I$_{J96}$, PAI II$_{J96}$, and PAIs I$_{536}$ to IV$_{536}$ was performed by investigating overlapping cosmid clones; the results of this analysis are discussed below (12, 78). A more detailed analysis of the nucleotide sequence of PAI I$_{CFT073}$ revealed the presence of 44 open reading frames (ORFs), four of which represent novel genes (32). Table 2 summarizes the identified virulence genes and putative loci present on PAIs of strains 536, J96, and CFT073.

By direct sequencing of a PAI I$_{536}$-specific, *hlyI*-positive cosmid library clone, a detailed analysis of the right part of PAI I$_{536}$ was performed. The homology search with the hemolysin nucleotide sequence of J96 and the naturally occurring plasmid pHly152 derived from *E. coli* PM152 revealed a very high degree of homology (96%) over the entire operon between these gene clusters (Table 2) (37). Interestingly, deletion of about 150 bp exists in the upstream region of the *hlyC* gene of PAI I$_{536}$ but not in that of PAI I$_{J96}$. While this region is flanked by 5-bp direct repeats (TGGAG) in strain J96, only one copy is present in strain 536, indicating the presence of a minideletion (62). In addition, strain 536 carries another *hly* copy on PAI II$_{536}$. Previously, it was demonstrated by deletion mutant analysis that the hemolytic activity of the PAI I-encoded HlyI is stronger than of the PAI II-encoded HlyII (33). The region upstream of *hlyC* of PAI II$_{536}$ has features in common with the corresponding pHly152 plasmid sequence (37, 46). Whether these sequence alterations in the upstream region of *hlyII* compared to *hlyI* contribute to the differential expression of the two hemolysin operons has still to be elucidated. Adjacent to the second copy of a *hly* operon in J96, *hlyII,* another toxin gene which encodes CNF1, could be identified (9, 78). The *cnf1* gene and the *hly* operon are frequently closely linked on the chromosome of UPEC isolates (23). Interestingly, while the coding sequence for *cnf1* is absent in strain 536, the sequences upstream and downstream of *cnf1* were present on PAI I$_{536}$ adjacent to the *hlyI* operon, arguing for another minideletion coding for CNF1 in the genome of strain 536 (Table 2). There is no evidence for *cnf1*-specific sequences in strain CFT073.

Another gene cluster which is often found in UPEC encodes P fimbriae, and these

Table 2. Putative virulence genes on PAIs of UPEC strains

PAI	ORF or clone	Database sequence with similarity	Accession no. of homologous sequence	Description of homologous sequence	Organism	G+C content of ORF or clone (%)
PAI I$_{536}$	pCos9–12	*hlyCABD*	M10133	Chromosomal hemolysin operon of PAI I$_{J96}$	*E. coli* J96	39.9
			M14107	Plasmid-located hemolysin operon of pHLY152	*E. coli*	
PAI I$_{536}$	9–12/3	*cnf1* upstream	X70670	Upstream region of CNF1	*E. coli* E-B35	43.6
PAI I$_{536}$	9–12/3 and 9–12/5	*cnf1* downstream	X70670	Downstream region of CNF1	*E. coli* E-B35	48
PAI II$_{536}$	pCos4–73	*hlyCABD*	M10133	Chromosomal hemolysin operon	*E. coli* J96	ND^a
PAI II$_{536}$	pCos4–73 (*prf*)	*prs*	X61238	P-related sequence	*E. coli* J96	42.2
PAI III$_{536}$	pCos1E-6	*sfaC* to *sfaH*	S59541	S fimbrial adhesin	*E. coli* 536	46.2
PAI IV$_{536}$	*fyuA*	*fyuA*	Z35104	Ferric yersiniabactin uptake	*Y. pestis*	54.1^b
PAI IV$_{536}$	*irp1* to *irp5*	*irp1* to *irp5*	AF091251	Iron-repressible proteins	*Y. pestis*	56.2^b
PAI I$_{J96}$	589/B^c	*hlyBD*	M10133	Chromosomal hemolysin operon	*E. coli* J96	ND
PAI I$_{96}$	pRHU845	*papG* to *papI*	X61239	P-pilus F13	*E. coli* J96	45.3
PAI I$_{96}$	DAR118^c	SsaB	M63481	Adhesin B, saliva binding protein	*Streptococcus sanguis*	NA^d
PAI II$_{J96}$	10–3^c	*hlyCABD*	M10133	Chromosomal hemolysin operon	*E. coli* J96	40.2
PAI II$_{J96}$	prsJ96	*prs*	X61238	P-related sequence	*E. coli* J96	40.8
PAI II$_{J96}$	9–15A^c	*hra*	U07174	Heat resistant agglutinin 1	*E. coli* O9:H10:K99	NA
PAI II$_{J96}$	9–8^c	Pmf	Z35428	*Proteus mirabilis* fimbriae (Pmf)	*Proteus mirabilis*	NA
PAI II$_{J96}$	10–3^c	*cnf1*	X70670	Cytotoxic necrotizing factor 1	*E. coli* E-B35	36.5^e
PAI I$_{CFT073}$	X^f	*hlyCABD*	M10133	Chromosomal hemolysin operon	*E. coli* J96	NA
PAI I$_{CFT073}$	X^f	*papG* to *papI*	X61239	P-pilus F13	*E. coli* J96	NA
PAI I$_{CFT073}$	L5/N	*prrA*	U85771	TonB-dependent outer membrane receptor	EPEC 2348/69	49.9
PAI I$_{CFT073}$	L6/N	*modD*	U85771	Molybdenum transport protein	EPEC 2348/69	51.5
PAI I$_{CFT073}$	L7/N	*orf2*	U85771	Similar to *H. influenzae* yc73 protein	EPEC 2348/69	55.7
PAI I$_{CFT073}$	L8/P	FepC	F64113	Ferric enterobactin transport ATP binding protein homolog	*H. influenzae*	50.6
PAI I$_{CFT073}$	R4	BfrA	U56084	Exogenous ferric siderophore receptor	*B. bronchiseptica*	51.6

^{a} ND, not determined.

^{b} The G+C content of the *fyuA* or *irp1* to *irp5* genes of *Y. pestis* is given.

^{c} The DNA sequence over the ORF or clone is not accessible in the data bank.

^{d} The G+C content could not be determined because the DNA sequence of the ORF or clone is not accessible in the data bank.

^{e} The G+C content of the *cnf1* gene of *E. coli* E-B35 is given (24).

^{f} No ORF names were given in the original description.

genes are very often linked to *hly* loci. Strain J96 carries two hemolysin determinants, which are associated with the adhesin gene clusters *pap* and *prs*. For strain CFT073, a linkage between the hemolysin gene cluster and a *pap* determinant was reported (32). In strain 536, the hemolysin and the P-related fimbrial (*prf*) gene cluster on PAI II$_{536}$ are closely linked. The *prf* determinant was shown to be highly homologous to the J96-specific *prs* and *pap* operons (Table 2). In strain 536, the *sfa* determinant, coding for S fimbriae, is located on a PAI (PAI III$_{536}$). With a few exceptions, PAI IV$_{536}$ is identical to the HPI of *Yersinia* which is discussed in chapter 5.

With more sequence information becoming available, unifying patterns are beginning to emerge for PAI analysis. Previously, a method called representational difference analysis (RDA), in which subtractive and kinetic enrichment was used to purify restriction endonuclease fragments present in one population of DNA fragments but not in another, was developed (52) (see chapter 2). RDA allows the identification of genetic differences and had already been successfully used with two closely related pathogenic *Neisseria* species, different *Vibrio cholerae* serogroups, and *Helicobacter pylori* strains (14, 16, 79). The method was used to identify genes present in the genome of strain 536 but absent from the genome of *E. coli* K-12. So far, nine PCR fragments which are specific for strain 536 have been isolated. Four were shown to be specific for the *hly* and *prf* loci of PAIs I$_{536}$ and II$_{536}$, and two others revealed homologies to the genes *waaL, waaV, waaY,* and *waaT.* These genes are involved in the assembly of the core lipopolysaccharide. Three PCR fragments, however, showed no homology to already known sequences (42). Further studies are necessary to demonstrate whether these fragments may be parts of PAIs III$_{536}$ and IV$_{536}$ or not yet identified PAI elements.

Sequence analysis of PAI-specific regions of UPEC strains revealed the presence of novel genes. In strain CFT073, four ORFs, *prrA, modD, yc73,* and *fepC,* that are located inside the left junction of the PAI may resemble a new iron transport system. Another iron acquisition gene homolog which may encode a homolog of an exogenous ferric siderophore receptor was identified inside the right junction of PAI I$_{CFT073}$ (32). Further investigations are necessary before their direct involvement in the virulence properties of UPEC can be confirmed. PAI-specific genes encoding toxin and adhesin determinants that were not known for UPEC were also identified for strain J96. Three PAI-specific regions of PAIs I$_{J96}$ and II$_{J96}$ showed significant homologies to adhesin gene clusters, namely, the *Proteus mirabilis* fimbriae (Pmf), heat-resistant agglutinin 1 of an enterotoxigenic *E. coli* (ETEC) strain, and a saliva binding protein of *Streptococcus sanguis* which is adjacent to the *hlyI* operon (Table 2) (25, 55, 56).

In contrast to already known and novel putative PAI-associated genes of UPEC mentioned above, the locations of other determinants encoding important virulence factors, such as capsules or aerobactin, are not known. Aerobactin (*aer*) genes, however, are often chromosomally encoded, and the association of the corresponding determinant with IS*1* elements strongly suggests a transposon-like or even a PAI-like structure of the *aer*-associated DNA region (82). Capsule antigens are encoded by a 20-kb stretch of DNA which, in one particular *E. coli* K1 strain, seems to be associated with the tRNA gene *pheV*. It is still speculative whether the *kps* gene cluster itself forms a PAI structure, as suggested in a recent article (19).

Regulatory Elements

Virulence-associated genes are not expressed constitutively; rather, their expression responds to changes in the environment. This is also true for genes located on PAIs, which are often tied in with regulatory networks. Thus, the expression of PAI-encoded virulence factors of UPEC, such as P and S fimbriae as well as alpha-hemolysin, is influenced by a number of regulators, whose genes are located on the "core chromosome." These regulators include the leucine-responsive regulatory protein (Lrp), the catabolite repression protein (Crp), the histone-like protein H-NS, and the RfaH factor (1, 2, 30, 59, 60). Following horizontal gene transfer, newly acquired sequences are under strong selective pressure, leading to changes of promoter and other regulatory sequences by point mutations to make them responsive to the already existing regulatory network. This has apparently been the case for virulence genes of UPEC.

On the other hand, regulatory genes are also located on PAIs. P and S fimbriae are regulated by two regulators, and the corresponding genes are located in the fimbrial operons themselves (3, 59, 60). It was shown for strain 536 that the regulators of P fimbriae (PrfB and PrfC) not only regulate P-fimbrial genes located on PAI II$_{536}$ but also are necessary for the activation of S fimbriae encoded by genes on PAI III$_{536}$. This process was termed "cross talk" between different PAIs (60). In addition, the DNA sequence of *ybtA* on PAI IV$_{536}$, which is identical to the *Yersinia* HPI, shows strong homology to regulators of the AraC family, which may also have an impact on the expression of other PAI and non-PAI genes. PAI II$_{536}$ is associated with the minor leucine-specific tRNA gene *leuX*. If *leuX* is expressed to a low level or is inactive, e.g., following deletion of PAI II$_{536}$ from the chromosome, the activity of a number of genes is modulated. Two-dimensional poly-acrylamide gel electrophoresis showed that the expression of more than 30 gene products appears to be PAI dependent and may be *leuX* regulated (65, 69, 70). The expression of the PAI-encoded virulence factor hemolysin, as well as of the non-PAI-encoded type 1 fimbriae, is modulated by *leuX* (11, 70). For type 1 fimbriae, the positive regulator FimB is repressed on the translational level in a *leuX* mutant background, leading to the downregulation of type 1 pili.

Different Types of Mobility Genes

The overall amount of horizontally transferred DNA in *E. coli* has been calculated to involve 755 of the 4,288 ORFs (17.6%) present in the genome of *E. coli* K-12 strain MG1655 (7, 49). It follows that horizontal transfer must have played a major role in the development of pathogenic enteric bacteria (3). Detailed sequence analysis of PAI-specific structures of UPEC revealed not only the presence of virulence-associated genes but also the occurrence of so-called mobility genes, indicating the involvement of horizontal gene transfer processes in the evolution of PAIs. In the following paragraph, integrase genes of bacteriophages, insertion (IS) elements, and transposases, as well as intron-specific structures on PAIs, are discussed.

PAIs of UPEC strains are often flanked by tRNA genes, which are also preferentially used as integration sites for bacteriophages (68). Interestingly, bacteriophage integrase genes and additional bacteriophage-specific sequences were found on PAIs of UPEC (11, 32, 78). As shown in Table 3, sequences of bacteriophage P4 were often identified in strains

Table 3. Mobility genes on PAIs of UPEC strains 536, J96 and CFT073

PAI	ORF or clone	Database sequence with similarity	Accession no. of homologous sequence	Description of homologous sequence	Organism with homologous sequence	% G+C content of ORF/clone
PAI I$_{536}$	9-12/2	IS911	X17613	Insertion sequence of IS3 group	Shigella dysenteriae	53.3
PAI I$_{536}$	9-12/2	IS1131	M82888	Insertion sequence	A. tumefaciens	53.1
PAI I$_{536}$	9-12/2	Maturase homolog	S43481	Maturase homolog	E. coli	48
PAI I$_{536}$	9-12/5	H-repeat gene	X77508	Intron-associated protein	E. coli	48
PAI I$_{536}$	pCos7-31	ΦR73int	M64113	ΦR73 integrase gene	Bacteriophage ΦR73, E. coli	44.8
PAI II$_{536}$	pCos10-21	P4int	X51522	P4 integrase gene	Bacteriophage P4, E. coli	43.7
PAI III$_{536}$	pCos1E6	DLP12int	M27155	Integrase gene of cryptic prophage DLP12	Bacteriophage DLP12, E. coli	49.8
PAI I$_{J96}$	4-18^a	IS911	U14003	Insertion sequence	E. coli	NA^b
PAI I$_{J96}$	4-27^a	IS630	X05955	Insertion sequence, unidentified reading frame	Shigella sonnei	NA
PAI I$_{J96}$	7-13^a	9.7K protein	X51522	Protein of unknown function	Bacteriophage P4, E. coli	NA
PAI II$_{J96}$	10-2^a	ORF1	D10543	ORF of IS element	Bacillus stearothermophilus	NA
PAI II$_{J96}$	12-6^a	ORF1	X78302	ORF1 of IS100	Y. pestis	NA
PAI II$_{J96}$	12-14^a	ORF2	X78302	ORF2 of IS100	Y. pestis	NA
PAI I$_{CFT073}$	HP1	IS600	P16940	IS600 hypothetical 31-kDa protein	Shigella sonnei	52.7
PAI I$_{CFT073}$	HP2	IS600	P16939	IS600 hypothetical 11-kDa protein	Shigella sonnei	53.7
PAI I$_{CFT073}$	R15		U06468	Putative transposase	E. coli	51.9
PAI I$_{CFT073}$	R14	IS629	P16942	Transposase	Shigella sonnei	53.6
PAI I$_{CFT073}$	R12	ISAE1	A47041	Transposase homolog	Alcaligenes eutrophus	51.6
PAI I$_{CFT073}$	R6		L49438	Transposase	Chelatobacter heinzii	54.2

^{a} The DNA sequence of the ORF or clone is not accessible in the data bank.
^{b} The G+C content could not be determined because the DNA sequence of the ORF or clone is not accessible in the data bank.

536, J96, and CFT073. In *E. coli* K-12 and in strain 536, DNA sequences corresponding to the P4 integrase gene occur immediately downstream of the *leuX* tRNA gene, which also served as the integration site for PAI II$_{536}$ (8, 66). An additional copy of the P4 integrase gene was found on PAI IV$_{536}$, which was originally identified as the HPI in *Y. enterocolitica*. Whereas the PAI II$_{536}$-based P4 integrase gene shows striking homology to the *E. coli* K-12 P4 integrase sequence, which is probably defective due to stop codons in the entire sequence, the P4 integrase sequence of PAI IV$_{536}$ seems to be intact. P4 integrase genes were found not only in *E. coli* PAIs but also in the *vap* (virulence-associated protein) regions of *Dichelobacter nodosus,* the principal causative agent of ovine foot rot (18). The high similarity of the integrases of different species suggests that these sequences may be transferred between distantly related bacteria. Further studies will show whether, in particular, the frequently found bacteriophage P4-specific sequences are involved in the acquisition of PAIs. A similar arrangement with integrase genes adjacent to tRNA genes could be demonstrated for PAIs I$_{536}$ and III$_{536}$. Next to the tRNA genes *selC* and *thrW,* which flank PAIs I$_{536}$ and III$_{536}$, respectively, sequences with homology to the ΦR73 *int* and DLP12 *int* were identified (12, 51). The *int*-specific sequence of PAI I$_{536}$ shows significant homologies to the *int* gene of the LEE$_{EDL933}$, the recently characterized PAI of enterohemorrhagic *E. coli* (EHEC) (64). It can therefore be concluded that integrase genes and other bacteriophage-specific sequences may have played an important role for the evolution of pathogenic bacteria and that their presence on PAIs is one of the main characteristics of PAIs.

Another example of mobility genes on PAIs is the presence of ORFs typical for IS elements and transposases. As summarized in Table 3, various ORFs of strains 536, J96, and CFT073 represent transposases or sequences of unknown function from IS elements. The origin of the PAI-located IS elements is not restricted to *E. coli* but also includes IS elements of other species, e.g., *Y. pestis, Agrobacterium tumefaciens,* and *Shigella* spp. (28, 67, 80). This implies that PAIs are targets for recombination and that foreign DNA has been inserted by mobile genetic elements.

Interestingly, PAI I$_{536}$ contains additional sequences which represent intron-specific DNA sequences. Group II introns were originally found in the organellar genomes of fungi and plants, but meanwhile they were also found in bacteria in the plasmid sequence of an ETEC strain (26, 48). The intron-specific sequences of PAI I$_{536}$ show homologies to the ETEC sequences. The intron seems to be inserted at the same location, the 3' end of the orf104 homolog, followed by domains V and VI and a maturase homolog sequence which is necessary for the splicing of group II introns.

PATHOGENICITY ISLANDS OF UROPATHOGENIC *E. COLI:* IMPLICATIONS FOR EVOLUTION

Four different categories of virulence factors are encoded by PAIs: adherence factors, toxins, iron uptake systems, and invasins including type III and IV secretory proteins. In UPEC all of these except invasins are PAI encoded. Evolutionary pressure to incorporate the respective genes, however, was presumably not caused by putative advantages to strains with the capacity to colonize the human urinary tract. It is not clear which driving forces lead to the development of *E. coli* strains with the properties of UPECs. One speculation is that UPECs represent *E. coli* variants specifically adapted to certain animals or to the human intestine. The fact that UPEC strains usually originate from the human intestine supports the latter assumption.

While most virulence factors of intestinal *E. coli* strains are plasmid or phage encoded, the determinants encoding the different virulence factors of UPEC are located on the chromosome (61). In this context, it is interesting that some of the PAI-located gene clusters of UPEC are also located on plasmids of fecal isolates, i.e., the alpha-hemolysin operon of strain PM152 (pHLY152). The toxin CNF1 is generally chromosomally encoded, but the *cnf2* gene, which codes for a very similar toxin of intestinal *E. coli,* is plasmid borne (63). One should also mention here that the gene clusters coding for the iron uptake system areobactin are plasmid as well as chromosomally located. Taking these data into consideration, it is tempting to speculate that PAIs of UPEC or at least parts of them could represent former plasmid-derived sequences.

DNA sequence analysis of PAIs from UPEC reveals that they represent heterogenous pieces of DNA. Accordingly, various (sometimes only partially) insertional sequences were detected in PAI-specific regions. PAIs even include introns, originally found in eukaryotic organisms and cryptic transposases. The occurrence of such diverse sequences in PAIs of UPEC strongly argues for a stepwise acquisition of these DNA fragments from very heterogenous sources, leading to the mosaic-like structure of the islands. Also, PAI sequences may be interrupted by K-12-specific sequence from different locations of the K-12 genome. The presence of sequences originating from plasmids and of phage-specific sequences such as cryptic integrase genes contributes to the mosaic-like structure concept of UPEC PAIs. In comparison, the iron uptake system yersiniabactin represents an unusually homogenous piece of DNA, which is also present in the genomes of other enterobacteria, e.g., *Yersinia, Salmonella,* and *Klebsiella* (74, 84). These PAIs are so far unique in enterobacteria, suggesting that they were acquired as one unit from an unknown donor, possibly via transducing phages.

It is obvious that tRNA genes play a key role in the development and function of PAIs. On one hand, the 3′ ends of tRNA genes often act as target sites for the integration of foreign DNA fragments. This is also true for UPEC PAIs, which are incorporated into particular tRNA genes. Most PAIs from UPEC are flanked by short direct-repeat DNA sequences which convert them into discrete regions of the genome (Fig. 2). Interestingly, *selC,* which encodes the selenocysteine-specific tRNA, also acts as the target for the LEE island of EPEC as well as EHEC and for the *Salmonella typhimurium* PAI SPI III (6, 64). In addition, *selC* carries the attachment site for bacteriophage ΦR73, suggesting that at least parts of the *selC*-associated PAIs have been acquired by transduction. The presence of a cryptic ΦR73-specific integrase gene on the *selC*-associated PAI I_{536} supports this hypothesis. The phenylalanine-specific tRNA genes *pheV* and *pheR*, as well as the asparagine-specific tRNA genes *asnT, asnW,* and *asnU,* are targets for the integration of PAIs in UPEC but also for the uptake of DNAs in other organisms (see below). Truncation of these tRNA genes by integration and/or deletion of PAIs would have no major consequences for translation, because both groups of genes code for tRNAs with identical anticodons. Furthermore, at least *leuX* acts as a small regulatory RNA because it modulates the expression of several genes including virulence loci (22). It is tempting to speculate that former phages and/or plasmids with PAI-associated genes may also carry tRNA genes to overcome the differences in codon usage between donor and recipient organisms and to allow a proper expression of the transferred genes with a larger number of codons

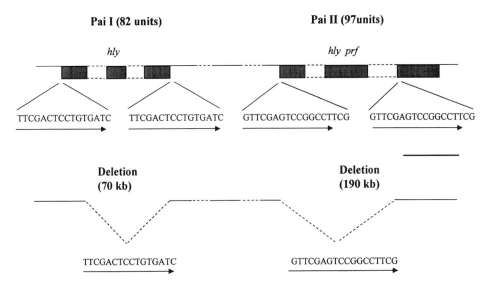

Figure 2. Deletion process of PAIs I_{536} and II_{536} involving the flanking direct-repeat sequences. Following deletion, one copy each of the direct repeats remains in the chromosome. The map positions and sizes of the PAIs are indicated.

recognized by the cotransferred tRNA compared to genes of the recipient organism. This assumption is corroborated by the fact that tRNA genes are often part of phage genomes, including those carrying Shiga toxin genes of EHEC (72).

The PAIs of UPEC have the tendency to be deleted from their host chromosomes with relatively high frequencies. Following deletion, one copy of the direct repeats remains in the chromosomes (Fig. 2). Similar mechanisms have been described for PAIs of *H. pylori, Staphylococcus aureus, Yersinia* spp., and others (13, 16, 50). Conjugative transposons show similar excision mechanisms (39). For other PAIs, however, a deletion following homologous recombination via IS elements located at the ends of or within PAIs has been described. These deletion events, on one hand, may reflect the general plasticity of the prokaryotic genome. On the other hand, deletions may represent special types of adaptation of microbes to certain environments. It was shown that UPEC strains isolated from patients with chronic UTI carry fewer virulence genes than do strains isolated from patients with acute infections (31). Deletion events may convert highly pathogenic strains found during the initial phase of an infection to moderately virulent strains during the chronic state of infection.

DNA sequence analysis showed that the genomes of prokaryotic organisms and possibly also of eukaryotes exhibit a mosaic-like structure composed of a core genome which is stable for long periods and newly acquired sequences. The newly acquired sequences often form blocks of DNA which may code for virulence but also code for other distinct properties such as secretion, degradation of xenobiotic compounds, metabolic functions, and resistance to antibiotics (49). We therefore termed these regions ''genomic islands'' because they represent newly acquired ''additional'' DNA in the ''ocean'' of species-specific genes. PAIs of UPEC are a good example of such genomic islands because they also

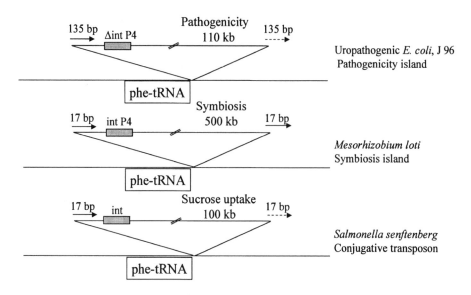

Figure 3. Presence of different genomic islands in phenylalanine-specific tRNA genes.

represent formerly transferred DNA and encode additional functions. As shown for the PAIs of UPEC J96, the PAI target sites, phenylalanine-specific tRNA loci, are also frequently used by other organisms for the incorporation of foreign DNA (Fig. 3). In a particular *E. coli* strain, the K1 capsule synthesis genes are located in the *pheV* locus (19). In EHEC strains, another LEE element, of 61 kb, was found next to the *pheR* locus (17). In the soil microorganism *Mesorhizobium loti,* a so-called symbiosis island, carrying the genes for nitrogen fixation, is located in the region occupied by PAI II$_{J96}$ (76). Indeed, this symbiosis island seems to be an integrated plasmid of 500 kb. In addition, in *Salmonella senftenberg* a conjugative transposon encoding sucrose uptake has the capacity to integrate into *pheV* and/or *pheR* genes (39).

PAIs of UPEC strains are excellent examples for the study of the evolution of prokaryotic genomes in pathogenic and nonpathogenic microbes. Since the discovery of PAIs in UPEC strains, several other examples of other genomic islands, spanning diverse physiological phenomena including nitrogen fixation systems and sucrose uptake, have been described. The principal mechanisms underlying these genetic processes resemble the basic mechanisms of UPEC to a striking extent.

Acknowledgments. We thank U. Dobrindt, K. Piechazceck and S. Khan for their permission to use unpublished data and S. Schubert and J. Heesemann for useful discussions. We gratefully acknowledge U. Hentschel for critically reading the manuscript. Part of our work was supported by the DFG Sonderforschungsbereich 479 (Erregervariabilität und Wirtsreaktionen bei infektiösen Krankheitsprozessen).

REFERENCES

1. **Atlung, T., and H. Ingmer.** 1997. H-NS: a modulator of environmentally regulated gene expression. *Mol. Microbiol.* **24:**7–17.

2. **Bailey M. J., C. Hughes, and V. Koronakis.** 1997. RfaH and the *ops* element, components of a novel system controlling bacterial transcription elongation. *Mol. Microbiol.* **26:**845–851.

3. **Barinaga, M.** 1996. A shared strategy for virulence. *Science* **272:**1261–1263.

4. **Berger, H., J. Hacker, A. Juarez, C. Hughes, and W. Goebel.** 1982. Cloning of the chromosomal determinants encoding hemolysin production and mannose-resistant hemagglutination in *Escherichia coli. J. Bacteriol.* **152:**1241–1247.

5. **Berlyn, M. K. B.** 1998. Linkage map of *Escherichia coli* K-12, edition 10: the traditional map. *Microbiol. Mol. Biol. Rev.* **62:**814–984.

6. **Blanc-Potard, A.-B., and E. A. Groisman.** 1997. The *Salmonella selC* locus contains a pathogenicity island mediating intramacrophage survival. *EMBO J.* **16:**5376–5385.

7. **Blattner, F. R., G. Plunkett III, C. A. Bloch, N. T. Perna, V. Burland, M. Riley, J. Collado-Vides, J. D. Glasner, C. K. Rode, G. F. Mayhew, J. Gregor, N. W. Davis, H. A. Kirkpatrick, M. A. Goeden, D. J. Rose, B. Mau, and Y. Shao.** 1997. The complete genome sequence of *Escherichia coli* K-12. *Science* **277:**1453–1474.

8. **Blum, G., M. Ott, A. Lischewski, A. Ritter, H. Imrich, H. Tschäpe, and J. Hacker.** 1994. Excision of large DNA regions termed pathogenicity islands from tRNA-specific loci in the chromosome of an *Escherichia coli* wild-type pathogen. *Infect. Immun.* **62:**606–614.

9. **Blum, G., V. Falbo, A. Caprioli, and J. Hacker.** 1995. Gene clusters encoding the cytotoxic necrotizing factor type 1, Prs-fimbriae and α-hemolysin form the pathogenicity island II of the uropathogenic *Escherichia coli* strain J96. *FEMS Microbiol. Lett.* **126:**189–196.

10. **Blum-Oehler, G., J. Heesemann, D. Kranzfelder, F. Scheutz, and J. Hacker.** 1997. Characterization of *Escherichia coli* serotype O12:K1:H7 isolates from an immunocompetent carrier with a history of spontaneous abortion and septicemia. *Eur. J. Clin. Microbiol. Infect. Dis.* **16:**153–155.

11. **Blum-Oehler, G., U. Dobrindt, N. Weiβ, B. Janke, S. Schubert, A. Rakin, J. Heesemann, R. Marre, and J. Hacker.** 1998. Pathogenicity islands of uropathogenic *Escherichia coli:* implications for the evolution of virulence. *Zentbl. Bakteriol. Suppl.* **29:**380–386.

12. **Blum-Oehler, G., G. Nagy, N. Weiβ, T. Steiner, and J. Hacker.** Unpublished data.

13. **Buchrieser, C., R. Brosch, S. Bach, A. Guiyoule, and E. Carniel.** 1998. The high-pathogenicity island of *Yersinia pseudotuberculosis* can be inserted into any of the three chromosomal *asn* tRNA genes. *Mol. Microbiol.* **30:**965–978.

14. **Calia, K. E., M. K. Waldor, and S. B. Calderwood.** 1998. Use of representational difference analysis to identify genomic differences between pathogenic strains of *Vibrio cholerae. Infect. Immun.* **66:**849–852.

15. **Carniel, E., I. Guilvout, and H. Prentice.** 1996. Characterization of a large chromosomal "high-pathogenicity island" in biotype 1B *Yersinia enterocolitica. J. Bacteriol.* **178:**6743–6751.

16. **Censini, S., C. Lange, Z. Xiang, J. E. Crabtree, P. Ghiara, M. Borodovsky, R. Rappuoli, and A. Covacci.** 1996. Cag, a pathogenicity island of *Helicobacter pylori,* encodes type I-specific and disease-associated virulence factors. *Proc. Natl. Acad. Sci. USA* **93:**14648–14653.

17. **Chakraborty, T.** Personal communication.

18. **Cheetham, B. F., D. B. Tattersall, G. A. Bloomfield, J. I. Rood, and M. E. Katz.** 1995. Identification of a gene encoding a bacteriophage-related integrase in a vap region of the *Dichelobacter nodosus* genome. *Gene* **162:**53–58.

19. **Cieslewicz, M., and E. Vimr.** 1997. Reduced polysialic acid capsule expression in *Escherichia coli* K1 mutants with chromosomal defects in *kps*F. *Mol. Microbiol.* **26:**237–249.

20. **Connell, H., M. Hedlund, W. Agace, and C. Svanborg.** 1997. Bacterial attachment to uro-epithelial cells: mechanisms and consequences. *Adv. Dent. Res.* **11:**50–58.

21. **Crosa, J. H.** 1989. Genetics and molecular biology of siderophore-mediated iron transport in bacteria. *Microbiol. Rev.* **53:**517–530.

22. **Dobrindt, U., P. S. Cohen, M. Utley, I. Mühldorfer, and J. Hacker.** 1998. The *leuX*-encoded tRNA5(Leu) but not the pathogenicity islands I and II influence the survival of the uropathogenic *Escherichia coli* strain 536 in CD-1 mouse bladder mucus in the stationary phase. *FEMS Microbiol. Lett.* **162:**135–141.

23. **Falbo, V., M. Famiglietti, and A. Caprioli.** 1992. Gene block encoding production of cytotoxic necrotizing factor 1 and hemolysin in *Escherichia coli* isolates from extraintestinal infections. *Infect. Immun.* **60:**2182–2187.

24. **Falbo, V., T. Pace, L. Picci, E. Pizzi, and A. Caprioli.** 1993. Isolation and nucleotide sequence of the gene encoding cytotoxic necrotizing factor 1 of *Escherichia coli. Infect. Immun.* **61:**4909–4914.

25. **Fenno, J. C., D. J. LeBlanc, and P. M. Fives-Taylor.** 1989. Nucleotide sequence analysis of a type 1 fimbrial gene of *Streptococcus sanguis* FW213. *Infect. Immun.* **57:**3527–3533.

26. **Ferat, J. L., M. Le Gouar, and F. Michel.** 1994. Multiple group II self-splicing introns in mobile DNA from *Escherichia coli. C. R. Acad. Sci. Ser. III* **317:**141–148.

27. **Fetherston, J. D., P. Schuetze, and R. D. Perry.** 1992. Loss of the pigmentation phenotype in *Yersinia pestis* is due to the spontaneous deletion of 102 kb of chromosomal DNA which is flanked by a repetitive element. *Mol. Microbiol.* **6:**2693–2704.

28. **Filippov, A. A., P. N. Oleinikov, V. L. Motin, O. A. Protsenko, and G. B. Smirnov.** 1995. Sequencing of two *Yersinia pestis* IS elements, IS285 and IS100. *Contrib. Microbiol. Immunol.* **13:**306–309.

29. **Flatau, G., E. Lemichez, M. Gauthier, P. Chardin, S. Paris, C. Fiorentini, and P. Boquet.** 1997. Toxin-induced activation of the G protein p21 Rho by deamidation of glutamine. *Nature* **387:**729–733.

30. **Forsman, K., B. Sonden, M. Goransson, and B. E. Uhlin.** 1992. Antirepression function in *Escherichia coli* for the cAMP-cAMP receptor protein transcriptional activator. *Proc. Natl. Acad. Sci. USA* **89:**9880–9884.

31. **Fünfstück, R., H. Tschäpe, G. Stein, H. Kunath, M. Bergner, and G. Wessel.** 1986. Virulence properties of *E. coli* strains in patients with chronic pyelonephritis. *Infection* **14:**3–8.

32. **Guyer, D. M., J.-S. Kao, and H. L. T. Mobley.** 1998. Genomic analysis of a pathogenicity island in uropathogenic *Escherichia coli* CFT073: distribution of homologous sequences among isolates from patients with pyelonephritis, cystitis, and catheter-associated bacteriuria and from fecal samples. *Infect. Immun.* **66:** 4411–4417.

33. **Hacker, J., S. Knapp, and W. Goebel.** 1983. Spontaneous deletions and flanking regions of the chromosomal inherited hemolysin determinant of an *Escherichia coli* O6 strain. *J. Bacteriol.* **154:**1145–1152.

34. **Hacker, J., L. Bender, M. Ott, J. Wingender, B. Lund, R. Marre, and W. Goebel.** 1990. Deletions of chromosomal regions coding for fimbriae and hemolysins occur *in vivo* and *in vitro* in various extraintestinal *Escherichia coli* isolates. *Microb. Pathog.* **8:**213–225.

35. **Hacker, J.** 1992. Role of fimbrial adhesins in the pathogenesis of *Escherichia coli* infections. *Can. J. Microbiol.* **38:**720–727.

36. **Hacker, J., G. Blum-Oehler, I. Mühldorfer, and H. Tschäpe.** 1997. Pathogenicity islands of virulent bacteria: structure, function and impact on microbial evolution. *Mol. Microbiol.* **23:**1089–1097.

37. **Hess, J., W. Wels, M. Vogel, and W. Goebel.** 1986. Nucleotide sequence of a plasmid-encoded hemolysin determinant and its comparison with a corresponding chromosomal hemolysin sequence. *FEMS Microbiol. Lett.* **34:**1–11.

38. **High, N. J., B. A. Hales, K. Jann, and G. J. Boulnois.** 1988. A block of urovirulence genes encoding multiple fimbriae and hemolysin in *Escherichia coli* O4:K12:H⁻. *Infect. Immun.* **56:**513–517.

39. **Hochhut, B., K. Jahreis, J. W. Lengeler, and K. Schmid.** 1997. CTn*scr94*, a conjugative transposon found in enterobacteria. *J. Bacteriol.* **179:**2097–2102.

40. **Huang, S. H., C. Wass, Q. Fu, N. V. Prasadarao, M. Stins, and K. S. Kim.** 1995. *Escherichia coli* invasion of brain microvascular endothelial cells in vitro and in vivo: molecular cloning and characterization of invasion gene *ibe10. Infect. Immun.* **63:**4470–4475.

41. **Hull, R. A., R. E. Gill, P. Hsu, B. H. Minshew, and S. Falkow.** 1981. Construction and expression of recombinant plasmids encoding type 1 or D-mannose-resistant pili from a urinary tract infection *Escherichia coli* isolate. *Infect. Immun.* **33:**933–938.

42. **Janke, B., J. Hacker, and G. Blum-Oehler.** Unpublished data.

43. **Johnson, J.** 1991. Virulence factors in *Escherichia coli* urinary tract infections. *Clin. Microbiol. Rev.* **4:** 80–128.

44. **Kao, J.-S., D. M. Stucker, J. W. Warren, and H. L. T. Mobley.** 1997. Pathogenicity island sequences of pyelonephritogenic *Escherichia coli* CFT073 are associated with virulent uropathogenic strains. *Infect. Immun.* **65:**2812–2820.

45. **Khan, S., and J. Hacker.** Unpublished data.

46. **Knapp, S., I. Then, W. Wels, G. Michel, H. Tschäpe, J. Hacker, and W. Goebel.** 1985. Analysis of the flanking regions from different haemolysin determinants of *Escherichia coli. Mol. Gen. Genet.* **200:**385–392.

47. **Knapp, S., J. Hacker, T. Jarchau, and W. Goebel.** 1986. Large unstable inserts in the chromosome affect virulence properties of uropathogenic *Escherichia coli* strain 536. *J. Bacteriol.* **168:**22–30.

48. **Knoop, V., and A. Brennicke.** 1994. Evidence for a group II intron in *Escherichia coli* inserted into a highly conserved reading frame associated with mobile DNA sequences. *Nucleic Acids Res.* **22:**1167–1171.

49. **Lawrence, J. G., and H. Ochman.** 1998. Molecular archaeology of the *Escherichia coli* genome. *Proc. Natl. Acad. Sci. USA* **95:**9413–9417.

50. **Lindsay J. A., A. Ruzin, H. F. Ross, N. Kurepina, and R. P. Novick.** 1998. The gene for toxic shock toxin is carried by a family of mobile pathogenicity islands in *Staphylococcus aureus. Mol. Microbiol.* **29:** 527–543.

51. **Lindsey, D. F., D. A. Mullin, and J. R. Walker.** 1989. Characterization of the cryptic lambdoid prophage DLP12 of *Escherichia coli* and overlap of the DLP12 integrase gene with the tRNA gene *argU. J. Bacteriol.* **171:**6197–6205.

52. **Lisitsyn, N., N. Lisitsyn, and M. Wigler.** 1993. Cloning of differences between two complex genomes. *Science* **259:**946–951.

53. **Low, D., V. David, D. Lark, G. Schoolnik, and S. Falkow.** 1984. Gene clusters governing the production of hemolysin and mannose-resistant hemagglutination are closely linked in *Escherichia coli* serotype O4 and O6 isolates from urinary tract infections. *Infect. Immun.* **43:**353–358.

54. **Ludwig, A., and W. Goebel.** 1991. Genetic determinants of cytolytic toxins from gram-negative bacteria, p. 117–146. *In* J. E. Alouf and J. H. Freers (ed.), *Sourcebook of Bacterial Protein Toxins.* Academic Press, Ltd., London, United Kingdom.

55. **Lutwyche, P., R. Rupps, J. Cavanagh, R. A. Warren, and D. E. Brooks.** 1994. Cloning, sequencing, and viscometric adhesion analysis of heat-resistant agglutinin 1, an integral membrane hemagglutinin from *Escherichia coli* O9 : H10 : K99. *Infect. Immun.* **62:**5020–5026.

56. **Massad, G., and H. L. Mobley.** 1994. Genetic organization and complete sequence of the *Proteus mirabilis pmf* fimbrial operon. *Gene* **150:**101–104.

57. **Meier, C., T. A. Oelschlaeger, H. Merkert, T. K. Korhonen, and J. Hacker.** 1996. Ability of *Escherichia coli* isolates that cause meningitis in newborns to invade epithelial and endothelial cells. *Infect. Immun.* **64:** 2391–2399.

58. **Mobley, H. L. T., D. M. Green, A. L. Trifillis, D. E. Johnson, G. R. Chippendale, C. V. Lockatell, B. D. Jones, and J. W. Warren.** 1990. Pyelonephritogenic *Escherichia coli* and killing of cultured human renal proximal tubular epithelial cells: role of hemolysin in some strains. *Infect. Immun.* **58:**1281–1289.

59. **Morschhäuser, J., B. E. Uhlin, and J. Hacker.** 1993. Transcriptional analysis and regulation of the *sfa* determinant coding for S fimbriae of pathogenic *Escherichia coli* strains. *Mol. Gen. Genet.* **238:**97–105.

60. **Morschhäuser, J., V. Vetter, L. Emödy, and J. Hacker.** 1994. Adhesin regulatory genes within large, unstable DNA regions of pathogenic *Escherichia coli:* cross-talk between different adhesin gene clusters. *Mol. Microbiol.* **11:**555–566.

61. **Mühldorfer, I., and J. Hacker.** 1994. Genetic aspects of *Escherichia coli* virulence. *Microb. Pathog.* **16:** 171–181.

62. **Nagy, G., J. Hacker, and G. Blum-Oehler.** Unpublished data.

63. **Oswald, E., M. Sugai, A. Labigne, H. C. Wu, C. Fiorentini, P. Bouquet, and A. D. O'Brien.** 1994. Cytotoxic necrotizing factor type 2 produced by virulent *Escherichia coli* modifies the small GTP-binding proteins Rho involved in assembly of actin stress fibers. *Proc. Natl. Acad. Sci. USA* **91:**3814–3818.

64. **Perna, N. T., G. F. Mayhew, G. Pósfai, S. Elliott, M. S. Donnenberg, J. B. Kaper, and F. R. Blattner.** 1998. Molecular evolution of a pathogenicity island from enterohemorrhagic *Escherichia coli* O157 : H7. *Infect. Immun.* **66:**3810–3817.

65. **Piechaczek, K., and J. Hacker.** Unpublished data.

66. **Pierson, L. S., III, and M. L. Kahn.** 1987. Integration of satellite bacteriophage P4 in *Escherichia coli.* DNA sequences of the phage and host regions involved in site-specific recombination. *J. Mol. Biol.* **196:** 487–496.

67. **Prere, M. F., M. Chandler, and O. Fayet.** 1990. Transposition in *Shigella dysenteriae:* isolation and analysis of IS*911,* a new member of the IS*3* group of insertion sequences. *J. Bacteriol.* **172:**4090–4099.

68. **Reiter, W.-D., P. Palm, and S. Yeats.** 1989. Transfer RNA genes frequently serve as integration sites for prokaryotic genetic elements. *Nucleic Acids Res.* **17:**1907–1914.

69. **Ritter, A., G. Blum, L. Emödy, M. Kerenyi, A. Böck, B. Neuhierl, W. Rabsch, F. Scheutz, and J. Hacker.** 1995. tRNA genes and pathogenicity islands: influence on virulence and metabolic properties of uropathogenic *Escherichia coli. Mol. Microbiol.* **17:**109–121.

70. **Ritter, A., D. L. Gally, P. B. Olsen, U. Dobrindt, A. Friedrich, P. Klemm, and J. Hacker.** 1997. The PAI-associated *leuX* specific tRNA5(Leu) affects type 1 fimbriation in pathogenic *Escherichia coli* by control of FimB recombinase expression. *Mol. Microbiol.* **25:**871–882.

71. **Schmidt, G., P. Sehr, M. Wilm, J. Selzer, M. Mann, and K. Aktories.** 1997. Gln 63 of Rho is deamidated by *Escherichia coli* cytotoxic necrotizing factor-1. *Nature* **387:**725–729.

72. **Schmidt, H., J. Scheef, C. Janetzki-Mittmann, M. Datz, and H. Karch.** 1997. An *ileX* tRNA gene is located close to the Shiga toxin II operon in enterohemorrhagic *Escherichia coli* O157 and non-O157 strains. *FEMS Microbiol. Lett.* **149:**39–44.

73. **Schmoll, T., H. Hoschützky, J. Morschhäuser, F. Lottspeich, K. Jann, and J. Hacker.** 1989. Analysis of genes coding for the sialic acid-binding adhesin and two other minor fimbrial subunits of the S-fimbrial adhesin determinant of *Escherichia coli. Mol. Microbiol.* **3:**1735–1744.

74. **Schubert, S., A. Rakin, H. Karch, E. Carniel, and J. Heesemann.** 1998. Prevalence of the "high-pathogenicity island" of *Yersinia* species among *Escherichia coli* strains that are pathogenic to humans. *Infect. Immun.* **66:**480–485.

75. **Schubert, S.** Personal communication.

76. **Sullivan, J. T., and C. W. Ronson.** 1998. Evolution of rhizobia by acquisition of a 500-kb symbiosis island that integrates into a phe-tRNA gene. *Proc. Natl. Acad. Sci. USA* **95:**5145–5149.

77. **Sussman, M.** 1997. Escherichia coli and human disease, p. 3–48. *In* M. Sussman (ed.), Escherichia coli: *Mechanisms of Virulence.* Cambridge University Press, Cambridge, United Kingdom.

78. **Swenson, D. L., N. O. Bukanov, D. E. Berg, and R. A. Welch.** 1996. Two pathogenicity islands in uropathogenic *Escherichia coli* J96: cosmid cloning and sample sequencing. *Infect. Immun.* **64:**3736–3743.

79. **Tinsley, C. R., and X. Nassif.** 1996. Analysis of the genetic differences between *Neisseria meningitidis* and *Neisseria gonorrhoeae:* two closely related bacteria expressing two different pathogenicities. *Proc. Natl. Acad. Sci. USA* **93:**11109–11114.

80. **Wabiko, H.** 1992. Sequence analysis of an insertion element, IS1131, isolated from the nopaline-type Ti plasmid of *Agrobacterium tumefaciens. Gene* **114:**229–233.

81. **Warren, J. W.** 1996. Clinical presentations and epidemiology of urinary tract infections, p. 3–27. *In* H. L. T. Mobley and J. W. Warren (ed.), *Urinary Tract Infections: Molecular Pathogenesis and Clinical Management.* American Society for Microbiology, Washington, D.C.

82. **Waters, V. L., and J. H. Crosa.** 1991. Colicin V virulence plasmids. *Microbiol. Rev.* **55:**437–450.

83. **Welch, R. A., R. Hull, and S. Falkow.** 1983. Molecular cloning and physical characterization of a chromosomal hemolysin from *Escherichia coli. Infect. Immun.* **42:**178–186.

84. **Zhang, D.-L., J. Hacker, and T. Oelschlaeger.** Unpublished data.

Pathogenicity Islands and Other Mobile Virulence Elements
Edited by J. B. Kaper and J. Hacker
© 1999 American Society for Microbiology, Washington, D.C.

Chapter 5

The High-Pathogenicity Island of Yersiniae

Alexander Rakin, Sören Schubert, Cosima Pelludat, Daniela Brem, and Jürgen Heesemann

Yersinia species are gram-negative rods that belong to the family of *Enterobacteriaceae*. According to biochemical and metabolic characteristics, DNA-DNA hybridization, and 16S rRNA sequencing results, the genus *Yersinia* comprises 11 different species. The G+C content of the DNA of the genus is 46 to 50 mol% (4). DNA hybridization studies revealed more than 90% intra- and interspecies relatedness between *Y. pestis* and *Y. pseudotuberculosis* and 20 to 55% between *Y. pseudotuberculosis* and the other *Yersinia* species (40, 49). A phylogenetic tree could be obtained from comparisons of genes coding for 16S rRNA (16S rDNA) of *Yersinia* species. Interestingly, the 16S rDNA sequence of *Y. pseudotuberculosis* was found to be identical to that of *Y. pestis* (49) (Fig. 1).

 Y. pestis, Y. pseudotuberculosis, and *Y. enterocolitica* are pathogens for humans, and *Y. ruckeri* is known as a fish pathogen (6). *Y. pestis,* the bacterial agent of bubonic plague, has been responsible for devastating epidemics throughout human history. This pathogen persists among certain wild rodent populations in many parts of the world (except Australia) and is transmitted by the bite of infected fleas. The blockage of the proventriculae of fleas by *Y. pestis* forces infected fleas to bite and subsequently regurgitate the infected blood meal into the bite site of a new host. The subsequent bacteremia in rodents completes the rodent-flea-rodent cycle essential for *Y. pestis* spread. The ecology, pathogenicity, and host range of *Y. pseudotuberculosis* and *Y. enterocolitica* differ fundamentally from those of *Y. pestis.* Both species are transmitted perorally by contaminated food or drinking water and subsequently invade Peyer's patches of the small bowel and multiply extracellularly. The bacteria then disseminate to mesenteric lymph nodes and occasionally via the bloodstream to the spleen, liver, and lungs, causing septicemic plague-like infections. Normally, infections with *Y. enterocolitica* or *Y. pseudotuberculosis* (yersiniosis) are self-limiting and benign. *Y. pseudotuberculosis* is widely distributed in nature in aquatic and animal reservoirs (rodents, cattle, swine, deer, and birds).

 Y. pseudotuberculosis strains can be divided into more than 10 serotypes, of which O:1, O:2, and O:3 are predominant in Europe. *Y. enterocolitica* comprises a biochemically and genetically heterogeneous group of organisms (6). About 40 different serotypes and

Alexander Rakin, Sören Schubert, Cosima Pelludat, Daniela Brem, and Jürgen Heesemann • Max von Pettenkofer-Institut für Hygiene und Mikrobiologie der Ludwig-Maximilians-Universität München, Pettenkoferstrasse 9a, 80336 Munich, Germany.

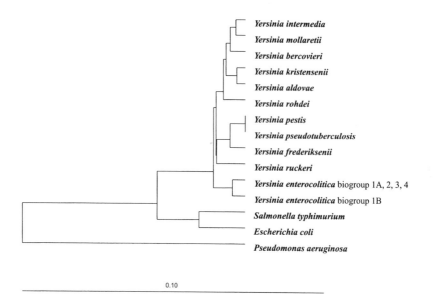

Figure 1. Phylogenetic tree calculated by neighbor-joining analysis (45) of 16S rRNA sequences with the *Pseudomonas aeruginosa* rRNA sequence as the outgroup. The distance matrix values were corrected by the Jukes-Cantor algorithm (32). The scale represents an evolutionary distance of 0.1 K_{nuc} (33).

six biogroups (1A, 1B, 2, 3, 4, and 5) have been defined. Biogroup 1A strains are nonpathogenic and are ecologically related to other nonpathogenic yersiniae. Previously, biogroup 1B strains (e.g., serotypes O:8, O:13, O:20, and O:21) were the dominant human isolates in the United States. However, European biogroup 4/serotype O:3 strains are currently frequently isolated in the United States. Interestingly, biogroup 1B strains are uncommon in Europe. According to 16S rDNA sequence analysis, biogroup 1B strains are distinct from biogroup 2 to 5 strains (Fig. 1). Obviously, two distinct phylogenetic groups of *Y. enterocolitica* exist: biogroup 1B comprises New World strains, and biogroups 2 to 5 include Old World or European strains. With respect to mouse virulence and ecology, *Y. enterocolitica* biogroup 1B strains resemble *Y. pseudotuberculosis* (high-pathogenicity group; 50% lethal dose $= 10^2$ to 10^3 microorganisms). The Old World *Y. enterocolitica* strains are less virulent for mice and are more host restricted than are biogroup 1B strains, and swine are the major reservoir. All enteropathogenic *Y. enterocolitica* strains produce heat-stable enterotoxins and thus are of higher diarrheagenic potential (causing gastroenteritis with occasional involvement of mesenteric lymphadenitis) than *Y. pseudotuberculosis* (which causes typical abdominal pain with mesenteric lymphadenitis). Old World *Y. enterocolitica* strains cause septicemia and liver abscesses in patients with iron overload or undergoing desferrioxamine treatment.

VIRULENCE DETERMINANTS OF *YERSINIA*

Although the three pathogenic *Yersinia* species differ greatly in their lifestyle, they have common strategies of pathogenesis, e.g., tropism for lymphatic tissue and extracellular

Table 1. Virulence-related genes of *Yersinia*

Determinant	Phenotype or function	Genes present in:		
		Y. pestis	*Y. pseudotuberculosis*	*Y. enterocolitica*
Chromosomal				
inv	Invasin, translocation by M cells	+[a]	+	+
ail	Attachment-invasin locus, serum resistance, cell adherence	+[a]	+	+
myf/psaA	Mucoid *Yersinia* fibrillae or pH6-antigen, cell adherence (?)	+	+	+
HPI (*irp/fyuA*)	HPI (36–43.4 kb) encoding yersiniabactin biosynthesis (Irp1 to Irp5, Irp9) and uptake (FyuA, Irp6, Irp7)	+	±[b]	±[b]
hms	Hemin storage or pigmentation locus, required for blocking proventriculae of fleas	+	+	−
Extrachromosomal				
pYV (pCD1)	70-kb *Yersinia* virulence plasmid			
virA, -B, -C, yopB, -D	Type III protein, secretion/translocation	+	+	+
yopE, -H, -M, -O, -P, -T	Yops with anti-host response function	+	+	+
yadA	*Yersinia* adhesin	+[a]	+	+
pYP (pPst, pPCP1)	9.5-kb plasmid	+	−	−
pla	Plasminogen activator, required for dissemination from flea bite site	+	−	−
pst	Pesticin, lysis of FyuA-positive bacteria	+	−	−
pim	Pesticin immunity	+	−	−
pFra (pMT1)	100-kb plasmid	+	−	−
caf	Fraction 1 (F1) capsule (antiphagocytic in mammalian host)	+	−	−
ymt	*Yersinia* mouse toxin/phospholipase D, required for erythrocyte lysis in flea proventriculae	+	−	−

[a] Inactive gene.
[b] ±, presence only in certain bio- or serogroups.

multiplication. As shown in Table 1, pathogenic yersiniae carry multiple sets of diverse pathogenicity- and transmission-related genes localized on the chromosome and on the plasmids (14, 37, 40). There are several genes for cell adhesion (*inv, ail, myf, psa,* and *yadA*), invasion (*inv*), evasion of the host immune response (virulence plasmid pYV, shared by all three *Yersinia* species), and plague pathogenesis and transmission (*hms, pla, ymt,* and *caf*). The high-pathogenicity group of yersiniae carries genes for the biosynthesis and uptake of the ferric iron-chelating substance (siderophore) yersiniabactin.

pgm LOCUS OF *Y. PESTIS*

Virulent *Y. pestis*, in contrast to other yersiniae, can adsorb large amounts of exogenous hemin at 26°C (40). *Y. pestis* strains that are unable to form pigmented colonies on a hemin agar (Pgm⁻ or Hms⁻ strains) are typically avirulent in mammalian hosts and are incapable of inducing block formation in a flea vector (5, 34). Hinnebusch et al. (29) have demonstrated that a pigmented (Pgm⁺ or Hms⁺) *Y. pestis* strain is capable of developing blockages in fleas while isogenic nonpigmented mutants cannot do so. The possible role of Hms in mammalian infection is less certain.

Hms-negative colonies arise with a high frequency (10^{-5}) in populations of *Y. pestis* and normally do not revert (22). Deletion of a 102-kb chromosomal *pgm* fragment that results in nonpigmented yersiniae might be mediated by homologous recombination between two IS*100* sequences flanking the *pgm* locus (Fig. 2). Such instability of the 102-kb chromosomal fragment, which is associated with virulence of *Y. pestis,* was the reason for denoting it a pathogenicity island (21). Nevertheless, deletions with other endpoints and sizes might occur within the 102-kb fragment (8). On the other hand, some *Y. pestis* strains give rise to Hms⁻ derivatives that are able to revert to the wild type (41). This is an indication of an additional mechanism that might regulate the expression of the hemin storage operon.

The 102-kb *pgm* locus is composed of two distinct parts (22), the *hms* part and the yersiniabactin (*ybt*) gene cluster, which contains genes responsible for the synthesis and

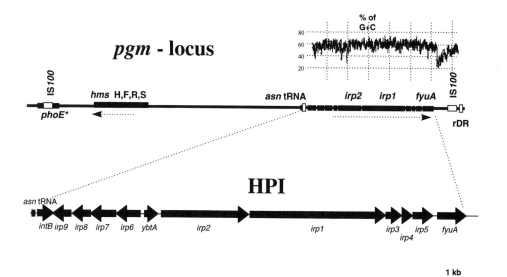

Figure 2. Pigmentation locus (*pgm*) and the HPI in *Y. pestis* (8, 11, 21). The graph above the *pgm* locus depicts the G+C content along the HPI sequence. Arrows show the positions of the genes and direction of transcription. *hms,* genes for hemin storage; *irp1* to irp9, iron-repressible genes involved in synthesis and uptake of the yersiniabactin; *asn* tRNA, asparagine-tRNA gene; *intB,* putative integrase gene; *ybtA,* yersiniabactin transcriptional activator gene; *fyuA,* yersiniabactin receptor gene; *phoE*,* phosphatase gene inactivated by IS*100* insertion; rDR, 17-bp direct repeat of the 3′ end of the *asn* tRNA.

uptake of the yersiniabactin (Fig. 2). These two parts seem to form a contiguous group only in *Y. pestis*, while the *hms* part is not adjacent to the *ybt* genes in *Y. pseudotuberculosis* and is absent in *Y. enterocolitica* (7) and yersiniabactin-positive *Escherichia coli* (46). Inactivation of the genes constituting the *ybt* gene cluster (*fyuA* in *Y. enterocolitica* and *psn* in *Y. pestis*, encoding yersiniabactin receptor or the biosynthetic genes *irp1, irp2, irp5* or *ybtE* in *Y. pestis*) results in a pronounced reduction of the virulence of these bacteria to laboratory animals (3, 21, 42). Inactivation of the *hms* genes, on the other hand, demonstrated the importance of these genes for survival of *Y. pestis* in fleas (29). The G+C content of the *hms* locus does not differ from that of the rest of the *Y. pestis* chromosome (46 to 48 mol%), while the G+C content of the *ybt* genes is significantly higher (57.5 mol%) (43). The *hms* part of the 102-kb chromosomal fragment of *Y. pestis* is not in the same linkage group with the yersiniabactin cluster and is not considered a high-pathogenicity island or part of such an island in this chapter.

THE HIGH-PATHOGENICITY ISLAND

Yersiniabactin-Related Genes

Survival and proliferation within the host depend on the ability of a pathogen to scavenge essential nutrients such as iron, which is bound by the host molecules ferritin, transferrin, and lactoferrin. Bacteria have developed an efficient strategy to obtain iron from these eukaryotic iron scavangers. They produce and secrete low-molecular-weight siderophores with extremely high affinities for ferric iron (36). Wake et al. (50) were the first to detect putative siderophore activity in *Y. pestis*, although Perry and Brubaker (39) were not able to detect any siderophore activity in *Yersinia*. The siderophore activity was subsequently rediscovered in yersiniae by Heesemann (27), and the siderophore was designated yersiniabactin (Ybt). Ybt purified from *Y. enterocolitica* has a molecular mass of 482 Da and contains aromatic and nonaromatic iron-chelating groups (24). Ybt displays relatively weak iron binding under in vitro culture conditions (30). Nevertheless, the siderophore activity was detected only in highly pathogenic yersiniae that are lethal for mice at low infectious doses: *Y. pestis*, *Y. pseudotuberculosis*, and *Y. enterocolitica* biotype 1B (New World strains); but it was not detected in low-pathogenicity *Y. enterocolitica* biotypes 2 to 5 (Old World strains) (13).

The yersiniabactin gene cluster responsible for the manifestation of lethality for mice was named the high-pathogenicity island (HPI) (11). The complete structure of the HPI is shown in Fig. 2. The functional "core" of the island consists of 12 genes. At least six genes encoding iron-repressible proteins (*irp1* to *irp5* and *irp9*) in *Y. enterocolitica* (*ybtE* and *ybtT* are *Y. pestis* synonyms for *irp4* and *irp5*, respectively) are involved in biosynthesis of the yersiniabactin (3, 8, 23, 38) (Table 2). The yersiniabactin receptor has a dual function; besides being a receptor for yersiniabactin, it is also a receptor for the *Y. pestis* bacteriocin pesticin (28, 35, 42). Therefore, loss of pesticin sensitivity correlates with loss of the yersiniabactin binding site and with inability of *Yersinia* to obtain sufficient iron for growth in the mammalian host environment. YbtA is the transcriptional regulator of the yersiniabactin regulon (20), IntB is a putative integrase (7), and Irp6 and Irp7 (YbtP and YbtQ in *Y. pestis*) (23) might be involved in the transport of the ferric yersiniabactin through the inner membrane, while Irp8 might be involved in signal transduction.

Table 2. Genes of the HPI

Y. enterocolitica gene (protein)	Y. pestis ortholog	Yersiniabactin production[a]	Possible function
intB	Int		Integration of the HPI
irp9	YbtS	+/−	Synthesis of salicylate
irp8	YbtX	+/−	Signal transducer
irp7	YbtQ	+/+++	Yersiniabactin transport
irp6	YbtP	+/+++	Yersiniabactin transport
ybtA	YbtA	+/−	Transcriptional regulator
irp2 (HMWP2)	HMWP2	+/−	Yersiniabactin peptide synthetase
irp1 (HMWP1)	HMWP1	+/−	Yersiniabactin polyketide synthetase
irp3	YbtU	Unknown	Unknown
irp4	YbtT	+/−	Thioesterase
irp5	YbtE	+/−	Salicyl-AMP ligase
fyuA	Psn	+/++	Yersiniabactin and pesticin receptor

[a] The first sign shows the wild-type reaction, and the second shows the effect of inactivation of the gene by reverse genetics. The semiquantitative estimation of the yersiniabactin production is designated +, + +, or + + +.

Carniel et al. described two iron-repressible proteins, HMWP1 (high-molecular-weight protein 1; 260 kDa, encoded by *irp1*) and HMWP2 (190 kDa, encoded by *irp2*) (12). The HMWPs were detected only in highly pathogenic *Yersinia* strains grown under iron limitation. Inactivation of *irp2* results in a considerable reduction of virulence to mice in *Y. pseudotuberculosis* O:1 (12). HMWP2 was found to be homologous to AngR (which is involved in anguibactin biosynthesis in *Vibrio anguillarum*) and is suspected to direct nonribosomal synthesis of small molecules such as antibiotics and siderophores. Inactivation of the *irp2* gene in *Y. enterocolitica* WA-314 results in its inability to produce detectable amounts of the yersiniabactin on Chrome-azurol S indicator plates. The *irp1* gene (coding for HMWP1 [38]), which is larger (9,486 kb), shares a unique motif with the polyketide synthases of *Streptomyces hygroscopicus* and *S. antibioticus* (1). *Y. enterocolitica* mutated in *irp1* was also unable to produce yersiniabactin.

Three additional open reading frames with the same transcriptional polarity could be defined on the yersiniabactin gene cluster (Fig. 2) (3, 38). Two of them, *irp4* and *irp5*, encode proteins with pronounced identity to a thioesterase-like protein from the anguibactin biosynthetic gene cluster of *V. anguillarum* (18) and EntE (2,3-dihydroxybenzoic acid-activating enzyme) from *E. coli* (48), respectively. Insertional inactivation of the *ybtE* gene in *Y. pestis* (ortholog of *irp5* in *Y. enterocolitica*) results in inability of the mutant to grow in iron-deficient medium at 37°C (3). *irp3* has no pronounced similarity to sequences in data libraries.

Structure and Mobility Characteristics of the HPI

The *fyuA* promoter contains a consensus Fur iron-repressor binding site (42) and a putative binding site for the yersiniabactin AraC-type transcriptional regulator YbtA (20). Transport of the ferric yersiniabactin is TonB dependent. Inactivation of the *fyuA* gene in yersiniae was followed by a significant reduction of virulence (21, 42).

The *ybtA* transcriptional regulator resides upstream of the yersiniabactin biosynthetic

genes (Fig. 2). YbtA belongs to the AraC family of transcriptional regulators and is proposed to be an iron-responsive regulator of the yersiniabactin receptor and synthetic genes
(20). Promoters of the *ybtA, fyuA,* and *irp2* genes possess inverted and directly repeated
structures that might present binding sites for YbtA. The *ybtA* promoter in *Y. enterocolitica*
IB strains is disrupted by an insertion of a 127-bp enterobacterial repetitive intergenic
consensus sequence (ERIC) (31). ERIC, also known as the intergenic repeated unit (IRU)
(47), is present in multiple copies in intergenic and untranslated regions upstream or
downstream of open reading frames in various genomes. Integration of the ERIC sequence
modifies the secondary structure of the *ybtA* promoter in *Y. enterocolitica* and thus dramatically affects its activity.

The open reading frame on the left extremity of the yersiniabactin cluster encodes a
basic protein with a 49.7% identity to the prophage P4 integrase (9). This integrase (IntB)
might be responsible for recognition and integration of the HPI. In *Y. enterocolitica* biotype
1B (serotypes O:8, O:13, O:20, and O:21), *intB* is inactivated by a G-to-T point mutation
leading to a stop codon. This mutation might result in a truncated and inactive IntB
polypeptide in these yersiniae.

The HPI is associated with the asparagine *asnT* RNA gene in *Y. enterocolitica* O:8
strain 8081 (11). The 3′ ends of tRNAs are frequently recognized as attachment sites for
integration of foreign DNA into bacterial genomes (10, 25, 44). Nevertheless, four identical
asn tRNA copies are present in the *E. coli* genome and at least three are present in *Yersinia*
(7). The HPI is integrated adjacent to the *asnT* RNA copy in all *Y. enterocolitica* IB strains
as well as in several HPI-positive *E. coli* strains of different pathotypes (46). In *Y. pestis*
and *Y. pseudotuberculosis,* the HPI is also associated with the *asn* tRNA. However, it
seems to utilize other *asn* tRNA copies in these species (7, 26).

Integration of prokaryotic genetic elements such as temperate phages and transmissible
plasmids occurs by a site-specific recombination between a short sequence on the element
and an identical sequence (attachment or target site) on the bacterial chromosome (44).
A recombination results in a duplication of the target site. A perfect 17-bp (imperfect 20-
bp) direct repeat, CCAGTCAGAGGAGCCAAaTT, can be recognized 5.6 kb downstream
of the *fyuA* gene on the *Y. pseudotuberculosis* and *Y. pestis* chromosomes and 12.5 kb
downstream of *fyuA* on the *Y. enterocolitica* chromosome. Primers designed for the sequences located upstream of the *asnT* RNA and downstream of the direct repeat of the
attachment site failed to amplify the whole HPI in *Y. enterocolitica* O8. The PCR was
also negative with *Y. enterocolitica* O:3, O:9, and O:5,27 isolates that do not contain the
island. The same primers successfully amplified a 16-bp recognition site in avirulent *Y.
enterocolitica* NF-O, O:5, biotype 1A strain. Thus, the *asnT* RNA attachment site of the
HPI is ''insertion free'' in an avirulent *Y. enterocolitica* O:5 isolate but has acquired
additional DNA insertions in human-pathogenic *Y. enterocolitica* isolates. A 17-bp junction fragment is proposed for the HPI in *Y. pseudotuberculosis* (7), and a 24-bp recognition
site is proposed in *Y. pestis* (26). In contrast to yersiniae, we were not able to detect a
duplication of the HPI attachment site in *E. coli.*

In several *E. coli* isolates, the HPI is also integrated adjacent to the *asnT* RNA gene,
as in *Y. enterocolitica* 1B (46). However, insertion of the HPI in *E. coli* isolates was
followed by a massive deletion of the adjacent DNA if compared to the physical map of
E. coli K-12 (Fig. 3). The HPI in *E. coli* terminates 1,227 bp downstream of the *fyuA* stop

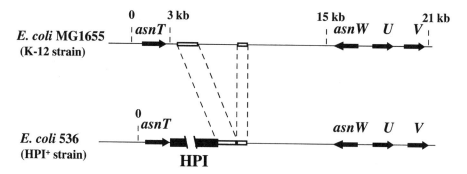

Figure 3. Comparison of the *asn* tRNA locus of the *E. coli* chromosome in HPI-negative *E. coli* K-12 strain MG1655 and HPI-positive uropathogenic *E. coli* 536. Arrows show the positions and directions of transcription of the *asn* tRNA genes. The shaded boxes indicate the positions of the HPI. Broken lines show the deletion of the *E. coli* chromosome (for abbreviations, see the legend to Fig. 2).

codon. It does not contain IS elements, and the right direct repeat is lost. This could be the result of a deletion(s) that occurred during integration of the island.

The organization of the functional ''core'' of the HPI associated with yersiniabactin uptake and synthesis is conserved in all island-positive carriers (7, 11) (Fig. 4). The sequence similarity of the genes constituting the island exceeds 98% (26, 38, 43). Neverthe-

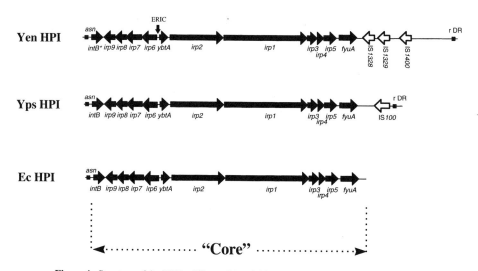

Figure 4. Structure of the HPI in different bacterial hosts. Black arrows show the positions of the genes and the directions of transcription. Open arrows depict the positions and orientations of the IS elements in HPIs. Yen HPI, *Y. enterocolitica* HPI; Yps HPI, *Y. pestis*/*Y. pseudotuberculosis* HPI; Ec HPI, Yps-type HPI found in *E. coli;* ERIC, position of integration of the ERIC sequence into the *ybtA* promoter in Yen HPI; *intB**, inactivation of a putative integrase gene in Yen HPI. For other abbreviations, see the legend to Fig. 2.

less, the presence of different insertion sequences as well as local differences in DNA sequences of the genes constituting the island makes it possible to distinguish two evolutionary groups of the HPI, i.e., the *Y. pseudotuberculosis-Y. pestis* (Yps HPI) and *Y. enterocolitica* (Yen HPI) lineages (43).

Distribution of the HPI

Several *E. coli* strains were known to be pesticin sensitive (19), and thus they possess the pesticin/yersiniabactin receptor. Moreover, they were found to harbor the HPI (43, 46). DNA comparison of the *fyuA* and *irp2* genes revealed a Yps-type HPI in *E. coli* (Fig. 4). This indicates a common ancestor of the island or a possible recent horizontal transfer between these two species. The integrase gene is not mutated in *E. coli*, but the right direct repeat is missing in the *E. coli* HPI.

Recently, the HPI was detected in other members of the family *Enterobacteriaceae*, e.g., in variety of pathotypes of *E. coli*, *Klebsiella*, *Enterobacter*, and *Citrobacter*. Particularly, strains isolated from blood cultures of patients suffering from septicemia and 70% of those isolated from urine samples from patients with urinary tract infections contained the island (46) (Fig. 5). However, HPI-positive *E. coli* strains are frequently isolated from stool samples from healthy individuals. Therefore, it remains unclear how the HPI contributes to the virulence of human-pathogenic *E. coli*. The HPI is not frequent in *E.*

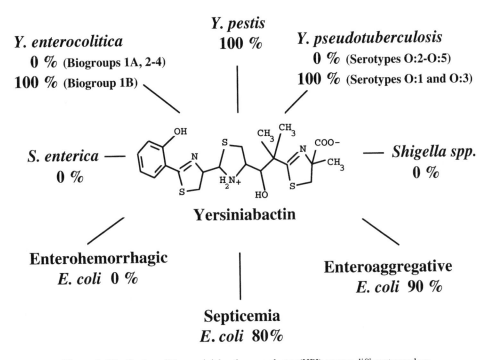

Figure 5. Distribution of the yersiniabactin gene cluster (HPI) among different members of the *Enterobacteriaceae.*

coli strains that are isolated from the natural environment. Therefore, one can speculate that acquisition of the HPI might be a factor in adaptation to a human host. The presence of an enterochelin siderophore system with much higher affinity to iron (15) in all HPI-positive *Enterobacteriaceae* family members indicates possible additional functions of the yersiniabactin. These functions could include modulation of cells of host defenses (2, 17), as has been demonstrated with other siderophores. On the other hand, the possible advantages of yersiniabactin over enterochelin under certain in vivo conditions cannot be excluded.

In most cases, the HPI is maintained in *E. coli* isolates as a complete physical entity. In 3% of HPI-positive *E. coli* isolates, deletions are found only in the *fyuA* region of the HPI (3' end). The HPI was found in 100% of *Y. pseudotuberculosis* O:1 strains and 50% of *Y. pseudotuberculosis* O:3 (O:3A) strains (43). In the latter group, the HPI has suffered a mass deletion of the *irp3* and *fyuA* genes. Therefore, these strains, like 3% of the *E. coli* isolates that have lost the *fyuA* extremity of the island, are not able to take up the yersiniabactin or even produce a full-sized siderophore molecule. Nevertheless, such strains are repeatedly isolated from nature, emphasizing a possible important role of the yersiniabactin precursor(s).

A different G+C content from that of the overall DNA composition of the host chromosome is thought to be a vital characteristic of pathogenicity islands (25). However, the G+C content is not uniform along the HPI. The functional ''core'' genes which are involved in yersiniabactin uptake and biosynthesis have a high G+C content (57.5 mol%) (Fig. 2), which is much higher than the G+C content of the chromosome of *E. coli* or *Yersinia* (46 to 50 mol%) (4). The sequences located downstream of the *fyuA* gene differ greatly in the two evolutionary groups and have a high A+T content (56 to 68 mol%). These AT-rich regions have acquired various insertion sequences. In the Yps HPI, one copy of the IS*100* mobile element is present. The variable AT-rich part of the Yen HPI is 7 kb larger than the variable AT-rich part of the Yps HPI. Three mobile elements, IS*1328*, IS*1329*, and IS*1400* (11), are present in this region.

The presence of insertion sequences on the HPI might result in DNA rearrangements in the 3' end of the island in *E. coli* and *Y. pseudotuberculosis* O:3. Pesticin-resistant mutants of *Y. enterocolitica* WA-314 that have acquired different-sized deletions were isolated (41). The deletions in this case could be promoted by one of the multiple insertion elements present on the Yen HPI. Precise excision of the HPI in *Y. enterocolitica* is not documented. The high frequency of homologous recombination between two IS*100* copies in *Y. pestis* or IS-promoted recombination in *Y. enterocolitica* might obscure the low-frequency site-specific excision of the HPI in yersiniae. Nevertheless, a precise excision with restoration of the original HPI attachment site was described in a *Y. pseudotuberculosis* O1 strain (7).

The finding of additional 5.6-kb (Yps HPI) or 12.8-kb (Yen HPI) AT-rich DNA regions in the HPI that have no obvious function poses questions about the possible mechanism of HPI dissemination. No genes that can be responsible for the self-transmissibility of the HPI were detected. Thus, the island might be mobilized passively by conjugative plasmids or transducing phages. Transduction by a full-head phage mechanism could explain the presence of additional and probably nonessential DNA in the HPI. Insertions of additional DNA mobile elements into Yen HPI could enlarge the HPI. Inactivation of the integrase gene in Yen HPI might explain exclusive dissemination of the *Y. pestis*-type island in *E. coli* (46).

Only the genes that are necessary for the expression of the iron acquisition function are recognized on the HPI. No genes that contribute otherwise to virulence could be detected on the HPI of either evolutionary lineage. Hence, the dominant function of the HPI is to provide bacteria with iron to improve their "fitness" in the rapidly changing environmental conditions.

CONCLUSIONS

The HPI that was detected primarily in yersiniae conforms to the criteria of a pathogenicity island (25). It contains a set of clustered genes associated with lethality of highly pathogenic yersiniae for mice. Its size is 36.1 kb for the Yps HPI and 43.4 kb for the Yen HPI. The HPI is a distinct genetic entity associated with *asn* tRNA genes. The HPI exploits a site-specific mechanism of integration and is flanked by 17-bp perfect (20-bp imperfect) direct repeats, which represent a duplication of the 3' end of the *asn* tRNA. A putative P4 prophage-type integrase could be responsible for the insertion of the HPI into its recognition site. The HPI can excise precisely in *Y. pseudotuberculosis* but not in *Y. enterocolitica*, where it undergoes deletions of different sizes that are probably mediated by multiple insertion sequences present on the island. The functional genes responsible for yersiniabactin uptake and synthesis ("core") have a higher G+C content (57.5 mol%) than do housekeeping genes of the host cell (46 to 50 mol%).

However, some characteristics specific to the HPI of *Yersinia* must be mentioned. (i) No determinants that directly contribute to pathogenicity could be defined on the island. The genes on the HPI are associated with pathogen propagation in the host rather than with direct damage to the host cells. Thus, the HPI can improve the "fitness" of pathogenic bacteria by being a factor in adaptation to the mammalian host. In addition to yersiniae and pathogenic *E. coli*, the HPI can be found in ca. 20% of the environmental isolates of *E. coli*. (ii) No genes that might be responsible for the HPI self-transmissibility could be defined on the island. This implies that the HPI might be passively transferred by transducing phages or conjugative plasmids. (iii) No genes that might be involved in self-replication could be defined on the island. Thus, the HPI does not present a replicon and can exist only as a part of another replicating unit. (iv) Two evolutionary lineages of the HPI can be distinguished, *Y. enterocolitica* 1B HPI and *Y. pestis*/*Y. pseudotuberculosis* HPI, with the latter also being disseminated among different pathotypes of *E. coli*. The Yen HPI has acquired several insertion sequences and its integrase is inactivated by a point mutation. Moreover, the expression of the yersiniabactin genes differs in the two lineages due to the integration of an ERIC sequence into the *ybtA* transcriptional activator. (v) The HPI is composed of two parts: a highly conserved functional "core" involved in uptake and synthesis of the yersiniabactin, and an AT-rich variable part that completely differs in islands of the two evolutionary lineages. The G+C content is not uniform along the island, being high (57.5%) for the core and low (32 to 44%) for the variable part. The variable part makes up 13% of the Yps HPI and 28% of the Yen HPI.

Considering the described characteristics of the HPI of yersiniae in toto, we would like to propose a definition of a pathogenicity island. A pathogenicity island can be defined as a nonreplicative, non-self-transmissible structural and functional genetic entity carrying virulence-associated sets of genes that utilizes a site-specific mechanism of integration into conserved target sites. Some of the characteristics of pathogenicity islands can be lost or modified in the process of evolution. Thus, a pathogenicity island can become a part of a specialized transducing phage, its integration abilities can be altered, or it can acquire IS insertions, etc. Nevertheless, the remaining features make it possible to distinguish a pathogenicity island from any other genetic element in the bacterial cell.

REFERENCES

1. **Aparicio, J. F., I. Molnar, T. Schwecke, A. Konig, S. F. Haydock, L. E. Khaw, J. Staunton, and P. F. Leadlay.** 1996. Organization of the biosynthetic gene cluster for rapamycin in *Streptomyces hygroscopicus:* analysis of the enzymatic domains in the modular polyketide synthase. *Gene* **169:**9–16.

2. **Autenrieth, I. B., E. Bohn, J. H. Ewald, and J. Heesemann.** 1995. Deferoxamine B but not deferoxamine G1 inhibits cytokine production in murine bone marrow macrophages. *J. Infect. Dis.* **172:**490–496.

3. **Bearden, S. W., J. D. Fetherston, and R. D. Perry.** 1997. Genetic organization of the yersiniabactin biosynthesis region and construction of avirulent mutants in *Yersinia pestis. Infect. Immun.* **65:**1659–1668.

4. **Bercovier, H., and H. H. Mollaret.** 1984. *Yersinia,* p. 498–506. *In* N. R. Krieg and J. G. Holt (ed.), *Bergey's Manual of Systematic Bacteriology,* vol. 1. The Williams & Wilkins, Co., Baltimore, Md.

5. **Bibikova, V. A.** 1977. Contemporary views on the interrelationships between fleas and the pathogens of human and animal diseases. *Annu. Rev. Entomol.* **22:**23–32.

6. **Bottone, E. J.** 1997. *Yersinia enterocolitica:* the charisma continues. *Clin. Microbiol. Rev.* **10:**257–276.

7. **Buchrieser, C., R. Brosch, S. Bach, A. Guiyoule, and E. Carniel.** 1998. The high-pathogenicity island of *Yersinia pseudotuberculosis* can be inserted into any of the three chromosomal *asn tRNA* genes. *Mol. Microbiol.* **30:**965–978.

8. **Buchrieser, C., M. Prentice, and E. Carniel.** 1998. The 102-kilobase unstable region of *Yersinia pestis* comprises a high-pathogenicity island linked to a pigmentation segment which undergoes internal rearrangement. *J. Bacteriol.* **180:**2321–2329.

9. **Burland, V., G. Plunkett III, H. J. Sofia, D. L. Daniels, and F. R. Blattner.** 1995. Analysis of the *Escherichia coli* genome VI: DNA sequence of the region from 92.8 through 100 minutes. *Nucleic Acids Res.* **23:**2105–2119.

10. **Campbell, A. M.** 1992. Chromosomal insertion sites for phages and plasmids. *J. Bacteriol.* **174:**7495–7499.

11. **Carniel, E., I. Guilvout, and M. Prentice.** 1996. Characterization of a large chromosomal "high-pathogenicity island" in biotype 1B *Yersinia enterocolitica. J. Bacteriol.* **178:**6743–6751.

12. **Carniel, E., A. Guiyoule, I. Guilvout, and O. Mercereau Puijalon.** 1992. Molecular cloning, iron-regulation and mutagenesis of the *irp2* gene encoding HMWP2, a protein specific for the highly pathogenic *Yersinia. Mol. Microbiol.* **6:**379–388.

13. **Carter, P. B.** 1975. Pathogenicity of *Yersinia enterocolitica* for mice. *Infect. Immun.* **11:**164–170.

14. **Cornelis, G. R., and H. Wolf-Watz.** 1997. The *Yersinia* Yop virulon: a bacterial system for subverting eukaryotic cells. *Mol. Microbiol.* **23:**861–867.

15. **Crosa, J. H.** 1989. Genetics and molecular biology of siderophore-mediated iron transport in bacteria. *Microbiol. Rev.* **53:**517–530.

16. **Emody, L., J. Heesemann, H. Wolf-Watz, M. Skurnik, G. Kapperud, P. O'Toole, and T. Wadstrom.** 1989. Binding to collagen by *Yersinia enterocolitica* and *Yersinia pseudotuberculosis:* evidence for *yopA*-mediated and chromosomally encoded mechanisms. *J. Bacteriol.* **171:**6674–6679.

17. **Ewald, J. H., J. Heesemann, H. Rüdiger, and I. B. Autenrieth.** 1994. Interaction of polymorphonuclear leukocytes with *Yersinia enterocolitica:* role of the *yersinia* virulence plasmid and modulation by the iron-chelator desferrioxamine B. *J. Infect. Dis.* **170:**140–150.

18. **Farrell, D. H., P. Mikesell, L. A. Actis, and J. H. Crosa.** 1990. A regulatory gene, *angR,* of the iron uptake system of *Vibrio anguillarum:* similarity with phage P22 *cro* and regulation by iron. *Gene* **86:**45–51.

19. **Ferber, D. M., J. M. Fowler, and R. R. Brubaker.** 1981. Mutations to tolerance and resistance to pesticin and colicins in *Escherichia coli* phi. *J. Bacteriol.* **146:**506–511.

20. **Fetherston, J. D., S. W. Bearden, and R. D. Perry.** 1996. YbtA, an AraC-type regulator of the *Yersinia pestis* pesticin/yersiniabactin receptor. *Mol. Microbiol.* **22:**315–325.

21. **Fetherston, J. D., J. W. Lillard, Jr., and R. D. Perry.** 1995. Analysis of the pesticin receptor from *Yersinia pestis:* role in iron-deficient growth and possible regulation by its siderophore. *J. Bacteriol.* **177:**1824–1833.

22. **Fetherston, J. D., and R. D. Perry.** 1994. The pigmentation locus of *Yersinia pestis* KIM6+ is flanked by an insertion sequence and includes the structural genes for pesticin sensitivity and HMWP2. *Mol. Microbiol.* **13:**697–708.

23. **Gehring, A. M., E. DeMoll, J. D. Fetherston, I. Mori, G. F. Mayhew, F. R. Blattner, C. T. Walsh, and R. D. Perry.** 1998. Iron acquisition in plague: modular logic in enzymatic biogenesis of yersiniabactin by *Yersinia pestis. Chem. Biol.* **5:**573–586.

24. **Haag, H., K. Hantke, H. Drechsel, I. Stojiljkovic, G. Jung, and H. Zähner.** 1993. Purification of yersiniabactin: a siderophore and a possible virulence factor of *Yersinia enterocolitica. J. Gen. Microbiol.* **139:** 2159–2165.

25. **Hacker, J., G. Blum Oehler, I. Muhldorfer, and H. Tschape.** 1997. Pathogenicity islands of virulent bacteria: structure, function and impact on microbial evolution. *Mol. Microbiol.* **23:**1089–1097.

26. **Hare, J. M., A. K. Wagner, and K. A. McDonough.** 1999. Independent acquisition and insertion into different chromosomal locations of the same pathogenicity island in *Yersinia pestis* and *Yersinia pseudotuberculosis. Mol. Microbiol.* **31:**291–303.

27. **Heesemann, J.** 1987. Chromosomal-encoded siderophores are required for mouse virulence of enteropathogenic *Yersinia* species. *FEMS Microbiol. Lett.* **48:**229–233.

28. **Heesemann, J., K. Hantke, T. Vocke, E. Saken, A. Rakin, I. Stojiljkovic, and R. Berner.** 1993. Virulence of *Yersinia enterocolitica* is closely associated with siderophore production, expression of an iron-repressible outer membrane protein of 65000 Da and pesticin sensitivity. *Mol. Microbiol.* **8:**397–408.

29. **Hinnebusch, B. J., R. D. Perry, and T. G. Schwan.** 1996. Role of the *Yersinia pestis* hemin storage *(hms)* locus in the transmission of plague by fleas. *Science* **273:**367–370.

30. **Hornung, J. M., H. A. Jones, and R. D. Perry.** 1996. The *hmu* locus of *Yersinia pestis* is essential for utilization of free haemin and haem-protein complexes as iron sources. *Mol. Microbiol.* **20:**725–739.

31. **Hulton, C. S., C. F. Higgins, and P. M. Sharp.** 1991. ERIC sequences: a novel family of repetitive elements in the genomes of *Escherichia coli, Salmonella typhimurium* and other enterobacteria. *Mol. Microbiol.* **5:** 825–834.

32. **Jukes, T. H., and C. R. Cantor.** 1969. Evolution of protein molecules, p. 32–132. *In* H. N. Munro (ed.), *Mammalian Protein Metabolism.* Academic Press, Inc., New York, N.Y.

33. **Kimura, M.** 1980. A simple method for estimating evolutionary rates of base substitutions through comparative studies of nucleotide sequences. *J. Mol. Evol.* **16:**111–120.

34. **Kutyrev, V. V., A. A. Filippov, O. S. Oparina, and O. A. Protsenko.** 1992. Analysis of *Yersinia pestis* chromosomal determinants Pgm⁺ and Pstˢ associated with virulence. *Microb. Pathog.* **12:**177–186.

35. **Lillard, J. W., Jr., J. D. Fetherston, L. Pedersen, M. L. Pendrak, and R. D. Perry.** 1997. Sequence and genetic analysis of the hemin storage *(hms)* system of *Yersinia pestis. Gene* **193:**13–21.

36. **Mietzner, T. A., and S. A. Morse.** 1994. The role of iron-binding proteins in the survival of pathogenic bacteria. *Annu. Rev. Nutr.* **14:**471–493.

37. **Miller, V. L., B. B. Finlay, and S. Falkow.** 1988. Factors essential for the penetration of mammalian cells by *Yersinia. Curr. Top. Microbiol. Immunol.* **138:**15–39.

38. **Pelludat, C., A. Rakin, C. A. Jacobi, S. Schubert, and J. Heesemann.** 1998. The yersiniabactin biosynthetic gene cluster of *Yersinia enterocolitica:* organization and siderophore-dependent regulation. *J. Bacteriol.* **180:**538–546.

39. **Perry, R. D., and R. R. Brubaker.** 1979. Accumulation of iron by yersiniae. *J. Bacteriol.* **137:**1290–1298.

40. **Perry, R. D., and J. D. Fetherston.** 1997. *Yersinia pestis*—etiologic agent of plague. *Clin. Microbiol. Rev.* **10:**35–66.

41. **Rakin, A., and J. Heesemann.** 1995. Yersiniabactin/pesticin receptor: a component of an iron uptake system of highly pathogenic *Yersinia. Contrib. Microbiol. Immunol.* **13:**244–247.

42. **Rakin, A., E. Saken, D. Harmsen, and J. Heesemann.** 1994. The pesticin receptor of *Yersinia enterocolitica:* a novel virulence factor with dual function. *Mol. Microbiol.* **13:**253–263.

43. **Rakin, A., P. Urbitsch, and J. Heesemann.** 1995. Evidence for two evolutionary lineages of highly pathogenic *Yersinia* species. *J. Bacteriol.* **177:**2292–2298.

44. **Reiter, W. D., P. Palm, and S. Yeats.** 1989. Transfer RNA genes frequently serve as integration sites for prokaryotic genetic elements. *Nucleic Acids Res.* **17:**1907–1914.

45. **Saitou, N., and M. Nei.** 1987. The neighbor-joining method: a new method for reconstructing phylogenetic trees. *Mol. Biol. Evol.* **4:**406–425.
46. **Schubert, S., A. Rakin, H. Karch, E. Carniel, and J. Heesemann.** 1998. Prevalence of the ''high-pathogenicity island'' of *Yersinia* species among *Escherichia coli* strains that are pathogenic to humans. *Infect. Immun.* **66:**480–485.
47. **Sharples, G. J., and R. G. Lloyd.** 1990. A novel repeated DNA sequence located in the intergenic regions of bacterial chromosomes. *Nucleic Acids Res.* **18:**6503–6508.
48. **Staab, J. F., M. F. Elkins, and C. F. Earhart.** 1989. Nucleotide sequence of the *Escherichia coli entE* gene. *FEMS Microbiol. Lett.* **50:**15–19.
49. **Trebesius, K., D. Harmsen, A. Rakin, J. Schmelz, and J. Heesemann.** 1998. Development of rRNA-targeted PCR and in situ hybridization with fluorescently labelled oligonucleotides for detection of *Yersinia* species. *J. Clin. Microbiol.* **36:**2557–2564.
50. **Wake, A., M. Misawa, and A. Matsui.** 1975. Siderochrome production by *Yersinia pestis* and its relation to virulence. *Infect. Immun.* **12:**1211–1213.

Pathogenicity Islands and Other Mobile Virulence Elements
Edited by J. B. Kaper and J. Hacker
© 1999 American Society for Microbiology, Washington, D.C.

Chapter 6

The 70-Kilobase Virulence Plasmid of Yersiniae

Maite Iriarte and Guy R. Cornelis

INTRODUCTION

Plague and Other Yersinioses

The *Yersinia* genus contains three species that are human pathogens, *Y. pestis, Y. pseudotuberculosis,* and *Y. enterocolitica. Y. pestis,* the agent of plague, is inoculated into the host by a flea bite and is drained to the regional lymph nodes, where it multiplies rapidly, causing the formation of the typical bubo (bubonic plague). The infection then spreads via the bloodstream and further localizes in the liver, spleen, and other organs. Septicemic plague is defined as infection in individuals with positive blood cultures but no apparent bubo. Pneumonic plague is a rare but more deadly form of plague that spreads via respiratory droplets transmitted by infected individuals (for a recent review, see reference 127).

Infections due to *Y. pseudotuberculosis* and *Y. enterocolitica* are acquired by ingestion of contaminated food. Like *Y. pestis, Y. pseudotuberculosis* is primarly a rodent pathogen, but it has also been associated with human infections and results in mesenteric adenitis and septicemia (for a review, see reference 37).

Y. enterocolitica is a common contaminant of pork meat (181, 191) and causes a self-limiting infection. Enterocolitis, the most common clinical form, occurs mainly in young children. A pseudoappendicular syndrome occurs primarily in older children and young adults. Postinfection complications include arthritis and erythema nodosum (for a review, see reference 44).

Taxonomy and Plasmids

Y. pseudotuberculosis is very closely related to *Y. pestis.* The main difference between the two species is the presence in *Y. pestis* of two additional plasmids: a large one encoding a capsule-like antigen called fraction 1 antigen (F1) and murine toxin (34, 95) and a small one encoding a plasminogen activator called Pla (169).

Y. enterocolitica is heterogeneous, with more than 70 serotypes and several biotypes (190; for reviews, see references 29 and 37). Pathogenic strains are restricted to a few bioserotypes, and these form two distinct groups: serotypes O:1,2,3, O:1,2, O:3, O:9, and

Maite Iriarte and Guy R. Cornelis • Microbial Pathogenesis Unit, Christian de Duve Institute of Cellular Pathology and Faculté de Médecine, Université Catholique de Louvain, B-1200 Brussels, Belgium.

O:5,27 (biotypes 2 to 5) are encountered worldwide, while serotypes O:4, O:8, O:13a,13b, O:18, O:20, and O:21 (biotype 1b) are encountered almost exclusively in North America (for reviews, see references 29, 37, and 190). The strains of the first group are less virulent than those of the second. The pathogenic *Y. enterocolitica* strains are thus divided into "low-virulence" strains and "high-virulence" or "American" strains. The main difference between these two groups resides in the capacity of the high-virulence strains to capture iron from the infected host (for a review, see reference 126).

Y. pestis, Y. pseudotuberculosis, and all pathogenic *Y. enterocolitica* strains harbor a 70-kb plasmid that is devoted to virulence. In *Y. enterocolitica,* this plasmid is called pYV (for "plasmid involved in *Yersinia* virulence") followed by the identification of the strain (59, 98). In *Y. pestis* and *Y. pseudotuberculosis,* the archetypes are called pCD1 (63) and pIB1 (26, 60) respectively. Most of this plasmid encodes the Yop virulon, a sophisticated virulence apparatus which is conserved in the three species and is considered an archetype of the so-called type III virulence systems encountered in several plant and animal pathogens (for reviews, see references 38, 39, and 82).

The Yop virulon endows *Yersinia* strains with the capacity to resist the nonspecific immune response of the host. In particular, it protects them from macrophage attack by destroying the phagocytic and signalling capacities of macrophages and finally by inducing apoptosis of these cells (109, 112, 156).

In this chapter, we describe the *Yersinia* 70-kb plasmid encoding the Yop virulon. First we describe the virulon, then we describe the organization of the pYVe227 plasmid of *Y. enterocolitica* W227, and finally we compare this plasmid to pCD1 and pIB1.

YOP VIRULON

Unravelling the Basic Model

When placed at 37°C in a medium deprived of Ca^{2+} ions, the 70-kb virulence plasmid governs the secretion of a set of proteins called Yops. These secreted Yops have no cytotoxicity on cultured cells, although live extracellular *Yersinia* organisms have such an activity (150). Cytotoxicity was nevertheless found to depend on the capacity of the bacterium to secrete YopE and YopD. However, YopE alone was found to be cytotoxic when microinjected into the cells. This led to the hypothesis that YopE is a cytotoxin that needs to be injected into the cytosol of the eukaryotic cells by a mechanism involving YopD in order to exert its effect (151). In 1994, this hypothesis was demonstrated by two different approaches. The first was based on immunofluorescence and confocal laser-scanning microscopy examinations (152), and the second was based on a reporter enzyme strategy introduced by Sory and Cornelis (170). The reporter system consisted of the calmodulin-activated adenylate cyclase domain (called Cya) of the *Bordetella pertussis* cyclolysin (62). Infection of a monolayer of eukaryotic cells by a recombinant *Y. enterocolitica* strain producing a Yop-Cya hybrid enzyme led to an accumulation of cyclic AMP (cAMP) in the cells. Since the enzyme is not functional in the bacterial cell and in the culture medium because of a lack of calmodulin, this accumulation of cAMP indicated the internalization of YopE-Cya into the cytosol of eukaryotic cells (170). Thus, extracellular *Yersinia* injects YopE into the cytosol of eukaryotic cells by a mechanism that involves at least one other Yop protein, YopD. YopH appeared later to be also injected into the

Table 1. Yop effectors

Protein	Size (kDa)	Activity and features	Relevant similarities	Reference(s)
YopE	22.9	Inhibition of phagocytosis; disruption of the cytoskeleton	ExoS (*P. aeruginosa*),[a] SptP/StpA (*Salmonella*)[b]	7, 151, 162, 170
YopH	51.0	Inhibition of phagocytosis; protein tyrosine phosphatase	Eukaryotic phosphatases SptP/StpA (*Salmonella*)[b]	8, 21, 25, 64, 130, 131, 149, 171, 179
YopM	41.6	Unknown; Leu-rich repeats	y4fR (*Rhizobium*),[c] IpaH (*Shigella*),[d] numerous proteoglycans, GPIb-α	24, 101, 102, 144
YpkA/YopO	81.7	Ser/Thr kinase	Eukaryotic Ser/Thr kinase, COT oncogene[e]	43, 57, 58, 86, 172
YopP/YopJ	29.9	Apoptosis induction; inhibition of TNF-α release	AvRxv (*X. campestris*),[f] AvrA (*Salmonella*)[f]	22, 109, 112, 172
YopT	35.5	Disruption of cytoskeleton	p76 (*H. somnus*)[g] (partial)	84

[a] Reference 195.
[b] References 11 and 88.
[c] Reference 54.
[d] Reference 73.
[e] Reference 75.
[f] Reference 70.
[g] Reference 36.

cytosol of the target cells (130, 171), and YopB appeared to be required for delivery of YopE and YopH, like YopD. These observations led to the present concept that Yops are a collection of intracellular effectors (including YopE and YopH) and proteins required for translocation of these effectors across the plasma membrane of eukaryotic cells (including YopB and YopD).

Most of the Yop proteins have now been sorted out by the two different approaches. Six Yops, YopE, YopH, YpkA/YopO, YopM, YopP/YopJ, and YopT (Table 1), appeared to be intracellular effectors (24, 67, 84, 87, 130, 152, 170, 171, 172). LcrV, a Yop with a different name (see below), is required for the extrusion of YopB and YopD from the bacterial cell (159) and hence, indirectly, for the delivery of the effectors. YopB, YopD, and LcrV will thus be considered translocator Yops. Another Yop, YopN, behaves as a plug closing the secretion channel (see below). A model of the interaction between *Yersinia* and the target cell is shown in Fig. 1.

Role of Adhesins

Yop delivery requires that living bacteria adhere to their target. In *Y. pseudotuberculosis,* the chromosome-encoded invasin (Inv) is the main adhesin promoting Yop translocation (130). In *Y. enterocolitica,* the pYVe227-encoded adhesin YadA (13, 86, 89, 90) is more important than Inv (170), but either YadA or Inv will suffice to initiate the contact between *Y. enterocolitica* and epithelial cells to allow subsequent translocation (27). The situation is not yet clear for *Y. pestis,* which lacks these two adhesins.

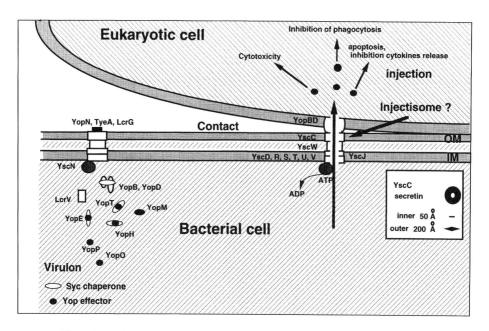

Figure 1. The basic model. When *Yersinia* organisms are placed at 37°C in a rich environment, the Ysc secretion apparatus is activated and a stock of Yop proteins is synthesized.
As long as there is no contact with a eukaryotic cell, a stop valve, possibly made of YopN,
TyeA, and LcrG, blocks the Ysc secretion channel. Upon contact with the eukaryotic
target cell, a sensor interacts with a receptor on the cell surface, resulting in the opening
of the secretion channel at the zone of contact. The Yops are then transported through
the secretion channels, and the Yop effectors are translocated across the plasma membrane,
guided by YopB and YopD. During their intrabacterial stage, Yops are capped with their
specific chaperone, presumably to prevent premature associations. Reprinted from reference 38 with permission of the publisher.

Syc Cytosolic Chaperones

At the first stages of the process, Yops appear to be cytosolic, and some of them are
associated with specific chaperones called Syc (for ''specific Yop chaperone'') (187; for
a review, see reference 189). Normal secretion of YopE, YopH, YopN, and YopT by a wild-
type *Yersinia* strain requires the presence of SycE, SycH, SycN, and SycT, respectively (84,
85, 186, 187) (Table 2). All these chaperones are small (14 to 15 kDa), acidic (pI 4.4 to

Table 2. Syc cytosolic chaperones

Protein	Size (kDa)	pI	Cognate Yop	Reference(s)
SycD/LcrH	19.0	4.5	YopB and YopD	117, 186
SycE/YerA	14.7	4.5	YopE	55, 187, 194
SycH	15.7	4.8	YopH	130, 186
SycT	15.1	4.4	YopT	84
SycN	13.6	5.2	YopN	45a, 85

5.2) proteins with a putative C-terminal amphiphilic α-helix, and they bind only to their partner Yop. SycE and SycH possess a conserved leucine repeat motif in this α-helical structure, where most of the hydrophobic residues, essentially leucines, are present on the same side of the helix. No chaperone has been found so far for YopO/YpkA, YopP/YopJ, YopK/YopQ, YopR, LcrV, or YopM. However, the region situated immediately upstream from *yopO-yopP* in the pYVe227 plasmid of *Y. enterocolitica* contains an open reading frame (ORF155) that forms an operon with *yopO/yopP* (86). The hydrophobic moment plot of the ORF155 product closely resembles that of the SycE, SycH, SycT, and SycN chaperones, and the C terminus is also predicted to form an α-helix. As with the other chaperones, the protein has an acidic isoelectric point (pI 4.5) (86). On the whole, it appears that the product of this ORF could act as a chaperone for YopO and/or YopP, but this hypothesis awaits further investigations.

Most of the research on Syc chaperones has focused so far on SycE and SycH. These two chaperones bind to their partner Yops at a unique site spanning roughly residues 20 to 70 (171). Surprisingly, when this site is removed, the Yop is still secreted, although maybe in reduced amounts, and the chaperone becomes dispensable for secretion (194). This suggests that it is the binding site itself that creates the need for the chaperone and thus that the chaperone somehow protects this site from premature associations which lead to degradation. In agreement with this hypothesis, SycE plays an antidegradation role: the half-life of YopE is longer in wild-type bacteria than in *sycE* mutant bacteria (33, 55). The antidegradation role of SycH is not as clear as that of SycE, because YopH can be detected in the cytosol of *sycH* mutant bacteria (186). In addition to this putative role of bodyguard, SycE acts as a secretion pilot, leading the YopE protein to the secretion locus (7). Finally, both SycE and SycH are also required for translocation of their partner Yop into eukaryotic cells (100, 171, 194) (see below).

SycD (called LcrH in *Y. pseudotuberculosis* and *Y. pestis*) (16, 142) is a bivalent chaperone serving both YopB and YopD (117, 186). In the absence of SycD, YopD and YopB are less detectable inside the bacterial cell (117, 186). SycD appears to be somewhat different from SycE and SycH in that it binds to several domains on YopB (117).

Recruitment for Export

To be secreted, Yops need to be specifically recognized by the secretion apparatus. Two secretion signals have been identified; the first lies in the amino terminus (7, 106, 108, 171) of the Yop protein or, rather, in the 5′ end of its RNA (7), and the second, weaker secretion signal, which was identified for YopE, corresponds to the SycE-binding site and is functional only in the presence of the SycE chaperone (33). The other Yops that have a specific chaperone (YopH, YopN, and YopT) are also likely to have this second secretion signal, but this has not been shown yet.

Ysc Secretion Apparatus

The Ysc secretion apparatus is complex and far from being completely characterized. Some elements have been shown to localize in the inner membrane and others in the outer membrane (Table 3). The system is assumed to be totally independent of the Sec machine (but this has not been formally proven) and is thought to form a continuous channel across

Table 3. Secretion apparatus

Protein	Size (kDa)	Features	Localization in bacteria[a]	Role in Yop secretion[b]	Reference(s)
YscA	3.8	Hydrophobic C-terminal domain	Unknown	−	107, 158
YscB	15.4		Cochaperone of YopN	NT	45a, 107
YscC	67.1	Signal sequence of 26 residues; member of the secretin family; forms pores of 200 Å with a central channel of 50 Å	OM	+	91, 107, 135
YscD	46.7	Hydrophobic domain (120–130 amino acids)	IM	+	107, 135
YscE	7.4	Hydrophobic C-terminal domain	Unknown	+	5, 107
YscF	9.4		Unknown	+	5, 107
YscG	12.9	Hydrophobic N-terminal domain	C/M	+	5, 107, 135
YopR	18.3	Encoded by *yscH*	Secreted	−	5, 107
YscI	12.6		Unknown	+	5, 107
YscJ	27.0	Lipoprotein; hydrophobic C-terminal domain followed by 3 positively charged residues; previously called YlpB	Unknown	+	5, 107
YscK	23.9	One hydrophobic domain	Unknown	+	5, 107
YscL	24.9		Unknown	+	107, 173
YscM1	12.3	Resembles YscM2 and YopH	Secreted	−	5, 107, 174
YscN	47.8	Contains Walker boxes A and B; putative ATPase	IM/C	+	15, 49, 193
YscO	19.0		Released in low Ca^{2+}	NT	15, 49, 86, 123
YscP	50.4		Released in low Ca^{2+}	NT	15, 49, 86, 124, 173
YscQ	34.4		Unknown	+	15, 49, 86
YscR	24.4	Four transmembrane domains and a large central cytoplasmic region	IM	+	15, 49, 86
YscS	9.6	Two putative transmembrane domains	Unknown (probably IM)	NT	15, 49, 86
YscT	28.4	Six putative transmembrane domains	Unknown (probably IM)	NT	15, 49, 86
YscU	40.3	Four transmembrane domains at the N terminus, with a large cytoplasmic C-terminal region	IM	+	6, 15, 49
YscX	13.6		Unknown	+	85
YscY	13.1		Unknown	+	85
YscV (LcrD)	77.8	Eight potential transmembrane domains; hydrophobic N-terminal half; hydrophilic C terminus predicted to protrude into the cytoplasm	IM	+	86, 133
YscW (VirG)	14.6	Lipoprotein ancillary to YscC secretin	Probably OM	+ (YopB, YopD, LcrV)	4

[a] IM, inner membrane; OM, outer membrane; C, cytosolic; M, membrane-associated protein.
[b] NT, not tested; +, required for secretion; −, not required for secretion.

the two bacterial membranes. We are still very far from assigning a role to each of the 29 components of the Ysc machine.

YscC (91, 107, 135) belongs to the family of secretins, a group of outer membrane proteins involved in the transport of various macromolecules and filamentous phages across the outer membrane. Like the other secretins, it exists as a very stable multimeric complex of about 600 kDa (91, 135) that forms a ring-shaped structure with an external diameter of about 200 Å and an apparent central pore of about 50 Å (91). The lipoprotein YscW (previously called VirG) (4) is required for efficient targeting of the YscC complex to the outer membrane (91). The Ysc apparatus contains another lipoprotein called YscJ.

Four proteins span the inner membrane: YscD (135), YscR (49), YscU (6), and YscV (formerly called LcrD) (133, 134). According to their sequences, two other proteins, YscS and YscT, are probably also inserted in the inner membrane. Finally, YscN is a 47.8-kDa protein with ATP-binding motifs (Walker boxes A and B) resembling the β catalytic subunit of F_0F_1 proton translocase and related ATPases (193).

Somewhat unexpectedly, the loci encoding the secretion apparatus also encode a few proteins that are themselves secreted by the machine. These are LcrQ/YscM, YopR (the product of *yscH*) (5), YopN (24, 52, 87), YscO (123), and YscP (124, 173). LcrQ/YscM is thought to be a regulator (see below), and YopN is considered an element of the plug closing down the channel and will be described below. YscO is necessary for secretion of all the Yops (123), but this is not the case for YscP (124) and YopR (5).

The Ysc machinery has several components that have homologs in the flagellum assembly apparatus, which suggests some relationship between the two structures (Fig. 2). This assumption has been strikingly supported by the recent electron microscopic observation of the type III apparatus of *Salmonella typhimurium* (93). This apparatus, evoking a syringe, resembles the basal body of a flagellum prolonged by a straight rod. This rod extends outside the bacterial cell, which indicates that the elements that allow secretion across the two bacterial membranes are only one part of a more complex supramolecular structure. In this context, it is not surprising that some Ysc proteins appear to be "secreted."

Translocator Yops: YopB, YopD, and LcrV

Of the 12 secreted Yops, only two, YopB and YopD, have hydrophobic domains (66), suggesting that they could interact with membranes. YopD is a 33.3-kDa protein with a central 31-amino-acid hydrophobic region (66). The Eisenberg plot analysis (46) suggests that it is a transmembrane protein (66). YopB is a 41.8-kDa protein with two central hydrophobic regions, separated by only 15 amino acids (66). It has a moderate level of similarity to proteins of the RTX family of alpha-hemolysins and leukotoxins (17, 178). YopB and YopD are encoded by the large *lcrGV sycD yopBD* operon (16, 115, 141, 142), which also encodes LcrG, LcrV, and SycD/LcrH, the chaperone of YopB and YopD.

YopB and YopD are both required for translocation of effector Yops across the eukaryotic cell membrane (24, 68, 84, 87, 151, 152, 170). The fact that YopB resembles toxins of the RTX family suggests that the translocation apparatus could involve some kind of a pore, where YopB would be the main element. The observation of Håkansson et al. (68) that *Yersinia* has a YopB- and contact-dependent lytic activity on sheep erythrocytes supports this hypothesis. This YopB-dependent lytic activity is higher when the effector

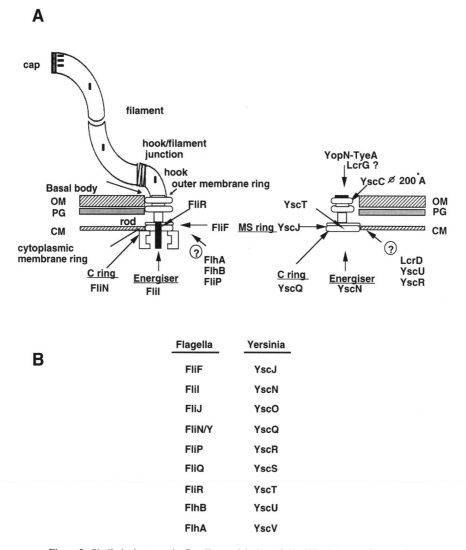

Figure 2. Similarity between the flagellum and the hypothetical *Yersinia* secretion translocation machinery. (A) Flagellum (left) and hypothetical Ysc secretion machinery (right). (B) Similarities between the Ysc secretion machinery and the proteins involved in the assembly of the flagellum (2, 19, 20, 31, 32, 103, 104, 110, 143).

yop genes are deleted, suggesting that the pore is normally filled with effectors during contact (68). By analysis of the protective effect of sugars of increasing size, Håkansson et al. (68) estimated that the internal diameter of the putative pore was between 12 and 35 Å, with the larger size being observed when YopK/YopQ is missing (79).

LcrV has been described as a regulatory protein involved in the calcium response, since a mutant with an in-frame deletion in *lcrV* was found to be Ca^{2+} independent and

Table 4. Proteins required for translocation of Yop effectors

Protein	Size (kDa)	Structural features	Role	References
YopB	41.8	Hydrophobic domains	Needed for translocation; needed for contact hemolysis; hypothetical constituent of a pore	24, 66, 67, 68, 71, 170
YopD	33.3	Central hydrophobic domain	Needed for translocation	24, 66, 72, 130, 170, 192
LcrV	37.2	Some polymorphism	Required for extrusion of YopB and YopD	142, 148, 159
LcrG	11.0	Forms dimers; heparin-binding domain	Required for efficient delivery of all Yop effectors; binds to heparin; involved in regulation of secretion	28, 120, 160, 164
YopK/YopQ	20.8	None	Controls translocation by modulating the size of the YopB-induced pore	79, 80
TyeA	10.8	Binds to YopN	Required for translocation of YopE and YopH but not for translocation of the other Yop effectors	52, 87, 185

downregulated in transcription of *yop* genes (16, 128, 141, 165, 177). However, other data indicate that LcrV could be a functional element of the translocation apparatus, since deletion of the entire *lcrV* gene abolishes the secretion of LcrV, YopB, and YopD but has no effect on the secretion of the other Yops (159). In agreement with these observations, LcrV interacts with both YopB and YopD proteins (159) as well as with LcrG (120, 159). From these observations, one can envision that LcrV is a third component of the delivery apparatus (121, 159). One could speculate that it forms some kind of a short pilus underneath YopB and YopD, but, as we have mentioned before, this function could also be fulfilled by the ''secreted'' Ysc proteins, such as YscO and YscP.

LcrG is an 11.0-kDa protein that is primarily cytosolic (120, 164). Like the other proteins encoded by the operon, it turned out to be also required for translocation (160). The proteins required for translocation are summarized in Table 4.

In Vivo Control of Yop Release by Cell Contact

When *Yersinia* organisms are incubated at 37°C in a Ca^{2+}-containing eukaryotic cell culture medium, they do not secrete Yops. Nevertheless, they inject Yops into the eukaryotic cells. This implies that contact with these cells somehow triggers the system and suggests that a particular bacterial ligand could be involved in this contact.

So far, however, no bacterial ligand interacting with eukaryotic cells has been identified. The isolation of Ca^{2+}-blind mutants, mutants that secrete Yops even in the presence of Ca^{2+} (197), allowed the identification of three proteins that are required to keep the channel

Table 5. Proteins involved in control of Yop release

Protein	Size (kDa)	Structural features	Role	References
YopN	32.6	Regions spanning 62–108 and 248–272 could form coiled-coil structures	Element of the putative plug closing the secretion channel; associated with TyeA	52, 87
TyeA	10.8	Binds to the second coiled-coil domain of YopN Binds to YopD	Element of the putative plug closing the secretion channel; associated with YopN; required for delivery of YopE and YopH but not for delivery of YopM, YopO, YopP, and YopT	52, 84, 87, 185
LcrG	11.0	Heparin-binding domains	Required for delivery of all effector Yops	28, 160, 164

closed in the presence of Ca^{2+}: YopN (24, 51, 52), LcrG (160, 164), and TyeA (87) (Table 5).

YopN is a 32.6-kDa protein encoded together with *ysc* gene products (52, 85, 86, 87, 185). In low-Ca^{2+} conditions, most of the YopN produced is released in the culture supernatant, while in the presence of Ca^{2+}, YopN is not released but is exposed at the bacterial surface (52, 87).

TyeA is a 10.8-kDa protein encoded by the gene immediately downstream of *yopN* (52, 87, 185). Like YopN, TyeA is loosely associated with the membrane, but, unlike YopN, it is not released after Ca^{2+} chelation. It has the capacity to bind to YopN (87) and was named TyeA by Iriarte et al. (87) because it plays a role in translocation of some Yop effectors. It is probably significant that YopN and TyeA are encoded by genes that are buried among *ysc* genes. It suggests that these two proteins belong to the Ysc secretion apparatus and eventually represent some kind of an external cap.

At variance with YopN and TyeA, LcrG is encoded by the operon devoted to the translocators (see above) and is required for translocation of all the effectors (160). The Ca^{2+}-blind phenotype of the mutant indicates that LcrG is also involved in the in vitro control of Yop release and suggests that LcrG could be localized at the bacterial surface. However, in spite of efforts made with both *Y. pestis* and *Y. enterocolitica*, it remains uncertain whether some LcrG is surface exposed (27, 120). One argument in favor of surface exposure of LcrG is that LcrG binds heparin and that heparin interferes with the translocation of YopE into HeLa cells (28).

Acting in the Eukaryotic Cell

Disturbing the eukaryotic cell to avoid the response that would clear *Yersinia* is the major goal of *Yersinia* pathogenesis. We have seen in the overview that six effectors have been identified so far (Table 1). Taking into account the information supplied by the sequence, it seems reasonable to assume that this list is now complete. We briefly mention the action of each of the effectors.

YopE (53, 108) is a 23-kDa cytotoxin that leads to disruption of the microfilament structure (151). Its exact enzyme activity and target are still unknown. Together with YopH, it blocks phagocytosis.

YopH (25, 105) is a powerful protein tyrosine phosphatase of 51.0 kDa (64). It contributes to the inhibition of bacterial uptake by dephosphorylation of p130^{cas} and focal adhesion kinase (FAK) and disruption of peripheral focal complexes (21, 131, 149). YopH inhibits phagocytosis by polymorphonuclear leukocytes and macrophages, mediated by complement receptors (157) or Fc receptors (48), respectively.

YopM (24, 43, 50, 102, 115) is a strongly acidic protein with an isoelectric point of 4.06 and a molecular mass of about 40 kDa. Unlike the other Yop effector proteins, which are well conserved among different *Yersinia* species, YopM is somewhat heterogeneous in size (23). Due to the presence of leucine-rich repeated motifs (LRRs), YopM shows similarity to many eukaryotic proteins, but its intracellular target and action remain unknown.

YpkA (YopO in *Y. enterocolitica*) is a protein kinase (57) which shows some similarity to the COT (cancer Osaka thyroid) oncogene product, a cytosolic serine/threonine protein kinase expressed in hematopoietic cells and implicated in signal transduction by growth factors (75). YpkA catalyzes the autophosphorylation of a serine residue in vitro. Infection of HeLa cells with a multiple *yop* mutant overproducing YpkA leads to a morphological alteration of the cells different from the alterations mediated by YopE and YopH. The cells round up but do not detach from the extracellular matrix. Inside the HeLa cells, the YpkA protein is targeted to the inner surface of the plasma membrane (67). No target protein of YpkA/YopO has been identified yet.

YopP (YopJ in *Y. pestis* and *Y. pseudotuberculosis*) is a 32.5-kDa protein encoded by the same operon as YpkA/YopO (43). It induces the apoptosis of murine macrophages (109, 112) but not of other cell types such as epithelial cells or fibroblasts (109, 112, 154, 155, 156). Injection of YopP into macrophages also leads to a significant reduction in the release of tumor necrosis factor alpha (TNF-α), a proinflammatory cytokine that plays a central role in the development of the immune and inflammatory responses to infection (22, 122). This reduction probably results from the inhibition of NF-κB activation by YopP/YopJ (154, 161). YopP/YopJ also inhibits ERK1/2, p38, and JNK mitogen-activated protein kinase activity (22, 122, 155). One can thus speculate that YopP would act upstream or at the junction of cascades leading to apoptosis on one hand and to the inhibition of TNF-α on the other hand. In addition, YopP/YopJ prevents the release of interleukin-8 by T84 epithelial cells (161, 163).

YopT is a 35.5-kDa Yop protein that has been described and characterized recently (84). It induces a cytotoxic effect in HeLa cells and macrophages. This effect consists of the disruption of the actin filaments and the alteration of the cell cytoskeleton.

Regulation of Transcription of the Virulon Genes

Transcription of the *ysc* genes and the *yop* genes is strongly induced at 37°C. This thermoregulation results from the interplay between the transcriptional activator VirF (LcrF in *Y. pestis* and *Y. pseudotuberculosis*) and chromatin structure. Transcription of the *yop* genes, but not the *ysc* genes, is repressed by Ca^{2+} or by mutations in the secretion apparatus. This second regulation is a feedback inhibition mechanism exerted by the closed secretion apparatus on transcription of the genes encoding the proteins to be secreted (for reviews, see references 60, 176, and 177).

VirF/LcrF is a 30.9-kDa basic protein that belongs to the AraC family of regulators (41, 77, 78, 96, 167). It binds to a 40-bp region localized immediately upstream from the RNA polymerase binding site on the *yopE, yopH, virC,* and *lcrGV sycD yopBD* promoters (188). These VirF-binding sites are located in an AT-rich region and appear either isolated or repeated in opposite orientation. They contain the 13-bp consensus sequence TTTTa-GYcTtTat (188). In *Y. enterocolitica,* the *virF* gene itself is strongly thermoregulated, and VirF is active only at 37°C.

By analogy to the secreted anti-sigma factor involved in the regulation of flagellum synthesis (83, 94), Rimpiläinen et al. (145) suggested that feedback inhibition could be mediated by a repressor that is normally expelled via the Yop secretion machinery. They suggested that in *Y. pseudotuberculosis,* LcrQ, a 12.4-kDa secreted protein encoded by the last gene of the *virC* locus, could be this hypothetical regulator because overproduction of this protein abolishes Yop production. In *Y. enterocolitica,* there are two homologs of LcrQ: YscM1 and YscM2 (5, 174). How LcrQ or YscM1 and YscM2 work is still unknown, but their mode of action is probably indirect.

pYVe227 PLASMID OF Y. ENTEROCOLITICA SEROTYPE O:9

Overview of the Plasmid

The pYVe227 plasmid of *Y. enterocolitica* W227 (42) has been completely sequenced (86). The circular map given in Fig. 3A highlights the genes encoding the Yop virulon, and the color code classifies the genes according to the part of the virulon they encode: adherence, secretion, translocation, intracellular effectors, and control of Yop release. The more detailed linear map (86) presented in Fig. 3B gives a clear view of the relative size of the genes and shows the most important transcriptional units. Tables 6 and 7 summarize the putative promoters and terminators identified in the pYVe227 plasmid.

Altogether, the genes encoding the Yop virulon occupy about two-thirds of the plasmid, with only two IS elements interspersed among the *yop* and *syc* genes (86). The other one-third of the plasmid, localized between the replication origin and the partition site, which underwent some genetic rearrangements during evolution, contains only three genes that are or could be involved in pathogenicity: *yadA* and two newly identified genes, *yomA* and *pprA* (86). The rest of this region consists of the replication and partition genes, the remains of a transfer operon, a transposon encoding arsenic resistance (see below), and four complete or vestigial IS elements, most of which belong to the IS*3* family. All the predicted elements and proteins encoded by the pYVe227 plasmid are summarized in Tables 8 through 10.

Genes Comprising the Virulon: a Pathogenicity Island on a Plasmid?

The secretion apparatus is composed of 29 genes organized in four main loci (Fig. 3), *virA* (*yopN, tyeA, sycN, yscXYV, lcrR*), *virB* (*yscNOPQRSTU*), *virG* (monocistronic, now called *yscW*), and *virC* (*yscABCDEFGHIJKLM*) (4, 5, 6, 85, 86, 107; for a review, see reference 39). *yscV* was initially described in *Y. pestis* as *lcrD* (*lcr* for "low calcium response") (133, 134). The *virB* and *virC* loci constitute two large operons transcribed in

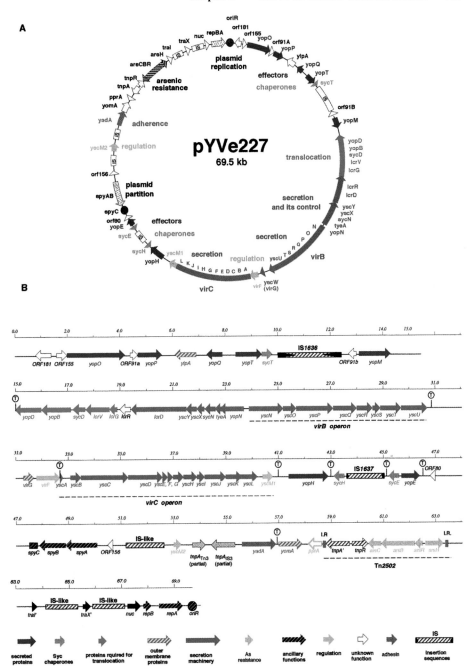

Figure 3. Detailed genetic map of the pYVe227 plasmid of *Y. enterocolitica* W22703 (86). The genes are colored according to the part of the apparatus they encode. Genes in green encode the Ysc secretion machinery and its control, genes in light blue encode the translocation machinery, genes in dark blue encode the effector Yops and their chaperones, genes in orange are involved in regulation of gene expression, the gene in khaki encodes an adhesin, and genes in mustard encode arsenic resistance proteins.

Table 6. Promoters identified in pYVe227

Gene or operon	Sequence of promoter[a]			Reference
	− 35	− 10	S.D.	
yopE		TAAGAT	AAGGGA	108
yopH	AAGAAA	TATAGT	AAGGAGG	105
virC	ACAC	TAAAAT	GAAGA	107

[a] S.D., Shine-Dalgarno sequence.

the same direction and separated by *yscW* and the regulatory gene *virF*. *virA* is transcribed divergently, and it is not clear whether it also constitutes a single operon. The proteins required for translocation of the effectors across the eukaryotic cell membrane, YopB, YopD, their chaperone SycD, LcrV, and LcrG, are all encoded by the same operon, which is located next to *virA* and transcribed in the same orientation (66, 86). Thus, the secretion-translocation apparatus is encoded by 35 contiguous genes including the regulatory gene *virF*. The compact character of this virulence genome suggests that these genes encode some kind of a complex structure and that a long evolutionary process has been brought to completion.

At variance with the genes encoding the secretion-translocation apparatus, the genes encoding the effectors and their chaperones appear to be more dispersed, suggesting that they were recruited more recently in the virulon (Fig. 3). In pYVe227, the four chaperones SycE, SycH, SycD, and SycT are encoded next to their cognate gene. *sycN* is separated from *yopN* by *tyeA,* but the latter also encodes a protein that interacts with YopN (85, 87). Between *yopP* and *yopQ* lies the gene encoding the outer membrane lipoprotein YlpA (35). YlpA is highly homologous to the TraT proteins encoded by a number of bacterial plasmids. These proteins are known to be involved in serum resistance (111) and inhibition of phagocytosis by macrophages (1), but YlpA does not seem to confer these properties (35). The only element suggesting that *ylpA* could play a role in virulence is the fact that it is regulated like the other *yop* genes (35).

In summary, a very compact group of 35 genes encoding the secretion-translocation

Table 7. Terminators identified in pYVe227

Gene or operon	Sequence of putative transcriptional terminator	Reference
virB	AACCAAACATCCTTTCTTTCACGAAAGAAAGGATGTTTGGTTTT	6
yopH	TATTTATTCCTATGAGTAAATA	105
	TAAACCTCAACTAAAGTAAGCAATTAGTTGAGGTTTA	
	AAATTAAAAGTTATGTGTCTACTTTTACTTT	
	GACGATGATCATCGTC	
virF	AACAGTATTATTCGCCGCTGGATGGCAATAATATGTT	41
	TTAATAATCAAGATAGCTTATCTGGCTTATTAA	
lcrGVH yopBD	TTGGTTAGTTAATTAACCGAAAGTTTT	66
sycE	AAAAGTTAACACCAAGTTGGAATGTTGACTTTT	86
yopE	AACAAGGGGGTAGTGTTTCCCCCTTTTT	86
yadA	AAAACACCGATTACGATTATGTAATCGGTGTTTT	86

Table 8. Functional and phenotypic classification of the predicted proteins encoded by pYVe227

Function	No.	Protein(s)
Yop virulon		
Secreted proteins	13	YopE, YopH, YopM, YopO, YopP, YopT, YopB, YopD, YopN, YopQ, YopR, LcrV, YscM1
Yop effectors translocated into eukaryotic cells	6	YopE, YopH, YopM, YopO, YopP, YopT
Proteins required for intracellular delivery of Yop effectors but not for Yop secretion	5	YopB, YopD, LcrV, LcrG (all effectors), TyeA (delivery of YopE and YopH only)
Proteins involved in control of Yop release	3	YopN, TyeA, LcrG.
Proteins required for secretion	15	YscC, YscD, YscE, YscF, YscG, YscI, YscK, YscL, YscN, YscQ, YscR, YscU, YscX, YscY, LcrD (could become YscV)
Lipoproteins of the Ysc secretion apparatus	1	YscW (previously called VirG), YscJ
Syc chaperones	5	SycE, SycH, SycD, SycT, SycN
Transcriptional regulator	1	VirF (AraC family)
Regulators with unknown mechanism of action	2	YscM1, YscM2
Unknown function	7	LcrR, YscA, YscB, YscO, YscP, YscS, YscT
Adhesin	1	YadA
Surface-exposed proteins		
Lipoprotein	1	YlpA
Outer membrane proteins	1	YomA
Ancillary functions		
Replication	2	RepA, RepB
Partition	2	SpyA, SpyB
Resistance to antimicrobial compounds	4	ArsC, ArsB, ArsR, ArsH
Unknown function		
With database homolog	7	ORF80, ORF155, YomA, PrpA, Nuc, TraX', TraI'
Without any database homolog	4	ORF181, ORF91A, ORF91B, ORF156

apparatus is flanked on either side by the genes encoding the Yop effectors and their chaperones. All the genes encoding the virulon are thus clustered, which evokes a pathogenicity island . . . on a plasmid.

Interestingly, the gene encoding the adhesin YadA, which is essential for the Yop virulon in *Y. enterocolitica* but not in *Y. pseudotuberculosis* or *Y. pestis,* is separated from the genes encoding the core of the apparatus, indicating that the adhesin may have been recruited more recently by the system (13, 86).

The DNA composition of the genes encoding the type III secretion system in several bacteria differs from the composition of the genomic DNA of the entire bacterium. This is not the case here. The average G+C content of the genes encoding the Yop virulon in *Y. enterocolitica* is 44.4% (86), which is not very different from the reported G+C content

Table 9. Putative ORFs of unknown function present in pYVe227

ORF	Size of product (kDa)	pI	Shine-Dalgarno sequence and start codon	Features	Relevant similarities (reference)
ORF181	20.3	9.9	$AGGAN_{10}ATG$		
ORF155	17.2	4.5	$AGAGN_7GTG$		ORF1 (*Y. pseudotuberculosis*) (58), ORF1 (*P. syringae*) (3)
ORF91A	10.1	8.9	$AGAGN_{10}ATG$		
ORF91B	10.5	10.2	$GGCCAN_6ATG$		
ORF156	17.7	8.4	$GAAGAN_6ATG$		
ORF80	8.8	6.8	$GGAGN_4ATG$		ORF83 (*M. tuberculosis*) (132)
YomA	32.3	9.9	$GGTGN_{10}ATG$	Putative signal sequence, eight transmembrane domains	ORFX (*Y. enterocolitica* O:3) (168), PagO (*S. typhimurium*) (65), YoaV (*B. subtilis*) (97), ORF (*Buchnera aphidicola*) (116)
PprA	16.2	10.5	$GGGAN_5ATG$, $GGGAN_2GTG$	Helix-turn-helix motif in C terminus	EvgA (*E. coli*) (183), BvgA (*B. pertussis*) (9, 10), LuxR (*V. fischeri*) (47)

of the *Y. enterocolitica* chromosome (46 to 50%) (30). This observation suggests that these genes have been in *Enterobacteriaceae,* if not in *Yersinia,* for a long time.

Ancillary Functions: Replication and Partition System

The replicon of the pYVe227 plasmid of *Y. enterocolitica* is of the RepFIIA type (archetype R100) (184). The replication machinery consists of two proteins, the RepA replicase and the RepB regulator, and an origin of replication (*oriR*) (184). The pYVe227 plasmid is incompatible with sex factor F (12) because they have a similar partition function (18). This function consists of two proteins, SpyA and SpyB (for "stability of pYV"), encoded by an operon (86). SpyA resembles SopA of the *Escherichia coli* F plasmid, a 388-residue protein with a DNA-dependent ATPase activity, involved in the autoregulation of the *sopAB* operon (114). SpyB resembles SopB of the F plasmid, a DNA-binding protein that specifically binds to the F-plasmid *sopC* locus (114) (Fig. 4). A sequence of 33 bp (ATTGGATATCCAGGTGACCGTGGTCCCAATTAC) is repeated twice, in the same order separated by 10 bp, 146 bp downstream from *spyB*. Nucleotides 13 to 29 of these repeats can be aligned with the consensus sequence of the 12 directed repeats that form the partition site *sopC* of F (74, 114) (Fig. 4). From these similarities, we infer that these repeats correspond to the partition site of the pYVe227 plasmid, and we called them *spyC*.

TraI′, TraX′, and Nuc, the Vestiges of a Transfer Operon

The virulence plasmid of *Yersinia* is not conjugative. However, the region situated between the *ars* transposon Tn*2502* and the *repBA* operon (coordinates 63.4 to 67.9) in

Table 10. Elements present in *Y. enterocolitica* pYVe227[a]

Gene	Start position (bp)	Stop position (bp)	Orientation	Protein size (kDa)	Accession no.	Function
oriR	53	203			M55182	pYV replication
ORF181	1434	889	−	20.3	AF054979	Unknown
ORF155	1616	2083	+	17.2	AF054978	Unknown
yopO	2091	4280	+	81.7	AF054978	Yop effector
ORF91a	4485	4760	+	10.1	AF054978	Unknown
yopP	4761	5627	+	29.9	AF023202	Yop effector
ylpA	6900	6151	−	26.6	M33786	Lipoprotein
yopQ	7918	7370	−	20.8	M33786	Control translocation
yopT	8439	9407	+	35.5	AF054981	Yop effector
sycT	9407	9799	+	15.1	AF054981	Chaperone of YopT
IS*1636*	10151	12470			AF080156	Unknown
ORF91b	13035	12760	−	10.5	AF080156	Unknown
yopM	13197	14300	+	41.6	Z69926	Yop effector
yopD	15994	15074	−	33.3	L06216	Translocator
yopB	17218	16013	−	41.8	L06216	Translocator
sycD	17702	17196	−	19.0	AF080155	Chaperone of YopB and YopD
lcrV	18679	17705	−	37.2	AF080155	Required for secretion of YopB and YopD
lcrG	18968	18681	−	11.0	AF022645	Control of Yop release; required for Yop delivery
lcrR	19450	19010	−	16.5	AF050104	Unknown
lcrD (*yscV*)	21561	19447	−	77.8	AF050104	Yop secretion
yscY	21892	21548	−	13.1	AF054977	Yop secretion
yscX	22257	21889	−	13.6	AF054977	Yop secretion
sycN	22625	22254	−	13.6	AF054977	Control of Yop release; chaperone of YopN
tyeA	22890	22612	−	10.8	AF033863	Control of Yop release; required for delivery of YopE and YopH
yopN	23752	22871	−	32.6	AF033863	Control of Yop release
yscN	23950	25269	+	47.8	UO2499	ATPase; Yop secretion
yscO	25266	25730	+	19.0	AF102990	Yop secretion
yscP	25730	27277	+	57.4	AF102990	Yop secretion
yscQ	27274	28197	+	34.4	AF102990	Yop secretion
yscR	28194	28847	+	24.4	AF102990	Yop secretion
yscS	28849	29115	+	9.6	AF102990	Yop secretion
yscT	29112	29897	+	28.4	AF102990	Yop secretion
yscU	29897	30961	+	40.3	U08019	Yop secretion
virG (*yscW*)	31537	31932	+	14.6	U21297	Lipoprotein; YscC localization
virF	32056	32871	+	30.8	M22781	Regulation
yscA	32949	33047	+	3.8	M74011	Unknown
yscB	33273	33686	+	15.4	M74011	Yop secretion (?)
yscC	33692	35515	+	67.1	M74011	Yop secretion
yscD	35512	36768	+	46.7	M74011	Yop secretion
yscE	36765	36965	+	7.4	M74011	Yop secretion
yscF	36966	37229	+	9.4	M74011	Yop secretion
yscG	37231	37578	+	12.9	M74011	Yop secretion
yscH	37575	38072	+	18.3	M74011	Secreted protein (YopR)
yscI	38073	38420	+	12.6	M74011	Yop secretion
yscJ	38427	39164	+	27.0	M74011	Yop secretion

(Table continues)

Table 10. *Continued*

Gene	Start position (bp)	Stop position (bp)	Orientation	Protein size (kDa)	Accession no.	Function
yscK	39161	39790	+	23.9	M74011	Yop secretion
yscL	39736	40407	+	24.9	M74011	Yop secretion
Intergenic	40407	40626			M74011	Unknown
yscM1	40626	40973	+	12.3	M74011	Regulation
yopH	41658	43064	+	51.0	M30457	Yop effector
sycH	43717	43292	−	15.7	U08222	Chaperone of YopH
IS*1637*	43913	45163			AF102990	Unknown
sycE	45717	45325	−	14.7	Z18539	Chaperone of YopE
yopE	45910	46569	+	22.9	M92066	Yop effector
ORF80	47243	47001	−	8.8	AF056093	Unknown
spyC	47898	47930			AF102990	pYV partition site
	47941	47973				
spyB	49085	48120	−	35.8	AF102990	pYV partition
spyA	50290	49082	−	45.2	AF102990	pYV partition
ORF156	50865	51335	+	17.7	AF102990	Unknown
IS-like	51335	53155			AF102990	Unknown
yscM2	53135	53497	+	12.0	U94827	Regulation
Intergenic	53497	55700			AF102990	Unknown
yadA	55753	57117	+	47.2	AF056092	Adhesin
yomA	57187	58062	+	32.3	AF056092	Unknown
pprA	58836	58384	−	16.2	AF054980	Unknown
tnpA'	59843	58992	−		U58366	Partial transposase, Tn*2502*
tnpR	60004	60583	+	21.2	U58366	Resolvase, Tn*2502*
arsC	61028	60603	−	15.8	U58366	Arsenic resistance
arsB	62330	61041	−	45.5	U58366	Arsenic resistance
arsR	62695	62342	−	13.5	U58366	Arsenic resistance
arsH	62781	63479	+	26.4	U58366	Arsenic resistance
traI'	63642	64091	+	16.3	AF102990	Unknown
IS-like	64091	65744			AF102990	Unknown
traX'	65744	66076	+	11.9	AF102990	Unknown
IS-like	66076	67432			AF102990	Unknown
nuc	67432	67974	+	19.7	AF102990	Unknown
repB	68112	68366	+	9.5	M55182	pYV replication
repA	68675	69541	+	33.5	M55182	pYV replication

[a] See reference 86.

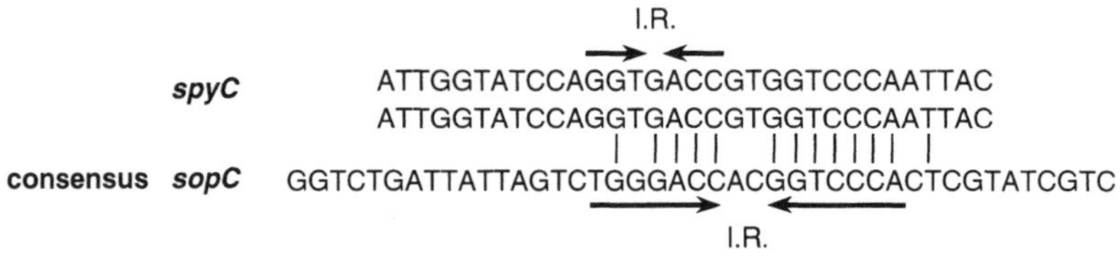

Figure 4. Partition site of the pYVe227 plasmid. Comparison between the sequence of the two direct repeats forming the *spyC* site of the pYVe227 plasmid and the consensus sequence derived from the 12 direct repeats of the *sopC* site of the *E. coli* F plasmid. The internal inverted repeats present in the central part of the direct repeats are indicated by two arrows and labeled I.R.

pYVe227 contains at least three partial ORFs whose products have homology to proteins encoded by *tra* operons involved in the conjugal transfer of plasmids (86). These partial ORFs are flanked by remains of insertion sequences (Fig. 5) (see below).

Translation of the region spanning coordinates 63.5 to 63.9 gives 158 amino acids that are 45.6% identical to the C terminus of TraI from F and R100 (196), an ATP-dependent DNA helicase of 1,765 amino acids. The conserved region includes two motifs (amino acids 1 to 5 and 21 to 37) seen in ATP- and GTP-binding proteins and in ATP-dependent DNA helicases such as UvrD, Rep, and RecD (76, 196). The *traI* vestige of pYVe227 is flanked by transposon Tn*2502* upstream (118) and by elements resembling insertion sequences downstream. The putative TraI represents only 1/10 of the complete protein encoded by F (Fig. 5) (86).

The region spanning coordinates 65.6 to 66.0 is an ORF encoding a putative protein of 110 amino acids that has significant similarity to the 248-amino-acid TraX protein encoded by R100 and F (50% identity in a 78-amino-acid overlap to TraX of F) (45) and is required for N-terminal acetylation of the F-pilin subunit (113). The pYV-encoded TraX also contains a lipid attachment motif (amino acids 52 to 72), but it is unlikely to be functional. The *traX* gene is probably a vestige of a larger operon that was disrupted by the insertion sequences and transposase-like elements situated immediately upstream and downstream (Fig. 5) (86).

The region spanning coordinates 67.3 to 67.8 encodes a protein of 180 amino acids that has 46.7% identity to the 177-amino-acid endonuclease (Nuc) encoded by the pKM101 plasmid of *Salmonella typhimurium* (86, 136) (Fig. 5) and 28.2% identity to an endonuclease of *Helicobacter pylori* (182). The start codon is preceded by a putative Shine-Dalgarno sequence (AGAGG).

An Operon Encoding Arsenic Resistance: Conquest of a New Ecological Niche?

The pYV plasmid of the low-virulence strains of *Y. enterocolitica* (O:1,2,3, O:1,2, O: 3, O:9, and O:5,27) contains a class II transposon, Tn*2502,* which confers resistance to arsenite and arsenate (118). This resistance involves four genes: three are the homologs to the *arsRBC* genes present on the *E. coli* chromosome, but the fourth, *arsH,* has no known homolog. ArsR is an arsenite-inducible transcriptional repressor, ArsB forms a transmembrane channel, and ArsC catalyzes the reduction of arsenate to arsenite, which is in turn expelled by the ArsB transport system. ArsH could act as a regulator, although this has never been shown. This is among the few examples of a virulence plasmid carrying resistance genes (118). The *ars* operon is not present on the pYV plasmid of the more virulent ''American'' strains (serotypes O:4, O:8, O:13a,13b, O:18, O:20, and O:21) of *Y. enterocolitica.* This suggests that the low-virulence strains, which are distributed worldwide, constitute a single clone that probably emerged quite recently. At present, pigs represent the major reservoir of pathogenic strains of *Y. enterocolitica,* and pork is recognized as the major source of human contamination (99, 181). Neyt et al. (118) speculated that the *ars* transposon might have favored the establishment of a strain of *Yersinia* in pigs. Arsenic compounds were largely used before World War II as therapeutic agents to protect pigs from diarrhea caused by *Serpulina hyodysenteriae.*

YomA, a Homolog of PagO from *S. typhimurium*

The region immediately downstream from *yadA* (coordinates 57.0 to 57.9) contains an ORF encoding a 291-amino-acid protein with a molecular mass of 32.3 kDa and a calcu-

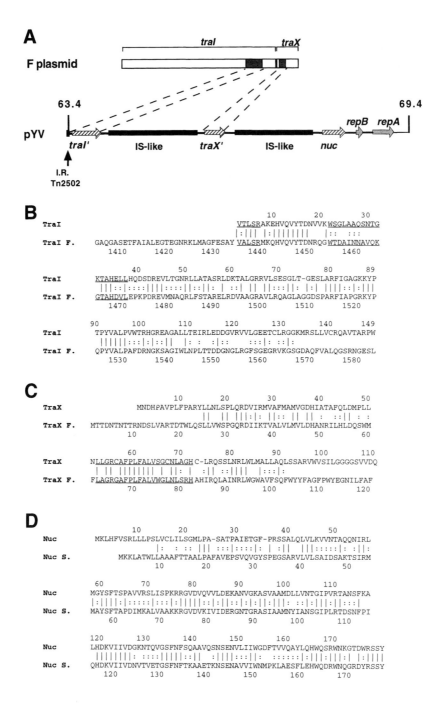

```
              10        20        30        40        50        60
YomA  MLMKNFLVILLFIMVSVTWGTTWLAMKLTVETIPPIFATGIRFMLAAPVLILISVLTKTR
      |::   : :||::||:|||||||||::|||||:||||||:||:| |  |:
PagO  MRKVSISILFMLVSLTWGTTWLAMRIAVETIPPVFATGMRFMFAAPFLIIIAWLRKKT
              10        20        30        40        50

              70        80        90       100       110       120
YomA  LLFPDGQKFFQLFVCIFYFSIPFSLMIYGETYVSPALASIIFSSMPVCVLFFSWLLLNER
      ||||  ||::||: :|||||:||||||||||||::||:|||::||| |: | | :|||
PagO  LLFPPGQRLFQFVICIFYFCIPFSLMIYGETYVNSGLAAIIFANMPVAVLIASVLFLNEK
              60        70        80        90       100       110

             130       140       150       160       170       180
YomA  VGIIAILGLVTSTVSLLAILFIETNIGSNNQWVGIISLVIAVIMHALVYVQCKKRSCSVS
      : :::| ||::::::| :||: |||:::::| ||::|: ||::||::|:||||||||||
PagO  AKLMQIAGLTIAITALTGILLEETNTSTESHWQGITALISAVLIHAIIYTQCKKRSCTVS
             120       130       140       150       160       170

             190       200       210       220       230       240
YomA  VLTFNAIPSLVAGILLCIVGWIAEQPVISKFSQQSLLSVIYLGIIAGVFGILCYFQLQNK
      |:|||||:|:|:||:|||: :||: |:|:||||| ||||||||| |||||||||||||:|
PagO  VITFNALPCLLAGLILSATGWFFERPQVSTFSVHSILATLYLGAFAGVFGILCYFALQQK
             180       190       200       210       220       230

             250       260       270       280       290
YomA  ASAFQRSTVFLVFPIIALLLDGYVYGRYFSLYSILLIIPLLTGVLLISLRK
      |:||| | |||:||:|: |::||: :| :||||||||::|::|:|
PagO  ANAFQASLVFLIFPLIAVSLEDYIYGYAISTHSMLLIIPLVIGIFLTLVARNLPVTSRCR
             240       250       260       270       280       290

PagO  DNSSQK
      300
```

Figure 6. Amino acid sequence alignment of YomA from pYVe227 (86) and PagO from *S. typhimurium* (65).

lated pI of 9.9 (86). The start codon is situated 69 bp downstream from the stop codon of *yadA* and 6 bp downstream from the *yadA* terminator. Sequence analysis of the protein predicts a putative signal sequence in the N terminus and eight transmembrane domains situated throughout the protein. The protein shows 57.7% identity to PagO, a *Salmonella typhimurium* protein encoded by a gene regulated by the PhoP-PhoQ system, which also controls type III secretion-dependent invasion genes of *S. typhimurium* (14, 125). It is also similar to YoaV of *Bacillus subtilis,* ORFX of *Buchnera aphidicola,* and YedA of *E. coli* (69, 97, 116). All the proteins of this family have approximately the same size and several putative transmembrane domains, but their function remains unknown. We called the *Y. enterocolitica* protein YomA (for ''*Yersinia* outer membrane protein A'') (86) (Fig. 6, Table 9, and data not shown).

Figure 5. Remains of a transfer operon. (A) Schematic representation of the region in pYVe227. The upper part of the panel represents the *traI* and *traX* region of the F plasmid. The lower panel indicates the region between coordinates 63.4 and 69.4. Solid boxes indicate insertion-like elements. The putative ORFs are shown by arrows. (B) Amino acid sequence alignment of the partial TraI protein encoded by the pYVe227 plamid and the corresponding part of TraI from the F plasmid. The conserved ATP- and GTP-binding domains are underlined. (C) Amino acid sequence alignment of the partial TraX protein encoded by the pYVe227 plamid and the corresponding part of TraX from F. The lipid attachment motif is underlined. (D) Amino acid sequence alignment of the Nuc endonuclease encoded by pYVe227 and Nuc encoded by pKM101 of *S. typhimurium* (Nuc S.).

According to the information available in the databases, the gene encoding YomA is not present in the 70-kb virulence plasmid of *Y. pseudotuberculosis* or *Y. pestis* and only a partial ORF encoding 166 amino acids with 100% identity to the N-terminus of YomA protein is found in the pYVe227 plasmid of *Y. enterocolitica* serotype O:3 (86, 168).

PprA, a Putative Transcriptional Activator?

DNA spanning coordinates 58.7 to 58.2 encodes a 150-amino-acid protein with a molecular mass of 16.2 kDa and a calculated pI of 10.5. Amino acids 62 to 116 of this hypothetical protein show some similarity to transcriptional activators of the family of two-component regulators, including EvgA of *E. coli* (38% identity and 63% similarity to amino acids 149 to 192) (183), BvgA of *Bordetella pertussis* (38% identity and 63% similarity to amino acids 86 to 140) (9, 10), and LuxR of *Vibrio fischeri* (47). The DNA-binding C-terminal helix-turn-helix motif is conserved in ORF150. However, the pYVe227 plasmid apparently does not encode the partner sensor protein. Since the DNA-binding C-terminal helix-turn-helix motif is conserved in this hypothetical protein, we called it PprA (for "pYV putative regulator A") (86) (Table 9).

ORF80, a Homolog of an *M. tuberculosis* ORF

DNA spanning coordinates 47.1 to 46.8 contains an ORF preceded by a putative Shine-Dalgarno sequence (GGAGN$_4$ATG) and encoding an 80-amino-acid protein with a molecular mass of 8.8 kDa and a calculated isoelectric point of 6.8, which shows significant similarity to the 83-amino-acid product of an ORF identified in the genome of *Mycobacterium tuberculosis* (86, 132) (Fig. 7 and Table 9). The role of this ORF in *Mycobacterium* is unknown, and the significance of the similarity remains unclear.

Insertion-Like Sequences

pYVe227 contains several insertion sequences, some of which are vestigial (86) (Fig. 3). Most of these belong to the IS*3* family, and they resemble IS*222* of *Pseudomonas aeruginosa*, (92), IS*1222* of *Enterobacter agglomerans* (175), IS*911* of *Shigella dysenteriae* (140), and IS*D1* of *Desulfovibrio vulgaris* (56). Elements of this family are 1.2 to 1.5 kb with imperfect terminal inverted repeats, and they generate a 3-bp duplication in the target DNA on insertion. They have a small ORF in phase 0 (ORFA) followed by a longer

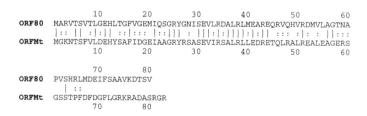

```
              10        20        30        40        50        60
ORF80   MARVTSVTLGEHLTGFVGEMIQSGRYGNISEVLRDALRLMEAREQRVQHVRDMVLAGTNA
        |::  ||  :|:||  ::|::: |::||| :  |||:|:||||:|:|| ::: :|: :  ||::::
ORFMt   MGKNTSFVLDEHYSAFIDGEIAAGRYRSASEVIRSALRLLEDRETQLRALREALEAGERS
              10        20        30        40        50        60

              70        80
ORF80   PVSHRLMDEIFSAAVKDTSV
        | ::
ORFMt   GSSTPFDFDGFLGRKRADASRGR
              70        80
```

Figure 7. Amino acid sequence alignment of the ORF80 product from pYVe227 (86) and the product of an ORF of 83 codons identified in the genome of *Mycobacterium tuberculosis* (132).

ORF in the -1 frame (ORFB). ORFB is the more highly conserved of the two within the group, and it has been proposed that it could carry the transposition-associated nicking-joining functions.

The region situated between *sycT* and *yopM* contains such an insertion sequence of approximately 2.1 kb (Fig. 3) (86). This element, called IS*1636,* is flanked by very long inverted repeats of 215 bp that generated direct repeats with a duplication of 3 bp (GTT) at the insertion site. The central part of the insertion sequence encodes two proteins, the ORFA and ORFB products, which are similar to the ORFA and ORFB products of the IS*D1* insertion sequence of *D. vulgaris* (56), to the ORF products encoded by IS*1222* of *Enterobacter agglomerans* (175), and to proteins encoded by other members of the IS*3* family.

The sequence between *sycE* and *sycH* (coordinates 43.9 to 45.1 of the pYVe227 plasmid) represents an IS called IS*1637*. It is flanked by two 36-bp imperfect inverted repeats that are very similar to those of IS*911*, and it is 70% identical to the 1,250-bp IS*911* of *Shigella dysenteriae* (140) (Fig. 3). The insertion of IS*1637* generated a 3-bp duplication of the target DNA on insertion (TTA) (86).

The 1,280-bp nucleotide IS*1638,* situated immediately upstream from *yscM2,* contains two putative ORFs with significant homology to the ORFA and ORFB present in the IS*3* elements and related to IS*D1* of *D. vulgaris* (56.1% identity) (56, 86). The region situated between *traI′* and *traX′* also shows some similarity to IS*D1* of *D. vulgaris* (56) and IS*222* of *Pseudomonas aeruginosa* (92). The region situated between *traX′* and *nuc* resembles a fragment of IS*911* from *Shigella dysenteriae* (140). No repeats were identified in these regions (86).

Finally, the region situated between *yscM2* and *yadA* contains two vestigial ORFs with significant similarity to the transposases of Tn*3* or IS*3* (Fig. 3) (86).

THE 70-kb PLASMID OF *Y. PSEUDOTUBERCULOSIS* AND *Y. PESTIS* AND EVOLUTIONARY ASPECTS

Overview

The virulence plasmid of *Y. pestis* has also been completely sequenced by two different groups (81, 129). The sequence of the *Y. pseudotuberculosis* pIB1 has not been published yet, but most of it is known (130). In general, the 70-kb plasmid is quite well conserved among the three species (18, 81, 86, 129, 137, 138, 139). All 35 genes of the secretion-translocation apparatus are present in the same order. The same effector genes are also present on the three plasmids but have been reshuffled. The ancillary functions of replication and partition of the three plasmids are also the same, indicating that they are derived from a common ancestor. There are variations in the other elements. A comparison of the three plasmids is shown in Fig. 8.

Major Inversions

The order of the genes is identical in pCD1 and pIB1, reinforcing the idea that *Y. pestis* and *Y. pseudotuberculosis* are extremely closely related. In contrast, half of the plasmid is inverted in pYVe227 (18). The inversion occurred between *yopH* and *sycH* on one side and between *ylpA* and *yopJ/yopK* on the other side. In addition, within the inverted half,

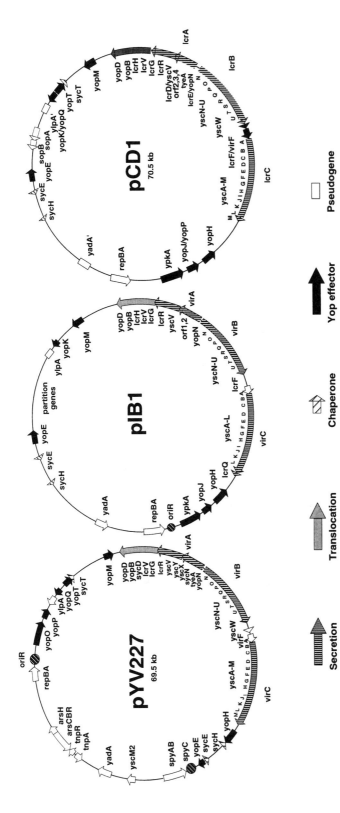
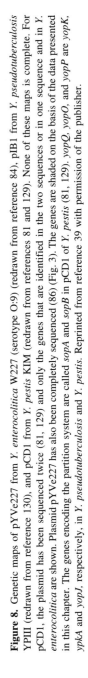

Figure 8. Genetic maps of pYVe227 from *Y. enterocolitica* W227 (serotype O:9) (redrawn from reference 130), and pCD1 from *Y. pseudotuberculosis* YPIII (redrawn from reference 84), pIB1 from *Y. pestis* KIM (redrawn from references 81 and 129). None of these maps is complete. For pCD1, the plasmid has been sequenced twice (81, 129) and only the genes that are identified in the two sequences or in one sequence and in *Y. enterocolitica* are shown. Plasmid pYVe227 has also been completely sequenced (86) (Fig. 3). The genes are shaded on the basis of the data presented in this chapter. The genes encoding the partition system are called *sopA* and *sopB* in pCD1 of *Y. pestis* (81, 129). *yopQ, yopO,* and *yopP* are *yopK, ypkA* and *yopJ,* respectively, in *Y. pseudotuberculosis* and *Y. pestis.* Reprinted from reference 39 with permission of the publisher.

114

the region containing the partition system, *yopE, sycE,* and *sycH,* suffered an inversion, putting it back in the original orientation. Surprisingly, the two major inversions are not bordered by transposable elements.

Minor Inversions

Minor rearrangements are also found in other regions of the 70-kb plasmid. The gene encoding YopM represents a nice illustration of such rearrangements. *yopM* itself shows some heterogeneity among different *Yersinia* isolates, probably because it encodes a protein with internal repetitions (23). In addition, the orientation of *yopM* varies. It is oriented clockwise in *Y. enterocolitica* but counterclockwise in *Y. pseudotuberculosis* and *Y. pestis.* The region upstream and downstream from *yopM* contains three long repeated sequences and putative ORFs (86, 144). Genetic recombinations between these repeats could explain the observed inversion of *yopM* (Fig. 9).

Localized Mutations

The *yadA* gene also underwent some modifications during evolution of the 70-kb plasmid. *yadA* varies in the different serotypes of *Y. enterocolitica,* resulting in proteins

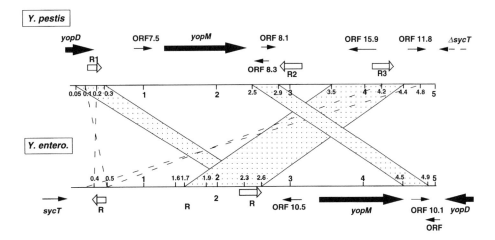

Figure 9. Comparison of the region encoding YopM in pCD1 (*Y. pestis*) and pYVe227 (*Y. enterocolitica*). The region situated upstream and downstream from *yopM* contains repeated sequences (represented by open arrow labeled R) that led to genetic rearrangement. The gene is oriented in the same direction as *yopD* in *Y. pestis* and *Y. pseudotuberculosis* (not shown) and in the opposite direction in *Y. enterocolitica.* The distance between the stop codon of *sycT* and the start codon of *yopM* is 3.4 kb in *Y. enterocolitica,* while the distance between the stop codon of *yopM* and the stop codon of *sycT* is 2.3 kb in *Y. pestis.* Putative ORFs identified upstream and downstream of *yopM* in the different species are shown by thin arrows labeled ORF followed by a number corresponding to the putative calculated molecular weight. The products of these ORFs have no match in the databases. The stippled areas indicate conserved regions between the downstream and upstream regions of *yopM.*

```
              A                               B
         1   10    20      30      40      50                          60      70      80
YadAO9  MTKDFKISVSAALISALFSSPYAFADD....YNGIPNLTAVQISPNADPALGQEY........................PVRPPVPGAGGLNCSAKGIHSIAIGATAEAAKQA
         ************************* **  *.***********        **                    ************ *** ****** ** ***** *
YadAO3  MTKDFKISVSAALISALFSSPYAFADD....YDGIPNLTAVQISPNADPALGLEY........................PVRPPVPGAGGLNASAKGIHSIAIGATAEAAKCA
         ************************   ******* **                                        * ** ** **** ** *****
YadAO8  MTKDFKISVSAALISALFSSPYAFANN.....DEV.HFTAVQISPNADPD.SHVV.....................IFQPAAEALGGTNALAKSIHSIAVGASAEAAKQA
         **********************     ****** **                               *    *** ***** ** *****
YadAPS  MTKDFKISVSAALISALFSSPYAFAEEPEDGNDGIPRLSAVQISPNVDPKLGVGLYPAKPILRQENPKLPPRGPQGPEKKRARLAEAIQPQVLGAGGLNARAKDPYSIAIGATAEAAKPA

              C                                    D
         90    100     110     120     130     140     150     160     170     180     190     200
YadAO9  AVAVGAGSIATGVNSVAIGPLSKALGDSAVTYGAASTAQKDGVAIGARASTSDTGVAVGFNSKADAKNSVAIGHSSHVAANHGYSIAIGDRSKTDRENSVSIGHESLNRQLTHLAAGTKD
         ***********************.**********************************************  ***  ** ****** **** **** ** ***** ** ***** **
YadAO3  AVAVGAGSIATGVNSVAIGPLSKALGDSAVTYGAASTAQKDGVAIGARASTSDTGVAVGFNSKADAKNSVAIGHSSHVAANHGYSIAIGDRSKTDRENSVSIGHESLNRQLTHLAAGTKD
         ***********************.**********************************************  ***  * *********** *********** *** ** ***** **
YadAO8  AVAVGAGSIATGVNSVAIGPLSKALGDSAVTYGAASTAQKDGVAIGARAFTSDTGVAVGFNSKVDAKNSVAIGHSSHVAVDHDYSIAIGDRSKTDRKNSVSIGHESLNRQLTHLAAGTKD
         ****  *****************.********************** *********** ***** ** ****  **  ** ** ** **** **** ** ***** ** ***** **
YadAPS  AVAVGSGSIATGVNSVAIGPLSKALGDSAVTYGASSTAQKDGVAIGARASASDTGVAVGFNSKVDAQNSVAIGHSSHVAADHGYSIAIGDHSKTDRENSVSIGHESLNRQLTHLAAGTED

         210     220     230     240     250     260     270     280     290     300     310     320
YadAO9  TDAVNVAQLKKEIEKTQENTNKKSAELLAKPNAYADNKSSSVLGIANNYTDSKSAETLENARKEAFAQSKDVLNMAKAHSNSVARTTLETAEEHANSVARTTLETAEEHANKKSAEALAS
         *********************.******  *****       **********  ****************** ****************************** *********** **
YadAO3  TDAVNVAQLKKEIEKTQENTNKRSAELLANANAYADNKSSSVLGIANNYTDSKSAETLENARKEAFAQSKDVLNMAKAHSNSVARTTLETAEEHANSVARTTLETAEEHANKKSAEALAS
         *****************  * ***   **************   * *** **************** * **** *********  *             *****  **
YadAO8  TDAVNVAQLKKEIEKTQVNANKKSAE...............VLGIANNYTDSKSAETLENARKEAFDLSNDALDMAKKHSNSVARTTLETAEEHPN..............KKSAETLAR
         ***********                           **********        ** **  *********** ** ***               ***** *
YadAPS  TDAVNVAQLKKEM..................................AETLENARKETLAQSNDVLDAAKKHSNSVARTTLETAEEHAN...............KKSAEALVS

         330     340     350     360     370     380     390     400     410     420     430     440
YadAO9  ANVYADSKSSHTLKTANSYTDVTVSNSTKKAIRESNQYTDHKFRQLDNRLDKLDTRVDKGLASSAALNSLFQPYGVGKVNFTAGVGGYRSSQALAIGSGYRVNENVALKP.VWLIGGSDV
         ***************************************************************************************************************     *****
YadAO3  ANVYADSKSSHTLKTANSYTDVTVSNSTKKAIRESNQYTDHKFRQLDNRLDKLDTRVDKGLASSAALNSLFQPYGVGKVNFTAGVGGYRSSQALAIGSGYRVNENVALKAGVAYAGSSDV
         ***************************************************************************************************************  ***********
YadAO8  ANVYADSKSSHTLQTANSYTDVTVSNSTKKAIRESNQYTDHKFRQLDNRLDKLDTRVDKGLASSAALNSLFQPYGVGKVNFTAGVGGYRSSQALAIGSGYRVNESVALKAGVAYAGSSDV
         ***** ******* ********************************************************************************************** ***********
YadAPS  AKVYADSNSSHTLKTANSYTDVTVSSSTKKAISESNQYTDHKFSQLDNRLDKLDKRVDKGLASSAALNSLFQPYGVGKVNFTAGVGGYRSSQALAIGSGYRVNESVALKAGVAYAGSSNV

         E
         450 454
YadAO9  MYNASFNIEW
         **********
YadAO3  MYNASFNIEW
         **********
YadAO8  MYNASFNIEW
         **********
YadAPS  MYNASFNIEW
```

Figure 10. Amino acid sequence alignment of YadA from *Y. enterocolitica* O:9 (YadAO9) (86), *Y. enterocolitica* O:3 (YadAO3), *Y. enterocolitica* O:8 (YadAO8), and *Y. pseudotuberculosis* (YadAPS). The three last sequences are from reference 168. The boxes and the bold letters indicate the different domains of the protein. (A) Signal sequence. (B) Residues required for adhesion to polymorphonuclear leukocytes and inhibition of the oxidative burst in *Y. enterocolitica* O:8. (C) Residues required for autoagglutination, collagen binding, and persistence in Peyer's patches of *Y. enterocolitica* O:3 and O:8. (D) Histidines 156 and 159 in *Y. enterocolitica* O:8, required for binding to different substrates and dissemination from Peyer's patches. (E) Residues required for anchoring to the outer membrane and polymer formation (146, 147, 166, 168, 180).

of different sizes (Fig. 10). Most importantly, the *yadA* gene of *Y. pestis* has a single-base-pair deletion that causes a shift in the reading frame of the gene and a reduction of the half-life of the mRNA, resulting in the loss of the protein (81, 139, 153, 168).

The information available in databases also indicates that *ylpA* is a pseudogene in *Y. pestis* (81, 129).

YscM2, YomA, PprA, and the ORF80 protein are not encoded by pCD1 (81, 86). According to the information available in the databases, the gene encoding YomA is also missing in pIB1 from *Y. pseudotuberculosis,* only a partial ORF encoding 166 amino acids with 100% identity to the N terminus of YomA protein is found in the pYV plasmid of *Y. enterocolitica* serotype O:3, and a short ORF encoding the first 53 amino acids of YomA is found in the pCD1 plasmid of *Y. pestis* (81, 86, 168). The available information does not allow us to draw conclusions about the presence of the genes encoding PprA and the ORF80 protein in pIB1.

Duplication

The pYVe227 plasmid from *Y. enterocolitica* contains two copies of *yscM* (174), a hypothetical player of the negative regulatory loop (145). In contrast, there is only one copy of the homolog *lcrQ* in *Y. pseudotuberculosis* and *Y. pestis*. Thus, *yscM* was presumably duplicated after *Y. pestis* and *Y. pseudotuberculosis* diverged (see below).

Lack of the *ars* Resistance Genes

As mentioned above, the pYV plasmid of low-virulence pathogenic *Y. enterocolitica* strains harbors a transposon encoding arsenite resistance (118). This transposon is absent from pIB1 and pCD1, which is is agreement with the hypothesis that it was recently acquired by a pYV plasmid from *Y. enterocolitica* (see above).

CONCLUSIONS

The three plasmids clearly have a common ancestor of the RepFII A type. pYVe227 is probably closer to this ancestor than are pIB1 and pCD1, because *yopH* and *sycH* are still associated and *yadA* and *ylpA* are intact (35, 86, 130).

The fact that the pYVe227 plasmid contains the remains of a transfer operon suggests that the plasmid was conjugative in origin. The *tra* genes that are still conserved, such as *ylpA*, homologous to *traT* and *nuc*, could have evolved to fulfill another, still unknown function.

As is generally the case for the large plasmids, the stability of the 70-kb plasmid is assured by a partition system. However, unlike large plasmids such as F, R1, and R438, the 70-kb plasmid does not have a system like *hok/sok, srnB,* or *pnd,* which kills plasmid-free segregants (61, 119). This observation is in perfect agreement with the fact that *Yersinia* easily gives pYV$^-$ segregants when plated at 37°C on a medium deprived of Ca^{2+} (18).

Acknowledgments. This work was supported by the Belgian Fonds National de la Recherche Scientifique Médicale (Convention 3.4595.97), the Direction générale de la Recherche Scientifique-Communauté Française de Belgique (Action de Recherche Concertée 94/99–172), and the Interuniversity Poles of Attraction Program—Belgian State, Prime Minister's Office, Federal Office for Scientific, Technical and Cultural Affairs (PAI 4/03).

REFERENCES

1. **Aguero, M. E., L. Aron, A. G. DeLuca, K. N. Timmis, and F. C. Cabello.** 1984. A plasmid-encoded outer membrane protein, TraT, enhances resistance of *Escherichia coli* to phagocytosis. *Infect. Immun.* **46:** 740–746.
2. **Albertini, A. M., T. Caramori, W. D. Crabb, F. Scoffone, and A. Galizzi.** 1991. The *flaA* locus of *Bacillus subtilis* is part of a large operon coding for flagellar structures, motility functions, and an ATPase-like polypeptide. *J. Bacteriol.* **173:**3573–3579.
3. **Alfano, J. R., H. S. Kim, T. P. Delaney, and A. Collmer.** 1997. Evidence that the *Pseudomonas syringae* pv. *syringae* hrp-linked *hrmA* gene encodes an Avr-like protein that acts in an hrp-dependent manner within tobacco cells. *Mol. Plant-Microbe Interact.* **10:**580–588.
4. **Allaoui, A., R. Scheen, C. L. Lambert de Rouvroit, and G. R. Cornelis.** 1995. VirG, a *Yersinia enterocoli-*

tica lipoprotein involved in Ca^{2+} dependency, is related to ExsB of *Pseudomonas aeruginosa. J. Bacteriol.* **177:**4230–4237.

5. **Allaoui, A., R. Schulte, and G. R. Cornelis.** 1995. Mutational analysis of the *Yersinia enterocolitica virC* operon: characterization of *yscE, F, G, I, J, K* required for Yop secretion and *yscH* encoding YopR. *Mol. Microbiol.* **18:**343–355.

6. **Allaoui, A., S. Woestyn, C. Sluiters, and G. R. Cornelis.** 1994. YscU, a *Yersinia enterocolitica* inner membrane protein involved in Yop secretion. *J. Bacteriol.* **176:**4534–4542.

7. **Anderson, D. M., and O. Schneewind.** 1997. A mRNA signal for the type III secretion of Yop proteins by *Yersinia enterocolitica. Science* **278:**1140–1143.

8. **Andersson, K., N. Carballeira, K.-E. Magnusson, C. Persson, O. Stendahl, H. Wolf-Watz, and M. Fällman.** 1996. YopH of *Yersinia pseudotuberculosis* interrupts early phosphotyrosine signalling associated with phagocytosis. Mol. Microbiol. **20:**1057–1069.

9. **Arico, B., J. F. Miller, C. Roy, S. Stibitz, D. Monack, S. Falkow, R. Gross, and R. Rappuoli.** 1989. Sequences required for expression of *Bordetella pertussis* virulence factors share homology with prokaryotic signal transduction proteins. *Proc. Natl. Acad. Sci. USA* **86:**6671–6675.

10. **Arico, B., V. Scarlato, D. M. Monack, S. Falkow, and R. Rappuoli.** 1991. Structural and genetic analysis of the *bvg* locus in *Bordetella* species. *Mol. Microbiol.* **5:**2481–2492.

11. **Arricau, N., D. Hermant, H. Waxin, and M. Y. Popoff.** 1997. Molecular characterization of the *Salmonella typhi* StpA protein that is related to both *Yersinia* YopE cytotoxin and YopH tyrosine phosphatase. *Res. Microbiol.* **148:**21–26.

12. **Bakour, R., Y. Laroche, and G. Cornelis.** 1983. Study of the incompatibility and replication of the 70-kb virulence plasmid of *Yersinia. Plasmid* **10:**279–289.

13. **Balligand, G., Y. Laroche, and G. Cornelis.** 1985. Genetic analysis of virulence plasmid from a serogroup 9 *Yersinia enterocolitica* strain: role of outer membrane protein P1 in resistance to human serum and autoagglutination. *Infect. Immun.* **48:**782–786.

14. **Belden, W. J., and S. I. Miller.** 1994. Further characterization of the PhoP regulon: identification of new PhoP-activated virulence loci. *Infect. Immun.* **62:**5095–5101.

15. **Bergman, T., K. Erickson, E. E. Galyov, C. Persson, and H. Wolf-Watz.** 1994. The *lcrB* (*yscN/U*) gene cluster of *Yersinia pseudotuberculosis* is involved in Yop secretion and shows high homology to the *spa* gene clusters of *Shigella flexneri* and *Salmonella typhimurium. J. Bacteriol.* **176:**2619–2626.

16. **Bergman, T., S. Hakansson, A. Forsberg, L. Norlander, A. Macellaro, A. Backman, I. Bolin, and H. Wolf-Watz.** 1991. Analysis of the V antigen *lcrGVH-yopBD* operon of *Yersinia pseudotuberculosis:* evidence for a regulatory role of LcrH and LcrV. *J. Bacteriol.* **173:**1607–1616.

17. **Bhakdi, S., N. Mackman, J. M. Nicaud, and I. B. Holland.** 1986. *Escherichia coli* hemolysin may damage target cell membranes by generating transmembrane pores. *Infect. Immun.* **52:**63–69.

18. **Biot, T., and G. R. Cornelis.** 1988. The replication, partition and *yop* regulation of the pYV plasmids are highly conserved in *Yersinia enterocolitica* and *Y. pseudotuberculosis. J. Gen. Microbiol.* **134:**1525–1534.

19. **Bischoff, D. S., and G. W. Ordal.** 1992. Identification and characterization of FliY, a novel component of the *Bacillus subtilis* flagellar switch complex. *Mol. Microbiol.* **6:**2715–2723.

20. **Bischoff, D. S., M. D. Weinreich, and G. W. Ordal.** 1992. Nucleotide sequences of *Bacillus subtilis* flagellar biosynthetic genes *fliP* and *fliQ* and identification of a novel flagellar gene, *fliZ. J. Bacteriol.* **174:**4017–4025.

21. **Black, D. S., and J. B. Bliska.** 1997. Identification of p130[Cas] as a substrate of *Yersinia* YopH (Yop51), a bacterial protein tyrosine phosphatase that translocates into mammalian cells and targets focal adhesions. *EMBO J.* **16:**2730–2744.

22. **Boland, A., and G. R. Cornelis.** 1998. Role of YopP in suppression of tumor necrosis factor alpha release by macrophages during *Yersinia* infection. *Infect. Immun.* **66:**1878–1884.

23. **Boland, A., S. Havaux, and G. R. Cornelis.** 1998. Heterogeneity of the *Yersinia* YopM protein. *Microb. Pathog.* **25:**343–348.

24. **Boland, A., M. P. Sory, M. Iriarte, C. Kerbourch, P. Wattiau, and G. R. Cornelis.** 1996. Status of YopM and YopN in the *Yersinia* Yop virulon: YopM of *Y. enterocolitica* is internalized inside the cytosol of PU5-1.8 macrophages by the YopB, D, N delivery apparatus. *EMBO J.* **15:**5191–5201.

25. **Bölin, I., A. Forsberg, L. Norlander, M. Skurnik, and H. Wolf-Watz.** 1988. Identification and mapping of the temperature-inducible, plasmid-encoded proteins of *Yersinia* spp. *Infect. Immun.* **56:**343–348.

26. **Bölin, I., and H. Wolf-Watz.** 1984. Molecular cloning of the temperature-inducible outer membrane protein 1 of *Yersinia pseudotuberculosis. Infect. Immun.* **43:**72–78.

27. **Boyd, A. P.** 1998. Unpublished data.

28. **Boyd, A. P., M.-P. Sory, M. Iriarte, and G. R. Cornelis.** 1998. Heparin interferes with translocation of Yop proteins into HeLa cells and binds to LcrG, a regulatory component of the *Yersinia* Yop apparatus. *Mol. Microbiol.* **27:**425–436.

29. **Brubaker, R. R.** 1991. Factors promoting acute and chronic diseases caused by yersiniae. *Clin. Microbiol. Rev.* **4:**309–324.

30. **Carniel, E., I. Guilvout, and M. Prentice.** 1996. Characterization of a large chromosomal "high pathogenicity island" in biotype 1B *Yersinia enterocolitica. J. Bacteriol.* **176:**6743–6751.

31. **Carpenter, P. B., and G. W. Ordal.** 1993. *Bacillus subtilis* FlhA: a flagellar protein related to a new family of signal-transducing receptors. *Mol. Microbiol.* **7:**735–743.

32. **Carpenter, P. B., A. R. Zuberi, and G. W. Ordal.** 1993. *Bacillus subtilis* flagellar proteins FliP, FliQ, FliR and FlhB are related to *Shigella flexneri* virulence factors. *Gene* **137:**243–245.

33. **Cheng, L. W., D. M. Anderson, and O. Schneewind.** 1997. Two independent type III secretion mechanisms for YopE in *Yersinia enterocolitica. Mol. Microbiol.* **24:**757–765.

34. **Cherepanov, P. A., T. G. Mikhailova, G. A. Farimova, N. M. Zakharova, Y. V. Ershov, and K. I. Volkovoi.** 1991. Cloning and detailed mapping of the Fra-Ymt region of the *Yersinia pestis* plasmid pFra. *Mol. Genet. Mikrobiol. Virusol.* **12:**19–26.

35. **China, B., T. Michiels, and G. R. Cornelis.** 1990. The pYV plasmid of *Yersinia* encodes a lipoprotein, YlpA, related to TraT. *Mol. Microbiol.* **4:**1585–1593.

36. **Cole, S. P., D. G. Guiney, and L. B. Corbeil.** 1993. Molecular analysis of a gene encoding a serum-resistance-associated 76 kDa surface antigen of *Haemophilus somnus. J. Gen. Microbiol.* **139:**2135–2143.

37. **Cornelis, G., Y. Laroche, G. Balligand, M.-P. Sory, and G. Wauters.** 1987. *Yersinia enterocolitica,* a primary model for bacterial invasiveness. *Rev. Infect. Dis.* **9:**64–87.

38. **Cornelis, G. R.** 1998. The *Yersinia* deadly kiss. *J. Bacteriol.* **180:**5495–5504.

39. **Cornelis, G. R., A. Boland, A. P. Boyd, C. Geuijen, M. Iriarte, C. Neyt, M.-P. Sory, and I. Stainier.** 1998. The virulence plasmid of *Yersinia,* an antihost genome. *Microbiol. Mol. Biol. Rev.* **62:**1315–1352.

40. **Cornelis, G. R., M. Iriarte, and M. P. Sory.** 1995. Environmental control of virulence functions and signal transduction in *Yersinia enterocolitica,* p. 95–110. *In* R. Rappuoli, V. Scarlato, and B. Arico (ed.), *Signal Transduction and Bacterial Virulence.* R. G. Landes, Co., Austin, Tex.

41. **Cornelis, G. R., C. Sluiters, C. L. Lambert de Rouvroit, and T. Michiels.** 1989. Homology between *virF,* the transcriptional activator of the *Yersinia* virulence regulon, and AraC, the *Escherichia coli* arabinose operon regulator. *J. Bacteriol.* **171:**254–262.

42. **Cornelis, G. R., M. P. Sory, Y. Laroche, and I. Derclaye.** 1986. Genetic analysis of the plasmid region controlling virulence in *Yersinia enterocolitica* O:9 by Mini-Mu insertions and *lac* gene fusions. *Microb. Pathog.* **1:**349–359.

43. **Cornelis, G. R., J. C. Vanooteghem, and C. Sluiters.** 1987. Transcription of the *yop* regulon from *Y. enterocolitica* requires trans acting pYV and chromosomal genes. *Microb. Pathog.* **2:**367–379.

44. **Cover, T. L., and R. C. Aber.** 1989. *Yersinia enterocolitica. N. Engl. J. Med.* **321:**16–24.

45. **Cram, D. S., S. M. Loh, K.-C. Cheah, and R. A. Skurray.** 1991. Sequence and conservation of genes at the distal end of the transfer region on plasmids F and R6-5. *Gene* **104:**85–90.

45a.**Day, J. B., and G. V. Plano.** 1998. A complex composed of SycN and YscB functions as a specific chaperone for YopN in *Yersinia pestis. Mol. Microbiol.* **30:**777–788.

46. **Eisenberg, D.** 1984. Three-dimensional structure of membrane and surface proteins. *Annu. Rev. Biochem.* **53:**595–623.

47. **Engebrecht, J., and M. Silverman.** 1987. Nucleotide sequence of the regulatory locus controlling expression of bacterial genes for bioluminescence. *Nucleic Acids Res.* **15:**10455–10467.

48. **Fallman, M., K. Andersson, S. Hakansson, K. E. Magnusson, O. Stendahl, and H. Wolf-Watz.** 1995. *Yersinia pseudotuberculosis* inhibits Fc receptor-mediated phagocytosis in J774 cells. *Infect. Immun.* **63:**3117–3124.

49. **Fields, K. A., G. V. Plano, and S. C. Straley.** 1994. A low-Ca^{2+} response (LCR) secretion (*ysc*) locus lies within the *lcrB* region of the LCR plasmid in *Yersinia pestis. J. Bacteriol.* **176:**569–579.

50. **Forsberg, A., I. Bolin, L. Norlander, and H. Wolf-Watz.** 1987. Molecular cloning and expression of calcium-regulated, plasmid-coded proteins of *Y. pseudotuberculosis. Microb. Pathog.* **2:**123–137.

51. **Forsberg, A., R. Rosqvist, and H. Wolf-Watz.** 1994. Regulation and polarized transfer of the *Yersinia* outer proteins (Yops) involved in antiphagocytosis. *Trends Microbiol.* **2:**14–19.

52. **Forsberg, A., A. M. Viitanen, M. Skurnik, and H. Wolf-Watz.** 1991. The surface-located YopN protein is involved in calcium signal transduction in *Yersinia pseudotuberculosis. Mol. Microbiol.* **5:**977–986.

53. **Forsberg, A., and H. Wolf-Watz.** 1988. The virulence protein Yop5 of *Yersinia pseudotuberculosis* is regulated at transcriptional level by plasmid-plB1-encoded trans-acting elements controlled by temperature and calcium. *Mol. Microbiol.* **2:**121–133.

54. **Freiberg, C., R. Fellay, A. Bairoch, W. J. Broughton, A. Rosenthal, and X. Perret.** 1997. Molecular basis of symbiosis between *Rhizobium* and legumes. *Nature* **387:**394–401.

55. **Frithz-Lindsten, E., R. Rosqvist, L. Johansson, and A. Forsberg.** 1995. The chaperone-like protein YerA of *Yersinia pseudotuberculosis* stabilizes YopE in the cytoplasm but is dispensable for targeting to the secretion loci. *Mol. Microbiol.* **16:**635–647.

56. **Fu, R. D., and G. Voordouw.** 1998. ISD1, an insertion element from the sulfate-reducing bacterium *Desulfovibrio vulgaris* Hildenborough: structure, transposition, and distribution. *Appl. Environ. Microbiol.* **64:**53–61.

57. **Galyov, E. E., S. Håkansson, A. Forsberg, and H. Wolf-Watz.** 1993. A secreted protein kinase of *Yersinia pseudotuberculosis* is an indispensable virulence determinant. *Nature* **361:**730–732.

58. **Galyov, E. E., S. Håkansson, and H. Wolf-Watz.** 1994. Characterization of the operon encoding the YpkA Ser/Thr protein kinase and the YopJ protein of *Yersinia pseudotuberculosis. J. Bacteriol.* **176:** 4543–4548.

59. **Gemski, P., J. R. Lazere, and T. Casey.** 1980. Plasmid associated with pathogenicity and calcium dependency of *Yersinia enterocolitica. Infect. Immun.* **27:**682–685.

60. **Gemski, P., J. R. Lazere, T. Casey, and J. A. Wohlmieter.** 1980. Presence of a virulence-associated plasmid in *Yersinia pseudotuberculosis. Infect. Immun.* **28:**1044–1047.

61. **Gerdes, K., A. Nielsen, P. Thorsted, and E. G. H. Wagner.** 1992. Mechanism of killer gene activation. Antisense RNA-dependent RNase III cleavage ensures rapid turnover of the stable Hork, SrnB, and PndA effector messenger RNAs. *J. Mol. Biol.* **226:**637–649.

62. **Glaser, P., H. Sakamoto, J. Bellalou, A. Ullmann, and A. Danchin.** 1988. Secretion of cyclolysin, the calmodulin-sensitive adenylate cyclase-haemolysin bifunctional protein of *Bordetella pertussis. EMBO J.* **7:**3997–4004.

63. **Goguen, J. D., J. Yother, and S. C. Straley.** 1984. Genetic analysis of the low calcium response in *Yersinia pestis* mu d1(Ap *lac*) insertion mutants. *J. Bacteriol.* **160:**842–848.

64. **Guan, K. L., and J. E. Dixon.** 1990. Protein tyrosine phosphatase activity of an essential virulence determinant in *Yersinia. Science* **249:**553–556.

65. **Gunn, J. S., W. J. Belden, and S. I. Miller.** 1997. Identification of PhoP-PhoQ activated genes within a duplicated region of the *Salmonella typhimurium* chromosome. GenBank accession no. AF013775.

66. **Håkansson, S., T. Bergman, J. C. Vanooteghem, G. Cornelis, and H. Wolf-Watz.** 1993. YopB and YopD constitute a novel class of *Yersinia* Yop proteins. *Infect. Immun.* **61:**71–80.

67. **Håkansson, S., E. E. Galyov, R. Rosqvist, and H. Wolf-Watz.** 1996. The *Yersinia* YpkA Ser/Thr kinase is translocated and subsequently targeted to the inner surface of the HeLa cell plasma membrane. *Mol. Microbiol.* **20:**593–603.

68. **Håkansson, S., K. Schesser, C. Persson, E. E. Galyov, R. Rosqvist, F. Homblé, and H. Wolf-Watz.** 1996. The YopB protein of *Yersinia pseudotuberculosis* is essential for the translocation of Yop effector proteins across the target cell plasma membrane and displays a contact dependent membrane disrupting activity. *EMBO J.* **15:**5812–5823.

69. **Hanck, T., N. Gerwin, and H. J. Fritz.** 1989. Nucleotide sequence of the dcm locus of Escherichia coli K12. *Nucleic Acids Res.* **17:**5844.

70. **Hardt, W.-D., and J. E. Galan.** 1997. A secreted *Salmonella* protein with homology to an avirulence determinant of plant pathogenic bacteria. *Proc. Natl. Acad. Sci. USA* **94:**9887–9892.

71. **Hartland, E. L., A. M. Bordun, and R. M. Robins Browne.** 1996. Contribution of YopB to virulence of *Yersinia enterocolitica. Infect. Immun.* **64:**2308–2314.

72. **Hartland, E. L., S. P. Green, W. A. Phillips, and R. M. Robins Browne.** 1994. Essential role of YopD in inhibition of the respiratory burst of macrophages by *Yersinia enterocolitica. Infect. Immun.* **62:** 4445–4453.

73. **Hartman, A. B., M. Venkatesan, E. V. Oaks, and J. M. Buysse.** 1990. Sequence and molecular characteri-

zation of a multicopy invasion plasmid antigen gene, *ipaH*, of *Shigella flexneri. J. Bacteriol.* **172:** 1905–1915.

74. **Herman, N. D., and T. D. Schneider.** 1992. High information conservation implies that at least three proteins bind independently to F plasmid *incD* repeats. *J. Bacteriol.* **174:**3558–3560.

75. **Higashi, T., H. Sasai, F. Suzuki, J. Miyoshi, T. Ohuchi, S. Taikai, T. Mori, and T. Kakunaga.** 1990. Hamster cell line suitable for transfection assay of transforming genes. *Proc. Natl. Acad. Sci. USA* **87:** 2409–2412.

76. **Hodgman, T. C.** 1988. A new superfamily of replicative proteins. *Nature* **333:**22–23.

77. **Hoe, N. P., and J. D. Goguen.** 1993. Temperature sensing in *Yersinia pestis:* translation of the LcrF activator protein is thermally regulated. *J. Bacteriol.* **175:**7901–7909.

78. **Hoe, N. P., F. C. Minion, and J. D. Goguen.** 1992. Temperature sensing in *Yersinia pestis:* regulation of *yopE* transcription by *lcrF. J. Bacteriol.* **174:**4275–4286.

79. **Holmström, A., J. Pettersson, R. Rosqvist, S. Håkansson, F. Tafazoli, M. Fallman, K. E. Magnusson, H. Wolf-Watz, and A. Forsberg.** 1997. YopK of *Yersinia pseudotuberculosis* controls translocation of Yop effectors across the eukaryotic cell membrane. *Mol. Microbiol.* **24:**73–91.

80. **Holmström, A., R. Rosqvist, H. Wolf-Watz, and A. Forsberg.** 1995. Virulence plasmid-encoded YopK is essential for *Yersinia pseudotuberculosis* to cause systemic infection in mice. *Infect. Immun.* **63:**2269–2276.

81. **Hu, P., J. Elliot, P. McCready, E. Skowronski, J. Garnes, A. Kobayashi, A. V. Carrano, R. Brubaker, and E. Garcia.** 1998. *Yersinia pestis* plasmid pCD1, complete plasmid sequence. GenBank accession no. AF053946.

82. **Hueck, C. J.** 1998. Type III protein secretion systems in bacterial pathogens of animals and plants. *Microbiol. Mol. Biol. Rev.* **62:**379–433.

83. **Hughes, K. T., K. L. Gillen, M. J. Semon, and J. E. Karlinsey.** 1993. Sensing structural intermediates in bacterial flagellar assembly by export of a negative regulator. *Science* **262:**1277–1280.

84. **Iriarte, M., and G. R. Cornelis.** 1998. YopT, a new *Yersinia* Yop effector protein, affects the cytoskeleton of host cells. *Mol. Microbiol.* **29:**915–929.

85. **Iriarte, M., and G. R. Cornelis.** 1999. Identification of SycN, YscX, and YscY, three new elements of the *Yersinia* Yop virulon. *J. Bacteriol.* **181:**675–680.

86. **Iriarte, M., I. Lambermont, C. Kerbourch, and G. R. Cornelis.** 1998. Complete sequence of the pYVe227 plasmid of *Yersinia enterocolitica* serotype O:9. GenBank accession no. AF102990.

87. **Iriarte, M., M. P. Sory, A. Boland, A. P. Boyd, S. D. Mills, I. Lambermont, and G. R. Cornelis.** 1998. TyeA, a protein involved in control of Yop release and in translocation of *Yersinia* Yop effectors. *EMBO J.* **17:**1907–1918.

88. **Kaniga, K., J. Uralil, J. B. Bliska, and J. E. Galan.** 1996. A secreted protein tyrosine phosphatase with modular effector domains in the bacterial pathogen *Salmonella typhimurium. Mol. Microbiol.* **21:**633–641.

89. **Kapperud, G., E. Namork, and H. J. Skarpeid.** 1985. Temperature-inducible surface fibrillae associated with the virulence plasmid of *Yersinia enterocolitica* and *Yersinia pseudotuberculosis. Infect. Immun.* **47:** 561–566.

90. **Kapperud, G., E. Namork, M. Skurnik, and T. Nesbakken.** 1987. Plasmid-mediated surface fibrillae of *Yersinia pseudotuberculosis* and *Yersinia enterocolitica:* relationship to the outer membrane protein YOP1 and possible importance for pathogenesis. *Infect. Immun.* **55:**2247–2254.

91. **Koster, M., W. Bitter, H. de Cock, A. Allaoui, G. R. Cornelis, and J. Tommassen.** 1997. The outer membrane component, YscC, of the Yop secretion machinery of *Yersinia enterocolitica* forms a ring-shaped multimeric complex. *Mol. Microbiol.* **26:**789–798.

92. **Kropinski, A. M., M. A. Farinha, and I. Jansons.** 1994. Nucleotide sequence of the *Pseudomonas aeruginosa* insertion sequence IS222: another member of the IS3 family. *Plasmid* **31:**222–228.

93. **Kubori, T., Y. Matsushima, D. Nakamura, J. Uralil, M. Lara-Tejero, A. Sukhan, J. E. Galan, and S.-I. Aizawa.** 1998. Supramolecular structure of the *Salmonella typhimurium* type III protein secretion system. *Science* **280:**602–605.

94. **Kutsukake, K.** 1994. Excretion of the anti-s factor through a flagellar substructure couples flagellar gene expression with flagellar assembly in *Salmonella typhimurium. Mol. Gen. Genet.* **243:**605–612.

95. **Kutyrev, V. V., Y. A. Popov, and O. A. Protsenko.** 1986. Pathogenicity plasmids of the plague microbe (*Yersinia pestis*). *Mol. Genet. Mikrobiol. Virusol.* **6:**3–11.

96. **Lambert de Rouvroit, C. L., C. Sluiters, and G. R. Cornelis.** 1992. Role of the transcriptional activator,

VirF, and temperature in the expression of the pYV plasmid genes of *Yersinia enterocolitica. Mol. Microbiol.* **6:**395–409.

97. **Lapidus, A., N. Galleron, A. Sorokin, and D. Ehrlich.** 1997. Sequence analysis of the *Bacillus subtilis* chromosome region between the *terC* and *odhAB* loci cloned in yeast artificial chromosome. GenBank accession no. AF027868.

98. **Laroche, Y., M. Van Bouchaute, and G. Cornelis.** 1984. A restriction map of virulence plasmid pVYE439-80 from a serogroup 9 *Yersinia enterocolitica* strain. *Plasmid* **12:**67–70.

99. **Lee, L. A., J. Taylor, G. P. Carter, B. Quinn, J. J. Farmer III, and R. V. Tauxe.** 1991. *Yersinia enterocolitica* O:3: an emerging cause of pediatric gastroenteritis in the United States. *J. Infect. Dis.* **163:** 660–663.

100. **Lee, V. T., D. M. Anderson, and O. Schneewind.** 1998. Targeting of *Yersinia* Yop proteins into the cytosol of HeLa cells: one-step translocation of YopE across bacterial and eukaryotic membranes is dependent on SycE chaperone. *Mol. Microbiol.* **28:**593–601.

101. **Leung, K. Y., B. S. Reisner, and S. C. Straley.** 1990. YopM inhibits platelet aggregation and is necessary for virulence of *Yersinia pestis* in mice. *Infect. Immun.* **58:**3262–3271.

102. **Leung, K. Y., and S. C. Straley.** 1989. The *yopM* gene of *Yersinia pestis* encodes a released protein having homology with the human platelet surface protein GPlb a. *J. Bacteriol.* **171:**4623–4632.

103. **Malakooti, J., B. Ely, and P. Matsumura.** 1994. Molecular characterization, nucleotide sequence, and expression of the *fliO, fliP, fliQ,* and *fliR* genes of *Escherichia coli. J. Bacteriol.* **176:**189–197.

104. **Malakooti, J., Y. Komeda, and P. Matsumura.** 1989. DNA sequence analysis, gene product identification, and localization of flagellar motor components of *Escherichia coli. J. Bacteriol.* **171:**2728–2734.

105. **Michiels, T., and G. Cornelis.** 1988. Nucleotide sequence and transcription analysis of *yop51* from *Yersinia enterocolitica* W22703. *Microb. Pathog.* **5:**449–459.

106. **Michiels, T., and G. R. Cornelis.** 1991. Secretion of hybrid proteins by the *Yersinia* Yop export system. *J. Bacteriol.* **173:**1677–1685.

107. **Michiels, T., J. C. Vanooteghem, C. L. Lambert de Rouvroit, B. China, A. Gustin, P. Boudry, and G. R. Cornelis.** 1991. Analysis of *virC,* an operon involved in the secretion of Yop proteins by *Yersinia enterocolitica. J. Bacteriol.* **173:**4994–5009.

108. **Michiels, T., P. Wattiau, R. Brasseur, J. M. Ruysschaert, and G. Cornelis.** 1990. Secretion of Yop proteins by yersiniae. *Infect. Immun.* **58:**2840–2849.

109. **Mills, S. D., A. Boland, M. P. Sory, P. Van der Smissen, C. Kerbourch, B. B. Finlay, and G. R. Cornelis.** 1997. *Yersinia enterocolitica* induces apoptosis in macrophages by a process requiring functional type III secretion and translocation mechanisms and involving YopP, presumably acting as an effector protein. *Proc. Natl. Acad. Sci. USA* **94:**12638–12643.

110. **Minamino, T., T. Iino, and K. Kutuskake.** 1994. Molecular characterization of the *Salmonella typhimurium flhB* operon and its protein products. *J. Bacteriol.* **176:**7630–7637.

111. **Moll, A., P. A. Manning, and K. N. Timmis.** 1980. Plasmid-determined resistance to serum bacterial activity: a major outer membrane protein, the *traT* gene product, is responsible for plasmid-specified serum resistance in *Escherichia coli. Infect. Immun.* **28:**359–367.

112. **Monack, D. M., J. Mecsas, N. Ghori, and S. Falkow.** 1997. *Yersinia* signals macrophages to undergo apoptosis and YopJ is necessary for this cell death. *Proc. Natl. Acad. Sci. USA* **94:**10385–10390.

113. **Moore, D., C. M. Hamilton, K. Manneewannakul, Y. Mintz, L. S. Frost, and K. Ippen-Ihler.** 1993. The *Escherichia coli* K-12 F plasmid gene *traX* is required for acetylation of F pilin. *J. Bacteriol.* **175:** 1375–1383.

114. **Mori, H., A. Kondo, A. Ohshima, T. Ogura, and S. Hiraga.** 1986. Structure and function of the F plasmid genes essential for partitioning. *J. Mol. Biol.* **192:**1–15.

115. **Mulder, B., T. Michiels, M. Simonet, M. P. Sory, and G. Cornelis.** 1989. Identification of additional virulence determinants on the pYV plasmid of *Yersinia enterocolitica* W227. *Infect. Immun.* **57:**2534–2541.

116. **Munson, M. A., and P. Baumann.** 1995. Swiss-Prot accession no. P42394.

117. **Neyt, C., and G. R. Cornelis.** 1999. Role of SycD, the chaperone of the *Yersinia* Yop translocators YopB and YopD. *Mol. Microbiol.* **31:**143–156.

118. **Neyt, C., M. Iriarte, V. Ha Thi, and G. R. Cornelis.** 1997. Virulence and arsenic resistance in yersiniae. *J. Bacteriol.* **179:**612–619.

119. **Nielsen, A. K., P. Thorsted, T. Thisted, E. G. H. Wagner, and K. Gerdes.** 1991. The rifampicin inducible

genes *srnB* from F and *pnd* from R483 are regulated by antisense RNAs and mediate plasmid maintenance by killing of plasmid-free segregants. *Mol. Microbiol.* **5:**1961–1973.

120. **Nilles, M. L., A. W. Williams, E. Skrzypek, and S. C. Straley.** 1997. *Yersinia pestis* LcrV forms a stable complex with LcrG and may have a secretion-related regulatory role in the low-Ca^{2+} response. *J. Bacteriol.* **179:**1307–1316.

121. **Nilles, M. L., K. A. Fields, and S. C. Straley.** 1998. The V antigen of *Yersinia pestis* regulates Yops vectorial targeting as well as Yops secretion through effects on YopB and LcrG. *J. Bacteriol.* **180:** 3410–3420.

122. **Palmer, L. E., S. Hobbie, J. E. Galan, and J. B. Bliska.** 1998. YopJ of *Yersinia pseudotuberculosis* is required for the inhibition of macrophage TNFa production and downregulation of the MAP kinases p38 and JNK. *Mol. Microbiol.* **27:**953–965.

123. **Payne, P. L., and S. C. Straley.** 1998. YscO of *Yersinia pestis* is a mobile core component of the Yop secretion system. *J. Bacteriol.* **180:**3882–3890.

124. **Payne, P. L., and S. C. Straley.** YscP of *Yersinia pestis* is a secreted component of the Yop secretion system. Submitted for publication.

125. **Pegues, D. A., M. J. Hantman, I. Behlau, and S. I. Miller.** 1995. PhoP/PhoQ transcriptional repression of *Salmonella typhimurium* invasion genes: evidence for a role in protein secretion. *Mol. Microbiol.* **17:** 169–181.

126. **Perry, R. D.** 1993. Acquisition and storage of inorganic iron and hemin by the yersiniae. *Trends Microbiol.* **1:**142–147.

127. **Perry, R. D., and J. D. Fetherston.** 1997. *Yersinia pestis*—etiological agent of plague. *Clin. Microbiol. Rev.* **10:**35–66.

128. **Perry, R. D., P. A. Harmon, W. S. Bowmer, and S. C. Straley.** 1986. A low-Ca^{2+} response operon encodes the V antigen of *Yersinia pestis. Infect. Immun.* **54:**428–434.

129. **Perry, R. D., S. C. Straley, J. D. Fetherston, D. J. Rose, J. Gregor, and F. R. Blattner.** 1998. DNA sequencing and analysis of the low-Ca^{2+} response plasmid pCD1 of *Yersinia pestis* KIM5. *Infect. Immun.* **66:**4611–4623.

130. **Persson, C., R. Nordfelth, A. Holmström, S. Håkansson, R. Rosqvist, and H. Wolf-Watz.** 1995. Cell-surface-bound *Yersinia* translocate the protein tyrosine phosphatase YopH by a polarized mechanism into the target cell. *Mol. Microbiol.* **18:**135–150.

131. **Persson, C., N. Carballeira, H. Wolf-Watz, and M. Fällman.** 1997. The PTPase YopH inhibits uptake of *Yersinia*, tyrosine phosphorylation of p130^{Cas} and FAK, and the associated accumulation of these proteins in peripheral focal adhesions. *EMBO J.* **16:**2307–2318.

132. **Philipp, W. J., S. Poulet, K. Eiglmeier, L. Pascopella, V. Balasubramanian, B. Heym, S. Bergh, B. R. Bloom, W. R. Jacobs, Jr., and S. T. Cole.** 1996. An integrated map of the genome of the tubercle bacillus, *Mycobacterium tuberculosis* H37Rv, and comparison with *Mycobacterium leprae. Proc. Natl. Acad. Sci. USA* **93:**3132–3137.

133. **Plano, G. V., S. S. Barve, and S. C. Straley.** 1991. LcrD, a membrane-bound regulator of the *Yersinia pestis* low-calcium response. *J. Bacteriol.* **173:**7293–7303.

134. **Plano, G. V., and S. C. Straley.** 1993. Multiple effects of *lcrD* mutations in *Yersinia pestis. J. Bacteriol.* **175:**3536–3545.

135. **Plano, G. V., and S. C. Straley.** 1995. Mutations in *yscC, yscD,* and *yscG* prevent high-level expression and secretion of V antigen and Yops in *Yersinia pestis. J. Bacteriol.* **177:**3843–3854.

136. **Pohiman, R. F., F. Lu, L. Wang, M. I. Moré, and S. C. Winans.** 1993. Genetic and biochemical analysis of an endonuclease encoded by the Inc plasmid pKM101. *Nucleic Acids Res.* **21:**4867–4872.

137. **Portnoy, D. A., and S. Falkow.** 1981. Virulence-associated plasmids from *Yersinia enterocolitica* and *Yersinia pestis. J. Bacteriol.* **148:**877–883.

138. **Portnoy, D. A., S. L. Moseley, and S. Falkow.** 1981. Characterization of plasmids and plasmid-associated determinants of *Yersinia enterocolitica* pathogenesis. *Infect. Immun.* **31:**775–782.

139. **Portnoy, D. A., H. Wolf-Watz, I. Bolin, A. B. Beeder, and S. Falkow.** 1984. Characterization of common virulence plasmids in *Yersinia* species and their role in the expression of outer membrane proteins. *Infect. Immun.* **43:**108–114.

140. **Prère, M. F., M. Chandler, and O. Fayet.** 1990. Transposition in *Shigella dysenteriae:* isolation and analysis of IS*911,* a new member of the IS*3* group of insertion sequences. *J. Bacteriol.* **172:**4090–4099.

141. **Price, S. B., C. Cowan, R. D. Perry, and S. C. Straley.** 1991. The *Yersinia pestis* V antigen is a regulatory

protein necessary for Ca^{2+}-dependent growth and maximal expression of low-Ca^{2+} response virulence genes. *J. Bacteriol.* **173:**2649–2657.

142. **Price, S. B., K. Y. Leung, S. S. Barve, and S. C. Straley.** 1989. Molecular analysis of *lcrGVH,* the V antigen operon of *Yersinia pestis. J. Bacteriol.* **171:**5646–5653.

143. **Ramakrishnan, G., J. L. Zhao, and A. Newton.** 1991. The cell cycle-regulated flagellar gene *flbF* of *Caulobacter crescentus* is homologous to a virulence locus (*lcrD*) of *Yersinia pestis. J. Bacteriol.* **173:** 7283–7292.

144. **Reisner, B. S., and S. C. Straley.** 1992. *Yersinia pestis* YopM: thrombin binding and overexpression. *Infect. Immun.* **60:**5242–5252.

145. **Rimpiläinen, M., A. Forsberg, and H. Wolf-Watz.** 1992. A novel protein, LcrQ, involved in the low-calcium response of *Yersinia pseudotuberculosis* shows extensive homology to YopH. *J. Bacteriol.* **174:** 3355–3363.

146. **Roggenkamp, A., H.-R. Neuberger, A. Flügel, T. Schmoll, and J. Heesemann.** 1995. Substitution of two histidine residues in YadA protein of *Yersinia enterocolitica* abrogates collagen binding, cell adherence and mouse virulence. *Mol. Microbiol.* **16:**1207–1219.

147. **Roggenkamp, A., K. Ruckdeschel, L. Leitritz, R. Schmitt, and J. Heesemann.** 1996. Deletion of amino acids 29 to 81 in adhesion protein YadA of *Yersinia enterocolitica* serotype O:8 results in selective abrogation of adherence to neutrophils. *Infect. Immun.* **64:**2506–2514.

148. **Roggenkamp, A., A. M. Geiger, L. Leitritz, A. Kessler, and J. Heesemann.** 1997. Passive immunity to infection with *Yersinia* spp. mediated by anti-recombinant V antigen is dependent on polymorphism of V antigen. *Infect. Immun.* **65:**446–451.

149. **Rosqvist, R., I. Bölin, and H. Wolf-Watz.** 1988. Inhibition of phagocytosis in *Yersinia pseudotuberculosis:* a virulence plasmid-encoded ability involving the Yop2b protein. *Infect. Immun.* **56:**2139–2143.

150. **Rosqvist, R., A. Forsberg, M. Rimpiläinen, T. Bergman, and H. Wolf-Watz.** 1990. The cytotoxic protein YopE of *Yersinia* obstructs the primary host defence. *Mol. Microbiol.* **4:**657–667.

151. **Rosqvist, R., A. Forsberg, and H. Wolf-Watz.** 1991. Intracellular targeting of the *Yersinia* YopE cytotoxin in mammalian cells induces actin microfilament disruption. *Infect. Immun.* **59:**4562–4569.

152. **Rosqvist, R., K.-E. Magnusson, and H. Wolf-Watz.** 1994. Target cell contact triggers expression and polarized transfer of *Yersinia* YopE cytotoxin into mammalian cells. *EMBO J.* **13:**964–972.

153. **Rosqvist, R., M. Skurnik, and H. Wolf-Watz.** 1988. Increased virulence of *Yersinia pseudotuberculosis* by two independent mutations. *Nature* **334:**522–525.

154. **Ruckdeschel, K., S. Harb, A. Roggenkamp, M. Hornef, R. Zumbihl, S. Kohler, J. Heesemann, and B. Rouot.** 1998. *Yersinia enterocolitica* impairs activation of transcription factor NF-kB: involvement in the induction of programmed cell death and in the suppression of the macrophage TNF-α production. *J. Exp. Med.* **187:**1069–1079.

155. **Ruckdeschel, K., J. Machold, A. Roggenkamps, S. Schubert, J. Pierre, R. Zumbihi, J. P. Liautard, J. Heesemann, and B. Rouot.** 1997. *Yersinia enterocolitica* promotes deactivation of macrophage mitogen-activated protein kinases extracellular signal-regulated kinase-1/2, p38, and c-Jun NH$_2$-terminal kinase. *J. Biol. Chem.* **272:**15920–15927.

156. **Ruckdeschel, K., A. Roggenkamp, V. Lafont, P. Mangeat, J. Heesemann, and B. Rouot.** 1997. Interaction of *Yersinia enterocolitica* with macrophages leads to macrophage cell death through apoptosis. *Infect. Immun.* **65:**4813–4821.

157. **Ruckdeschel, K., A. Roggenkamp, S. Schubert, and J. Heesemann.** 1996. Differential contribution of *Yersinia enterocolitica* virulence factors to evasion of microbicidal action of neutrophils. *Infect. Immun.* **64:**724–733.

158. **Sarker, M., and G. R. Cornelis.** Unpublished data.

159. **Sarker, M. R., C. Neyt, I. Stainier, and G. R. Cornelis.** 1998. The *Yersinia* Yop virulon: LcrV is required for extrusion of the translocators YopB and YopD. *J. Bacteriol.* **180:**1207–1214.

160. **Sarker, M. R., M.-P. Sory, A. P. Boyd, M. Iriarte, and G. R. Cornelis.** 1998. LcrG is required for efficient translocation of *Yersinia* Yop effector proteins into eukaryotic cells. *Infect. Immun.* **66:**2976–2979.

161. **Schesser, K., A.-K. Spiik, J.-M. Dukuzumuremyl, M. F. Neurath, S. Pettersson, and H. Wolf-Watz.** 1998. The *yopJ* locus is required for *Yersinia*-mediated inhibition of NF-kB activation and cytokine expression: YopJ contains a eukaryotic SH2-like domain that is essential for its repressive activity. *Mol. Microbiol.* **28:**1067–1079.

162. **Schesser, K., E. Frithz-Lindsten, and H. Wolf-Watz.** 1996. Delineation and mutational analysis of the

Yersinia pseudotuberculosis YopE domains which mediate translocation across bacterial and eukaryotic cellular membranes. *J. Bacteriol.* **178:**7227–7233.

163. **Schulte, R., P. Wattlau, E. L. Hartland, R. M. Robins Browne, and G. R. Cornelis.** 1996. Differential secretion of interleukin-8 by human epithelial cell lines upon entry of virulent or nonvirulent *Yersinia enterocolitica. Infect. Immun.* **64:**2106–2113.

164. **Skrzypek, E., and S. C. Straley.** 1993. LcrG, a secreted protein involved in negative regulation of the low-calcium response in *Yersinia pestis. J. Bacteriol.* **175:**3520–3528.

165. **Skrzypek, E., and S. C. Straley.** 1995. Differential effects of deletions in *lcrV* on secretion of V antigen, regulation of the low-Ca^{2+} response, and virulence of *Yersinia pestis. J. Bacteriol.* **177:**2530–2542.

166. **Skurnik, M., Y. El Tahir, M. Saarinen, S. Jalkanen, and P. Toivanen.** 1994. YadA mediates specific binding of enteropathogenic *Yersinia enterocolitica* to human intestinal submucosa. *Infect. Immun.* **62:** 1252–1261.

167. **Skurnik, M., and P. Toivanen.** 1992. LcrF is the temperature-regulated activator of the *yadA* gene of *Yersinia enterocolitica* and *Yersinia pseudotuberculosis. J. Bacteriol.* **174:**2047–2051.

168. **Skurnik, M., and H. Wolf-Watz.** 1989. Analysis of the *yopA* gene encoding the Yop1 virulence determinants of *Yersinia* spp. *Mol. Microbiol.* **3:**517–529.

169. **Sodeinde, O. A., and J. D. Goguen.** 1988. Genetic analysis of the 9.5-kilobase virulence plasmid of *Yersinia pestis. Infect. Immun.* **56:**2743–2748.

170. **Sory, M. P., and G. R. Cornelis.** 1994. Translocation of a hybrid YopE-adenylate cyclase from *Yersinia enterocolitica* into HeLa cells. *Mol. Microbiol.* **14:**583–594.

171. **Sory, M. P., A. Boland, I. Lambermont, and G. R. Cornelis.** 1995. Identification of the YopE and YopH domains required for secretion and internalization into the cytosol of macrophages, using the *cyaA* gene fusion approach. *Proc. Natl. Acad. Sci. USA* **92:**11998–12002.

172. **Sory, M. P., C. Kerbourch, and G. R. Cornelis.** Unpublished data.

173. **Stainier, I., and G. R. Cornelis.** Unpublished data.

174. **Stainier, I., M. Iriarte, and G. R. Cornelis.** 1997. YscM1 and YscM2, two *Yersinia enterocolitica* proteins causing down regulation of *yop* transcription. *Mol. Microbiol.* **26:**833–843.

175. **Steibl, H. D., and F. M. Lewecke.** 1995. IS1222: analysis and distribution of a new insertion sequence in *Enterobacter agglomerans* 339. *Gene* **156:**37–42.

176. **Straley, S. C., and R. D. Perry.** 1995. Environmental modulation of gene expression and pathogenesis in *Yersinia. Trends Microbiol.* **3:**310–317.

177. **Straley, S. C., G. V. Plano, E. Skrzypek, P. L. Haddix, and K. A. Fields.** 1993. Regulation by Ca^{2+} in the *Yersinia* low-Ca^{2+} response. *Mol. Microbiol.* **8:**1005–1010.

178. **Strathdee, C. A., and R. Y. Lo.** 1989. Cloning, nucleotide sequence, and characterization of genes encoding the secretion function of the *Pasteurella haemolytica* leukotoxin determinant. *J. Bacteriol.* **171:**916–928.

179. **Su, X. D., N. Taddei, M. Stefani, G. Ramponi, and P. Nordlund.** 1994. The crystal structure of a low-molecular-weight phosphotyrosine protein phosphatase. *Nature* **370:**575–578.

180. **Tamm, A., A. M. Tarkkanen, T. K. Korhonen, P. Kuusela, P. Toivanen, and M. Skurnik.** 1993. Hydrophobic domains affect the collagen-binding specificity and surface polymerization as well as the virulence potential of the YadA protein of *Yersinia enterocolitica. Mol. Microbiol.* **10:**995–1011.

181. **Tauxe, R. V., J. Vandepitte, G. Wauters, S. M. Martin, V. Goossens, P. De Mol, R. Van Noyen, and G. Thiers.** 1987. *Yersinia enterocolitica* infections and pork: the missing link. *Lancet* **ii:**1129–1132.

182. **Tomb, J.-F., O. White, A. R. Kerlavage, R. A. Clayton, G. G. Sutton, R. D. Fleischmann, et al.** 1997. The complete genome sequence of the gastric pathogen *Helicobacter pylori. Nature* **388:**539–547.

183. **Utsumi, R., S. Katayama, M. Taniguchi, T. Horie, M. Ikeda, S. Igaki, H. Nakagawa, A. Miwa, H. Tanabe, and M. Noda.** 1994. Newly identified genes involved in the signal transduction of *Escherichia coli* K-12. *Gene* **140:**73–77.

184. **Vanooteghem, J.-C., and G. R. Cornelis.** 1990. Structural and functional similarities between the replication region of the *Yersinia* virulence plasmid and the RepFIIA replicons. *J. Bacteriol.* **172:**3600–3608.

185. **Viitanen, A. M., P. Toivanen, and M. Skurnik.** 1990. The *lcrE* gene is part of an operon in the *lcr* region of *Yersinia enterocolitica* O:3. *J. Bacteriol.* **172:**3152–3162.

186. **Wattiau, P., B. Bernier, P. Deslee, T. Michiels, and G. R. Cornelis.** 1994. Individual chaperones required for Yop secretion by *Yersinia. Proc. Natl. Acad. Sci. USA* **91:**10493–10497.

187. **Wattiau, P., and G. R. Cornelis.** 1993. SycE, a chaperone-like protein of *Yersinia enterocolitica* involved in the secretion of YopE. *Mol. Microbiol.* **8:**123–131.

188. **Wattiau, P., and G. R. Cornelis.** 1994. Identification of DNA sequences recognized by VirF, the transcriptional activator of the *Yersinia yop* regulon. *J. Bacteriol.* **176:**3878–3884.

189. **Wattiau, P., S. Woestyn, and G. R. Cornelis.** 1996. Customized secretion chaperones in pathogenic bacteria. *Mol. Microbiol.* **20:**255–262.

190. **Wauters, G., S. Aleksic, J. Charlier, and G. Schulze.** 1991. Somatic and flagellar antigens of *Yersinia enterocolitica* and related species. *Contrib. Microbiol. Immunol.* **12:**239–243.

191. **Wauters, G., V. Goossens, M. Janssens, and J. Vandepitte.** 1988. New enrichment method for isolation of pathogenic *Yersinia enterocolitica* serogroup O:3 from pork. *Appl. Environ. Microbiol.* **54:**851–854.

192. **Williams, A. W., and S. C. Straley.** 1998. YopD of *Yersinia pestis* plays a role in negative regulation of the low-calcium response in addition to its role in translocation of Yops. *J. Bacteriol.* **180:**350–358.

193. **Woestyn, S., A. Allaoui, P. Wattiau, and G. R. Cornelis.** 1994. YscN, the putative energizer of the *Yersinia* Yop secretion machinery. *J. Bacteriol.* **176:**1561–1569.

194. **Woestyn, S., M. P. Sory, A. Boland, O. Lequenne, and G. R. Cornelis.** 1996. The cytosolic SycE and SycH chaperones of *Yersinia* protect the region of YopE and YopH involved in translocation across eukaryotic cell membranes. *Mol. Microbiol.* **20:**1261–1271.

195. **Yahr, T. L., J. Goranson, and D. W. Frank.** 1996. Exoenzyme S of *Pseudomonas aeruginosa* secreted by a type III secretion pathway. *Mol. Microbiol.* **22:**991–1003.

196. **Yoshioka, Y., Y. Fujita, and E. Ohtsubo.** 1990. Nucleotide sequence of the promoter-distal region of the *tra* operon of plasmid R100, including *traI* (DNA helicase I) and *traD* genes. *J. Mol. Biol.* **214:**39–53.

197. **Yother, J., and J. D. Goguen.** 1985. Isolation and characterization of Ca^{2+}-blind mutants of *Yersinia pestis. J. Bacteriol.* **164:**704–711.

Pathogenicity Islands and Other Mobile Virulence Elements
Edited by J. B. Kaper and J. Hacker
© 1999 American Society for Microbiology, Washington, D.C.

Chapter 7

Pathogenicity Islands and the Evolution of *Salmonella* Virulence

Eduardo A. Groisman, Anne-Béatrice Blanc-Potard, and Keiichi Uchiya

The salmonellae are gram-negative bacteria which are responsible for a variety of disease syndromes in humans and domesticated animals. There is a single species in the genus *Salmonella—Salmonella enterica*—which encompasses >2,300 serotypes. *Salmonella* serotypes are defined by the flagellar and lipopolysaccharide antigens, and this classification does not reflect genetic relatedness within the species, host specificity, or type of disease. For example, subspecies I includes serovar Typhi, a human-adapted serotype that is the causal agent of typhoid fever; serovar Typhimurium, which is responsible for gastroenteritis in humans and a typhoid-like disease in mice; and the bacteremia-causing serovar Choleraesuis. The salmonellae are responsible for an estimated 16 million annual cases of typhoid fever, primarily in developing countries, and untold millions of cases of gastroenteritis in both industrialized and developing countries.

The salmonellae are typically acquired through the consumption of contaminated water or food, and they experience a number of environments during the course of infection (83). They endure the acidic pH of the stomach before adhering to and entering the cells that line the epithelium of the small intestine. The invasive microorganisms destined to cause systemic disease can survive in blood and are genetically equipped to replicate within the macrophages of the liver and spleen, and the microorganisms that cause chronic infection often "hide" in the gallbladder.

In this chapter, we discuss the structure and function of *Salmonella*-specific DNA segments that play a role in virulence. These DNA segments are of different lengths (i.e., from 1.6 to 40 kb), vary in their distribution among the salmonellae, and play distinct roles during infection. The vast majority of these sequences are located in the chromosome, but some reside within the large virulence plasmid present in certain *Salmonella* serovars. The properties of SPI-1 through SPI-5 are listed in Table 1.

THE SPI-1 PATHOGENICITY ISLAND

Genetic Structure and Organization

SPI-1 is a 40-kb DNA segment located at 63 min on the *S. enterica* serovar Typhimurium chromosome. It is flanked by two housekeeping genes, *fhlA* and *mutS* (102), and

Eduardo A. Groisman, Anne-Béatrice Blanc-Potard, and Keiichi Uchiya • Department of Molecular Microbiology, Howard Hughes Medical Institute, Washington University School of Medicine, St. Louis, MO 63110.

Table 1. *Salmonella* PAIs

PAI	Size (kb)	Location (min)	Role in virulence
SPI-1	40	63	Invasion of epithelial cells, macrophage apoptosis
SPI-2	40	30.7	Intracellular proliferation, systemic disease
SPI-3	17	81	Intramacrophage survival
SPI-4	25	92	Intramacrophage survival
SPI-5	7	20	Enteropathogenesis

this distinguishes it from other pathogenicity islands (PAIs), which are typically adjacent to tRNA genes. While the mechanism by which SPI-1 integrated into the *Salmonella* chromosome remains unknown, an IS*3* element is present at the right end of SPI-1 (4). SPI-1 sequences have been detected in all *Salmonella* subspecies tested, indicating that this island is ancestral to the genus (46, 108). SPI-1 appears to be genetically stable in the laboratory; however, environmental isolates belonging to serovars Senftenberg and Litchfield were found to harbor large deletions encompassing several SPI-1 genes (54).

SPI-1 contains at least 31 genes which code for a type III secretion apparatus, its effector proteins and corresponding chaperones, and regulatory factors (Fig. 1). The SPI-1 type III system, designated Inv-Spa, is similar to that encoded within the virulence plasmid of *Shigella flexneri* and, to a lesser extent, to the type III secretion apparatuses of pathogenic *Yersinia* strains (see reference 79) for a review of type III secretion systems). The organization of the *Salmonella spa, sip,* and *prg* genes is remarkably highly conserved with the corresponding gene clusters in the *Shigella* plasmid (58, 85, 86, 110). As expected, the degree of similarity between the *Salmonella* and *Shigella* components of the secretion apparatus is higher than that for secreted proteins (58, 79, 93). However, the *Shigella* plasmid is an unlikely source of SPI-1 genes because *Shigella* is a relatively recent pathogen.

Function of SPI-1-Encoded Proteins

The type III secretion system encoded within SPI-1 mediates the translocation of several proteins into eukaryotic cells. The translocated proteins modulate different host functions,

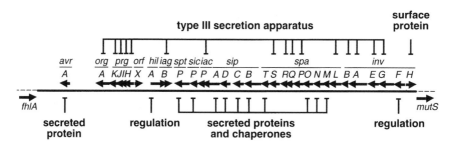

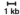
1 kb

Figure 1. Physical and genetic map of the SPI-1 PAI of *S. enterica.*

including membrane ruffling and interference with signal transduction pathways. These proteins are responsible for the ability of *Salmonella* to enter nonphagocytic cells and to promote apoptosis in macrophages.

Structural Components of the SPI-1 Secretion Apparatus

The type III secretion machinery is organized in a supramolecular structure that is distinct from the flagellar apparatus and which spans both the inner and outer membranes of the *Salmonella* envelope (90). This includes a base resembling the flagellar basal body, with two upper and two lower rings, and a complex structure resembling a needle (80 nm long, 13 nm wide) on the cell surface. InvG, PrgH, and PrgK are the most abundant proteins in highly purified preparations of the needle complexes, which are absent from strains carrying mutations in the *invG, prgH,* or *prgK* gene (90).

InvG exhibits similarity to the PulD family of specialized Sec-independent translocases (84) and is the only component that exhibits similarity to type II secretion systems. In a recombinant *Escherichia coli* strain, InvG forms an oligomeric ring-like structure that is 15 nm wide (30), the same size calculated for the needle. It has been proposed that localization of InvG to the outer membrane is dependent upon the InvH protein (30, 32), a situation that would be unique for *Salmonella* because InvH homologs have not been identified in other type III systems. PrgH and PrgK are predicted to be membrane lipoproteins (13, 110). A *prgH*::Tn*phoA* mutant exhibits defects in the protein profile of culture supernatants, indicating that *prgH*, or a downstream gene, is required for secretion (110).

The InvA, SpaP, SpaQ, and SpaR proteins are predicted to localize to the inner membrane (47, 58) and might be components of the basal structure of the secretion machinery. InvA has eight potential membrane-spanning domains and a cytoplasmic hydrophilic C-terminal region (47). Complementation experiments, as well as the use of chimeric proteins with *Shigella* and *Yersinia* homologs, suggest that the N-terminal region of InvA serves as a membrane anchor or may be involved in the formation of a pore in the inner membrane whereas the specificity determinants may be located at the carboxy terminus (52). Based on secondary-structure predictions and sequence similarity to membrane-associated proteins, the SpaP, SpaQ, and SpaR proteins might be inner membrane proteins. These proteins are required for secretion of the SipB, SipC, and SpaN proteins (25, 58); however, the particular contribution of SpaP, SpaQ, and SpaR to secretion remains unknown.

The SpaL protein (also known as InvC) exhibits similarity to the catalytic subunit of the F_0F_1 ATPase family of proteins and shows ATP-hydrolyzing activity that is dependent on the presence of an intact Walker A nucleotide binding motif (35). *spaL* mutants are defective for secretion of the SpaN (also known as InvJ) and SopE (27, 69) proteins, suggesting that SpaL may provide energy to the export apparatus and that ATP hydrolysis may be required for protein translocation. The SpaS protein might also be involved in energizing the system, because it contains a motif that defines a group of mitochondrial proteins responsible for energy transfer (58); however, the role of SpaS in the SPI-1 secretion system remains to be determined.

Secreted Proteins

Several proteins exported via the Inv-Spa system are found in culture supernatants, and a subset of them are directly translocated into the cytoplasm of epithelial cells. There is a hierarchy in the set of secreted proteins because some of them are required for the secretion and/or translocation of other proteins. Like the substrates of other type III systems, the proteins secreted via the Inv-Spa system lack a cleavable N-terminal signal sequence.

Secreted proteins required for secretion and/or translocation of other proteins (SpaN, SpaO, SipD, SipB, and SipC). The SpaN and SpaO proteins (28, 58) are required for secretion of all substrates by the SPI-1 secretory system, and thus they can be considered part of the export apparatus (25). The SpaN protein contains a Walker A nucleotide binding motif, which does not appear to be necessary for invasion (28). The SipD protein acts downstream of SpaN and SpaO because it modulates secretion of the SipA, SipB, and SipC proteins but not of the SpaN and SpaO proteins (25, 85). The SipD protein is also likely to be secreted, but analysis of culture supernatants gave ambiguous results due to the similar molecular weights of the SipD and SpaN proteins (25, 85). The SipB and SipC proteins (also known as SspB and SspC, respectively), which are translocated into the cytoplasm of cultured epithelial cells, are themselves required for the translocation (but not secretion) of certain effector proteins into the host cell and may therefore be considered translocases (26).

Secreted proteins with effector functions (SptP, AvrA, SipA, SopB, SopD, SopE, and SipB). At least six proteins are translocated into cultured epithelial cells by the SPI-1 secretion system (42, 48, 68, 134). This is in addition to the SipB and SipC proteins, which function as protein translocases but are also detected in the cytosol of host cells. SipA was originally believed to be secreted but not translocated. However, it is not involved in the export process itself (26, 27), and recent evidence indicates that it can bind actin and may participate in membrane ruffling (135).

The SptP protein exhibits similarity to two bacterial toxins in the N-terminal domain and to tyrosine phosphatases in the C-terminal region (87). Microinjection of purified SptP protein resulted in reversible disruption of the actin cytoskeleton (42). A similar result was obtained after microinjection of either half of the SptP protein, suggesting that SptP is organized in two independent domains that affect similar cellular functions. The SptP protein exhibits tyrosine phosphatase activity, which is dependent on a conserved Cys residue in the putative active site. It has been proposed that SptP modulates intracellular host cell signaling rather than a signal transduction pathway in *Salmonella,* because the bacteria are largely devoid of tyrosine phosphate (87). The cellular target of the SptP protein remains unknown, and candidate target molecules are components of the signaling cascades involving the small GTP binding protein Rho. An *sptP* mutant retained the ability to disrupt actin (42) and to invade cultured epithelial cells, suggesting that disruption of the host cell cytoskeleton may be mediated by several *Salmonella* proteins, some of which may have redundant functions. In addition, inactivation of *sptP* impaired the ability of *Salmonella* to colonize the spleen in orally infected mice (87).

The SopB and SopE proteins were first identified in serovar Dublin by analysis of the culture supernatants of a mutant deficient in the secretion of flagellin and Sip proteins (48, 134). Curiously, SopB and SopE are encoded outside SPI-1: *sopB* is part of the SPI-5 PAI at 20 min in the Dublin chromosome (133), and *sopE* is part of a cryptic bacteriophage located at 61 min in the Typhimurium chromosome (69). The Typhimurium SopB homolog (i.e., SigD) was identified during a search for invasion loci mapping outside SPI-1 (78). This is surprising because neither SopB nor the *Shigella* SopB homolog (IpgD) is required for invasion (2, 48).

The SopB protein promotes fluid secretion and inflammatory responses in the infected ileum (48). It has recently been shown that purified SopB protein has inositol phosphate phosphatase activity (107). This activity may account for the increase in the intracellular levels of inositol 1,4,5,6-tetrakisphosphate resulting from *Salmonella* infection of human intestinal epithelial cells (34). Since this molecule promotes chloride secretion in *Salmonella*-infected cells, SopB may be responsible for the fluid secretion and diarrhea that accompany *Salmonella* infection. A *sopD* mutant exhibits the same phenotype as a *sopB* mutant (48), but the biochemical function of the SopD protein remains unknown.

The SopE protein promotes efficient bacterial entry into nonphagocytic cells but it is not required for virulence in mice (69, 134). Transient expression or microinjection of SopE into epithelial cells stimulates membrane ruffling and cytoskeletal reorganization, morphological changes that promote the internalization of an invasion-defective *Salmonella* strain (67). In addition, SopE expression stimulates the activation of the mitogen-activated protein kinase JNK. SopE-mediated ruffling and nuclear responses require the function of the Rho-like GTPases Rac-1 and CDC42. In vitro, SopE stimulates GDP-GTP nucleotide exchange by interacting directly with these proteins (67). Hence, SopE can directly activate Rho GTPase signaling pathways that are required for nuclear and cytoskeletal responses.

The AvrA protein displays sequence similarity to an avirulence factor from the plant pathogen *Xanthomonas campestris* pv. vesicatoria. This suggests that AvrA might be involved in a hypersensitive-type response, which in plants activates a defense mechanism that leads to cell death in specific hosts (68). Consistent with this notion, the *avrA* gene is absent from certain host-specific *Salmonella* serovars (68) and the AvrA homolog in *Yersinia* has been implicated in apoptosis (103, 104). However, an *avrA* mutant behaves like wild-type *Salmonella* in invasion of epithelial cells and mouse virulence (68). Thus, demonstration of the ability of AvrA to induce a hypersensitive-type response will require the identification of a nonpermissive host in which AvrA could exert its putative avirulence function by interacting with specific resistance gene products.

In addition to its role as effector translocase, the SipB protein has been recently shown to bind and activate proapoptotic protease caspase 1 (77). These data indicate that the inability of *sipB* mutants to induce macrophage apoptosis (21, 77) is due to the absence of a direct effector function of SipB on macrophage cytotoxicity rather than to the lack of translocation of another effector protein.

Chaperones

Substrate proteins of type III secretion systems are often associated with specific chaperones, which are typically encoded in the vicinity of the cognate substrate protein genes and are required for the stabilization and/or translocation of these proteins. The SPI-1-encoded SicP, SpaM, and SpaT proteins exhibit features common to type III secretion chaperones, including high charge, small size, and potential to form α-helices. SicP appears to be an SptP chaperone because it binds directly to the N-terminal region of SptP and because a null mutation in *sicP* causes degradation of the SptP protein (41). SpaM/InvI is a candidate chaperone for SpaN and SpaO, because a mutation in *spaM* prevents secretion of these proteins (43). The SpaT (also known as SicA) protein might be a chaperone for the SipB and SipC proteins (86), because the *Shigella* SpaT homolog (IpgC) is a chaperone that stabilizes the IpaB and IpaC proteins (99). In addition, the SigD/SopB protein, which is encoded outside of SPI-1, may use SigE/PipC as a chaperone, since this protein exhibits features common to chaperones and is required for SigD secretion (78, 133).

SPI-1 Proteins of Unknown Function

InvH is a membrane-associated protein that is required for both efficient adherence and entry into epithelial cells. Originally thought to function as an adhesin (4), InvH has been recently implicated in the secretion of SipC and possibly of SipA and SipD (128). This could be because InvH mediates the proper localization of InvG in the outer membrane (30, 32). The InvE protein (51), which exhibits sequence similarity to the *Yersinia* YopN protein, appears to regulate the secretion process, because an *invE* mutant secreted the SpaN protein only upon exposure to cultured epithelial cells (136). Finally, the IacP protein belongs to the family of acyl carrier proteins and has been proposed to be involved in the posttranslational modification of exported proteins (85).

Role in Virulence

The major role of SPI-1 is to govern bacterial entry into nonphagocytic cells. However, SPI-1 genes have also been implicated in inflammation and macrophage apoptosis.

Role in Invasion

The SPI-1 island is required for invasion in several *Salmonella* serovars including Typhimurium, Typhi, Enteritidis, Gallinarum, and Dublin (46, 76). Most of the SPI-1 genes are required to induce the membrane ruffling and cytoskeletal reorganization of the host cell which precede bacterial internalization. On the other hand, the *invB, sipA, sptP,* and *avrA* genes are dispensable for invasion, which has been attributed to SPI-1 genes having redundant functions. The role of *prgI, prgJ, iagB,* and *iacP* in invasion has not been investigated.

M cells play a pivotal role in the pathogenesis of serovar Typhimurium, because they are the primary site of bacterial entry into the mouse intestine. Noninvasive mutants harboring defects in SPI-1 genes are generally unable to invade and destroy M cells of ileal Peyer's patches in a murine ligated-intestinal-loop model (23, 82, 111). On the other hand, *invG* and *invH* mutants, which are less invasive in cultured cells, have no detectable defect in a rabbit ileal-loop invasion assay (96). It has been proposed that *Salmonella* can invade M cells by an *inv*-independent mechanism, because *invA* and *invG* mutants retain the ability to invade M cells in some experiments (24). The use of different invasion mechanisms is dependent on the inoculum composition, which might modulate the expression of invasion genes (23).

Role in Adherence

Except for *invH*, SPI-1 genes do not appear to be required for adherence to epithelial cells (4), indicating that attachment and entry are genetically separate events. The extent of the defects of *invH* mutants is different for different *Salmonella* serovars (4), and some *invH* mutants of serovar Enteritidis are deficient for invasion but not adherence (120).

Role in Inflammation

The SopB/SigD and InvH proteins have been implicated in the induction of fluid secretion and inflammatory responses in the infected ileum, provoked by the migration of polymorphonuclear leukocytes into the intestinal mucosa and the gut lumen (128). The interaction of *Salmonella* with epithelial cells elicits transepithelial signaling to polymorphonuclear leukocytes, and mutations in SPI-1 genes prevented the organism from eliciting such a response in a cell culture model of human intestinal epithelium (97).

Role in Macrophage Cytotoxicity

When grown under conditions that promote invasiveness (see below), *Salmonella* is cytotoxic for both cultured and bone marrow-derived macrophages, inducing apoptosis in these cells (21, 105). This effect is dependent on the SPI-1 type III secretion system and several of its secreted proteins, because mutants defective in the *invA, invG, spaN, spaO, sipB, sipC,* or *sipD* gene are not cytotoxic. Interestingly, IpaB, the *Shigella* homolog of SipB, has been implicated in *Shigella*-induced apoptosis (137), and SipB can partially rescue an *ipaB* mutant for this property (76). As described above, the SipB protein can bind and activate the proapoptotic protease caspase 1 (77). It remains controversial whether *Salmonella* needs to be internalized by the macrophages to promote apoptosis (21, 105). On the other hand, apoptosis of human colon epithelial cells was found to result from infection by *S. enterica* serovar Dublin in a process that required a functional *invA* gene and the ability to replicate within host cells (88). The significance of macrophage and epithelial cell apoptosis in the pathogenesis of salmonellosis remains to be established.

Role in Mouse Virulence

Mutants defective in *invA, orgA, invG, sipC, sipD, hilA, invF,* or *spaR* are attenuated 30- to 100-fold when administered to mice orally but are as virulent as wild-type *Salmonella* if inoculated intraperitoneally (44, 82, 111). This is consistent with the notion that these SPI-1 genes are required for passage through the intestinal epithelium and Peyer's patches but not for later stages of the infection process. One possible exception is the *prgH* gene, because a *prgH*::Tn*phoA* mutant has a 50% lethal dose (LD_{50}) that is 10 times higher than that of wild-type *Salmonella* whether mice are inoculated orally or intraperitoneally (13). This result is surprising because mutations in other components of the Inv/Spa secretion apparatus are not attenuated by the intraperitoneal route. One possible interpretation for this result is that the *prgH*::Tn*phoA* mutation is interfering with the proper function of the type III secretion apparatus encoded within the SPI-2 island, which is required for systemic infection (see below). Complementation studies and the use of nonpolar mutations should clarify this issue. Finally, inactivation of SPI-1 effector proteins has rather minor effects on virulence attenuation (42, 68, 85, 134), which have been attributed to redundancy in the functions provided by these proteins.

Regulation of SPI-1 Genes

The ability of *Salmonella* to invade epithelial cells is affected by growth conditions (82, 92). Expression of the *orgA, invF, prgH, prgK, sipC,* and *sipA* genes is increased under low-oxygen, high-osmolarity, and low-pH conditions (6), which are believed to mimic the gut environment experienced by *Salmonella*. These invasion genes are regulated by a cascade of transcriptional regulators encoded within and outside SPI-1 (Fig. 2). SPI-1 genes are organized in several transcriptional units: *avrA, prgHIJK, orfX, hilAiagB,* the *sipABCD* operon that might extend through *sptP,* a large operon including genes from *invF* through *spaT,* and *invH* (Fig. 1).

Regulation of Invasion Gene Expression

The coordinate regulation of invasion genes by environmental conditions is mediated by HilA (6), a protein that exhibits similarity to the DNA binding domain of the OmpR/ToxR family of transcriptional activators (5). While HilA is required for transcrip-

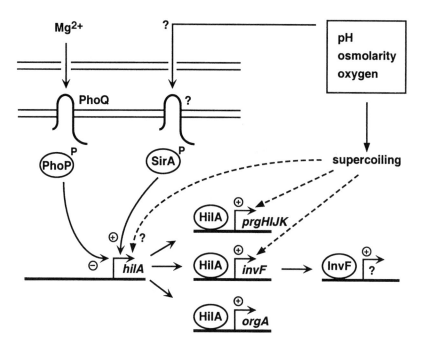

Figure 2. Model for transcriptional control of invasion genes by regulatory proteins encoded within and outside SPI-1.

tion of several invasion genes (5, 6), binding of the HilA protein to SPI-1 gene promoters has not been demonstrated. One of the HilA-regulated genes is *invF* (5, 6), which encodes a protein of the AraC family of transcriptional activators (84). The *invF* gene is required for invasion, but the targets of InvF regulation remain unknown (84). It is unlikely that HilA senses environmental cues per se, because it contains neither a domain that could be involved in signal sensing nor a phosphoryl acceptor domain that could be phosphorylated by a sensor protein. Thus, it appears that environmental cues sensed by various regulatory systems control the expression of the HilA protein, which then activates the transcription of invasion determinants.

HilA is negatively regulated by the PhoP-PhoQ two-component system (6), which is encoded outside SPI-1 and regulates gene expression in response to environmental Mg^{2+} concentrations (50). Expression of *hilA* and HilA-regulated genes is repressed in a *phoQ* mutant that promotes increased transcription of PhoP-activated genes and decreased expression of PhoP-repressed genes (6, 13, 110). This mutant is defective for epithelial-cell invasion and secretion of Sip proteins (13, 110). Invasion genes, being PhoP-repressed loci, are expected to be expressed in millimolar concentrations of Mg^{2+}, a condition that *Salmonella* would encounter in extracellular environments. However, transcriptional regulation of *hilA* or other invasion genes by Mg^{2+} has not been demonstrated.

On the other hand, HilA is positively regulated by SirA, a protein that belongs to the family of response regulators of the two-component systems (81). The SirA protein, which is also encoded outside SPI-1, is essential for both secretion of Sip/Ssp proteins and invasion of epithelial cells (81). SirA positively regulates expression of the SopB/SigD protein, which is secreted by the SPI-1 type III secretion system but is encoded outside of SPI-1 (81). The cognate sensor for the SirA protein and the signals that control its activity have not been identified. In addition, two loci, *sirB* and *sirC,* that are able to complement a *sirA* mutant have been isolated, but their role in the SirA-HilA regulatory cascade remains to be established (81).

Environmental parameters known to affect the level of DNA supercoiling—oxygen tension, osmolarity, and pH—regulate invasion gene expression. Consistent with a role of DNA supercoiling in invasion gene expression, inhibition of DNA gyrase activity by novobiocin treatment (which reduces the level of negative supercoiling) decreases the transcription of *invA* in serovar Typhimurium (45) and of *invG* and *prgH* in serovar Typhi (91). This effect might be through the *hilA* promoter, which controls expression of these genes.

Regulation of the SPI-1 Type III Secretion System by Contact with Epithelial Cells

Translocation of proteins by the SPI-1 type III secretion system into the cytoplasm of cultured epithelial cells is induced by growing bacteria under conditions that promote *Salmonella* invasiveness and is mediated by extracellular bacteria, since cytochalasin D, which inhibits bacterial invasion, does not prevent protein translocation (25, 26, 48, 134). In addition, secretion of SpaN/InvJ is stimulated by the presence of epithelial cells and/or serum (136). However, recent experiments indicate that contact with eukaryotic cells is not required for secretion of the SpiC protein (31). Indeed, secretion of SpiC and SpaN could be promoted in laboratory-grown bacteria by shifting the culture from pH 6.0 to 8.0 (31), a condition believed to mimic the passage from the acidic environment of the stomach to the mildly alkaline environment of the small intestine.

The interaction of *Salmonella* with cultured cells also leads to the transient assembly of bacterial surface structures called invasomes (53). These structures are different from flagella or pili and have a diameter of 60 nm and a length of 0.3 to 1 μm (53). Although the components of the invasome have not been identified, it has been proposed that the SPI-1 secretion system and/or its substrates are part of it because formation of this structure was affected by mutations in several SPI-1 genes (43, 53). However, this view has been recently challenged because appendage formation has been observed in strains harboring mutations in the Inv-Spa secretion system (112).

THE SPI-2 PATHOGENICITY ISLAND

Genetic Structure and Organization

The SPI-2 island was independently discovered during the characterization of a *Salmonella*-specific clone (109) and of a set of mutants defective in causing systemic infection in BALB/c mice (116). SPI-2 is located at 30.7 min on the serovar Typhimurium chromosome and is flanked by the *pykF* gene and the *valV* tRNA gene (72). Sequences hybridizing to the center and to the *valV* end of the 40-kb SPI-2 have been detected in seven of the eight subspecific groups of *S. enterica* (72, 108), the exception being strains of *S. bongori,* which is the most divergent subspecific group of *Salmonella.* On the other hand, a probe corresponding to the *pykF* end of SPI-2 gave a positive signal with two of three *S. bongori*

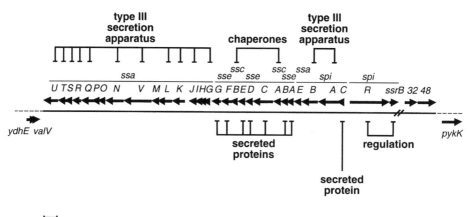

Figure 3. Physical and genetic map of the SPI-2 PAI of *S. enterica.*

isolates and was negative for all isolates of *S. enterica* subspecies IIIa and IV (72). The latter region may have an independent origin and may not be involved in virulence, since attenuating mutations have not been recovered in the 13-kb segment proximal to *pykF* (116).

SPI-2 contains at least 32 genes which code for a type III secretion apparatus, its putative effector proteins and corresponding chaperones, and a two-component regulatory system (22, 72, 74, 75, 109, 116, 125) (Fig. 3). The SPI-2 type III system, designated Spi-Ssa, is most closely related to the type III system encoded within the locus of enterocyte effacement PAI of enteropathogenic *E. coli* (37). Moreover, it is clearly distinct from the Inv-Spa system encoded within SPI-1, suggesting the Inv-Spa and Spi-Ssa systems were independently acquired by *Salmonella* (as opposed to the *spi-ssa* locus arising by gene duplication of the *inv-spa* region, which is ancestral to the species [108]).

Function of SPI-2-Encoded Proteins

The function of most SPI-2-encoded type III system proteins, effectors, and chaperones is based solely on the phenotype exhibited by related proteins from other type III systems, and a direct role in protein secretion and/or translocation is yet to be demonstrated (22, 74, 75, 109, 116, 125). The biochemical characterization of the Spi-Ssa system has been hampered because in vitro conditions allowing the expression and translocation of SPI-2-encoded effectors have not been defined. However, recent work has established that the SpiC protein is an effector and that SpiA is a component of the type III secretion apparatus necessary for translocation of the SpiC protein into the host cell cytosol (123).

The *ssaG, ssaJ, ssaK, ssaL, ssaV, ssaN, ssaO, ssaQ, ssaR, ssaS, ssaT, ssaU, spiA,* and *spiB/ssaD* gene products exhibit sequence similarity to various components of type III secretion systems (22, 74, 75, 109, 125). The *sscA* and *sscB* gene products may be effector chaperones (75) because they exhibit sequence similarity to the *Yersinia* chaperone SycD (129) and to the *Shigella* chaperone IppI (7), respectively. It has been suggested that *sseA, sseB, sseC, sseD, sseE, sseF,* and *sseG* encode effectors of the Spi-Ssa system, because they appear to be cotranscribed and because some of the encoded products display sequence similarity to known effectors of the type III system present in enteropathogenic *E. coli* strains (22, 75). Specifically, the *sseB, sseC,* and *sseD* gene products exhibit weak similarity to the EspA, EspD, and EspB proteins, respectively. The EspA protein of enteropathogenic *E. coli* can form surface appendages and is involved in host signaling (89), and together with EspB (131), it has been implicated in protein translocation.

The SPI-2 genes *spiC, ssaH, ssaI, ssaM, ssaO,* and *ssaP* do not exhibit sequence identity to known components of other type III secretion systems, raising the possibility that these genes encode effectors specific to SPI-2. This seems to be the case for the SpiC protein, which has been detected in the cytosol of macrophages infected with wild-type *Salmonella* but not in the cytosol of macrophages infected with a mutant defective in the type III secretion gene *spiA* (123). The SpiC protein appears to be responsible for the ability of *Salmonella* to alter intracellular trafficking, because a *spiC* mutant could not inhibit phagosome-endosome fusion. Moreover, purified SpiC protein inhibited vesicle fusion in a defined in vitro system (123). The 127-amino-acid SpiC does not have homologs in the sequence databases, and the mechanism by which it inhibits vesicle fusion is presently unclear.

Spi-Ssa provides the first example of a type III system that functions from within a cell, as opposed to classical type III systems, which deliver proteins by extracellularly located microorganisms (79). Because *Salmonella* remains within a membrane-bound vacuole inside host cells, Ochman et al. (109) originally suggested that proteins translocated via the Spi-Ssa system across the phagosomal membrane and into the host cytosol may inhibit phagosome-lysosome fusion or phagosome acidification. The inability of *spiA* and *spiC* mutants to affect intracellular trafficking supports this hypothesis.

Role in Virulence

Mutants defective in SPI-2 genes were first recovered during a screening for genes defective in causing systemic disease (73). The majority of SPI-2 mutants are highly attenuated for virulence in mice and in their ability to grow within mammalian cells.

Role in Mouse Virulence

Mutants harboring insertions in the SPI-2 type III secretion genes are attenuated in mice whether they are inoculated orally, intravenously, or intraperitoneally. The LD_{50} of such mutants is typically 5 orders of magnitude higher than that of wild-type *Salmonella* for intraperitoneally inoculated mice (22, 73, 75, 109, 116). This indicates that the SPI-2 island is necessary to cause systemic disease and distinguishes it from SPI-1, inactivation of which attenuates virulence only in animals inoculated by the oral route.

The attenuating effects of mutations in the two-component regulatory genes *ssrA*/*spiR* and *ssrB* were as strong as those in components of the Spi-Ssa secretion apparatus (75, 109, 116). Likewise, inactivation of the effector genes *spiC* (123), *sseA, sseB,* and *sseC* prevented *Salmonella* from causing a lethal infection in mice (75). In contrast, mutation of other putative effector genes had weak (*sseF* and *sseG*) or no (*sseE*) attenuating effect (75).

The SPI-2 island appears to confer the ability to proliferate in host tissues, because mutants defective in the regulatory gene *spiR*/*ssrA* or in the putative effector gene *sseB* failed to accumulate in the mesenteric lymph nodes and could not be detected in the liver or spleen 3 days after oral administration (22). Moreover, the numbers of an *ssaL* mutant bacteria did not change 16 h after intraperitoneal inoculation whereas those of wild-type *Salmonella* continually increased until the animal died (115). Failure of the *ssaL* mutant to accumulate in the spleen has been attributed to its inability to replicate within host cells rather than to an increased susceptibility to host microbicidal mechanisms (115). The virulence phenotypes exhibited by SPI-2 mutants are similar to those exhibited by strains defective in the plasmid-encoded *spv* genes (63). However, competition experiments with single and double mutants defective in SPI-2 and/or *spv* genes suggest that these two loci govern distinct virulence pathways (115).

Role in Intracellular Proliferation

The SPI-2 island was first proposed to mediate survival and proliferation within host cells because a *spiA* mutant did not replicate within J774 macrophages as well as wild-type *Salmonella* did (109). While this view was transiently challenged (74), it has now been corroborated and extended with the demonstration that several SPI-2 mutants are also defective in survival and replication within RAW 264.7 macrophages, periodate-elicited peritoneal macrophages from C3H/HeN mice, and HEp-2 cells (22, 75). Moreover, *S. bongori*, which lacks SPI-2 genes (72, 108), is unable to survive within J774 macrophages (124).

Role of SPI-2 in Epithelial Cell Invasion and Resistance to Antimicrobial Compounds

It has been hypothesized that the Spi-Ssa type III secretion system interacts with the Inv-Spa system, because certain SPI-2 mutants showed a 10-fold reduction in their ability to invade HEp-2 cells (74). These noninvasive mutants failed to secrete the SPI-1-encoded SipC protein and exhibited reduced cytotoxicity toward macrophages, phenotypes that are dependent on a functional Inv-Spa type III system. Further characterization of this phenomenon indicated that transcription of the SPI-1 genes *sipC, prgK,* and *hilA* was reduced in the invasion-defective SPI-2 mutants (33).

However, the SPI-1 and SPI-2 type III systems are unlikely to interact under normal physiological conditions because (i) the phenotypic defect of the *ssaV* mutations was allele specific and invasion of a nonpolar *ssaV* mutant was the same as that exhibited by wild-type *Salmonella* (33, 74); (ii) plasmids harboring wild-type copies of the *ssaTU* genes could not restore SpiC secretion to an *ssaT* mutant (33); and (iii) the SPI-1 and SPI-2 genes are expressed under different conditions, which makes it rather unlikely that their respective type III components would coexist in a given tissue. Thus, this phenomenon most probably results from a dominant negative effect of the aberrant proteins produced in certain SPI-2 mutant strains.

Finally, interference with the flagellar assembly, which requires a distinct set of type III system components, could be responsible for the presence of a flagellin-derived fragment in the culture supernatants of *spiA* and *spiR/ssrA* mutants (109) but not in supernatants of other SPI-2 mutants (74). Likewise, the hypersusceptibility of certain SPI-2 mutants to polymyxin, gentamicin, and serum complement (33, 74) is most probably due to the disruption of the cell wall, resulting from the production of aberrant proteins.

Regulation of SPI-2 Genes

The SPI-2 island encodes a two-component system that consists of the putative sensor SpiR-SsaA and the response regulator SsrB (22, 109, 116). The 920-amino-acid SpiR/

SsrA has two predicted transmembrane domains that define a putative periplasmic domain of approximately 265 residues, which is presumably involved in sensing host signals, and a 600-amino-acid cytoplasmic region that exhibits sequence identity to sensor kinases and is most closely related to the C-terminal region of the RscC protein of *E. coli* (121). SpiR belongs to the subset of sensor kinases harboring a transmitter domain that is followed by a consensus receiver domain and a C-terminal domain. In these sensor kinases, sequential phosphorylation of these domains takes place before transfer of the phosphate to the cognate response regulator.

Transcription of the *ssaJ, ssaN, spiA,* and *sseB* genes is induced within macrophages in a SpiR-dependent manner (22). Bafilomycin A1 treatment, which prevents phagosome acidification, decreased the expression of these genes. On the other hand, transcription of the regulatory gene *spiR/ssrB* was induced within macrophages in a SpiR-independent manner and was only mildly affected by bafilomycin A1 treatment (22). Transcription of *spiR* is promoted early and precedes that of *ssaJ* and *spiA* (22). While the signal sensed by the SpiR protein remains unknown, expression of the *sseA* gene was detected in minimal but not in rich media (75). Transcription of *sseA* required a functional *spiR* gene but was unaltered in strains with mutations in *ssaJ* and *ssaT,* which encode components of the type III secretion system (22, 75).

THE SPI-3 PATHOGENICITY ISLAND

Genetic Structure and Organization

SPI-3 is a 17-kb segment located downstream of the *selC* tRNA gene at 81 min on the serovar Typhimurium chromosome (15). *selC* is the site of insertion of two PAIs and a retronphage in *E. coli* (18, 80, 98). SPI-3 was discovered when the *Salmonella selC* locus was examined for the presence of horizontally acquired sequences (15). Even though SPI-3 appears to be genetically stable, the distribution of SPI-3 sequences varies among the salmonellae: the right end of the island is present in all eight subspecies of the genus, whereas a four-gene cluster bracketed by remnants of insertion sequences located at the center of SPI-3 is found only in some of the subspecies (16). This suggests that evolution of SPI-3 sequences occurred via a multistep process.

Function of SPI-3-Encoded Proteins

SPI-3 harbors 10 open reading frames that appear to be organized in six transcriptional units (16). These include the *mgtCB* operon, which encodes a high-affinity Mg^{2+} transporter (MgtB) and a protein of unknown biochemical function (MgtC) (117). The MgtC protein is required for growth in low Mg^{2+} and is predicted to localize to the inner membrane, suggesting that it could mediate the transport of Mg^{2+} (15). The *Salmonella mgtC* gene confers the ability to grow in low Mg^{2+} upon *E. coli* K-12, which does have an *mgtC* gene (15). However, MgtC neither mediates the transport of Ni^{2+} or Co^{2+} by itself (17, 106) nor is necessary for membrane insertion or transport function of the MgtB protein (122). The hypothesis that MgtC is a transporter specific for Mg^{2+} (rather than Ni^{2+} or Co^{2+}) has not been tested but seems rather unlikely.

SPI-3 encodes a protein, designated MisL, that exhibits similarity in its C-terminal domain to the immunoglobulin A1 protease family of autotransported proteins, which have thus far been found only in pathogenic bacteria. These proteins consist of an N-terminal effector domain and a C-terminal conserved domain that forms a pore in the outer membrane through which the N-terminal domain is translocated (71). The highest degree of similarity is found between MisL and the AIDA-I protein from diffusely adherent *E. coli* (14) and the VirG protein from *Shigella flexneri* (55).

The MarT protein might be a regulator because it exhibits similarity in its N-terminal domain to the cytoplasmic domain of the ToxR protein from *Vibrio cholerae* (101). Like ToxR, MarT contains a potential transmembrane domain in its central region. However, the MarT protein has different amino acids at three of four positions shown to be important for ToxR function (16), raising the possibility that it plays a role other than transcriptional regulation. Also, the SugR protein might be involved in energy transfer, because it exhibits similarity to a putative ATP binding protein encoded in the genome of a clinical isolate of *E. coli* (95) and it contains an imperfect nucleotide-binding Walker A motif.

Role in Virulence

The *mgtC* gene is required for both intramacrophage survival and virulence in mice (15). MgtC mediates intramacrophage survival in the absence of the MgtB protein. This indicates that MgtC function does not require MgtB, a view supported by the identification of an *mgtC* homolog in the genome of *Mycobacterium tuberculosis,* which does not harbor *mgtB*. Addition of Mg^{2+} to macrophage tissue culture media can partially rescue the macrophage growth defect of the *mgtC* mutant (15), suggesting that the *Salmonella*-containing phagosome is a low-Mg^{2+} environment, which is consistent with the transcriptional induction of PhoP-activated genes in host cells (3, 49, 70, 125).

The *sugR, rhuM, misL, fidL, marT, slsA,* and *mgtB* genes appear to be dispensable for intramacrophage survival and invasion of epithelial cells (16). Because some of these genes have a restricted distribution within the salmonellae, they might be involved in other processes such as host specificity or chronic infection.

Regulation of SPI-3 Genes

Transcription of the *mgtCB* operon is induced in low-Mg^{2+} media via the PhoP-PhoQ two-component regulatory system (50, 118). However, regulation by PhoP is not a general feature of SPI-3 genes, because transcription of the *sugR, rhuM, misL,* and *marT* genes does not require the PhoP regulatory protein when bacteria are grown under laboratory conditions (16). Despite its similarity to the regulatory protein ToxR, MarT does not appear to control expression of the *sugR, rhuM, misL,* and *mgtC* genes or its own expression.

THE SPI-4 PATHOGENICITY ISLAND

SPI-4 is a 25-kb segment located downstream from a tRNA-like gene at 92 min on the serovar Typhimurium chromosome (132). SPI-4 harbors 18 open reading frames that might constitute a single operon. The products of three of them—ORF-C, ORF-D, and ORF-R—exhibit similarity to proteins involved in the secretion of toxins (132). However, there is no experimental data to support the hypothesis that these genes encode a type I secretion system involved in toxin secretion. A mutant harboring a transposon insertion in the ORF-L gene is defective in its ability to survive within macrophages (10, 38), yet it is unclear whether the ORF-L gene itself or a downstream gene is responsible for this phenotype. Surprisingly, 11 of the SPI-4-encoded proteins—ORF-F through ORF-P—are related to one another. This suggests that this region has been subjected to extensive recombination processes resulting in the partial duplication of some of these sequences.

THE SPI-5 PATHOGENICITY ISLAND

Genetic Structure, Organization, and Regulation

SPI-5 is a 7-kb island (or islet, depending on the definition used) located downstream from the *serT* tRNA gene at the 20-min region on the serovar Dublin chromosome (133). SPI-5 encodes six potential proteins, which include SopB, an inositol phosphate phosphatase secreted by the Inv-Spa type III secretion system (48, 107), and PipC, a small acidic protein proposed to be the SopB chaperone. SPI-5 also encodes a putative membrane protein, PipD, with sequence similarity to *Lactobacillus* dipeptidases, as well as three proteins of unknown function (133). The *sopB/sigD* and *pipC/sigE* genes exhibit sequence similarity to the *ipgD* and *ipgE* genes, which are located in the *Shigella* virulence plasmid next to the type III secretion structural *mxi* and *spa* genes. SPI-5-hybridizing sequences have been detected in the serotypes Typhimurium, Enteritidis, Choleraesuis, Gallinarum, and Pullorum (133). Expression of the *sigDE* genes is dependent on the SirA protein but does not require the HilA protein (78). This is surprising because the SirA protein regulates the transcription of several SPI-1 genes via HilA (81).

Role in Virulence

Insertions in the *sopB, pipA, pipB,* or *pipD* genes reduce fluid secretion and the inflammatory responses in a bovine ligated-ileal-loop model (134). In contrast, these mutants retain the ability to cause systemic disease in mice, since bacteria were recovered in similar numbers to those of the wild-type strain from the spleens and livers of inoculated animals (133). The specific contribution of these genes remains to be determined, because *sopB, pipC, pipB,* and *pipA* appear to be cotranscribed and complementation experiments have not been reported. Even though *pipD* is part of a separate transcriptional unit, a *pipD* mutant exhibits a virulence defect similar to that in strains with mutations in the *sopB* operon. None of the SPI-5 mutants exhibit invasion defects in serovar Dublin (133); however, a *sigE* (i.e., *pipC*) mutant of serovar Typhimurium was 10-fold reduced in invasion (78).

PATHOGENICITY ISLETS

Several other *Salmonella*-specific sequences have been implicated in virulence. These regions are typically smaller than SPI-1 and SPI-2 and have been referred to as pathogenicity islets (59). For example, the *sifA* gene is required to form filamentous structures in lysosomal vacuoles and to cause a lethal infection in mice (119). The 1.1-kb *sifA* gene is part of a 1.6-kb *Salmonella*-specific DNA segment located at 27 min on the serovar Typhimurium chromosome. This segment is flanked by 14-bp direct repeats and surrounded by the *potB* and *potC* genes, which correspond to the *potABCD* operon of *E. coli* K-12. The housekeeping *potABCD* operon, which mediates polyamine transport in *E. coli* K-12, is dispensable for mouse virulence in *Salmonella* (119).

At 25 min on the chromosome of serovar Typhimurium is a gene, *msgA*, that is required for the ability to replicate within macrophages and to cause a lethal infection in mice (65). The *msgA* gene encodes a 79-amino-acid protein that exhibits 36% sequence identity to a DNA damage-inducible protein of *E. coli* K-12 and 24 to 31% identity to bacteriophage-encoded SOS proteins. *msgA*-hybridizing sequences have been detected in serovars Typhi, Paratyphi A, Paratyphi C, and Enteriditis, as well as in the genomes of *Shigella sonnei*, *Shigella flexneri*, *Citrobacter freundii*, and *Klebsiella pneumoniae* but not in *E. coli*, *Vibrio cholerae*, *Yersinia enterocolitica*, *Morganella morganii*, or *Providencia stuartii* (65). The *msgA* gene is located 3 kb upstream of *pagC*, a gene that exhibits a narrower phylogenetic distribution than *msgA*, suggesting independent acquisition of these sequences (65). Mutants harboring transposon insertions in *pagC* are attenuated for virulence (100), but a strain with a deletion in *pagC* is fully virulent (66).

Five fimbrial loci have been identified in *Salmonella*, four of which are located in the chromosome: *fim*, *agfA*, *lpf*, and *ser* (12). These fimbrial genes exhibit a different distribution within the salmonellae. *fim* and *agf* are found in all serovars tested as well as in isolates of *S. bongori*. In contrast, *sef* and *lpf* exhibit a sporadic distribution (9). Inactivation of individual fimbrial loci reduces mouse virulence only moderately, but a mutant of Typhimurium defective in all fimbrial operons (including the plasmid-located *pef* [see below]) had an increased LD_{50} and a reduced capacity to colonize the intestinal lumen (127). A combination of horizontal gene transfer and deletion events seems to be responsible for the distribution of the *sef* and *lpf* fimbrial genes among the salmonellae (9). Since the adhesive properties of *Salmonella* are determined, in part, by the particular combination of fimbrial genes, this raises the possibility of these surface appendages conferring the particular host range of *Salmonella* subspecies and serovars (11). However, further experiments are required to demonstrate this hypothesis and rule out the possibility that the observed combinations of fimbrial loci arose by chance.

Finally, several promoters recovered by in vivo expression technology correspond to *Salmonella*-specific gene clusters (29). These gene clusters appear to have been acquired by horizontal gene transfer based on their phyologenetic distribution and their association with mobile genetic elements or linkage to tRNA-like genes. Deletion of some of these gene clusters reduced the ability of the resulting strains to compete with the wild-type parent during mixed infections (29). However, the identity of these *Salmonella*-specific genes, as well as the role they play in pathogenesis, remains unknown.

VIRULENCE PLASMID

Most pathogenic nontyphoidal serovars of *Salmonella* harbor a large plasmid that is required for virulence. While the size and genetic content of these plasmids vary among these serovars, they all contain five genes—*spvRABCD*—in a highly conserved 7.8-kb region (62). This five-gene cluster is necessary and sufficient to cause a lethal infection in mice (61). In serovar Typhimurium, the *spv* genes are necessary for proliferation but not for protection of the microorganisms from being killed (64). Infection of calves with the serovar Dublin demonstrated that the *spvR* gene is required for causing diarrhea and for growth within monocytes (94). The virulence plasmid also contains a fimbrial operon, designated *pef*, outside the 7.8-kb region that is essential for virulence (40).

The *spvR* gene, which is located upstream of the *spvABCD* genes, encodes a positive regulator that is necessary for transcription of the *spvABCD* operon (63). The *spvR* gene encodes a transcriptional activator of the LysR family. On the other hand, the *spvABCD* operon encodes proteins that do not exhibit sequence similarity to known proteins and their biochemical function remains unknown. Subcellular-localization studies showed that the SpvA protein localized to the outer membrane, the SpvB protein was present in both the cytoplasm and the inner membrane, the SpvC protein resided in the cytoplasm, and, interestingly, the SpvD protein was found in the supernatant (36).

The SpvR protein binds to the promoter regions of the *spvA* and *spvR* genes and activates the transcription of both genes (56). Expression of the *spvABCD* operon is also dependent on the stationary-phase-specific sigma factor RpoS (60). The *spvR* gene is transcribed at a basal level in the absence of both *spvR* and *rpoS,* while *spvA* expression is absolutely dependent on a functional *spvR* gene (19). However, expression of *spvR* increases during postexponential growth and *rpoS* is required for optimal transcription (1), suggesting that RpoS is the preferred sigma factor at the *spvR* promoter. Recently, the histone-like protein H-NS, which negatively controls the levels of RpoS, was shown to regulate *spv* gene expression independently of its function in controlling RpoS levels (114).

Expression of the *spv* genes is induced when the bacteria are in stationary growth phase or cultivated under a number of stress conditions, including iron limitation and low pH (126). Interestingly, expression of these genes is induced after phagocytosis of *Salmonella* by macrophages, intestinal epithelial cells, and hepatocytes, within the first hour after internalization (20, 39, 113). The recent demonstration that *spv* genes were maximally induced during exponential growth in a defined medium that mimics the intracellular environment of mammalian cells suggests that nutrient deprivation associated with the intracellular environment can induce *spv* expression and that cessation of growth may not be the most relevant inducing signal for *spv* gene expression (130).

REGULATING THE EXPRESSION OF HORIZONTALLY ACQUIRED SEQUENCES

The incorporation of PAIs allows a microorganism to gain access to new niches. However, for the incorporated sequences to be useful, their expression must take place at the correct time and place during infection and must be coordinated with that of the rest of the genome. Thus, while several transcriptional regulators are encoded within the SPI-1, SPI-2, and SPI-3 islands and in the virulence plasmid, expression of PAI genes is typically controlled by ancestral regulatory proteins.

The best example is provided by the PhoP-PhoQ system, which positively governs the expression of the *mgtC* gene in SPI-3 (50) and the *spvB* gene in the virulence plasmid (70) and negatively regulates the *prgH* gene in SPI-1 (13). The PhoP-PhoQ system is present in both pathogenic and nonpathogenic bacterial species, where it governs the adaptation to low-Mg^{2+} environments, and it has been hypothesized that these horizontally acquired sequences are regulated by the PhoP-PhoQ system because *Salmonella* determines its cellular location by examining the Mg^{2+} concentration in its surroundings (57). As discussed above, the ancestral SirA response regulator and the RpoS sigma factor also control the expression of various horizontally acquired sequences.

The presence of two distinct type III secretion systems (three if one considers the flagellum assembly components as a type III system) raises a fundamental question of what determines the specificity of a type III system so that only the effectors specific to the system are exported. One possibility is that the secretion apparatuses recognize still undefined features of the secreted proteins. While this hypothesis cannot be completely ruled out at present, it seems rather unlikely because components of the secretion machinery appear to be interchangeable among type III systems used by extracellular microorganisms. Alternatively, specificity may be achieved by the coordinate regulation of the effector and secretion apparatus genes: effector proteins encoded within SPI-1 would not be exported by the Spi-Ssa system, because no SPI-1 effectors would be made under conditions in which the Spi-Ssa system is made. Likewise, SPI-2-encoded effectors would not be present when the Inv-Spa system is produced. This model predicts that ectopic expression of effector proteins may result in inappropriate secretion and translocation of the effector proteins.

CONCLUSIONS

A large number of genes have been implicated in *Salmonella* virulence (59), many of which are specific to the genus and some of which are found only in particular serovars. Since diverging from *E. coli* some 100 million years ago, *Salmonella* has acquired several PAIs which rendered it a pathogen and expanded its ecological niche (8, 59). Incorporation of SPI-1, which conferred the ability to invade host cells, was essential for the successful colonization of intestinal tissues. The subsequent acquisition of the SPI-3 gene *mgtC* allowed replication in low-Mg^{2+} environments, including the host cell phagosome. SPI-2 was introduced later in the evolution of *Salmonella* and conferred upon the microorganism the ability to proliferate within host cells and to cause systemic disease. Other *Salmonella*-specific sequences may specify host range, govern other aspects of infection, or mediate growth in nonhost environments.

Acknowledgments. Work in our laboratory is supported by grants from the National Institutes of Health, the U.S. Department of Agriculture, the Cystic Fibrosis Foundation, and the North American Treaty Organization. E.A.G. is an Associate Investigator of the Howard Hughes Medical Institute.

REFERENCES

1. **Abe, A., H. Matsui, H. Danbara, K. Tanaka, H. Takahashi, and K. Kawahara.** 1994. Regulation of *spvR* gene expression of *Salmonella* virulence plasmid pKDSC50 in *Salmonella choleraesuis* serovar Choleraesuis. *Mol. Microbiol.* **12:**779–787.
2. **Allaoui, A., P. J. Sansonetti, and C. Parsot.** 1993. MxiD, an outer membrane protein necessary for the secretion of the *Shigella flexneri* Ipa invasins. *Mol. Microbiol.* **7:**59–68.
3. **Alpuche-Aranda, C. M., J. A. Swanson, W. P. Loomis, and S. I. Miller.** 1992. *Salmonella typhimurium* activates virulence gene transcription within acidified macrophage phagosomes. *Proc. Natl. Acad. Sci. USA* **89:**10079–10083.
4. **Altmeyer, R. M., J. K. McNern, J. C. Bossio, I. Rosenshine, B. B. Finlay, and J. E. Galán.** 1993. Cloning and molecular characterization of a gene involved in *Salmonella* adherence and invasion of cultured epithelial cells. *Mol. Microbiol.* **7:**89–98.
5. **Bajaj, V., C. Hwang, and C. A. Lee.** 1995. *hilA* is a novel *ompR/toxR* family member that activates the expression of *Salmonella typhimurium* invasion genes. *Mol. Microbiol.* **18:**715–727.
6. **Bajaj, V., R. L. Lucas, C. Hwang, and C. A. Lee.** 1996. Co-ordinate regulation of *Salmonella typhimurium* invasion genes by environmental and regulatory factors is mediated by control of *hilA* expression. *Mol. Microbiol.* **22:**703–714.

7. **Baudry, B., M. Kaczorek, and P. J. Sansonetti.** 1988. Nucleotide sequence of the invasion plasmid antigen B and C genes (ipaB and ipaC) of *Shigella flexneri*. *Microb. Pathog.* **4:**345–357.

8. **Bäumler, A. J.** 1997. The record of horizontal gene transfer in *Salmonella. Trends Microbiol.* **5:**318–322.

9. **Bäumler, A. J., A. J. Gilde, R. M. Tsolis, A. W. M. van der Velden, B. M. M. Ahmer, and F. Heffron.** 1997. Contribution of horizontal gene transfer and deletion events to development of distinctive patterns of fimbrial operons during evolution of *Salmonella* serotypes. *J. Bacteriol.* **179:**317–322.

10. **Bäumler, A. J., J. G. Kusters, I. Stojiljkovic, and F. Heffron.** 1994. *Salmonella typhimurium* loci involved in survival within macrophages. *Infect. Immun.* **62:**1623–1630.

11. **Bäumler, A. J., R. M. Tsolis, T. A. Ficht, and L. G. Adams.** 1998. Evolution of host adaptation in *Salmonella enterica. Infect. Immun.* **66:**4579–4587.

12. **Bäumler, A. J., R. M. Tsolis, and F. Heffron.** 1997. Fimbrial adhesins of *Salmonella typhimurium.* Role in bacterial interactions with epithelial cells. *Adv. Exp. Med. Biol.* **412:**149–158.

13. **Behlau, I., and S. I. Miller.** 1993. A PhoP-repressed gene promotes *Salmonella typhimurium* invasion of epithelial cells. *J. Bacteriol.* **175:**4475–4484.

14. **Benz, I., and M. A. Schmidt.** 1992. AIDA-I, the adhesin involved in diffuse adherence of the diarrhoeagenic *Escherichia coli* strain 2787 (O126:H27), is synthesized via a precursor molecule. *Mol. Microbiol.* **6:** 1539–1546.

15. **Blanc-Potard, A.-B., and E. A. Groisman.** 1997. The *Salmonella selC* locus contains a pathogenicity island mediating intramacrophage survival. *EMBO J.* **16:**5376–5385.

16. **Blanc-Potard, A.-B., F. Solomon, J. Kayser, and E. A. Groisman.** 1999. The SPI-3 pathogenicity island of *Salmonella enterica. J. Bacteriol.* **181:**998–1004.

17. **Blanc-Potard, A. B., and E. A. Groisman.** Unpublished results.

18. **Blum, G., M. Ott, A. Lischewski, A. Ritter, H. Imrich, H. Tschäpe, and J. Hacker.** 1994. Excision of large DNA regions termed pathogenicity islands from tRNA-specific loci in the chromosome of an *Escherichia coli* wild-type pathogen. *Infect. Immun.* **62:**606–614.

19. **Chen, C. Y., N. A. Buchmeier, S. Libby, F. C. Fang, M. Krause, and D. G. Guiney.** 1995. Central regulatory role for the RpoS sigma factor in expression of *Salmonella dublin* plasmid virulence genes. *J. Bacteriol.* **177:**5303–5309.

20. **Chen, C. Y., L. Eckmann, S. J. Libby, F. C. Fang, S. Okamoto, M. F. Kagnoff, J. Fierer, and D. G. Guiney.** 1996. Expression of *Salmonella typhimurium rpoS* and *rpoS*-dependent genes in the intracellular environment of eukaryotic cells. *Infect. Immun.* **64:**4739–4743.

21. **Chen, L. M., K. Kaniga, and J. E. Galán.** 1996. *Salmonella* spp. are cytotoxic for cultured macrophages. *Mol. Microbiol.* **21:**1101–1115.

22. **Cirillo, D. M., R. H. Valdivia, D. M. Monack, and S. Falkow.** 1998. Macrophage-dependent induction of the *Salmonella* pathogenicity island 2 type III secretion system and its role in intracellular survival. *Mol. Microbiol.* **30:**175–188.

23. **Clark, M. A., B. H. Hirst, and M. A. Jepson.** 1998. Inoculum composition and *Salmonella* pathogenicity island 1 regulate M-cell invasion and epithelial destruction by *Salmonella typhimurium. Infect. Immun.* **66:**724–731.

24. **Clark, M. A., K. A. Reed, J. Lodge, J. Stephen, B. H. Hirst, and M. A. Jepson.** 1996. Invasion of murine intestinal M cells by *Salmonella typhimurium inv* mutants severely deficient for invasion of cultured cells. *Infect. Immun.* **64:**4363–4368.

25. **Collazo, C. M., and J. E. Galán.** 1996. Requirement for exported proteins in secretion through the invasion-associated type III system of *Salmonella typhimurium. Infect. Immun.* **64:**3524–3531.

26. **Collazo, C. M., and J. E. Galán.** 1997. The invasion-associated type III system of *Salmonella typhimurium* directs the translocation of Sip proteins into the host cell. *Mol. Microbiol.* **24:**747–756.

27. **Collazo, C. M., and J. E. Galán.** 1997. The invasion-associated type-III protein secretion system in *Salmonella*—a review. *Gene* **192:**51–59.

28. **Collazo, C. M., M. K. Zierler, and J. E. Galán.** 1995. Functional analysis of the *Salmonella typhimurium* invasion genes *invI* and *invJ* and identification of a target of the protein secretion apparatus encoded in the *inv* locus. *Mol. Microbiol.* **15:**25–38.

29. **Conner, C. P., D. M. Heithoff, S. M. Julio, R. L. Sinsheimer, and M. J. Mahan.** 1998. Differential patterns of acquired virulence genes distinguish *Salmonella* strains. *Proc. Natl. Acad. Sci. USA* **95:** 4641–4645.

30. **Crago, A. M., and V. Koronakis.** 1998. *Salmonella* InvG forms a ring-like multimer that requires the InvH lipoprotein for outer membrane localization. *Mol. Microbiol.* **30:**47–56.

31. **Daefler, S.** 1999. Type III secretion by *Salmonella typhimurium* does not require contact with a eukaryotic host. *Mol. Microbiol.* **31:**45–51.

32. **Daefler, S., and M. Russel.** 1998. The *Salmonella typhimurium* InvH protein is an outer membrane lipoprotein required for the proper localization of InvG. *Mol. Microbiol.* **28:**1367–1380.

33. **Deiwick, J., T. Nikolaus, J. E. Shea, C. Gleeson, D. W. Holden, and M. Hensel.** 1998. Mutations in *Salmonella* pathogenicity island 2 (SPI2) genes affecting transcription of SPI1 genes and resistance to antimicrobial agents. *J. Bacteriol.* **180:**4775–4780.

34. **Eckmann, L., M. T. Rudolf, A. Ptasznik, C. Schultz, T. Jiang, N. Wolfson, R. Tsien, J. Fierer, S. B. Shears, M. F. Kagnoff, and A. E. Traynor-Kaplan.** 1997. D-*myo*-Inositol 1,4,5,6-tetrakisphosphate produced in human intestinal epithelial cells in response to *Salmonella* invasion inhibits phosphoinositide 3-kinase signaling pathways. *Proc. Natl. Acad. Sci. USA* **94:**14456–14460.

35. **Eichelberg, K., C. C. Ginocchio, and J. E. Galán.** 1994. Molecular and functional characterization of the *Salmonella typhimurium* invasion genes *invB* and *invC:* homology of InvC to the F_0F_1 ATPase family of proteins. *J. Bacteriol.* **176:**4501–4510.

36. **El-Gedaily, A., G. Paesold, and M. Krause.** 1997. Expression profile and subcellular location of the plasmid-encoded virulence (Spv) proteins in wild-type *Salmonella dublin. Infect. Immun.* **65:**3406–3411.

37. **Elliott, S. J., L. A. Wainwright, T. K. McDaniel, K. G. Jarvis, Y. K. Deng, L. C. Lai, B. P. McNamara, M. S. Donnenberg, and J. B. Kaper.** 1998. The complete sequence of the locus of enterocyte effacement (LEE) from enteropathogenic *Escherichia coli* E2348/69. *Mol. Microbiol.* **28:**1–4.

38. **Fields, P. I., R. V. Swanson, C. G. Haidaris, and F. Heffron.** 1986. Mutants of *Salmonella typhimurium* that cannot survive within the macrophage are avirulent. *Proc. Natl. Acad. Sci. USA* **83:**5189–5193.

39. **Fierer, J., L. Eckmann, F. Fang, C. Pfeifer, B. B. Finlay, and D. Guiney.** 1993. Expression of the *Salmonella* virulence plasmid gene *spvB* in cultured macrophages and nonphagocytic cells. *Infect. Immun.* **61:**5231–5236.

40. **Friedrich, M. J., N. E. Kinsey, J. Vila, and R. J. Kadner.** 1993. Nucleotide sequence of a 13.9 kb segment of the 90 kb virulence plasmid of *Salmonella typhimurium:* the presence of fimbrial biosynthetic genes. *Mol. Microbiol.* **8:**543–558.

41. **Fu, Y., and J. E. Galán.** 1998. Identification of a specific chaperone for SptP, a substrate of the centisome 63 type III secretion system of *Salmonella typhimurium. J. Bacteriol.* **180:**3393–3399.

42. **Fu, Y., and J. E. Galán.** 1998. The *Salmonella typhimurium* tyrosine phosphatase SptP is translocated into host cells and disrupts the actin cytoskeleton. *Mol. Microbiol.* **27:**359–368.

43. **Galán, J. E.** 1996. Molecular genetic bases of *Salmonella* entry into host cells. *Mol. Microbiol.* **20:**263–272.

44. **Galán, J. E., and R. Curtiss.** 1989. Cloning and molecular characterization of genes whose products allow *Salmonella typhimurium* to penetrate tissue culture cells. *Proc. Natl. Acad. Sci. USA* **86:**6383–6387.

45. **Galán, J. E., and R. Curtiss III.** 1990. Expression of *Salmonella typhimurium* genes required for invasion is regulated by changes in DNA supercoiling. *Infect. Immun.* **58:**1879–1885.

46. **Galán, J. E., and R. Curtiss III.** 1991. Distribution of the *invA, -B, -C,* and *-D* genes of *Salmonella typhimurium* among other *Salmonella* serovars: *invA* mutants of *Salmonella typhi* are deficient for entry into mammalian cells. *Infect. Immun.* **59:**2901–2908.

47. **Galán, J. E., C. Ginocchio, and P. Costeas.** 1992. Molecular and functional characterization of the *Salmonella* invasion gene *invA:* homology of InvA to members of a new protein family. *J. Bacteriol.* **174:**4338–4349.

48. **Galyov, E. E., M. W. Wood, R. Rosqvist, P. B. Mullan, P. R. Watson, S. Hedges, and T. S. Wallis.** 1997. A secreted effector protein of *Salmonella dublin* is translocated into eukaryotic cells and mediates inflammation and fluid secretion in infected ileal mucosa. *Mol. Microbiol.* **25:**903–912.

49. **Garcia-del Portillo, F., J. W. Foster, M. E. Maguire, and B. B. Finlay.** 1992. Characterization of the micro-environment of *Salmonella typhimurium*-containing vacuoles within MDCK epithelial cells. *Mol. Microbiol.* **6:**3289–3297.

50. **García-Véscovi, E., F. C. Soncini, and E. A. Groisman.** 1996. Mg^{2+} as an extracellular signal: environmental regulation of *Salmonella* virulence. *Cell* **84:**165–174.

51. **Ginocchio, C., J. Pace, and J. E. Galán.** 1992. Identification and molecular characterization of a *Salmonella typhimurium* gene involved in triggering the internalization of salmonellae into cultured epithelial cells. *Proc. Natl. Acad. Sci. USA* **89:**5976–5980.

52. **Ginocchio, C. C., and J. E. Galán.** 1995. Functional conservation among members of the *Salmonella typhimurium* InvA family of proteins. *Infect. Immun.* **63:**729–732.

53. **Ginocchio, C. C., S. B. Olmsted, C. L. Wells, and J. E. Galán.** 1994. Contact with epithelial cells induces the formation of surface appendages on *Salmonella typhimurium. Cell* **76:**717–724.

54. **Ginocchio, C. C., K. Rahn, R. C. Clarke, and J. E. Galán.** 1997. Naturally occurring deletions in the centisome 63 pathogenicity island of environmental isolates of *Salmonella* spp. *Infect. Immun.* **65:** 1267–1272.

55. **Goldberg, M. B., O. Barzu, C. Parsot, and P. J. Sansonetti.** 1993. Unipolar localization and ATPase activity of IcsA, a *Shigella flexneri* protein involved in intracellular movement. *J. Bacteriol.* **175:** 2189–2196.

56. **Grob, P., and D. G. Guiney.** 1996. In vitro binding of the *Salmonella dublin* virulence plasmid regulatory protein SpvR to the promoter regions of *spvA* and *spvR. J. Bacteriol.* **178:**1813–1820.

57. **Groisman, E. A.** 1998. The ins and outs of virulence gene expression: Mg^{2+} as a regulatory signal. *Bioessays* **20:**96–101.

58. **Groisman, E. A., and H. Ochman.** 1993. Cognate gene clusters govern invasion of host epithelial cells by *Salmonella typhimurium* and *Shigella flexneri. EMBO J.* **12:**3779–3787.

59. **Groisman, E. A., and H. Ochman.** 1997. How *Salmonella* became a pathogen. *Trends Microbiol.* **5:** 343–349.

60. **Guiney, D. G., S. Libby, F. C. Fang, M. Krause, and J. Fierer.** 1995. Growth-phase regulation of plasmid virulence genes in *Salmonella. Trends Microbiol.* **3:**275–279.

61. **Gulig, P. A., A. L. Caldwell, and V. A. Chiodo.** 1992. Identification, genetic analysis and DNA sequence of a 7.8-kb virulence region of the *Salmonella typhimurium* virulence plasmid. *Mol. Microbiol.* **6:**1395–1411.

62. **Gulig, P. A., H. Danbara, D. G. Guiney, A. J. Lax, F. Norel, and M. Rhen.** 1993. Molecular analysis of *spv* virulence genes of the *Salmonella* virulence plasmids. *Mol. Microbiol.* **7:**825–830.

63. **Gulig, P. A., and T. J. Doyle.** 1993. The *Salmonella typhimurium* virulence plasmid increases the growth rate of salmonellae in mice. *Infect. Immun.* **61:**504–511.

64. **Gulig, P. A., T. J. Doyle, J. A. Hughes, and H. Matsui.** 1998. Analysis of host cells associated with the Spv-mediated increased intracellular growth rate of *Salmonella typhimurium* in mice. *Infect. Immun.* **66:** 2471–2485.

65. **Gunn, J. S., C. M. Alpuche-Aranda, W. P. Loomis, W. J. Belden, and S. I. Miller.** 1995. Characterization of the *Salmonella typhimurium* pagC/pagD chromosomal region. *J. Bacteriol.* **177:**5040–5047.

66. **Gunn, J. S., W. J. Belden, and S. I. Miller.** 1998. Identification of phoP-phoQ activated genes within a duplicated region of the *Salmonella typhimurium* chromosome. *Microb. Pathog.* **25:**77–90.

67. **Hardt, W.-D., L.-M. Chen, K. E. Schuebel, X. R. Bustelo, and J. E. Galán.** 1998. S. *typhimurium* encodes an activator of Rho GTPases that induces membrane ruffling and nuclear responses in host cells. *Cell* **93:**815–826.

68. **Hardt, W.-D., and J. E. Galán.** 1997. A secreted *Salmonella* protein with homology to an avirulence determinant of plant pathogenic bacteria. *Proc. Natl. Acad. Sci. USA* **94:**9887–9892.

69. **Hardt, W.-D., H. Urlaub, and J. E. Galán.** 1998. A substrate of the centisome 63 type III protein secretion system of *Salmonella typhimurium* is encoded by a cryptic bacteriophage. *Proc. Natl. Acad. Sci. USA* **95:** 2574–2579.

70. **Heithoff, D. M., C. P. Conner, P. C. Hanna, S. M. Julio, U. Hentschel, and M. J. Mahan.** 1997. Bacterial infection as assessed by *in vivo* gene expression. *Proc. Natl. Acad. Sci. USA* **94:**934–939.

71. **Henderson, I. R., F. Navarro-García, and J. P. Nataro.** 1998. The great escape: structure and function of the autotransporter family. *Trends Microbiol.* **6:**370–378.

72. **Hensel, M., J. E. Shea, A. J. Bäumler, C. Gleeson, F. Blattner, and D. W. Holden.** 1997. Analysis of the boundaries of *Salmonella* pathogenicity island 2 and the corresponding chromosomal region of *Escherichia coli* K-12. *J. Bacteriol.* **179:**1105–1111.

73. **Hensel, M., J. E. Shea, C. Gleeson, M. D. Jones, E. Dalton, and D. W. Holden.** 1995. Simultaneous identification of bacterial virulence genes by negative selection. *Science* **269:**400–403.

74. **Hensel, M., J. E. Shea, B. Raupach, D. Monack, S. Falkow, C. Gleeson, T. Kubo, and D. F. Holden.** 1997. Functional analysis of *ssaJ* and the *ssaK/u* operon, 13 genes encoding components of the type III secretion apparatus of *Salmonella* pathogenicity island 2. *Mol. Microbiol.* **24:**155–167.

75. **Hensel, M., J. E. Shea, S. R. Waterman, R. Mundy, T. Nikolaus, G. Banks, A. Vazquez-Torres, C. Gleeson, F. C. Fang, and D. W. Holden.** 1998. Genes encoding putative effector proteins of the type III

secretion system of *Salmonella* pathogenicity island 2 are required for bacterial virulence and proliferation in macrophages. *Mol. Microbiol.* **30**:163–174.

76. **Hermant, D., R. Ménard, N. Arricau, C. Parsot, and M. Y. Popoff.** 1995. Functional conservation of the *Salmonella* and *Shigella* effectors of entry into epithelial cells. *Mol. Microbiol.* **17**:781–789.

77. **Hersh, D., D. M. Monack, M. R. Smith, N. Ghori, S. Falkow, and A. Zychlinsky.** 1999. The *Salmonella* invasin SipB induces macrophage apoptosis by binding to caspase-1. *Proc. Natl. Acad. Sci. USA* **96**: 2396–2401.

78. **Hong, K. H., and V. L. Miller.** 1998. Identification of a novel *Salmonella* invasion locus homologous to *Shigella ipgDE. J. Bacteriol.* **180**:1793–1802.

79. **Hueck, C. J.** 1998. Type III protein secretion systems in bacterial pathogens of animals and plants. *Microbiol. Mol. Biol. Rev.* **62**:379–433.

80. **Inouye, S., M. G. Sunshine, E. W. Six and M. Inouye.** 1991. Retronphage ϕR73: an *E. coli* phage that contains a retroelement and integrates into a tRNA gene. *Science* **252**:969–971.

81. **Johnston, C., D. A. Pegues, C. J. Hueck, C. A. Lee, and S. I. Miller.** 1996. Transcriptional activation of *Salmonella typhimurium* invasion genes by a member of the phosphorylated response-regulator superfamily. *Mol. Microbiol.* **22**:715–727.

82. **Jones, B. D., and S. Falkow.** 1994. Identification and characterization of a *Salmonella typhimurium* oxygen-regulated gene required for bacterial internalization. *Infect. Immun.* **62**:3745–3752.

83. **Jones, B. D., and S. Falkow.** 1996. Salmonellosis: host immune responses and bacterial virulence determinants. *Annu. Rev. Immunol.* **14**:533–561.

84. **Kaniga, K., J. C. Bossio, and J. E. Galán.** 1994. The *Salmonella typhimurium* invasion genes *invF* and *invG* encode homologues of the AraC and PulD family of proteins. *Mol. Microbiol.* **13**:555–568.

85. **Kaniga, K., D. Trollinger, and J. E. Galán.** 1995. Identification of two targets of the type III protein secretion system encoded by the *inv* and *spa* loci of *Salmonella typhimurium* that have homology to the *Shigella* IpaD and IpaA proteins. *J. Bacteriol.* **177**:7078–7085.

86. **Kaniga, K., S. Tucker, D. Trollinger, and J. E. Galán.** 1995. Homologs of the *Shigella* IpaB and IpaC invasins are required for *Salmonella typhimurium* entry into cultured epithelial cells. *J. Bacteriol.* **177**: 3965–3971.

87. **Kaniga, K., J. Uralil, J. B. Bliska, and J. E. Galán.** 1996. A secreted protein tyrosine phosphatase with modular effector domains in the bacterial pathogen *Salmonella typhimurium. Mol. Microbiol.* **21**:633–641.

88. **Kim, J. M., L. Eckmann, T. C. Savidge, D. C. Lowe, T. Witthoft, and M. F. Kagnoff.** 1998. Apoptosis of human intestinal epithelial cells after bacterial invasion. *J. Clin. Invest.* **102**:1815–1823.

89. **Knutton, S., I. Rosenshine, M. J. Pallen, I. Nisan, B. C. Neves, C. Bain, C. Wolff, G. Dougan, and G. Frankel.** 1998. A novel EspA-associated surface organelle of enteropathogenic *Escherichia coli* involved in protein translocation into epithelial cells. *EMBO J.* **17**:2166–2176.

90. **Kubori, T., Y. Matsushima, D. Nakamura, J. Uralil, M. Lara-Tejero, A. Sukhan, J. E. Galán, and S.-I. Aizawa.** 1998. Supramolecular structure of the *Salmonella typhimurium* type III protein secretion system. *Science* **280**:602–605.

91. **Leclerc, G. J., C. Tartera, and E. S. Metcalf.** 1998. Environmental regulation of *Salmonella typhi* invasion-defective mutants. *Infect. Immun.* **66**:682–691.

92. **Lee, C. A., and S. Falkow.** 1990. The ability of *Salmonella* to enter mammalian cells is affected by bacterial growth state. *Proc. Natl. Acad. Sci. USA* **87**:4304–4308.

93. **Li, J., H. Ochman, E. A. Groisman, E. F. Boyd, F. Solomon, K. Nelson, and R. K. Selander.** 1995. Relationship between evolutionary rate and cellular location among the Inv/Spa invasion proteins of *Salmonella enterica. Proc. Natl. Acad. Sci. USA* **92**:7252–7256.

94. **Libby, S. J., L. G. Adams, T. A. Ficht, C. Allen, H. A. Whitford, N. A. Buchmeier, S. Bossie, and D. G. Guiney.** 1997. The *spv* genes on the *Salmonella dublin* virulence plasmid are required for severe enteritis and systemic infection in the natural host. *Infect. Immun.* **65**:1786–1792.

95. **Lim, D.** 1992. Structure and biosynthesis of unbranched multicopy single-stranded DNA by reverse transcriptase in a clinical *Escherichia coli* isolate. *Mol. Microbiol.* **6**:3531–3542.

96. **Lodge, J., G. R. Douce, I. I. Amin, A. J. Bolton, G. D. Martin, S. Chatfield, G. Dougan, N. L. Brown, and J. Stephen.** 1995. Biological and genetic characterization of Tn*phoA* mutants of *Salmonella typhimurium* TML in the context of gastroenteritis. *Infect. Immun.* **63**:762–769.

97. **McCormick, B. A., S. I. Miller, D. Carnes, and J. L. Madara.** 1995. Transepithelial signaling to neutrophils by salmonellae: a novel virulence mechanism for gastroenteritis. *Infect. Immun.* **63**:2302–2309.

98. **McDaniel, T. K., K. G. Jarvis, M. S. Donnenberg, and J. B. Kaper.** 1995. A genetic locus of enterocyte effacement conserved among diverse enterobacterial pathogens. *Proc. Natl. Acad. Sci. USA* **92:**1664–1668.

99. **Menard, R., P. Sansonetti, C. Parsot, and T. Vasselon.** 1994. Extracellular association and cytoplasmic partitioning of the IpaB and IpaC invasins of *S. flexneri. Cell* **79:**515–525.

100. **Miller, S. I., A. M. Kukral, and J. J. Mekalanos.** 1989. A two-component regulatory system (*phoP phoQ*) controls *Salmonella typhimurium* virulence. *Proc. Natl. Acad. Sci. USA* **86:**5054–5058.

101. **Miller, V. L., R. K. Taylor, and J. J. Mekalanos.** 1987. Cholera toxin transcriptional activator ToxR is a transmembrane DNA binding protein. *Cell* **48:**271–279.

102. **Mills, D. M., V. Bajaj, and C. A. Lee.** 1995. A 40 kilobase chromosomal fragment encoding *Salmonella typhimurium* invasion genes is absent from the corresponding region of the *Escherichia coli* K-12 chromosome. *Mol. Microbiol.* **15:**749–759.

103. **Mills, S. D., A. Boland, M. P. Sory, P. van der Smissen, C. Kerbourch, B. B. Finlay, and G. R. Cornelis.** 1997. *Yersinia enterocolitica* induces apoptosis in macrophages by a process requiring functional type III secretion and translocation mechanisms and involving YopP, presumably acting as an effector protein. *Proc. Natl. Acad. Sci. USA* **94:**12638–12643.

104. **Monack, D. M., J. Mecsas, N. Ghori, and S. Falkow.** 1997. *Yersinia* signals macrophages to undergo apoptosis and YopJ is necessary for this cell death. *Proc. Natl. Acad. Sci. USA* **94:**10385–10390.

105. **Monack, D. M., B. Raupach, A. E. Hromockyj, and S. Falkow.** 1996. *Salmonella typhimurium* invasion induces apoptosis in infected macrophages. *Proc. Natl. Acad. Sci. USA* **93:**9833–9838.

106. **Moncrief, M. B. C., and M. E. Maguire.** 1998. Magnesium and the role of *mgtC* in growth of *Salmonella typhimurium. Infect. Immun.* **66:**3802–3809.

107. **Norris, F. A., M. P. Wilson, T. S. Wallis, E. E. Galyov, and P. W. Majerus.** 1998. SopB, a protein required for virulence of *Salmonella dublin,* is an inositol phosphate phosphatase. *Proc. Natl. Acad. Sci. USA* **95:**14057–14059.

108. **Ochman, H., and E. A. Groisman.** 1996. Distribution of pathogenicity islands in *Salmonella. Infect. Immun.* **64:**5410–5412.

109. **Ochman, H., F. C. Soncini, F. Solomon, and E. A. Groisman.** 1996. Identification of a pathogenicity island required for *Salmonella* survival in host cells. *Proc. Natl. Acad. Sci. USA* **93:**7800–7804.

110. **Pegues, D. A., M. J. Hantman, I. Behlau, and S. I. Miller.** 1995. PhoP/PhoQ transcriptional repression of *Salmonella typhimurium* invasion genes: evidence for a role in protein secretion. *Mol. Microbiol.* **17:** 169–181.

111. **Penheiter, K. L., N. Mathur, D. Giles, T. Fahlen, and B. D. Jones.** 1997. Non-invasive *Salmonella typhimurium* mutants are avirulent because of an inability to enter and destroy M cells of ileal Peyer's patches. *Mol. Microbiol.* **24:**697–709.

112. **Reed, K. A., M. A. Clark, T. A. Booth, C. J. Hueck, S. I. Miller, B. H. Hirst, and M. A. Jepson.** 1998. Cell-contact-stimulated formation of filamentous appendages by *Salmonella typhimurium* does not depend on the type III secretion system encoded by *Salmonella* pathogenicity island 1. *Infect. Immun.* **66:** 2007–2017.

113. **Rhen, M., P. Riikonen, and S. Taira.** 1993. Transcriptional regulation of *Salmonella enterica* virulence plasmid genes in cultured macrophages. *Mol. Microbiol.* **10:**45–56.

114. **Robbe-Saule, V., F. Schaeffer, L. Kowarz, and F. Norel.** 1997. Relationships between H-NS, σ^S, SpvR and growth phase in the control of *spvR,* the regulatory gene of the *Salmonella* plasmid virulence operon. *Mol. Gen. Genet.* **256:**333–347.

115. **Shea, J. E., C. R. Beuzon, C. Gleeson, R. Mundy, and D. W. Holden.** 1999. Influence of the *Salmonella typhimurium* pathogenicity island 2 type III secretion system on bacterial growth in the mouse. *Infect. Immun.* **67:**213–219.

116. **Shea, J. E., M. Hensel, C. Gleeson, and D. W. Holden.** 1996. Identification of a virulence locus encoding a second type III secretion system in *Salmonella typhimurium. Proc. Natl. Acad. Sci. USA* **93:**2593–2597.

117. **Snavely, M. D., C. G. Miller, and M. E. Maguire.** 1991. The *mgtB* Mg^{2+} transport locus of *Salmonella typhimurium* encodes a P-type ATPase. *J. Biol. Chem.* **266:**815–823.

118. **Soncini, F. C., E. García Véscovi, F. Solomon, and E. A. Groisman.** 1996. Molecular basis of the magnesium deprivation response in *Salmonella typhimurium:* identification of PhoP-regulated genes. *J. Bacteriol.* **178:**5092–5099.

119. **Stein, M. A., K. Y. Leung, M. Zwick, F. García-del Portillo, and B. B. Finlay.** 1996. Identification of a

Salmonella virulence gene required for formation of filamentous structures containing lysosomal membrane glycoproteins within epithelial cells. *Mol. Microbiol.* **20:**151–164.

120. **Stone, B. J., C. M. Garcia, J. L. Badger, T. Hassett, R. I. F. Smith, and V. L. Miller.** 1992. Identification of novel loci affecting entry of *Salmonella enteritidis* into eukaryotic cells. *J. Bacteriol.* **174:**3945–3952.

121. **Stout, V., and S. Gottesman.** 1990. RcsB and RcsC: a two-component regulator of capsule synthesis in *Escherichia coli. J. Bacteriol.* **172:**659–669.

122. **Tao, T., M. D. Snavely, S. G. Farr, and M. E. Maguire.** 1995. Magnesium transport in *Salmonella typhimurium: mgtA* encodes a P-type ATPase and is regulated by Mg^{2+} in a manner similar to that of the *mgtB* P-type ATPase. *J. Bacteriol.* **177:**2654–2662.

123. **Uchiya, K., M. A. Barbieri, K. Funato, A. H. Shah, P. D. Stahl, and E. A. Groisman.** Inhibition of cellular trafficking by a *Salmonella* virulence protein. Submitted for publication.

124. **Uchiya, K., and E. A. Groisman.** Unpublished results.

125. **Valdivia, R. H., and S. Falkow.** 1997. Fluorescence-based isolation of bacterial genes expressed within host cells. *Science* **277:**2007–2010.

126. **Valone, S. E., G. K. Chikami, and V. L. Miller.** 1993. Stress induction of the virulence proteins (SpvA, -B, and -C) from native plasmid pSDL2 of *Salmonella dublin. Infect. Immun.* **61:**705–713.

127. **Van der Velden, A. W. M., A. J. Bäumler, R. M. Tsolis, and F. Heffron.** 1998. Multiple fimbrial adhesins are required for full virulence of *Salmonella typhimurium* in mice. *Infect. Immun.* **66:**2803–2808.

128. **Watson, P. R., E. E. Galyov, S. M. Paulin, P. W. Jones, and T. S. Wallis.** 1998. Mutation of *invH,* but not *stn,* reduces *Salmonella*-induced enteritis in cattle. *Infect. Immun.* **66:**1432–1438.

129. **Wattiau, P., B. Bernier, P. Deslée, T. Michiels, and G. R. Cornelis.** 1994. Individual chaperones required for Yop secretion by *Yersinia. Proc. Natl. Acad. Sci. USA* **91:**10493–10497.

130. **Wilson, J. A., T. J. Doyle, and P. A. Gulig.** 1997. Exponential-phase expression of *spvA* of the *Salmonella typhimurium* virulence plasmid: induction in intracellular salts medium and intracellularly in mice and cultured mammalian cells. *Microbiology* **143:**3827–3839.

131. **Wolff, C., I. Nisan, E. Hanski, G. Frankel, and I. Rosenshine.** 1998. Protein translocation into host epithelial cells by infecting enteropathogenic *Escherichia coli. Mol. Microbiol.* **28:**143–156.

132. **Wong, K.-K., M. McClelland, L. C. Stillwell, E. C. Sisk, S. J. Thurston, and J. D. Saffer.** 1998. Identification and sequence analysis of a 27-kilobase chromosomal fragment containing a *Salmonella* pathogenicity island located at 92 minutes on the chromosome map of *Salmonella enterica* serovar typhimurium LT2. *Infect. Immun.* **66:**3365–3371.

133. **Wood, M. W., M. A. Jones, P. R. Watson, S. Hedges, T. S. Wallis, and E. E. Galyov.** 1998. Identification of a pathogenicity island required for *Salmonella* enteropathogenicity. *Mol. Microbiol.* **29:**883–891.

134. **Wood, M. W., R. Rosqvist, P. B. Mullan, M. H. Edwards, and E. E. Galyov.** 1996. SopE, a secreted protein of *Salmonella dublin,* is translocated into the target eukaryotic cell via a *sip*-dependent mechanism and promotes bacterial entry. *Mol. Microbiol.* **22:**327–338.

135. **Zhou, D., M. S. Mooseker, and J. E. Galán.** 1999. Role of the *S. typhimurium* actin-binding protein SipA in bacterial internalization. *Science* **283:**2092–2095.

136. **Zierler, M. K., and J. E. Galán.** 1995. Contact with cultured epithelial cells stimulates secretion of *Salmonella typhimurium* invasion protein InvJ. *Infect. Immun.* **63:**4024–4028.

137. **Zychlinsky, A., B. Kenny, R. Ménard, M.-C. Prévost, I. B. Holland, and P. J. Sansonetti.** 1994. IpaB mediates macrophage apoptosis induced by *Shigella flexneri. Mol. Microbiol.* **11:**619–627.

Pathogenicity Islands and Other Mobile Virulence Elements
Edited by J. B. Kaper and J. Hacker
© 1999 American Society for Microbiology, Washington, D.C.

Chapter 8

The Virulence Plasmid of Shigellae: an Archipelago of Pathogenicity Islands?

Claude Parsot and Philippe J. Sansonetti

SHIGELLA AND SHIGELLOSIS

Bacteria of the genus *Shigella* are the causative agents of shigellosis. Characteristic symptoms of this disease include fever, severe abdominal cramps, and diarrhea containing blood and mucus. The only natural hosts of *Shigella* are humans and monkeys; infections are localized in the colon and restricted to the outermost layer of the intestinal wall, where they elicit a strong inflammatory reaction. Transmission of *Shigella* occurs through the fecal-oral route or by the ingestion of contaminated foods or water (106). The infectious dose is very low, since ingestion of as few as 10 bacteria may cause symptomatic infections (30). There are 200 millions cases of shigellosis every year, killing about 650,000 people, mostly children in developing countries.

Shigella strains are gram-negative, nonsporulating, nonencapsulated, facultative aerobic, nonmotile, straight rods that belong to the family *Enterobacteriaceae* and to the tribe *Escherichiaeae*. The genus *Shigella* is divided into four groups (designated species), *S. boydii, S. dysenteriae, S. flexneri,* and *S. sonnei,* on the basis of their capacity to ferment different sugars and on their O-antigen serotypes. Actually, there is a continuum of biotypes and bioserotypes between typical *Shigella* and *Escherichia* species, and the so-called enteroinvasive *E. coli* (EIEC) strains are responsible for a disease similar to shigellosis (29). *E. coli* and the four groups of *Shigella* are so closely related that they constitute a single species, and the decision to maintain *Shigella* and *E. coli* as separate entities was made only in the interest of epidemiology and clinical medicine.

ENTRY INTO EPITHELIAL CELLS AND INTERCELLULAR DISSEMINATION

The various aspects of *Shigella* pathogenicity have been extensively reviewed (76a) and are not discussed in detail here. Essential virulence attributes of *Shigella* are the abilities to enter into (34, 47) and disseminate within (65) epithelial cells, as well as the ability to induce apoptosis in macrophages (21, 110). The cellular biology and genetic

---

Claude Parsot and Philippe J. Sansonetti • Unité de Pathogénie Microbienne Moléculaire, Unité INSERM U389, Institut Pasteur, 25 rue du Dr. Roux, 75724 Paris Cedex 15, France.

studies of entry and dissemination have been performed mainly with *S. flexneri,* but most conclusions derived from these studies probably also apply to other *Shigella* species and to EIEC.

Bacteria enter through the basolateral pole rather than through the apical pole of epithelial cells (61, 67). Contact of bacteria with the epithelial cell surface induces massive rearrangements of the cytoskeleton, which results in localized membrane ruffles leading to bacterial uptake (1, 22, 96). Once internalized by the cell, bacteria lyse the membrane of the endosomal vacuole and gain access to the cell cytoplasm, where they multiply with a generation time of about 40 min (82). Intracellular bacteria move within the cytoplasm of infected cells (65) via polymerization of actin filaments at one pole of the bacterium (15, 43, 50, 69). This movement generates the formation of membranous protrusions which contain a bacterium at their tip and can be engulfed by adjacent cells. Once the protrusion has entered into a cell, the two cellular membranes that surround the bacterium are lysed. This allows bacteria to disseminate from cell to cell without being exposed to the external milieu (4, 64).

FAMILY OF RELATED VIRULENCE PLASMIDS

Evidence for the essential role of a large plasmid in bacterial virulence came from the observation that a plasmid of about 200 kb was present in invasive isolates of *Shigella* and EIEC and that deletions within or loss of this plasmid abolished the ability of bacteria to enter epithelial cells (37, 79, 80, 85). Moreover, mobilization of the large plasmid from *S. flexneri* to *E. coli* K-12 gave rise to an *E. coli* strain that was able to enter HeLa cells (77).

Large plasmids from strains of different species and even of different serotypes within the same species exhibit different restriction patterns; however, hybridization experiments indicate that homologous sequences are present throughout the different plasmids (78). The plasmids that have been studied the most extensively are pMYSH600 and pWR100 from *S. flexneri* YSH6000 and M90T of serotype 2a and 5, respectively. The *Sal*I fragments, designated A to T, of pMYSH6000 (230 kb) were ordered to yield the first restriction map of a virulence plasmid (87), and genes were designated according to the *Sal*I fragment on which they were carried on pMYSH6000; e.g., genes present on *Sal*I fragments B, F, and G were designated *virB, virF,* and *virG,* respectively. The *Sal*I fragments of pWR100 (about 200 kb) are different from those of pMYSH6000, and there are differences in the respective positions of some genes on the two plasmids; for example, *virG (icsA)* is located 40 kb downstream from *virB* on pMYSH6000, whereas it is located 45 kb upstream from *virB* on pWR100. Therefore, in addition to differences in the physical map, there are differences in the genetic organization of these plasmids. On the other hand, genes that have been characterized from different plasmids have almost identical sequences. These observations suggest that virulence plasmids are made up of conserved building blocks and that some differences between various plasmids might be the result of shuffling of these building blocks. However, none of the virulence plasmids has been completely sequenced and, to date, there are no differences between the flanking regions of any gene that has been characterized on two plasmids. Therefore, identification of the putative building blocks is based mostly on differences in their G+C content and the involvement of the encoded protein(s) in different functions.

For the sake of clarity, we refer to the virulence plasmid as a generic entity even though, as indicated above, there are differences between plasmids from different origins. The available sequence data cover approximately 70 kb, which represents about one-third of the virulence plasmid. This review focuses on genes carried by the virulence plasmid that are or might be involved in the pathogenicity of *Shigella*. The virulence plasmid is an IncFII replicon (51, 91), and functions involved in plasmid maintenance and stability have been recently described (70).

ENTRY REGION

Screening of recombinant cosmids introduced into a strain that had been cured of the virulence plasmid and transposon mutagenesis of the wild-type strain were used to identify genes involved in entry into epithelial cells (44, 53, 84, 87). The insert present in cosmids that conferred entry to the virulence plasmid-cured strain contained a common region of 37 kb, and the transposon insertions in derivatives of the wild-type strain that were deficient for entry were mapped to a 30-kb fragment of the same region. Since then, this 30-kb fragment, or part of it, has been sequenced from the virulence plasmids pMYSH6000 and pWR100 of *S. flexneri* (3–7, 9, 12, 20, 100, 102, 103) and from those of *S. dysenteriae* (108) and *S. sonnei* (10, 104). There are only minute differences between genes sequenced from different plasmids.

The entry region contains 35 genes, from *virB* to *orf11* (Fig. 1), which are organized in large transcriptional units, with promoters located upstream from *virB, icsB, ipgC, ipgD, spa47,* and probably *mxiE*. Characterization of the phenotype of mutants obtained after transposon mutagenesis or constructed by allelic replacement indicated that (i) the *virB* (*invE, ipaR*) gene codes for the activator that is required for transcription of the *ipa, mxi,* and *spa* operons (2, 20, 104); (ii) the region extending from *ipgD* to *spa40* codes mostly for the Mxi-Spa type III secretion machinery (3, 5–9, 86, 103); and (iii) the region extending from *icsB* to *ipgG* codes mostly for proteins secreted by this secretion machinery (the IpaA to IpaD proteins) and a cytoplasmic chaperone (IpgC) (4, 12, 60, 83, 96, 100, 102). The *ipgA, ipgB, ipgG,* and *ipgE* genes and the *mxiH, mxiI, mxiK, mxiL, mxiM,* and *mxiE* genes have not been inactivated yet, and their role in entry or in secretion is not established. Several genes of the entry region, *icsB, ipaA, ipgD, ipgF, spa15,* and *orf10,* are not absolutely required for entry into cultured cells (3, 4, 59, 83, 86). However, inactivation of *ipaA* reduces the efficiency of entry into epithelial cells (96) and inactivation of *icsB* decreases the ability to lyse the membrane of the protrusions during intercellular dissemination (4). In contrast, inactivation of *ipgD, ipgF, spa15,* and *orf10* has no effect on either entry or dissemination (3, 86). Secretion of Ipa proteins is induced upon contact of bacteria with host cells (57, 105). IpaB and IpaC form a complex in the extracellular medium (60), and latex beads coated with this complex are internalized by epithelial cells, which suggests that IpaB and IpaC are the main effectors of entry into epithelial cells (57).

As indicated above, the limits of the entry region were defined by the site of transposon insertions that did not affect entry into epithelial cells (87). Such insertions were identified downstream from *virB* and within *orf10* (84, 86), which suggests that the entire region is contained within the DNA fragment extending from *virB* to *spa40*. No features characteristic of mobile genetic elements were detected within the 500-bp sequences located downstream from either *virB* or *spa40*. Since some genes located within the entry region are

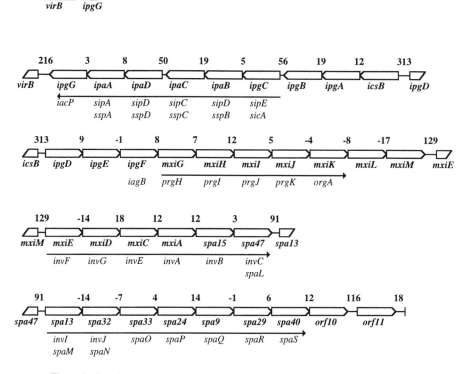

Figure 1. Genetic organization of the entry region. The 31-kb entry region of the *Shigella* virulence plasmid is shown in a discontinuous manner, and the gene order reads from top to bottom and from left to right. *Shigella* genes are shown by open arrows (not to scale), and their names are indicated in bold type. Numbers indicate the size (in base pairs) of intergenic regions. Homologous genes present in the SPI-1 region at centisome 68 of the *Salmonella* chromosome (see references 33 and 56 for reviews) are indicated in standard characters below the *Shigella* genes; gene clusters are indicated by thin arrows.

not absolutely required for entry, the region might be larger than that defined by the transposon mutagenesis and additional sequence information is required to define its exact boundaries. Several lines of evidence suggest that the entry region corresponds to a functional unit: (i) the G+C content of the region (34.1%) is remarkably homogeneous and much lower than that of the chromosome and other regions of the virulence plasmid; (ii) the genetic organization is compact, with only a few nucleotides between the various genes; (iii) all the genes of the entry region are under the same transcriptional control (i.e., their transcription absolutely requires VirB) (2, 94, 95, 104); (iv) inactivation of most genes of the region leads to a noninvasive phenotype; (v) unlike most other genes identified on the virulence plasmid, genes of the entry region are not separated by insertion (IS) sequences; and (vi) most genes of the entry region (25 of 35) have a counterpart in the SPI-1 (*Salmonella* pathogenicity island 1) region located at centisome 63 on the *Salmonella* chromosome (Fig. 1) (see references 33 and 56 for reviews). These observations suggest that the entry region of the virulence plasmid corresponds to a pathogenicity island (PAI) that was acquired by *Shigella* through horizontal gene transfer.

GENES INVOLVED IN ACTIN-BASED MOTILITY OF INTRACELLULAR BACTERIA

Three genes carried by the virulence plasmid have been implicated in the ability of *Shigella* to move within the cytoplasm of infected cells: *icsA* (*virG*), *sopA* (*icsP*), and *virK* (Fig. 2). Two of these genes, *icsA* and *virK,* were identified by screening transposon-induced mutants for their inability to form plaques on confluent monolayers of epithelial cells (64).

The *icsA* (*virG*) mutants are unable to induce actin polymerization at the pole of intracellular bacteria and therefore to move within infected cells and to spread from cell to cell (15, 50). The *icsA* gene encodes a 120-kDa outer membrane protein (48) that is enriched in the bacterial pole opposite the septation furrow (35). Surface presentation of IcsA, which is independent of the Mxi-Spa secretion machinery, involves an N-terminal signal sequence for export of the precursor through the inner membrane and a C-terminal auto-transporter domain that inserts into the outer membrane and allows the N-terminal domain to translocate across and to remain anchored within the outer membrane (93). The G+C content of the *icsA* coding sequence is 41.0%. Beginning 76 bp downstream from the stop codon of *icsA,* there is a 70-bp fragment that corresponds to an internal part of IS2. Located 528 bp upstream from *icsA* and transcribed in the opposite orientation lies the *virA* gene, which encodes a protein secreted by the Mxi-Spa secretion machinery (see below). Despite a possible role of VirA in cell-to-cell spread (97), the difference in G+C content of *icsA* (41.0%) and *virA* (35.2%) suggests that these two genes were acquired independently and that their proximity on the virulence plasmid might be fortuitous. Expression of *icsA* in *E. coli* gave rise to recombinant strains that were able to move in extracts of *Xenopus* oocytes, indicating that IcsA is sufficient to induce actin polymerization and bacterial movement (36, 45).

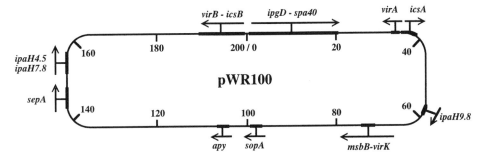

Figure 2. Schematic genetic map of pWR100, the virulence plasmid of *S. flexneri* M90T. The virulence plasmid is shown in a circular form, on which the position of genes is indicated by thick lines and their direction of transcription is indicated by arrows. The positions of *virF, ipaH1.4, ipaH2.5, phoN,* and *senA* have not been determined. Numbers refer to the coordinates on the plasmid, in kilobases.

During growth of bacteria in laboratory media, about 50% of the total amount of IcsA is released into the culture medium as a 95-kDa molecular species designated IcsAα (32, 35). Cleavage of surface-exposed IcsA to yield IcsAα is due to SopA (IcsP), an outer membrane protease of the OmpT family that is also encoded by the virulence plasmid (31, 90). The G+C content of the *sopA* coding sequence is 37.6%. A DNA fragment corresponding to the first 156 bp of IS*629* is located 34 bp downstream from the *sopA* stop codon, and no genes or IS elements were detected immediately upstream from *sopA*. The role of IcsA cleavage in the ability of bacteria to move intracellularly is controversial; inactivation of *sopA* on the virulence plasmid of M90T reduced the spreading ability of the mutant (31), whereas a similar mutation on the virulence plasmid of 2457T increased the motility of the mutant (90) and abolition of IcsA cleavage by modification of the cleavage site on IcsA did not affect spreading in YSH6000 (32).

Transposon insertion in the *virK* gene decreases the ability of bacteria to move within infected cells and to induce actin polymerization around intracellular bacteria (62). This defect appears to be the consequence of a reduced production of IcsA in *virK* mutants. Since transcription of the *icsA* gene is not affected in *virK* mutants, it has been proposed that VirK could be required for the stability of IcsA. Sequence analysis indicates that the start codon of *virK* is located 4 bp downstream from the stop codon of an open reading frame (ORF; OrfA), whose product exhibits sequence similarity to proteins involved in sugar-phosphate metabolism, and that the stop codon of *virK* is located 63 bp upstream from the start codon of another ORF (OrfB), whose product exhibits extensive sequence similarity to the product of the *msbB* gene of *E. coli* (70). A DNA fragment related to IS*630* is located 130 bp downstream from the stop codon of OrfB. This genetic organization and the similar G+C content of OrfA (44% G+C), *virK* (42% G+C), and OrfB (43% G+C) suggest that the region might correspond to an operon. The similarity of the products of OrfA and OrfB to proteins involved in lipopolysaccharide biosynthesis suggests that the virulence plasmid might encode proteins that modify the surface of the bacterium, and the phenotype of the *virK* mutant suggests that these modifications might be required for the proper localization or conformation of IcsA. However, no differences have yet been detected in the lipopolysaccharide produced by bacteria containing or not containing a virulence plasmid.

THE *virF* GENE

The *virF* gene, the first gene of the virulence plasmid to have been cloned and sequenced (74, 75), has a G+C content of 30.4%. The stop codon of *virF* is immediately followed by a 40-bp fragment that is identical to an internal fragment of IS*100* from *Yersinia*. VirF is a 30-kDa protein that belongs to the AraC family of transcriptional activators and is required for expression of genes of the entry region as well as *icsA* (76). Actually, VirF positively controls the transcription of *virB,* whose product activates the transcription of the *ipa, mxi,* and *spa* operons of the entry region (2, 42, 94, 104).

Expression of genes of the entry region is regulated by the growth temperature, these genes being expressed at 37°C but not at 30°C (54). Screening of transposon-induced mutants for an increased expression of entry genes at 30°C led to the identification of the chromosmally located *virR* gene (55), which encodes the H-NS (H1) protein. H-NS is a major component of the nucleoid and is involved in the regulation of a variety of genes

(28, 41). The current model proposes that binding of H-NS to the *virB* promoter at low temperature prevents its activation by VirF (94, 95).

THE *ipaH* GENES AND *virA*

Using plasmid antigen-specific rabbit sera to screen a λgt11 library constructed from the DNA of a derivative of pWR100, Buysse et al. (19) identified a gene, designated *ipaH,* that encodes a 60-kDa protein. Southern blot analysis indicated that several copies of the *ipaH* genes are present on the virulence plasmid (Fig. 2); these copies were designated *ipaH1.4, ipaH2.5, ipaH4.5, ipaH7.8,* and *ipaH9.8,* according to the size of the *Hin*dIII fragments that hybridized with a probe corresponding to the 3′ part of *ipaH7.8* (38). The region corresponding to the last 300 codons of each *ipaH* gene is almost identical in the five *ipaH* copies and represents the characteristic feature of the *ipaH* family (101). The stop codon of both *ipaH2.5* and *ipaH4.5* corresponds to one extremity of IS*629* (99), and there are slight differences between the very last codons of *ipaH7.8, ipaH1.4,* and *ipaH9.8.* The constant 3′ region is preceded by related but different 5′ regions that encode mostly repeats of the 20-residue motif LxxLPxxLPxxLxxLxxxxNx (101). The *ipaH7.8, ipaH4.5,* and *ipaH9.8* genes contain six, eight, and five repeats, respectively (25, 38, 101), and the number of repeats in *ipaH4.5* and *ipaH1.4* is unknown since these genes have not been entirely sequenced (101). The *ipaH7.8* and *ipaH4.5* genes are located in the same region and transcribed in the same orientation; the 427-bp fragment separating the stop codon of *ipaH7.8* from the start codon of *ipaH4.5* contains remnants of IS*2* and IS*629.* The G+C content of *ipaH* genes is around 46%. No genetic studies have been performed to investigate the role of *ipaH* genes in entry or intracellular dissemination. The repeated units of IpaH proteins are similar to the 13 repeats that constitute the major part of YopM. This 41-kDa protein encoded by the *Yersinia* virulence plasmid is secreted by the type III secretion machinery encoded by the same plasmid (49) and is translocated by extracellular *Yersinia* into the cytoplasmic compartment of infected cells (17). Upon characterization of proteins secreted by *Shigella,* Demers et al. (25) found that IpaH9.8 is secreted by the Mxi-Spa secretion machinery.

The *ipaH* genes are poorly expressed by bacteria growing in laboratory media, and their transcription is induced under conditions that increase the activity of the secretion machinery (25), i.e., upon entry into epithelial cells (58, 105), by addition of Congo red to the growth medium (11, 66), and in an *ipaD* mutant (58). A similar regulation was also found for *virA,* another gene carried by the virulence plasmid and encoding a protein secreted by the Mxi-Spa secretion machinery (25). In contrast, transcription of the *ipaB-CDA* and *mxi* operon is not regulated by the activity of the Mxi-Spa secretion machinery (25). The mechanism of control of *ipaH* and *virA* transcription by the activity of the Mxi-Spa secretion machinery might involve secretion of a negative regulator by the secretion machinery, as previously described for FlgM in *Salmonella* (40, 46) and LcrQ in *Yersinia* (68).

As indicated above, *virA* encodes a protein secreted by the Mxi-Spa secretion machinery (25, 97). Its start codon is located 533 bp upstream from that of *icsA* (*virG*), and its stop codon is located 126 bp upstream from an incomplete IS*629.* Inactivation of *virA* in strain YSH6000 led to a fivefold decrease in the efficiency of entry into MK2 cells (97), whereas inactivation of *virA* in strain M90T had no effect on the efficiency of entry into HeLa or

Caco-2 cells (25). These relatively minor discrepancies might be due to differences in the *Shigella* strains or in the epithelial cells used in the different studies. In both cases, inactivation of *virA* led to a decreased transcription of the upstream *icsA* gene; this effect could not be complemented by a plasmid expressing a wild-type copy of *virA* and might be due to changes in the topology of the DNA induced by insertion of the transposon or the suicide plasmid used to inactivate *virA*.

THE *sepA* GENE

The *sepA* gene (48.7% G+C) is located 40 kb downstream from *virB* on pWR100 and encodes a 146-kDa precursor protein that is converted into the mature secreted protein of 110 kDa after two cleavage events which remove an N-terminal signal sequence and a C-terminal autotransporter domain. Inactivation of *sepA* affects neither entry into nor dissemination within epithelial cells, but the *sepA* mutant exhibited an attenuated virulence in the rabbit ligated-ileal-loop model (13). SepA belongs to a family of proteins that are characterized by their extracellular localization, their mode of secretion (which involves a C-terminal autotransporter domain), the size of the mature protein (about 100 kDa), the similarity exhibited by the sequences of their first 500 residues, and the presence within this conserved region of the motif GDSGSP that is part of the active site of various serine proteases. Indeed, proteolytic activity has been documented for several members of this family, including SepA (14). SepA homologs such as PssA from Shiga toxin-producing *E. coli* (27) and EspP from enterohemorrhagic *E. coli* (18) are also encoded by virulence plasmids and are flanked by sequences related to IS*600*, IS*911*, IS*203*, and IS*1*. Approximately 50 bp downstream from the *sepA* stop codon is a 50-bp fragment that is identical to a fragment located 1.1 kb downstream from the *espP* gene and might correspond to the remnant of an IS element. Two genes, *she* and *sigA*, that encode proteins related to SepA are present on the chromosome of *S. flexneri* 2a strains; these genes, together with sequences related to IS*2*, IS*600*, and IS*629*, are part of a 51-kb region that has been proposed to be a PAI (71).

THE *apy* AND *phoN* GENES

Two different genes, designated *apy* and *phoN-Sf*, encoding periplasmic phosphatases of about 25 kDa have been cloned from the virulence plasmid of two *S. flexneri* isolates of serotype 2a (16, 98). The coding sequences of both genes have a G+C content of 42.2%. The sequence of PhoN-Sf exhibits 80% identity to the sequence of PhoN from *Providencia stuartii* and 75% identity to that of PhoC from *Morganella morganii* but only 50% identity to the sequence of Apy, which strongly suggests that the *apy* and *phoN-Sf* genes did not arise by duplication within *Shigella* but were acquired independently from different sources. A *phoN-Sf* gene was detected in all *Shigella* species; however, it was present in only 50% of the strains tested (98). The virulence plasmid pWR100 of the *S. flexneri* 5 isolate M90T contains two genes encoding active periplasmic phosphatases, one of which is identical to *apy* (26). The sequences flanking *phoN-Sf* have not been published. Sequence analysis of the region located 3′ of *apy* reveals the presence of a 50-bp fragment related to IS*629*. The *apy* gene has not been inactivated yet, and a *phoN-Sf* mutant is not affected in its ability to invade and disseminate in epithelial cells (98).

Periplasmic phosphatases with a broad substrate specificity, such as Apy and PhoN-Sf, might be involved in the drop of intracellular ATP levels that follows the entry of *Shigella* into macrophages (81) and epithelial cells (52).

THE *senA* GENE

To identify the gene(s) responsible for the enterotoxin-like activity detected in the culture supernatant of EIEC strains, Tn*phoA* mutants expressing iron-regulated alkaline phosphatase recombinant proteins were screened in the Ussing chamber assay (63). Complementation studies of a mutant that exhibited a reduced enterotoxic activity led to the characterization of the *senA* gene, encoding a 63-kDa protein. Although *senA* was not the gene in which Tn*phoA* was inserted in the original mutant, inactivation of *senA* in the wild-type strain reduced the enterotoxic activity to 50% of that of the wild type. Southern blot analysis indicated that *senA* was present in most isolates of EIEC as well as members of all *Shigella* species. The *senA* gene was characterized in an *S. flexneri* strain and was found to be identical to that of EIEC. A *senA* probe did not hybrize to the DNA of an *S. flexneri* strain that had lost the virulence plasmid, suggesting that *senA* is carried by the virulence plasmid. The G+C content of the *senA* coding sequence is 35.7%, and no IS-like sequences were detected in the immediate vicinity of *senA*. The deduced sequence of SenA does not exhibit a signal sequence and does not have sequence similarity to other proteins. The mode of secretion of SenA and its role in pathogenicity have yet to be characterized (63).

CONCLUDING REMARKS

So far, all the proteins identified as or proposed to be effectors of the specific interactions that occur between *Shigella* and host cells are encoded by the virulence plasmid. These include (i) the IpaA to IpaD proteins and the Mxi-Spa secretion machinery, which are required for entry into epithelial cells, induction of apoptosis in infected macrophages, and contact hemolysis; (ii) possibly other proteins secreted by the Mxi-Spa secretion machinery, such as IpgD, IpaH, and VirA, which are candidates for *Shigella* proteins that might be translocated into eukaryotic cells as described for some proteins secreted by the type III secretion machinery of *Yersinia* and *Salmonella* (17, 23, 73, 92, 107); (iii) IcsA, which appears to be the only bacterial protein that is directly involved in the movement of intracellular bacteria; and (iv) SepA and SenA, which might play a role during infection of the host but whose function remains to be characterized.

The plasmid appears to carry regions of different origins, as suggested by differences in their G+C content, ranging from 30% for *virF* to 49% for *sepA*. Except for genes located in the entry region, which are clustered in large transcription units and are not linked to IS elements, most of the other genes identified so far do not belong to large operons and are flanked by often incomplete IS elements. Additional sequence information is required to define more precisely each of these regions and the possible involvement of these IS elements in the construction of the plasmid.

The entry region has most probably been acquired en bloc by horizontal gene transfer, as suggested by its low G+C content (34.1%). The similar G+C content of *virA* (35.2%) and the fact that the encoded protein is secreted by the Mxi-Spa secretion machinery suggest that *virA* might have the same origin as the entry region. In contrast, the G+C content of *ipaH* genes, which also encode proteins secreted by the Mxi-Spa secretion machinery, is much higher (47%) than that of the entry region (see above), and this suggests that *ipaH* genes might have a different origin. Secretion of proteins of heterologous origin by type III secretion machineries has been documented in several cases (39, 72). Therefore, it is conceivable that horizontal transfers of genetic information might have allowed bacteria to enhance their repertoire of proteins secreted by their type III secretion machinery. Since it is difficult to imagine that genes encoding proteins that are secreted by a type III secretion machinery could provide a selective advantage in the absence of genes encoding the secretion machinery, *ipaH* genes might have been acquired after those of the entry region. However, two regions encoding a type III secretion machinery might have coexisted at some time in *Shigella,* as is the case now in *Salmonella* (89), and hypotheses on the relative order of acquisition of the entry region and *ipaH* genes are highly speculative.

The G+C content of *icsA* is different from that of the entry region, which suggests that they do not have the same origin. Acquisition of *icsA,* by allowing a more efficient spreading of bacteria within infected cells, might have provided a selective advantage to some ''ancestral'' *Shigella* strains that were already able to enter cells and to escape from the endocytic vacuole. Assuming that a protein allowing spreading within infected cells would not provide any selective advantage unless bacteria can reach the cell cytoplasm, acquisition of *icsA* might also have been posterior to that of the entry region. However, IcsA might be involved in another function not yet identified, such as adhesion, which could have been beneficial even for extracellular bacteria.

Control of transcription of entry genes by temperature should allow bacteria to express these genes strictly when they have reached their host, which might be particularly important since expression of entry genes leads to plasmid instability (88). Integration of the virulence plasmid into the chromosome, which inactivates the production of cystathionine-γ-synthase, also leads to the silencing of the virulence plasmid genes (109). The DNA topology resulting from integration of the plasmid might increase the binding of H-NS to the *virB* promoter and thereby decrease the ability of this promoter to be activated by VirF (24). The plasmid can excise from the chromosome to give rise to strains that are indistinguishable from the parental strain. Integration has thus been proposed as a means of ensuring maintenance of the plasmid, which is not self-transmissible, and of down-regulating the expression of the virulence-associated genes (109). Alternatively, the integrated state might be viewed as a pro-PAI, an evolutionary intermediate between an autonomously replicating plasmid and a chromosomal fragment.

REFERENCES

1. **Adam, T., M. Arpin, M.-C. Prévost, P. Gounon, and P. J. Sansonetti.** 1995. Cytoskeletal rearrangements during entry of *Shigella flexneri* into HeLa cells. *J. Cell Biol.* **129:**367–381.
2. **Adler, B., C. Sasakawa, T. Tobe, S. Makino, K. Komatsu, and M. Yoshikawa.** 1989. A dual transcriptional activation system for the 230 kb plasmid genes coding for virulence-associated antigens of *Shigella flexneri. Mol. Microbiol.* **3:**627–635.
3. **Allaoui, A., R. Ménard, P. J. Sansonetti, and C. Parsot.** 1993. Characterization of the *Shigella flexneri ipgD* and *ipgF* genes, which are located in the proximal part of the *mxi* locus. *Infect. Immun.* **61:**1707–1714.
4. **Allaoui, A., J. Mounier, M.-C. Prévost, P. J. Sansonetti, and C. Parsot.** 1992. *icsB:* a *Shigella flexneri* virulence gene necessary for the lysis of protrusions during intercellular spread. *Mol. Microbiol.* **6:**1605–1616.

5. **Allaoui, A., P. J. Sansonetti, R. Ménard, S. Barzu, J. Mounier, A. Phalipon, and C. Parsot.** 1995. MxiG, a membrane protein required for secretion of *Shigella* invasins: involvement in entry into epithelial cells and in intracellular dissemination. *Mol. Microbiol.* **17:**461–470.

6. **Allaoui, A., P. J. Sansonetti, and C. Parsot.** 1992. MxiJ, a lipoprotein involved in secretion of *Shigella* Ipa invasins, is homologous to YscJ, a secretion factor of the *Yersinia* Yop proteins. *J. Bacteriol.* **174:** 7661–7669.

7. **Allaoui, A., P. J. Sansonetti, and C. Parsot.** 1993. MxiD: an outer membrane protein necessary for the secretion of the *Shigella flexneri* Ipa invasins. *Mol. Microbiol.* **7:**59–68.

8. **Andrews, G. P., A. E. Hromockyj, C. Coker, and A. T. Maurelli.** 1991. Two novel virulence loci, *mxiA* and *mxiB*, in *Shigella flexneri* 2a facilitate excretion of invasion plasmid antigens. *Infect. Immun.* **59:** 1997–2005.

9. **Andrews, G. P., and A. T. Maurelli.** 1992. *mxiA* of *Shigella flexneri* 2a, which facilitates export of invasion plasmid antigens, encodes a homolog of the low-calcium response protein, LcrD, of *Yersinia pestis. Infect. Immun.* **60:**3287–3295.

10. **Arakawa, E., J. I. Kato, K. I. Ito, and H. Watanabe.** Accession no. D50601.

11. **Bahrani, F. K., P. J. Sansonetti, and C. Parsot.** 1997. Secretion of Ipa proteins by *Shigella flexneri:* inducer molecules and kinetics of activation. *Infect. Immun.* **65:**4005–4010.

12. **Baudry, B., M. Kaczorek, and P. J. Sansonetti.** 1988. Nucleotide sequence of the invasion plasmid antigen B and C genes (*ipaB* and *ipaC*) of *Shigella flexneri. Microb. Pathog.* **4:**345–357.

13. **Benjelloun-Touimi, Z., P. J. Sansonetti, and C. Parsot.** 1995. SepA, the major extracellular protein of *Shigella flexneri:* autonomous secretion and involvement in tissue invasion. *Mol. Microbiol.* **17:**123–125.

14. **Benjelloun-Touimi, Z., M. Si Tahar, C. Montecucco, P. J. Sansonetti, and C. Parsot.** 1998. SepA, the 110 kDa protein secreted by *Shigella flexneri:* two-domain structure and proteolytic activity. *Microbiology* **144:**1815–1822.

15. **Bernardini, M. L., J. Mounier, H. d'Hauteville, M. Coquis-Rodon, and P. J. Sansonetti.** 1989. Identification of *icsA*, a plasmid locus of *Shigella flexneri* that governs bacterial intra- and intercellular spread through interaction with F-actin. *Proc. Natl. Acad. Sci. USA* **86:**3867–3871.

16. **Bhargava, T., S. Datta, V. Ramachandran, R. Ramakrishnan, K. Sankaran, and Y. V. B. K. Subrahmanyam.** 1995. Virulent *Shigella* codes for a soluble apyrase: identification, characterization and cloning of the gene. *Curr. Sci.* **68:**293–300.

17. **Boland, A., M.-P. Sory, M. Iriarte, C. Kerbourch, P. Wattiau, and G. Cornelis.** 1996. Status of YopM and YopN in the *Yersinia* Yop virulon: YopM of *Y. enterocolitica* is internalized inside the cytosol of PU5-1.8 macrophages by the YopB, D, N delivery apparatus. *EMBO. J.* **15:**5191–5201.

18. **Brunder, W., H. Schmidt, and H. Karch.** 1997. EspP, a novel extracellular serine protease of enterohaemorrhagic *Escherichia coli* O157:H7 cleaves human coagulation factor V. *Mol. Microbiol.* **24:**767–778.

19. **Buysse, J. M., C. K. Stover, E. V. Oaks, M. Venkatesan, and D. J. Kopecko.** 1987. Molecular cloning of invasion plasmid antigen (*ipa*) genes from *Shigella flexneri:* analysis of *ipa* gene products and genetic mapping. *J. Bacteriol.* **169:**2561–2569.

20. **Buysse, J. M., M. Venkatesan, J. Mills, and E. V. Oaks.** 1990. Molecular characterization of a *trans*-acting, positive effector (*ipaR*) of invasion plasmid antigen synthesis in *Shigella flexneri* serotype 5. *Microb. Pathog.* **8:**197–211.

21. **Chen, Y., M. R. Smith, K. Thirumalai, and A. Zychlinsky.** 1996. A bacterial invasin induces macrophage apoptosis by binding directly to ICE. *EMBO J.* **15:**3853–3860.

22. **Clerc, P., and P. J. Sansonetti.** 1987. Entry of *Shigella flexneri* into HeLa cells: evidence for directed phagocytosis involving actin polymerization and myosin accumulation. *Infect. Immun.* **55:**2681–2688.

23. **Collazo, C. M., and J. E. Galan.** 1997. The invasion-associated type III system of *Salmonella typhimurium* directs the translocation of Sip proteins into the host cell. *Mol. Microbiol.* **24:**747–756.

24. **Colonna, B., M. Casalino, P. A. Fradiani, C. Zagaglia, S. Naitza, L. Leoni, G. Prosseda, A. Coppo, P. Ghelardini, and M. Nicoletti.** 1995. H-NS regulation of virulence gene expression in enteroinvasive *Escherichia coli* harboring the virulence plasmid integrated into the host chromosome. *J. Bacteriol.* **177:** 4703–4712.

25. **Demers, B., P. J. Sansonetti, and C. Parsot.** 1998. Induction of type III secretion in *Shigella flexneri* is associated with differential control of transcription of genes encoding secreted proteins. *EMBO J.* **17:** 2894–2903.

26. **Demers, B., P. J. Sansonetti, and C. Parsot.** Unpublished data.

27. **Djafari, S., F. Ebel, C. Deibel, S. Krämer, M. Hudel, and T. Chakraborty.** 1997. Characterization of an exported protease from Shiga toxin-producing *Escherichia coli*. *Mol. Microbiol.* **25**:771–784.
28. **Dorman, C. J., N. Ni Bhriain, and C. F. Higgins.** 1990. DNA supercoiling and environmental regulation of virulence gene expression in *Shigella flexneri*. *Nature* **344**:789–792.
29. **DuPont, H. L., S. B. Formal, R. B. Hornick, M. J. Snyder, J. B. Libonati, D. G. Sheahan, E. H. LaBrec, and J. P. Kalas.** 1971. Pathogenesis of *Escherichia coli* diarrhea. *N. Engl. J. Med.* **285**:1–9.
30. **DuPont, H. L., M. M. Levine, R. B. Hornick, and S. B. Formal.** 1989. Inoculum size in shigellosis and implications for expected mode of transmission. *J. Infect. Dis.* **159**:1126–1128.
31. **Egile, C., H. d'Hauteville, C. Parsot, and P. J. Sansonetti.** 1997. SopA, the outer membrane protease responsible for polar localization of IcsA in *Shigella flexneri*. *Mol. Microbiol.* **23**:1063–1073.
32. **Fukuda, I., T. Suzuki, H. Munakata, N. Hayashi, E. Katayama, M. Yoshikawa, and C. Sasakawa.** 1995. Cleavage of *Shigella* surface protein VirG occurs at a specific site, but the secretion is not essential for intracellular spreading. *J. Bacteriol.* **177**:1719–1726.
33. **Galan, J. E.** 1996. Molecular genetic bases of *Salmonella* entry into host cells. *Mol. Microbiol.* **20**:263–271.
34. **Gerber, D. F., and H. M. S. Watkins.** 1961. Growth of shigellae in monolayer tissue cultures. *J. Bacteriol.* **82**:815–822.
35. **Goldberg, M. B., O. Bârzu, C. Parsot, and P. J. Sansonetti.** 1993. Unipolar localization and ATPase activity of IcsA, a *Shigella flexneri* protein involved in intracellular movement. *J. Bacteriol.* **175**:2189–2196.
36. **Goldberg, M. B., and A. J. Theriot.** 1995. *Shigella flexneri* surface protein IcsA is sufficient to direct actin-based motility. *Proc. Natl. Acad. Sci. USA* **92**:6572–6576.
37. **Harris, J. R., I. K. Wachmuth, B. R. Davies, and M. L. Cohen.** 1982. High-molecular-weight plasmid correlates with *Escherichia coli* enteroinvasiveness. *Infect. Immun.* **37**:1295–1298.
38. **Hartman, A. B., M. M. Venkatesan, E. V. Oaks, and J. M. Buysse.** 1990. Sequence and molecular characterization of a multicopy invasion plasmid antigen gene, *ipaH*, of *Shigella flexneri*. *J. Bacteriol.* **172**:1905–1915.
39. **Hermant, D., R. Ménard, N. Arricau, C. Parsot, and M. Y. Popoff.** 1995. Functional conservation of the *Salmonella* and *Shigella* effectors of entry into epithelial cells. *Mol. Microbiol.* **17**:781–789.
40. **Hughes, K. T., K. L. Gillen, M. J. Semon, and J. E. Karlinsey.** 1993. Sensing structural intermediates in bacterial flagellar assembly by export of a negative regulator. *Science* **262**:1277–1280.
41. **Hulton, C. S. J., A. Seirafi, J. C. D. Hinton, J. M. Sidebotham, L. Waddell, G. D. Pavitt, T. Owen-Hughes, A. Spassky, H. Buc, and C. F. Higgins.** 1990. Histone-like protein H1 (H-NS), DNA supercoiling, and gene expression in bacteria. *Cell* **63**:631–642.
42. **Jost, B. H., and B. Adler.** 1993. Site of transcriptional activation of *virB* on the large plasmid of *Shigella flexneri* 2a by VirF, a member of the AraC family of transcriptional activators. *Microb. Pathog.* **14**:481–488.
43. **Kadurugamuwa, J. L., M. Rhode, J. Wehland, and K. M. Timmis.** 1991. Intercellular spread of *Shigella flexneri* through a monolayer mediated by membranous protrusions and associated with reorganization of the cytoskeletal protein vinculin. *Infect. Immun.* **59**:3463–3471.
44. **Kato, J., K. Ito, A. Nakamura, and H. Watanabe.** 1989. Cloning of regions required for contact hemolysis and entry into LLC-MK2 cells from *Shigella sonnei* form I plasmid: *virF* is a positive regulator gene for these phenotypes. *Infect. Immun.* **57**:1391–1398.
45. **Kocks, C., J. B. Marchand, E. Gouin, H. d'Hauteville, P. J. Sansonetti, M.-F. Carlier, and P. Cossart.** 1995. The unrelated proteins ActA of *Listeria monocytogenes* and IcsA of *Shigella flexneri* are sufficient to confer actin-based motility on *Listeria innocua* and *Escherichia coli*, respectively. *Mol. Microbiol.* **18**:413–423.
46. **Kutsukake, K., S. Iyoda, K. Ohnishi, and T. Iino.** 1994. Genetic and molecular analysis of the interaction between the flagellum-specific sigma factors in *Salmonella typhimurium*. *EMBO J.* **13**:4568–4576.
47. **LaBrec, E. H., H. Schneider, T. J. Magnani, and S. B. Formal.** 1964. Epithelial cell penetration as an essential step in the pathogenesis of bacillary dysentery. *J. Bacteriol.* **88**:1503–1518.
48. **Lett, M. C., C. Sasakawa, K. Kamata, T. Kurata, and M. Yoshikawa.** 1989. *virG*, a plasmid-coded virulence gene of *Shigella flexneri*: identification of the VirG protein and determination of the complete coding sequence. *J. Bacteriol.* **171**:353–359.
49. **Leung, K. Y., and S. C. Straley.** 1989. The *yopM* gene of *Yersinia pestis* encodes a released protein having homology with the human platelet surface protein GP1b. *J. Bacteriol.* **171**:4623–4632.
50. **Makino, S., C. Sasakawa, K. Kamata, T. Kurata, and M. Yoshikawa.** 1986. A genetic determinant

required for continuous reinfection of adjacent cells on large plasmid in *Shigella flexneri* 2a. *Cell* **46:** 551–555.

51. **Makino, S. I., C. Sasakawa, and M. Yoshikawa.** 1988. Genetic relatedness of the basic replicon of the virulence plasmid in shigellae and enteroinvasive *Escherichia coli. Microb. Pathog.* **5:**276–274.

52. **Mantis, N., M.-C. Prévost, and P. J. Sansonetti.** 1996. Analysis of epithelial cell stress response during infection by *Shigella flexneri. Infect. Immun.* **64:**2474–2482.

53. **Maurelli, A. T., B. Baudry, H. d'Hauteville, T. L. Hale, and P. J. Sansonetti.** 1985. Cloning of plasmid DNA sequences involved in invasion of HeLa cells by *Shigella flexneri. Infect. Immun.* **49:**164–171.

54. **Maurelli, A. T., B. Blackmon, and R. Curtiss.** 1984. Temperature-dependent expression of virulence genes in *Shigella* species. *Infect. Immun.* **43:**195–201.

55. **Maurelli, A. T., and P. J. Sansonetti.** 1988. Identification of a chromosomal gene controlling temperature-regulated expression of *Shigella* virulence. *Proc. Natl. Acad. Sci. USA* **85:**2820–2824.

56. **Mecas, J., and E. J. Strauss.** 1996. Molecular mechanisms of bacterial virulence: type III secretion and pathogenicity islands. *Emerging Infect. Dis.* **2:**271–288.

57. **Ménard, R., M. Prévost, P. Gounon, P. J. Sansonetti, and C. Dehio.** 1996. The secreted Ipa complex of *Shigella flexneri* promotes entry into mammalian cells. *Proc. Natl. Acad. Sci. USA* **93:**1254–1258.

58. **Ménard, R., P. J. Sansonetti, and C. Parsot.** 1994. The secretion of the *Shigella flexneri* Ipa invasins is activated by epithelial cells and controlled by IpaB and IpaD. *EMBO J.* **13:**5293–5302.

59. **Ménard, R., P. J. Sansonetti, and C. Parsot.** 1993. Nonpolar mutagenesis of the *ipa* genes defines IpaB, IpaC, and IpaD as effectors of *Shigella flexneri* entry into epithelial cells. *J. Bacteriol.* **175:**5899–5906.

60. **Ménard, R., P. J. Sansonetti, C. Parsot, and T. Vasselon.** 1994. Extracellular association and cytoplasmic partitioning of the IpaB and IpaC invasins of *Shigella flexneri. Cell* **79:**515–525.

61. **Mounier, J., T. Vasselon, R. Hellio, M. Lesourd, and P. J. Sansonetti.** 1992. *Shigella flexneri* enters human colonic Caco-2 epithelial cells through the basolateral pole. *Infect. Immun.* **60:**237–248.

62. **Nakata, N., C. Sasakawa, N. Okada, T. Tobe, I. Fukuda, T. Suzuki, K. Komatsu, and M. Yoshikawa.** 1992. Identification and characterization of *virK*, a virulence-associated large plasmid gene essential for intercellular spreading of *Shigella flexneri. Mol. Microbiol.* **6:**2387–2395.

63. **Nataro, J. P., J. Seriwatana, A. Fasano, D. R. Maneval, L. D. Guers, F. Noriega, F. Dobovsky, M. M. Levine, and J. G. Morris.** 1995. Identification and cloning of a novel plasmid-encoded enterotoxin of enteroinvasive *Escherichia coli* and *Shigella* strains. *Infect. Immun.* **63:**4721–4728.

64. **Oaks, E. V., M. E. Wingfield, and S. B. Formal.** 1985. Plaque formation by virulent *Shigella flexneri. Infect. Immun.* **48:**124–129.

65. **Ogawa, H., A. Nakamura, and R. Nakaya.** 1968. Cinemicrographic study of tissue culture infected with *Shigella flexneri. Jpn. J. Med. Sci. Biol.* **21:**259–273.

66. **Parsot, C., R. Ménard, P. Gounon, and P. J. Sansonetti.** 1995. Enhanced secretion through the *Shigella flexneri* Mxi-Spa translocon leads to assembly of extracellular proteins into macromolecular structures. *Mol. Microbiol.* **16:**291–300.

67. **Perdomo, O. J. J., P. Gounon, and P. J. Sansonetti.** 1994. Polymorphonuclear leukocyte transmigration promotes invasion of colonic epithelial monolayer by *Shigella flexneri. J. Clin. Investig.* **93:**633–643.

68. **Pettersson, J., R. Nordfelth, E. Dubinina, T. Bergman, M. Gustafsson, K. E. Magnusson, and H. Wolf-Watz.** 1996. Modulation of virulence factor expression by pathogen target cell contact. *Science* **273:** 1231–1233.

69. **Prévost, M. C., M. Lesourd, M. Arpin, F. Vernel, J. Mounier, R. Hellio, and P. J. Sansonetti.** 1992. Unipolar reorganization of F-actin layer at bacterial division and bundling of actin filaments by plastin correlate with movement of *Shigella flexneri* within HeLa cells. *Infect. Immun.* **60:**4088–4099.

70. **Radnedge, L., M. A. Davis, B. Youngren, and S. J. Austin.** 1997. Plasmid maintenance functions of the large virulence plasmid of *Shigella flexneri. J. Bacteriol.* **179:**3670–3675.

71. **Rajakumar, K., C. Sasakawa, and B. Adler.** 1997. Use of a novel approach, termed island probing, identifies the *Shigella flexneri she* pathogenicity island which encodes a homolog of the immunoglobulin A protease-like family of proteins. *Infect. Immun.* **65:**4606–4614.

72. **Rosqvist, R., S. Hakansson, A. Forsberg, and H. Wolf-Watz.** 1995. Functional conservation of the secretion and translocation machinery for virulence proteins of yersiniae, salmonellae and shigellae. *EMBO J.* **14:**4187–4195.

73. **Rosqvist, R., K.-E. Magnusson, and H. Wolf-Watz.** 1994. Target cell contact triggers expression and polarized transfer of *Yersinia* YopE cytotoxin into mammalian cells. *EMBO J.* **13:**964–972.

74. **Sakai, T., C. Sasakawa, S. Makino, K. Kamata, and M. Yoshikawa.** 1986. Molecular cloning of a genetic determinant for Congo red binding ability which is essential for the virulence of *Shigella flexneri*. *Infect. Immun.* **51:**476–482.

75. **Sakai, T., C. Sasakawa, S. Makino, and M. Yoshikawa.** 1986. DNA sequence and product analysis of the *virF* locus responsible for Congo red binding and cell invasion in *Shigella flexneri* 2a. *Infect. Immun.* **54:**395–402.

76. **Sakai, T., C. Sasakawa, and M. Yoshikawa.** 1988. Expression of four virulence antigens of *Shigella flexneri* is positively regulated at the transcriptional level by the 30 kiloDalton VirF protein. *Mol. Microbiol.* **2:**589–597.

76a.**Sansonetti, P. J. (ed.).** 1992. Pathogenesis of shigellosis. *Curr. Top Microbiol. Immunol.* **180:**1–137.

77. **Sansonetti, P. J., T. L. Hale, G. J. Dammin, C. Kapfer, H. H. Collins, Jr, and S. B. Formal.** 1983. Alterations in the pathogenicity of *Escherichia coli* K-12 after transfer of plasmid and chromosomal genes from *Shigella flexneri*. *Infect. Immun.* **39:**1392–1402.

78. **Sansonetti, P. J., H. d'Hauteville, C. Ecobichon, and C. Pourcel.** 1983. Molecular comparison of virulence plasmids in *Shigella* and enteroinvasive *Escherichia coli*. *Ann. Inst. Pasteur Microbiol.* **134A:** 295–318.

79. **Sansonetti, P. J., D. J. Kopecko, and S. B. Formal.** 1981. *Shigella sonnei* plasmids: evidence that a large plasmid is necessary for virulence. *Infect. Immun.* **34:**75–83.

80. **Sansonetti, P. J., D. J. Kopecko, and S. B. Formal.** 1982. Involvement of a plasmid in the invasive ability of *Shigella flexneri*. *Infect. Immun.* **35:**852–860.

81. **Sansonetti, P. J., and J. Mounier.** 1987. Metabolic events mediating early killing of host cells infected by *Shigella flexneri*. *Microb. Pathog.* **3:**53–61.

82. **Sansonetti, P. J., A. Ryter, P. Clerc, A. T. Maurelli, and J. Mounier.** 1986. Multiplication of *Shigella flexneri* within HeLa cells: lysis of the phagocytic vacuole and plasmid-mediated contact hemolysis. *Infect. Immun.* **51:**461–469.

83. **Sasakawa, C., B. Adler, T. Tobe, V. Okada, S. Nagai, K. Komatsu, and M. Yoshikawa.** 1989. Functional organization and nucleotide sequence of virulence region 2 on the large virulence plasmid of *Shigella flexneri* 2a. *Mol. Microbiol.* **3:**1191–1201.

84. **Sasakawa, C., K. Kamata, T. Sakai, S. Makino, M. Yamada, N. Okada, and M. Yoshikawa.** 1988. Virulence-associated genetic regions comprising 31 kilobases of the 230-kilobase plasmid in *Shigella flexneri* 2a. *J. Bacteriol.* **170:**2480–2484.

85. **Sasakawa, C., K. Kamata, T. Sakai, S. Y. Murayama, S. Makino, and M. Yoshikawa.** 1986. Molecular alterations of the 140-megadalton plasmid associated with loss of virulence and Congo red binding activity in *Shigella flexneri*. *Infect. Immun.* **51:**470–475.

86. **Sasakawa, C., K. Komatsu, T. Tobe, T. Suzuki, and M. Yoshikawa.** 1993. Eight genes in region 5 that form an operon are essential for invasion of epithelial cells by *Shigella flexneri* 2a. *J. Bacteriol.* **175:** 2334–2346.

87. **Sasakawa, C., S. Makino, K. Kamata, and M. Yoshikawa.** 1986. Isolation, characterization, and mapping of Tn*5* insertions into the 140-megadalton invasion plasmid defective in the mouse Sereny test in *Shigella flexneri* 2a. *Infect. Immun.* **54:**32–36.

88. **Schuch, R., and A. Maurelli.** 1997. Virulence plasmid instability in *Shigella flexneri* 2a is induced by virulence gene expression. *Infect. Immun.* **65:**3686–3692.

89. **Shea, J. E., M. Hensel, C. Gleeson, M. D. Jones, E. Dalton, and D. W. Holden.** 1996. Identification of a virulence locus encoding a second type III secretion system in *Salmonella typhimurium*. *Proc. Natl. Acad. Sci. USA* **93:**2593–2597.

90. **Shere, K. D., S. Sallustio, T. G. Manessis, T. G. d'Aversa, and M. B. Goldberg.** 1997. Disruption of IcsP, the major *Shigella* protease that cleaves IcsA, accelerates actin-based motility. *Mol. Microbiol.* **25:** 451–462.

91. **Silva, R. M., S. Saadi, and W. K. Maas.** 1988. A basic replicon of virulence associated plasmids of *Shigella* spp. and enteroinvasive *Escherichia coli* is homologous with a basic replicon in plasmids of IncF groups. *Infect. Immun.* **56:**836–842.

92. **Sory, M.-P., and G. R. Cornelis.** 1994. Translocation of an hybrid YopE-adenylate-cyclase from *Yersinia enterocolitica* into HeLa cells. *Mol. Microbiol* **14:**583–594.

93. **Suzuki, T., M. C. Lett, and C. Sasakawa.** 1995. Extracellular transport of VirG protein in *Shigella*. *J. Biol. Chem.* **270:**30874–30880.

94. **Tobe, T., S. Nagai, N. Okada, B. Adler, M. Yoshikawa, and C. Sasakawa.** 1991. Temperature-regulated expression of invasion genes in *Shigella flexneri* is controlled through the transcriptional activation of the *virB* gene on the large plasmid. *Mol. Microbiol.* **5:**887–893.

95. **Tobe, T., M. Yoshikawa, T. Mizuno, and C. Sasakawa.** 1993. Transcriptional control of the invasion regulatory gene *virB* of *Shigella flexneri:* activation by VirF and repression by H-NS. *J. Bacteriol.* **175:** 6142–6149.

96. **Tran Van Nhieu, G., A. Ben-Ze'ev, and P. J. Sansonetti.** 1997. Modulation of bacterial entry into epithelial cells by association between vinculin and the *Shigella* IpaA invasin. *EMBO J.* **16:**2717–2729.

97. **Uchiya, K. I., T. Tobe, K. Komatsu, T. Suzuki, M. Watarai, I. Fukuda, M. Yoshikama, and C. Sasakawa.** 1995. Identification of a novel virulence gene, *virA,* on the large plasmid of *Shigella,* involved in invasion and intercellular spreading. *Mol. Microbiol.* **17:**241–250.

98. **Uchiya, K. I., M. Tohsuji, T. Nikai, H. Sugihara, and C. Sasakawa.** 1996. Identification and characterization of *phoN-Sf,* a gene on the large plasmid of *Shigella flexneri* 2a encoding a nonspecific phosphatase. *J. Bacteriol.* **178:**4548–4554.

99. **Venkatesan, M. M., W. A. Alexander, and C. Fernandez-Prada.** 1996. A *Shigella flexneri* invasion gene, *ipgH,* with homology to IS629 and sequences encoding bacterial sugar phosphate transport proteins. *Gene* **175:**23–27.

100. **Venkatesan, M. M., and J. M. Buysse.** 1991. Nucleotide sequence of invasion plasmid antigen gene *ipaA* from *Shigella flexneri* 5. *Nucleic Acids Res.* **18:**1648.

101. **Venkatesan, M. M., J. M. Buysse, and A. B. Hartman.** 1991. Sequence variation in two *ipaH* genes of *Shigella flexneri* 5 and homology to the LRG-like family of proteins. *Mol. Microbiol.* **5:**2435–2445.

102. **Venkatesan, M. M., J. M. Buysse, and D. J. Kopecko.** 1988. Characterization of invasion plasmid antigen genes (*ipaBCD*) from *Shigella flexneri. Proc. Natl. Acad. Sci. USA* **85:**9317–9321.

103. **Venkatesan, M. M., J. M. Buysse, and E. V. Oaks.** 1992. Surface presentation of *Shigella flexneri* invasion plasmid antigens requires the products of the *spa* locus. *J. Bacteriol.* **174:**1990–2001.

104. **Watanabe, H., E. Arakawa, K. I. Ito, J. I. Kato, and A. Nakamura.** 1990. Genetic analysis of an invasion region by use of a Tn*3-lac* transposon and identification of a second positive regulator gene, *invE,* for cell invasion of *Shigella sonnei:* significant homology of InvE with ParB of plasmid P1. *J. Bacteriol.* **172:**619–629.

105. **Watarai, M., T. Tobe, M. Yoshikawa, and C. Sasakawa.** 1995. Contact of *Shigella* with host cells triggers release of Ipa invasins and is an essential function of invasiveness. *EMBO J.* **14:**2461–2470.

106. **Wharton, M., R. A. Spiegel, J. M. Horan, R. V. Tauxe, J. G. Wells, N. Barg, J. Herndon, R. A. Meriwether, J. Newton MacCormack, and R. H. Levine.** 1990. A large outbreak of antibiotic-resistant shigellosis at a mass gathering. *J. Infect. Dis.* **162:**1324–1328.

107. **Wood, M. W., R. Rosqvist, P. B. Mullan, M. H. Edwards, and E. E. Galyov.** 1996. SopE, a secreted protein of *Salmonella dublin,* is translocated into the target eukaryotic cell via a *sip*-dependent mechanism and promotes bacterial entry. *Mol. Microbiol.* **22:**327–338.

108. **Yao, R., and S. Palchaudhuri.** 1992. Nucleotide sequence and transcriptional regulation of a positive regulatory gene of *Shigella dysenteriae. Infect. Immun.* **60:**1163–1169.

109. **Zagaglia, C., M. Casalino, B. Colonna, C. Conti, A. Calconi, and M. Nicoletti.** 1991. Virulence plasmids of enteroinvasive *Escherichia coli* and *Shigella flexneri* integrate into a specific site on the host chromosome: integration greatly reduces expression of plasmid-carried virulence genes. *Infect. Immun.* **59:**792–799.

110. **Zychlinsky, A., M. C. Prevost, and P. J. Sansonetti.** 1992. *Shigella flexneri* induces apoptosis in infected macrophages. *Nature* **358:**167–168.

Pathogenicity Islands and Other Mobile Virulence Elements
Edited by J. B. Kaper and J. Hacker
© 1999 American Society for Microbiology, Washington, D.C.

Chapter 9

Pathogenicity Islands and Other Mobile Virulence Elements of *Vibrio cholerae*

David K. R. Karaolis and James B. Kaper

INTRODUCTION

Cholera is an ancient diarrheal disease that causes significant morbidity and mortality (10, 80). An estimated 120,000 individuals, mostly children, die each year from cholera. Cholera is a major world health concern because of its ability to occur in epidemic and pandemic forms involving many countries and extending over many years. In the last decade of the 20th century, the current cholera pandemic has reached a wider distribution than any other pandemic in the 20th century. Cholera is acquired by ingesting food or water contaminated with the bacterium *Vibrio cholerae*. The majority of *V. cholerae* strains are harmless estuarine microorganisms; however, specific strains have adapted to causing human disease through the ability to effectively colonize the small intestine and release a potent enterotoxin. This toxin acts on intestinal cells and results in voluminous secretory diarrhea, leading to severe fluid loss and ultimately to death if untreated.

Epidemic and Pandemic Cholera

There have been seven pandemics of cholera since the early 19th century. Little is known about the characteristics of strains responsible for the first four pandemics; however, the fifth, sixth, and seventh pandemics are known to have been caused by *V. cholerae* serogroup O1 strains. In areas of endemic infection such as Bangladesh and India, although a variety of O1 and non-O1 strains may coexist, each with a similar epidemiological opportunity, only a few clones (typically of the O1 serogroup) have been responsible for large epidemics. The genetic basis underlying this ability is not well understood; however, several known virulence gene clusters present in these strains could also play roles in endemicity, epidemicity, and pandemicity.

The sixth pandemic is thought to have begun in 1899 and continued to cause significant disease through 1923 (80). Except for a large epidemic in Egypt in 1947 (97), cholera caused by strains of the sixth pandemic clone remained confined to Asia from the mid-

David K. R. Karaolis • Division of Hospital Epidemiology, University of Maryland School of Medicine, Baltimore, MD 21201. ***James B. Kaper*** • Center for Vaccine Development and Department of Microbiology and Immunology, University of Maryland School of Medicine, Baltimore, MD 21201.

1920s until the start of the seventh pandemic. Numerous studies involving DNA sequencing, hybridization, ribotyping, and multilocus enzyme electrophoresis analysis of epidemic "classical" *V. cholerae* O1 strains that were isolated between 1921 and 1970 have shown a clonal relationship among these strains and have further shown that these strains are distinct from other *V. cholerae* strains such as those from the seventh-pandemic clone (15, 19, 25, 53, 56, 76, 81). The classical strains isolated after the end of the sixth pandemic could be thought of as remnants of the main sixth-pandemic clone. The current (seventh) pandemic began on the island of Sulawesi in Indonesia in 1961 (8, 47). The clone rapidly spread to neighboring countries and replaced the previously established sixth-pandemic strain in India within a year, while in Bangladesh the seventh-pandemic clone became the dominant form in 1968 (91). The reason why the seventh-pandemic clone replaced the sixth-pandemic clone is not well understood, but the strains responsible for the seventh pandemic could potentially possess genetic factors which provide some selective advantage.

VIBRIO CHOLERAE

V. cholerae Genome

The genome of *V. cholerae* had long been assumed to consist of a single circular chromosome, but recently it was shown that *V. cholerae* actually contains two unique chromosomes (107). The larger chromosome is ca. 2.4 Mb and contains the genes encoding 16S rRNA, the *rfa* region encoding the lipopolysaccharide (LPS), the *toxR* genes encoding the ToxR global regulator, and the *Vibrio* pathogenicity island (VPI) (see below). The smaller chromosome is ca. 1.6 Mb and contains the *hlyA* gene cluster (see below), among other genes. The smaller replicon was termed a chromosome rather than a megaplasmid since it represents 40% of the entire genome by size and was found in all strains of all biotypes and serotypes examined. Each replicon contains unique genes, with the only duplication seen so far being the presence of the CTX phage element (see below) in both replicons of the classical biotype. The approximate G+C content of the genome is 47 to 49%, which will be confirmed when the genomic sequence of *V. cholerae* is completed in 1999. The genomic sequence will also establish whether the two chromosomes vary significantly in G+C content.

The genome contains a variety of potentially mobile genetic elements including plasmids, bacteriophages, and pathogenicity islands (PAIs), which are reviewed in this chapter. We also describe recent exciting and provocative discoveries that the PAIs in epidemic *V. cholerae* can be acquired by horizontal gene transfer by bacteriophages.

Subtyping

V. cholerae is not homogeneous with regard to pathogenic potential. Specifically, important distinctions within the species are made on the basis of production of cholera enterotoxin (CT), serogroup, and potential for epidemic spread. Some *V. cholerae* strains are members of the normal, free-living (autochthonous) bacterial flora in estuarine environments (26). Other strains possess specific genes encoding virulence factors that allow this organism to colonize the human intestinal tract and cause severe, potentially life-threatening diarrheal disease. The genes encoding the most important virulence factors, CT and the toxin-coregulated pilus (TCP), are not usually present in *V. cholerae* strains that are commonly isolated from the environment. The most important pathogenic members of this species (members of the *V. cholerae* O1 serogroup) are subdivided still further.

Serogroups and Serotypes

Serologically, *V. cholerae* is a diverse species, and to date over 150 different O antigens (serogroups) have been identified. O antigens are thermostable polysaccharides that are part of the bacterial LPS (reviewed in reference 64). The O1 serogroup was the first somatic antigen identified and is traditionally the serogroup associated with epidemic and pandemic cholera.

Unlike other enteric species, for which the term "serotype" usually signifies an assortment of O and H (flagellar) antigens, "serotype" in *V. cholerae* usually refers to different antigenic forms of the O1 antigen. A flagellar antigen is present, but because of common H epitopes among all *Vibrio* species, the value of this antigen for identification is limited. *V. cholerae* O1 strains are subdivided into three serotypes: Ogawa, Inaba, and Hikojima (rare). Antigenic shifts of Ogawa to Inaba and Inaba to Ogawa have been reported, and antigenic shifts within epidemics have also been reported (64).

Biotypes: Classical and El Tor

Traditionally, *V. cholerae* O1 strains are further divided into two biotypes, classical and El Tor. Strains of the sixth pandemic are of the classical biotype, while seventh-pandemic strains are of the El Tor biotype. The basis underlying the distinction between classical and El Tor strains has been questioned, since many of the traits used to distinguish sixth-pandemic (classical) strains from seventh-pandemic (El Tor) strains have now been shown to be variable (54).

Originally, at the start of the seventh pandemic, the isolated strains were distinguished from sixth-pandemic (classical) strains by their ability to hemolyze sheep and goat erythrocytes (28). However, as the seventh pandemic progressed, more strains have been isolated which show variations in hemolytic activity. In fact, as early as 1963, seventh-pandemic strains which were nonhemolytic were being isolated (30). Environmental non-O1 *V. cholerae* strains are usually hemolytic and carry the hemolysin (*hlyA*) gene (71), while sixth-pandemic strains are defective due to an 11-bp deletion in *hlyA* (4, 82). Thus, sixth-pandemic strains could be thought of as having a nonfunctional remnant of *hlyA*, suggesting that this property is required for the environmental niche of the organisms but not for human pathogenesis. Other tests to aid in the distinction between sixth- and seventh-pandemic strains, such as phage typing, have not resulted in wide use due to variations in phage susceptibility (86). Other inconsistencies have been found in phenotypes traditionally used to distinguish between these biotypes, including hemagglutination of chicken erythrocytes (27), Voges-Proskauer reactions (27), and susceptibility to polymyxin B (9, 31). More recently, clear-cut differences in DNA sequences encoding virulence factors have allowed a better distinction between the two biotypes; e.g., the *tcpA* gene, encoding the major subunit of the TCP (see below), differs in 18% of nucleotides between El Tor and classical strains (85). The variability of the biochemical tests described above, the gradual progression of phenotypic traits of seventh-pandemic strains toward those of sixth-pandemic strains, and the great discriminating power of DNA sequence-based tests suggest that the current classification of "biotypes" may need to be revised.

Genetic Relationship of the Sixth (Classical) and Seventh (El Tor) Pandemic Strains

Evidence suggests that the seventh-pandemic clone may not have evolved directly from a sixth-pandemic strain (54), and the full genetic relationship between these pandemic clones is still not well established. Some multilocus enzyme electrophoresis data indicates that these clones are not directly related and are separate from nontoxigenic non-O1 isolates (90), while other data suggests that toxigenic and nontoxigenic *V. cholerae* O1 strains are indistinguishable (5, 15). Ribotyping suggests that sixth- and seventh-pandemic isolates are distinguishable and represent distinct clones (53, 56, 81).

Emergence of *V. cholerae* O139 Bengal

Beginning in late 1992 and continuing into 1993, epidemic cholera was reported in India and Bangladesh that was caused not by *V. cholerae* O1 but by *V. cholerae* expressing a distinctly different surface antigen, which was identified as belonging to the O139 serogroup (3, 16, 83). This was the first description in the literature of a highly virulent *V. cholerae* non-O1 strain that had the ability to cause epidemic disease. The emergence, rapid spread, and initial dominance of this O139 strain over established O1 strains led to the suggestion that this strain could be responsible for the next (eighth) pandemic of cholera. In contrast to nearly all non-O1 strains, CT production is a feature of these O139 isolates. The designation *V. cholerae* O139 Bengal was given to this strain to signify its isolation from coastal cities along the Bay of Bengal (95).

The O139 Bengal strain possesses most, if not all, of the known *V. cholerae* O1 El Tor virulence factors (2). After *V. cholerae* O139 emerged, two hypotheses were advanced to explain this phenomenon. The first hypothesis held that a non-O1 strain had acquired genes encoding CT and other essential virulence factors to gain virulence. The second hypothesis proposed that a *V. cholerae* O1 strain had lost genes encoding the O1 antigen and gained genes encoding the O139 antigen. The second hypothesis proved correct, and work from a number of laboratories has shown that *V. cholerae* O139 and the seventh-pandemic *V. cholerae* O1 El Tor strains share many properties (reviewed by Waldor et al. [110]), including (i) agglutination of chicken erythrocytes, (ii) resistance to polymyxin B, (iii) in vitro growth conditions for the expression of virulence factors, (iv) identically sized restriction fragments for genes which have known polymorphisms, (v) identical electrophoretic types by multilocus enzyme electrophoresis analysis, (vi) tandem duplication of the CTX genetic element (see below), and (vii) identical chromosomal location of the CTX genetic element. However, in contrast to seventh-pandemic strains, O139 Bengal was encapsulated and was resistant to the vibriostatic agent O/129, sulfamethoxazole, trimethoprim, streptomycin, and furazolidone (110). As described below, these resistances are encoded on a 62-kb self-transmissible integrating element and the O139 antigen and capsule are encoded on a 35-kb region of DNA that was introduced into the O1 chromosome, thereby replacing a 22-kb region that encoded the O1 antigen.

After the initial isolation of O139 Bengal and its dominance over O1 strains, the numbers of cases due to this novel strain gradually decreased, with seventh-pandemic (O1) strains again becoming the predominant form (24). What had been expected to be the eighth global pandemic of cholera never progressed much beyond India and Bangladesh.

However, recent evidence from the Indian subcontinent suggests that the incidence of O139 is again on the increase (72).

Virulence Factors

CT

The clinical appearance of cholera involves explosive watery diarrhea and significant dehydration due to fluid and electrolyte loss. One property of epidemic *V. cholerae* strains is their ability to produce CT, which is directly responsible for the majority of diarrhea and fluid loss. CT binds to specific receptors on the intestinal mucosal cells and stimulates adenylate cyclase activity, causing secretion of Cl^- and malabsorption of Na^+. Water follows this ionic gradient into the gut lumen, resulting in voluminous watery diarrhea. Additional effects of CT on the enteric nervous system and prostaglandin synthesis also contribute to diarrhea (reviewed in references 50 and 92).

CT is the prototype of the A-B toxin family. Five copies of the B subunit bind a single copy of the A subunit (holotoxin), after which binding of the B subunit to the GM1 receptor on the eukaryotic cell allows the holotoxin to enter the cell. Neither subunit individually has any major effect in animal or cell culture systems. CT shares structural, functional, immunological, and 80% sequence relatedness with the *Escherichia coli* heat-labile toxin which is usually, if not exclusively, plasmid encoded (50).

All epidemic strains of *V. cholerae* contain *ctxAB* genes, which encode CT. As discussed below, the *ctxAB* locus is carried by a lysogenic filamentous bacteriophage that is similar to phage M13 in structure (108). Comparisons show that the *ctx* sequences are highly conserved among *V. cholerae* strains; however, nucleotide differences that have been observed have been used to distinguish major pathogenic forms. Analysis of *ctxB* from many *V. cholerae* O1 strains isolated in 29 countries over 70 years revealed only three nucleotide changes, each resulting in an amino acid substitution (76). In this study, genotype 1 contained sixth-pandemic classical strains and U.S. Gulf Coast strains, genotype 2 contained Australian El Tor strains, and genotype 3 contained seventh-pandemic El Tor strains. These findings suggest a reservoir of toxigenic *V. cholerae* in the U.S. Gulf Coast and in Australia. These foci may reflect strains responsible for previous pandemics or merely strains which have epidemic and pandemic potential but do not result in large-scale disease due to the high level of sanitation in these countries.

The Toxin-Coregulated Pilus

In 1987, Taylor et al. (104) reported the discovery of a pilus colonization factor in *V. cholerae* O1 strains which was composed of long filaments 7 nm in diameter and up to 15 μm in length which extrude from the cells. These structures, the TCP, were seen to aggregate into bundles apparently due to the hydrophobic nature of the pilus subunit. This bundled appearance is typical of other type IV pili such as the bundle-forming pilus of *E. coli* (32), and TCP has substantial sequence homology to other type IV pili (94). Synthesis of TCP is complex and incompletely understood; up to 15 open reading frames (ORFs) are found in the *tcp* gene cluster (63). The major protein forming the pilus structure (TcpA) is encoded by the *tcpA* gene and is 20.5 kDa in size.

The TCP is an essential colonization factor of *V. cholerae*. *tcpA* mutants have a 50% lethal dose in the suckling-mouse model that is 5 log units higher than that of the wild-type parent (104). Antibodies to TcpA protect mice from *V. cholerae* challenge (93, 102).

Conclusive proof of the importance of TCP in human disease was shown in volunteer studies, where *tcpA* mutants failed to cause disease or colonize volunteers (38, 103).

The ToxR Regulon

Specific strains of *V. cholerae* have the ability to exist in both the environment and the human intestine. The ability of these strains to respond to specific signals in both these environments is part of a complex regulon which, ultimately, is coordinately regulated under ToxR, a 32-kDa transmembrane protein which controls the growth of the organism and the expression of its most extensively studied virulence factors in vivo (69). The activity of ToxR is enhanced by the ToxS protein, a 19-kDa transmembrane protein that is thought to interact with and stabilize ToxR (20). In addition to CT, ToxR regulates the expression of at least 17 genes, some of which are involved in the production of important virulence factors including the TCP colonization factor (104) and the accessory colonization factor (ACF) (79). Although ToxR can directly bind to cloned *ctx* genes in an *E. coli* background, most if not all genes in the ToxR regulon are directly controlled by ToxT, which is a 32-kDa protein that has homology to the family of AraC transcriptional activators (21). A regulatory cascade exists in which ToxR controls the expression of the *toxT* gene, which in turn regulates other genes in the ToxR regulon. An additional layer of complexity was recently added by the discovery that TcpP and TcpH are also important regulators of virulence gene expression, including expression of *tcpA* and *ctx* (14, 37).

Other Potential Virulence Factors

The importance of the *ctx, tcpA,* and *toxR* genes has been definitively established by the study of isogenic mutants in volunteers (reviewed in reference 50). A variety of other potential virulence factors have been described for this organism, including other fimbriae, outer membrane proteins, toxins, colonization factors, and proteases. However, the evidence for the importance of these factors in human disease is much weaker than the evidence supporting the role of *ctx, tcpA,* and *toxR*. Some of these factors are briefly reviewed here in the context of other mobile genetic elements, but a comprehensive review of *V. cholerae* virulence factors is presented elsewhere (50).

MOBILE GENETIC ELEMENTS

The severe secretory diarrhea and fluid loss characteristic of cholera infection depend on the ingestion of specific *V. cholerae* strains which have the ability to colonize the small intestine and secrete toxin, in particular CT. Like many bacterial pathogens which possess clusters of virulence genes (PAIs) (13, 34, 35), epidemic *V. cholerae* strains possess virulence genes that are clustered into genetic elements which are integral to the pathogenesis and epidemic potential of the organism.

CTX Genetic Element

Epidemic strains of *V. cholerae* O1 can contain multiple copies of the *ctxAB* locus which are contained on a large element called the CTX element. In particular, sixth-pandemic classical strains contain two copies, which have recently been shown to be located on two separate chromosomes (107), and while most seventh-pandemic El Tor strains contain only a single copy, approximately 30% of El Tor strains contain two or

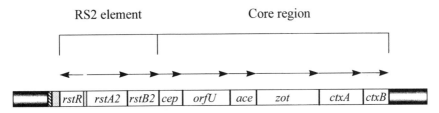

Figure 1. Schematic map of the CTXΦ genome integrated in the *V. cholerae* chromosome.

more tandem copies (66, 67). CT, Zot, and Ace are encoded by genes on a 4.5-kb region of the *V. cholerae* chromosome termed the core region (33). In addition, the core region encodes a peptide termed Cep (core-encoded pilin), which has similarity to a pilin produced by *Aeromonas hydrophilia* (78), and also contains a gene, *orfU,* which until recently had no demonstrated function (106, 108). Flanking the core region are one or more sets of genes contained on a 2.7-kb sequence called the RS element (Fig. 1). The RS element encodes a site-specific recombination system (78), and until recently, the CTX element was thought to comprise a site-specific transposon that was able to integrate into specific sites of the *V. cholerae* chromosome.

Discovery of CTXΦ

In 1996, Waldor and Mekalanos demonstrated that the CTX element was transmissible (108). In their study, a strain containing a kanamycin resistance gene in place of *ctxAB* was able to transfer this resistance plus the entire CTX element to other strains (108). The transfer was not dependent on cell-to-cell contact, since cell-free culture supernatants transferred the resistance phenotype, suggesting that CTX transfer occurred via transduction. Examination by electron microscopy of concentrated culture supernatants obtained from an El Tor strain grown under conditions in which no TCP structures are expressed revealed "bundled" filaments, leading to the conclusion that these filaments represent a filamentous phage, which was termed CTXΦ. DNA obtained from these preparations showed the presence of a 6.9-kb single-stranded DNA genome that contained the entire CTX element. These investigators also showed that, like other filamentous phages, the genome of CTXΦ forms a plasmid replicative form in the cell.

Analysis of the sequence, structure, and function of the CTXΦ-encoded proteins reveals similarity to multiple filamentous phage proteins. The Zot protein has sequence similarity to the *E. coli* phage M13 gene I product, which is required for phage assembly (57, 89). Functional analysis of *zot* has shown it to be required for CTXΦ transduction, since *zot* mutants were unable to transfer CTXΦ (108). Similar results for *orfU* show that it also is required for CTXΦ transduction (108), and given its location on the CTXΦ genome compared to phage M13, *orfU* appears to be similar to gene III, which encodes a minor coat protein involved in binding phage to the F pilus (70). Although no function has been shown experimentally, Cep appears to be homologous to the gene VIII major coat protein of M13 (70), while Ace, in addition to its potential role as a toxin (106), appears to be homologous to the gene VI protein of *Pseudomonas aeruginosa* phage Pf1 (39, 108).

The RS element of CTXΦ has been shown to contain three ORFs, and it is this region which is involved in the regulation, replication, and integration of CTXΦ into the chromosome (109). Within the RS element, RstR resembles a family of transcriptional repressors and has been shown to influence the expression of the adjacent and oppositely transcribed *rstA* gene, which appears to play a role in replication, while RstB plays a role in integration of the element. There are two variants of the RS element in *V. cholerae* strains. The RS element adjacent to the core region in all CTXΦ genomes is termed RS2 and encodes RstR, RstA, and RstB. RS1, which is adjacent to RS2 in the chromosomally integrated form of CTXΦ, encodes RstR, RstA, RstB, and the additional protein RstC, which has no known function. Although the RS1 form has not been found to be part of the phage particle, it may still play a role, together with RS2, in the genetics of phage production.

Transfer studies have demonstrated that the receptor for CTXΦ is the TCP structure (108). As discussed above, expression of TcpA, a major protein of TCP, is essential for intestinal colonization. Although TcpA plays a clear role in virulence in both biotypes, there are differences in the expression of TcpA between classical and El Tor strains, which are not well understood. The efficiency of transfer of CTXΦ varies with the production of TCP. In vitro culture conditions for optimal TCP expression by classical strains are well defined, and in vitro transfer of CTXΦ to classical strains occurs at high frequency. However, in vitro culture conditions for optimal TCP expression by El Tor strains are not as well defined, and in vitro transfer of the phage to El Tor strains occurs at low frequency (108). In vivo transfer of CTXΦ to El Tor strains in the mouse intestine occurs at a much higher level of efficiency, presumably due to the optimized expression of TCP in vivo under conditions that have not yet been reproduced in vitro.

The *V. cholerae* Pathogenicity Island

A second distinguishing characteristic of epidemic and pandemic strains is their ability to colonize the human intestine. This property is associated with the production of TCP, which functions both as an essential colonization factor (38, 104) and as the CTXΦ receptor (108). Thus, for *V. cholerae* to colonize and to become toxigenic following infection by CTXΦ, it must first express TCP. The genes encoding the TCP structure are part of a large PAI called the VPI (*V. cholerae* pathogenicity island). For this reason, we and others have proposed that the VPI is one of the initial genetic factors that must be present for the emergence of epidemic and pandemic cholera.

Identification of the VPI

Studies of the genetic relationship between *V. cholerae* strains and the genetic factors that contribute to the epidemic ability of specific *V. cholerae* strains have provided evidence suggesting that the sixth- and seventh-pandemic strains (classical and El Tor, respectively) may be derived from nontoxigenic strains and that horizontal gene transfer in *V. cholerae* results in the emergence of new epidemic forms (54). In an extension of these studies, the prevalence and variation of two genes (*aldA* and *tagA*) under ToxR control were investigated (52). The *aldA* gene encodes a cytoplasmic coenzyme A-independent aldehyde dehydrogenase (77), whereas the adjacent and oppositely transcribed *tagA* encodes a lipoprotein (36). The prevalence of *aldA* and *tagA* was studied in a large number of *V. cholerae* strains (pathogenic and nonpathogenic) whose isolations were temporally (1931 to 1994) and geographically widespread. The results showed that *aldA* and *tagA* were associated with epidemic strains, in particular CT-positive strains, and absent from nonpathogenic isolates. Further characterization demonstrated that the *aldA-tagA* region

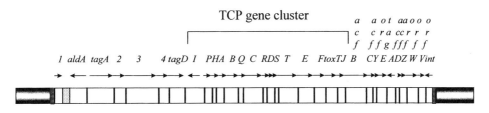

Figure 2. Schematic map of the VPIΦ genome integrated in the *V. cholerae* chromosome.

was linked to the TCP-ACF gene cluster (~10 kb away), which was known to be important for virulence and was associated with epidemic strains (59, 105). This particular region of the chromosome was found to be part of a larger locus (40 kb) which was associated with epidemic strains. The characteristics of this locus, i.e., large, absent from nonpathogenic strains, with a G+C content strikingly different from the rest of the chromosome (35 versus ca. 48%), possession of genes associated with virulence (TCP-ACF cluster), regulation of virulence (*toxT* and *tcpPH*) and mobility (*int* and *orfl*), and insertion into a sequence homologous to a phage attachment (*att*) site adjacent to a tRNA-like gene (*ssrA*), suggested that it was a PAI and so it was named the *V. cholerae* pathogenicity island (VPI) (Fig. 2) (52).

Genes Located in the VPI

As noted above, the *tcp* gene cluster encodes a critical intestinal colonization factor for *V. cholerae*. Downstream of this cluster is a group of genes called *acf,* which encode the accessory colonization factor (ACF) (79) (Fig. 2). Mutations in several of the genes in this cluster were demonstrated to affect the level of colonization in an infant-mouse model and to play potential roles in chemotaxis and motility (23, 43, 79). Towards the end of the *tcp* cluster is the *toxT* gene, which encodes a transcriptional activator that is an important component of the ToxR regulatory cascade, as described above. On the opposite side of the *tcp* gene cluster are the *tcpP* and *tcpH* genes, which have recently been shown to encode regulators that are required for the transcription of *toxT* (14, 37).

There are a number of VPI-located genes for which no function has yet been described. Many ToxR-activated genes which at present play no obvious role in an infant-mouse model of cholera infection have been given the *tag* designation (79). Several of these genes have been studied and shown to be located on the VPI. The TagA gene product was found to encode a lipoprotein with homology to the *E. coli* K99 pilus biogenesis determinant FanD (36). TagD was reported to have sequence similarity to a protein involved in fimbria synthesis in *Streptococcus sanguis* (42), and TagE has some sequence similarity to *Staphylococcus simulans* lysostaphin (58). The gene adjacent to and oppositely transcribed to *tagA* was found to encode an aldehyde dehydrogenase (*aldA*); however, mutants with mutations in this gene, although it has a known function, were unaffected in their colonization in an infant-mouse model (77). Several genes on the VPI whose roles in virulence and mechanism of regulation are unknown have been identified; these include the *orfYZWV* genes of the ACF cluster (79) and the recently described *orf1234* genes at the left end of the VPI (52). Although virulence functions for these genes have yet to be described, the control of some by the ToxR-ToxT regulatory system and the location of all on the VPI suggest that they may play important roles in the virulence of epidemic *V. cholerae.*

Discovery of VPIΦ

In the study which led to the identification of the VPI (52), we had identified an El Tor strain which apparently had lost its VPI. This strain was CT positive and had an altered *att* site compared to other VPI-negative strains, suggesting that it once possessed the VPI to allow CTXΦ infection. This finding suggested the VPI was a mobile element, and while investigating this possibility, we recently discovered that the VPI is located on a novel bacteriophage (55). In these studies, phage preparations from the *V. cholerae* El Tor strain N16961 and classical strain 395 were examined for the presence of VPI genes by PCR analysis, which detected the VPI-located genes *orf1, tcpA, toxT,* and *int*. PCR did not detect flanking DNA immediately outside the left and right ends of the VPI. In addition, PCR did not detect the chromosomal genes *ompT* (encoding an outer membrane protein) and *rfaD* (involved in LPS synthesis), which are also outside the VPI. The finding of VPI genes in cell-free, DNase- and RNase-treated phage preparations suggested that the VPI was protected by a protein coat and was most probably located on a bacteriophage which we have called VPIΦ. Analysis of the genome of this phage suggests that it contains a single-stranded DNA genome and, once in the cell, has the ability to form a double-stranded plasmid replicative form.

Phage preparations of several epidemic strains were examined by electron microscopy. Phage preparations from classical strain 395 revealed structures that resembled TCP. These structures bound anti-TcpA antibodies which were visualized with colloidal gold-conjugated goat anti-rabbit antibodies. Strain CVD110 is an El Tor strain with *ctxA, zot, ace,* and *orfU* deleted and is unable to produce CTXΦ (68). Phage preparations of CVD110 demonstrated numerous phage particles, some of which formed a ''braided'' network of filaments, and examination of wild-type El Tor strain N16961 by immunoelectron microscopy with anti-TcpA antibodies showed numerous gold particles bound to filamentous phage, similar to those seen with strain 395.

Our data showing that the VPI is the genome of a phage, together with previous suggestions that type IV pili resemble filamentous bacteriophages (40), led us to hypothesize that TCP and its major protein subunit (TcpA) might in fact be a VPIΦ coat protein. PCR analysis of phage preparations from two independent TcpA mutants did not detect VPI genes, whereas genes of CTXΦ, which still should be made in these strains, were identified. The PCR analysis suggested that VPIΦ production by both mutants was restored when each strain was supplied with TcpA encoded on a plasmid. The lack of VPI genes in phage preparations of TcpA mutants suggested that TcpA was required for VPIΦ production. Immunoprecipitation studies were then performed on wild-type and TcpA mutant strains. In these studies, a VPIΦ–rabbit anti-TCP antibody complex was bound by mouse anti-rabbit immunoglobulin G–agarose beads. This complex was selectively removed from the reaction mixture and analyzed by PCR, which showed the presence of VPI genes in the phage-antibody complex from the wild-type strain but not in complexes from the TcpA mutants and not in reaction mixtures that did not contain anti-TcpA. These results provided further independent evidence that TcpA is a major coat protein of VPIΦ.

Transfer of VPIΦ

The evidence suggesting that the VPI was the genome of a phage containing genes associated with mobility (e.g., *orf1* and *int*), together with the finding that TcpA was a major coat protein of the phage, led us to perform studies investigating whether VPIΦ can transfer between strains (55). In these studies, we marked the VPI of N16961 Str by the insertion of *aphA-3* (encoding Kan[r] and Neo[r]), creating strain DK238. With DK238 as a donor, transfer experiments with the non-O1 (serogroup O10) strain DK236 (Nal[r]) as the recipient were performed. Incubation of whole cells or cell-free phage preparations of the donor and recipient strains followed by plating on appropriate selective media produced Nal[r] Neo[r] colonies, suggesting that transduction mediated the transfer of the VPI into the VPI-negative recipient. Subsequent analysis showed that the VPI had integrated into the same chromosomal site as other VPI-positive strains (52, 55).

Surprisingly, not all VPI-positive strains tested appear to be capable of serving as donors, since no transfer of VPIΦ was observed when the classical strain 395Str[r] (with VPI marked with *aphA-3* in the same manner as N16961) was used as the donor. This may indicate that classical strains either lack the appropriate mechanism for VPIΦ infection or transfer VPIΦ under different conditions from those used by El Tor strains. Interestingly, not all VPI-negative strains could act as recipients for VPIΦ. No transfer was observed when DK238 was used as the donor and the nontoxigenic VPI-negative strain DK237 (serogroup O1) was used as the recipient. These results suggest that there are differences in the ability of the VPI-negative nontoxigenic strains to be infected by VPIΦ and acquire VPI, and they highlight the potential for strains of different serogroups (other than O1) to acquire VPI and CT and become potentially virulent with epidemic and pandemic potential.

Other Bacteriophages

Bacteriophages in *V. cholerae* have been studied for many decades (reviewed in reference 48 and 86). However, until the last few years, most studies used phages merely as typing reagents to distinguish among different *V. cholerae* strains, and attempts to link phages and virulence were unsuccessful. Transduction of various chromosomal markers by the CP-T1 phage and the generation of both insertion and deletion mutations by VcA1, VcA2, and VcA3 phages have been demonstrated (reviewed in reference 48). One class of *V. cholerae* phages studied over the years was the kappa family of O1 bacteriophages.

In 1995, Reidl and Mekalanos (84) described the K139 phage of the kappa family and presented evidence linking this phage and virulence. The temperate K139 phage was originally discovered in an O139 strain, but phage genes were subsequently shown to be present in many, but not all, virulent O1 strains (84). The K139 genome is a 35-kb double-stranded linear DNA molecule which circularizes and integrates into a specific *attB* site located between the *flaA* and *flaC* genes of O1 El Tor (73). One gene in the K139 genome, *glo,* encodes a 137-amino-acid periplasmic protein that constitutes a phage exclusion system (73). Comparison of isogenic *glo*[+] and *glo* K139-lysogenic strains in infant mice revealed no differences in intestinal colonization, but the number of bacteria required to kill infant mice was 10- to 100-fold higher for the *glo* mutants.

In addition to the CTX and VPI filamentous phages described above, several other filamentous phages of *V. cholerae* have been reported (88). Phage 493 was isolated from an O139 strain, and homologous phage sequences are present in most O139 strains but not in O1 strains (45). The genome is a 9.3-kb closed circular single-stranded molecule, and the phage receptor is the mannose-sensitive hemagglutinin (46). Interestingly, the susceptibility of El Tor strains to this phage varies with the year of isolation, suggesting that phage 493 may play a role in the population dynamics of *V. cholerae*. Another phage, VSK, was also isolated from an O139 strain; it has a 7-kb single-stranded DNA genome and replicates by using a double-stranded DNA intermediate (51). The fs1 and fs2 phages were also originally isolated from an O139 strain, and each phage has been found in a variety of O1 and O139 strains (22, 96). These phages have single-stranded genomes of 6.4 (fs1) and 8.5 (fs2) kb. Unlike CTX and VPI phages, none of these filamentous phages have been linked to gene transfer or virulence.

Plasmids

Plasmids encoding resistance to a variety of antibiotics have been found in *V. cholerae* strains isolated throughout the world (reviewed in reference 48). Generally, these R factors are large (110 to 170 kb) and self-transmissible and belong to the C incompatibility group. Up to seven different resistances have been found to be encoded on a single plasmid.

Another plasmid that has been studied for many years is the P factor, which is ca. 68 kb and is present in a single copy per cell (reviewed in references 48 and 49). The P factor is capable of mobilizing chromosomal genes, although it is much less efficient than the F factor of *E. coli*. The occurrence of the P factor among wild-type *V. cholerae* strains is extremely rare (49). Interestingly, possession of the P plasmid markedly attenuates *V. cholerae* strains and decreases intestinal colonization by ca. 5 log units (7).

A 4.7-kb cryptic plasmid present in all *ctx*$^+$ *V. cholerae* strains was recently character-ized by Rubin et al. (87). Interestingly, *V. cholerae* strains contain this plasmid in both extrachromosomal and chromosomally integrated forms, and the chromosomal insertion site is immediately upstream of the CTX prophage. This plasmid is tandemly duplicated in the chromosome, and it was speculated that the extrachromosomal form may have arisen from homologous recombination between directly repeated copies. Sequence analysis of this plasmid (called pTLC, for "toxin-linked cryptic") reveals an ORF encoding a protein similar to the replication initiation protein (pII) of *E. coli* F-specific filamentous phages. Mutation of this gene (called *cri*, for "cryptic replication initiation") resulted in failure of this plasmid to replicate or integrate. Since the CTXΦ genome lacks a homolog of gene II/X that is found in other filamentous phages, the authors suggest that the *cri* gene product is required for CTXΦ replication.

When integrated into the chromosome, pTLC is located only 842 bp upstream of the CTXΦ genome. Recently, Lin et al. (61) described a gene cluster (*rtxABCD*) encoding a toxin that resembles members of the RTX (repeats in toxin) family of toxins, which includes the hemolysin of uropathogenic *E. coli* and the adenylate cyclase of *Bordetella pertussis*. This *rtx* gene cluster is located 693 bp downstream of the *rstB* gene of the CTX element in O1 El Tor and O139 strains. In classical strains, the *rtx* gene cluster has undergone a deletion of 7,869 bp relative to El Tor strains. Thus, this region of the *V. cholerae* chromosome is very dynamic, since it contains a filamentous phage, an element that can exist as both an extrachromosomal plasmid and an integrated element, and a large toxin gene cluster that has undergone a major deletion in one biotype of *V. cholerae* O1.

The Conjugal Self-Transmissible Integrating Element

As noted above, *V. cholerae* O139 shares many characteristics with *V. cholerae* O1 El Tor. However, one important difference besides the O antigen is a distinct set of antibiotic resistances. O139 strains are resistant to sulfamethoxazole, trimethoprim, streptomycin, and furazolidone. (The resistance of O139 to the vibriostatic compound O/129 is probably due to the trimethoprim-resistant dihydrofolate reductase [110].) Waldor et al. (110) showed that resistance to the first three antibiotics is mediated by a 62-kb self-transmissible, chromosomally integrating genetic element, which they called the SXT element. The initial characterization of this element indicated that it was a conjugative transposon similar to those seen in *Bacteroides* (see chapter 17). However, more recent data indicates that chromosomal integration of this element does not resemble transposition but is strikingly similar to site-specific recombination found in phage lambda (41). The authors have therefore recently renamed it CONSTIN, for "conjugal self-transmissible integrating element."

CONSTIN can be transferred between *V. cholerae* strains and *E. coli* strains, but an extrachromosomal state could not be detected by conventional plasmid extraction techniques (110). Rather than inserting at random sites in the chromosome, the element specifically inserted into the *prfC* gene of *E. coli,* which encodes peptide chain release factor 3 (RF3), a GTP-binding protein which plays a role in the termination of protein synthesis (41). The integration site in *V. cholerae* is a *prfC* homolog. The integrated element is flanked on each side by a 17-bp sequence corresponding to the sequence encoding amino acids 18 to 23 of RF3. This 17-bp site is presumed to represent the core of a CONSTIN attachment (*att*) site, similar to the *att* sites of bacteriophages that integrate in a site-specific manner. Since lambda and similar bacteriophages integrate and excise from the chromosome via a circular extrachromosomal intermediate, the authors used PCR to test whether the CONSTIN element could form a similar intermediate. By designing primers that read out of the integrated element across the putative *att* sites, they showed that a circular extrachromosomal form of this element was also present in strains harboring the integrated form. The PCR product contained a single 17-bp *att* sequence that was predicted to be formed by circularization of the right (*attR*) and left (*attL*) ends of the integrated element. Finally, they showed that this element encoded a protein with significant similarity to the integrase family of site-specific recombinases. Mutation of this gene (*int*) abolished excision and circularization of this element as well as transfer into other strains.

CONSTIN can be transferred to both classical and El Tor strains of the O1 serogroup and has also been detected in recent clinical El Tor isolates (110). It is possible, although it has not yet been demonstrated, that this element transfers unlinked chromosomal genes among *V. cholerae* strains. Given the mobility and natural distribution of this element as well as its demonstrated ability to transfer antibiotic resistances, it is possible that CONSTIN has played a role in the emergence of new *V. cholerae* strains in the recent past or could play such a role in the future.

The VCR Integron

Barker et al. (6) described a repeated 123- to 126-bp sequence that was present in nine copies in the locus encoding the mannose- and fucose-resistant hemagglutinin. This sequence, called VCR (for "*V. cholerae* repetitive DNA sequence"), was shown by Southern hybridization to occur in at least 60 to 100 copies in the *V. cholerae* chromosome. The multiple VCR elements were proposed to constitute a mega-integron by Clark et al. (17), and proof of this hypothesis was recently obtained by Mazel et al. (65). Integrons are gene expression elements that can capture and disseminate heterologous genes (gene cassettes). The insertion of a gene cassette involves a site-specific recombination between the circularized cassette and the recipient integron. Insertion of a gene cassette into an integron can convert a nonfunctional gene into a functional gene. The essential elements in this gene acquisition system are an integrase gene (*int*) (related to the integrase genes of temperate bacteriophages) and a linked attachment site (*attI*). Integrons were initially discovered because of their role in disseminating antibiotic resistance genes. Mazel et al. (65) cloned an integrase gene from *V. cholerae* with 45 to 50% identity to previously described integron integrases and demonstrated that a cloned *V. cholerae* ORF adjacent to a VCR element could be inserted into an integron in *E. coli*.

The VCR cassette is present in strains of *V. mimicus* and *V. parahaemolyticus,* as well as in a strain of *V. metschnikovii* isolated in 1888 (65). Interestingly, these sequences are not dispersed throughout the *V. cholerae* genome but are all present in a single 300-kb *Not*I fragment in an El Tor strain (6). The G+C content of the ORFs associated with VCR elements (33 to 45%) suggests that these genes were recruited from other microbial sources. In addition to the genes encoding the mannose- and fucose-resistant hemagglutinin, VCR elements flank the gene encoding a heat-stable enterotoxin present in many non-O1 *V. cholerae* strains and occasional O1 strains (74). The demonstration of a functional integron system and the association of genes encoding a potential adherence factor and enterotoxin suggest that integrons have played a role in the acquisition of virulence factor genes and the evolution of *V. cholerae* as a pathogen.

O-Antigen Synthesis Region

The emergence of *V. cholerae* O139 in 1992 was an unprecedented event in the history of cholera. Before this event, epidemic and pandemic cholera was caused only by strains of the O1 serogroup, of the classical or El Tor biotype. As noted above, the major difference between the two O serogroups is the acquisition of new genes encoding the O139 O antigen and capsule. Work from several groups has shown that a 22-kb DNA region encoding the O1 antigen (*rfb* region) has been replaced by a 35-kb region of novel DNA encoding the O139 surface polysaccharides (11, 12, 18, 98, 101). The replacement DNA included 29 ORFs encoding O antigen and capsule biosynthesis (*wbf* genes), regulation of O antigen length (*wzz* or *otnB*), capsule transport (*wbtF* or *otnA*), and other functions (reviewed by Stroeher et al. [99]). The 22-kb deletion and 35-kb substitution responsible for the conversion of O1 to O139 are markedly different from the minor genetic changes responsible for antigenic shifts between the Ogawa and Inaba serotypes. Serotype conversions between the Ogawa and Inaba serotypes within the O1 serogroup are due to mutations in a single gene, *wbeT*; mutations as small as the deletion of a single nucleotide can bring about this seroconversion (100).

The region encoding the O139 polysaccharides was apparently introduced into an El Tor O1 strain by horizontal transfer, although the origin of these genes and the mechanism of transfer are unknown. Given that the genes flanking the *rfb* regions are essentially identical between O1 and O139 strains and that all of the O1 *rfb* region has been precisely deleted, a logical hypothesis is that the entire region was introduced into an O1 strain en bloc from a non-O1 strain via homologous recombination. However, hybridization of the O139 *rfb* and capsule genes to a variety of non-O1 *V. cholerae* strains and *Vibrio* species other than *V. cholerae* did not reveal the presence of this entire region in any single potential donor strain. The *wzm* (formerly *otnA*) and *wzz* (formerly *otnB*) genes hybridize to strains of the O69 and O141 serogroups, but sequence analysis indicates that the O139 DNA has not been directly acquired from these serogroups (12). Probes for the *wbfW* and *wbfX* genes hybridize to a wide range of non-O1 strains, while a *wbfR* probe hybridizes to *V. damsela* but not to any non-O1 *V. cholerae* strains tested (18). The G+C composition of the region provides little insight, since the majority of the O139 genes have a G+C content between 42 and 49%, although several ORFs have G+C contents of around 30% (99). An insertion sequence, IS*1358,* is present within both O1 and O139 *rfb* clusters, and it has been speculated that this element played a role in insertion of the O139 *rfb* region, although evidence for a role other than providing conserved sequences for homologous recombination is lacking (99). The mode of transfer, whether by phages, plasmids, or conjugative transposons, is unknown.

The *rfb* region encoding the O antigen makes a major contribution to the virulence of *V. cholerae*. Mutations in the *rfb* region result in attenuation of virulence in animal models (44), but a more dramatic example of this contribution can be seen in the epidemiology of cholera in Bangladesh, when the O139 serogroup first emerged. Prior to the emergence of O139, the majority of cholera cases in Bangladesh and other countries with endemic infection were in individuals younger than 15 years, since substantial immunity is acquired by adulthood. However, when O139 emerged, the majority of cases were in individuals older than 15 years, since their preexisting immunity to *V. cholerae* O1 apparently provided no protection against *V. cholerae* O139 (1). After many people had acquired immunity to O139, the majority of cases were again found in individuals younger than 15 years. These results are consistent with a variety of evidence showing that the LPS antigen is the most important determinant of immunity in cholera (reviewed in reference 50).

The Hemolysin-Lipase Region

The gene encoding the El Tor hemolysin (*hlyA*) was first cloned some 15 years ago. Recently, it has been shown that several genes flanking *hlyA* encode products that can damage host cells, suggesting that this region may be a PAI (29, 75). Upstream of *hlyA* and divergently transcribed is the *lec* gene, encoding a lecithinase/phospholipase (29). Downstream of *hlyA* are the *lipA* and *lipB* genes, whose predicted products have strong homology to lipase genes of *Pseudomonas* spp. Downstream of the *lipAB* genes is the *prtV* gene, encoding a predicted 102-kDa metalloprotease (75). Between *hlyA* and *lipA* is the *hlyB* gene, which encodes a predicted chemotactic transducer that could potentially monitor the nutrient status of the surrounding environment and signal the bacteria to move accordingly (75). These genes are all contained in a 12-kb region that is located on the smaller of the two *V. cholerae* chromosomes (107). The full extent of this region is not known, since the available sequence information does not extend beyond the *lec* and *prtV* genes at each end.

The contribution of this region to disease due to *V. cholerae* is not known. A number of animal studies have implicated the El Tor hemolysin as a virulence factor of *V. cholerae*, perhaps as an enterotoxin (reviewed in reference 50). However, a volunteer study comparing Δ*ctx* strains mutated in the gene encoding the hemolysin did not show obvious differences in human disease with regard to diarrheal attack rate or stool volume (60). A *lec* mutant was unaltered in activity in rabbit ligated-ileal-loop assays (29), and neither *lipA* nor *prtV* mutants were attenuated in the infant-mouse model (75). No genes with obvious homology to phage or insertion elements are present in the available sequence. Thus, the designation of the hemolysin-lipase region as a true PAI awaits further evidence.

CONCLUSIONS

The concept that mobile genetic elements play a crucial role in the pathogenesis of disease due to *V. cholerae* has emerged only in the last 3 years. It was only in the last year that the *V. cholerae* genome was discovered to contain two chromosomes rather than the single chromosome that had long been assumed. In the past decade, a completely new form of epidemic *V. cholerae* has emerged, *V. cholerae* O139. Also in the past decade, cholera struck South America, the one continent previously untouched by this disease in the 20th century, in an epidemic that is the largest ever recorded. These new discoveries and new developments have occurred with a pathogen that has been extensively studied since the latter part of the 19th century.

The two major virulence factors so far described for *V. cholerae* are CT and TCP. Remarkably, both of these have recently been shown to be encoded on genomes of transferable phages, discoveries which provide new information about the mechanisms involved in the emergence of epidemic and pandemic *V. cholerae*. A phage origin has been hypothesized for many PAIs, but it was only recently shown that a toxin-encoding PAI in *Staphylococcus aureus* is actually the genome of a phage (see chapter 14) (62). VPIΦ and CTXΦ of *V. cholerae,* as well as phages of other bacterial species which confer virulence properties and pathogenic potential to the host bacterium, could be referred to as ''pathophages.'' Given the recent finding that the VPI is the genome of a phage, future studies may reveal its bacterial receptor, the role of VPI-encoded proteins in phage assembly and infectivity, and the mechanism by which VPIΦ can serve as both a colonization factor and a bacteriophage. The requirement in bacterial disease for a virus encoding a protein receptor for another virus which then infects the same bacterial cell is a novel finding and suggests that this phenomenon may be more common in nature.

Although the results suggest that the VPI and CTX element can potentially be transferred and present in multiple serogroups of *V. cholerae,* the pathogenic potential of such recipient strains has not yet been studied, and it is not known whether the addition of only these two elements is sufficient to convert an avirulent *V. cholerae* strain to a virulent strain. The contributions of other bacteriophages, the VCR integron, CONSTIN, and other mobile virulence determinants to the evolution of this pathogen are also unknown. The determination of the genomic sequence of *V. cholerae* will undoubtedly reveal additional virulence factors, PAIs, and other mobile virulence elements. The dual role of *V. cholerae* as a member of the normal bacterial flora in estuarine aquatic environments and as a potentially lethal human intestinal pathogen no doubt requires numerous mechanisms for gene regulation and exchange. The recent findings described in this chapter should lead to future studies that will help us understand the emergence, pathogenesis, and spread of cholera, a disease which still surprises and challenges us after a century of study.

Acknowledgments. This work is supported by NIH grant AI-19716 (J.B.K.). D.K.R.K. is a recipient of a Burroughs Wellcome Career Award in the Biomedical Sciences.

REFERENCES

1. **Albert, M. J.** 1996. Epidemiology and molecular biology of *Vibrio cholerae* O139 Bengal. *Indian J. Med. Res.* **104:**14–27.

2. **Albert, M. J.** 1994. *Vibrio cholerae* O139 Bengal. *J. Clin. Microbiol.* **32:**2345–2349.

3. **Albert, M. J., A. K. Siddique, M. S. Islam, A. S. G. Faruque, M. Ansaruzzaman, S. M. Faruque, and R. B. Sack.** 1993. A large outbreak of clinical cholera due to *Vibrio cholerae* non-O1 in Bangladesh. *Lancet* **341:**704.

4. **Alm, R. A., U. H. Stroeher, and P. A. Manning.** 1988. Extracellular proteins of *Vibrio cholerae:* nucleotide sequence of the structural gene (*hlyA*) for the haemolysin of the haemolytic El Tor strain O17 and characterization of the *hlyA* mutation in the non-haemolytic classical strain 569B. *Mol. Microbiol.* **2:**481–488.

5. **Almeida, R. J., D. N. Cameron, W. L. Cook, and I. K. Wachsmuth.** 1992. Vibriophage VcA-3 as an epidemic strain marker for the U.S. Gulf Coast *Vibrio cholerae* O1 clone. *J. Clin. Microbiol.* **30:**300–304.

6. **Barker, A., C. A. Clark, and P. A. Manning.** 1994. Identification of VCR, a repeated sequence associated with a locus encoding a hemagglutinin in *Vibrio cholerae* O1. *J. Bacteriol.* **176:**5450–5458.

7. **Bartowsky, E. J., S. R. Attridge, C. J. Thomas, G. Mayrhofer, and P. A. Manning.** 1990. Role of the P plasmid in attenuation of *Vibrio cholerae* O1. *Infect. Immun.* **58:**3129–3134.

8. **Barua, D.** 1972. The global epidemiology of cholera in recent years. *Proc. R. Soc. Med.* **65:**423–428.

9. **Barua, D., and C. Z. Gomez.** 1967. Observations on some tests commonly employed for the characterization of El Tor vibrios. *Bull. W. H. O.* **37:**800–803.

10. **Benenson, A. S.** 1995. Cholera, p. 94–100. *In* A. S. Benenson (ed.), *Control of Communicable Diseases in Man,* 16th ed. American Public Health Association, New York, N.Y.

11. **Bik, E. M., A. E. Bunschoten, R. D. Gouw, and F. R. Mooi.** 1995. Genesis of the novel epidemic *Vibrio cholerae* O139 strain: evidence for horizontal transfer of genes involved in polysaccharide synthesis. *EMBO J.* **14:**209–216.

12. **Bik, E. M., A. E. Bunscoten, R. J. L. Willems, A. C. Y. Chang, and F. R. Mooi.** 1996. Genetic organization and functional analysis of the *otn* DNA essential for cell-wall polysaccharide synthesis in *Vibrio cholerae* O139. *Mol. Microbiol.* **20:**799–811.

13. **Blum, G., M. Ott, A. Lischewski, A. Ritter, H. Imrich, H. Tschape, and J. Hacker.** 1994. Excision of large DNA regions termed pathogenicity islands from tRNA-specific loci in the chromosome of an *Escherichia coli* wild-type pathogen. *Infect. Immun.* **62:**606–614.

14. **Carroll, P. A., K. T. Tashima, M. B. Rogers, V. J. DiRita, and S. B. Calderwood.** 1997. Phase variation in *tcpH* modulates expression of the ToxR regulon in *Vibrio cholerae. Mol. Microbiol.* **25:**1099–1111.

15. **Chen, F., G. M. Evins, W. L. Cook, R. Almeida, N. Hargrett-Bean, and I. K. Wachsmuth.** 1991. Genetic diversity among toxigenic and nontoxigenic *Vibrio cholerae* O1 isolated from the western hemisphere. *Epidemiol. Infect.* **107:**225–233.

16. **Cholera Working Group International Centre for Diarrhaeal Diseases Research, Bangladesh.** 1993. Large epidemic of cholera-like disease in Bangladesh caused by *Vibrio cholerae* O139 synonym Bengal. *Lancet* **342:**387–390.

17. **Clark, C. A., L. Purins, P. Kaewrakon, and P. A. Manning.** 1997. VCR repetitive sequence elements in the *Vibrio cholerae* chromosome constitute a mega-integron. *Mol. Microbiol.* **26:**1137–1138.

18. **Comstock, L. E., J. A. Johnson, J. M. Michalski, J. G. Morris, Jr., and J. B. Kaper.** 1996. Cloning and sequence of a region encoding a surface polysaccharide of *Vibrio cholerae* O139 and characterization of the insertion site in the chromosome of *V. cholerae* O1. *Mol. Microbiol.* **19:**815–826.

19. **Cook, W. L., K. Wachsmuth, S. R. Johnson, K. A. Birkness, and A. R. Samadi.** 1984. Persistence of plasmids, cholera toxin genes, and prophage DNA in classical *Vibrio cholerae* O1. *Infect. Immun.* **45:**222–226.

20. **DiRita, V. J., and J. J. Mekalanos.** 1991. Periplasmic interaction between two membrane regulatory proteins, ToxR and ToxS, results in signal transduction and transcriptional activation. *Cell* **64:**29–37.

21. **DiRita, V. J., C. Parsot, G. Jander, and J. J. Mekalanos.** 1991. Regulatory cascade controls virulence in *Vibrio cholerae. Proc. Natl. Acad. Sci. USA* **88:**5403–5407.

22. **Ehara, M., S. Shimodori, F. Kojima, Y. Ichinose, T. Hirayama, M. J. Albert, K. Supawat, Y. Honma, M. Iwanaga, and K. Amako.** 1997. Characterization of filamentous phages of *Vibrio cholerae* O139 and O1. *FEMS Microbiol. Lett.* **154:**293–301.

23. **Everiss, K. D., K. J. Hughes, M. E. Kovach, and K. M. Peterson.** 1994. The *Vibrio cholerae acfB*

colonization determinant encodes an inner membrane protein that is related to a family of signal-transducing proteins. *Infect. Immun.* **62:**3289–3298.

24. **Faruque, A. S. G., G. J. Fuchs, and M. J. Albert.** 1996. Changing epidemiology of cholera due to *Vibrio cholerae* O1 and O139 Bengal in Dhaka, Bangladesh. *Epidemiol. Infect.* **116:**275–278.

25. **Faruque, S. M., A. R. M. A. Alim, M. M. Rahman, A. K. Siddique, R. B. Sack, and M. J. Albert.** 1993. Clonal relationships among classical *Vibrio cholerae* O1 strains isolated between 1961 and 1992 in Bangladesh. *J. Clin. Microbiol.* **31:**2513–2516.

26. **Faruque, S. M., M. J. Albert, and J. J. Mekalanos.** 1998. Epidemiology, genetics, and ecology of toxigenic *Vibrio cholerae. Microbiol. Mol. Biol. Rev.* **62:**1301–1314.

27. **Feeley, J. C.** 1965. Classification of *Vibrio cholerae* (*Vibrio comma*), including El Tor vibrios, by intrasub-specific characteristics. *J. Bacteriol.* **89:**665–678.

28. **Felsenfeld, O., S. Mukerjee, and N. Nasunya.** 1962. Some characteristics of El Tor vibrios isolated from the 1961–62 epidemics. *J. Trop. Med. Hyg.* **65:**200–202.

29. **Fiore, A. E., J. M. Michalski, R. G. Russell, C. L. Sears, and J. B. Kaper.** 1997. Cloning, characterization, and chromosomal mapping of a phospholipase (lecithinase) produced by *Vibrio cholerae. Infect. Immun.* **65:**3112–3117.

30. **Gallut, J.** 1974. The cholera vibrios, p. 17–40. *In* D. Barua and W. Burrows (ed.), *Cholera.* The W. B. Saunders Co., Philadelphia, Pa.

31. **Gangarosa, E. J., A. Sanati, H. Saghari, and J. C. Feeley.** 1967. Multiple serotypes of *Vibrio cholerae* isolated from a case of cholera. *Lancet* **i:**646–648.

32. **Girón, J. A., A. S. Y. Ho, and G. K. Schoolnick.** 1991. An inducible bundle-forming pilus of enteropatho-genic *Escherichia coli. Science* **254:**710–713.

33. **Goldberg, I., and J. J. Mekalanos.** 1986. Effect of a *recA* mutation on cholera toxin gene amplification and deletion events. *J. Bacteriol.* **165:**723–731.

34. **Hacker, J., L. Bender, M. Ott, J. Wingender, B. Lund, R. Marre, and W. Goebel.** 1990. Deletions of chromosomal regions coding for fimbriae and hemolysins occur in vivo and in vitro in various extraintestinal *Escherichia coli* isolates. *Microb. Pathog.* **8:**213–225.

35. **Hacker, J., G. Blum-Oehler, I. Muhldorfer, and H. Tschape.** 1997. Pathogenicity islands of virulent bacteria: structure, function and impact on microbial evolution. *Mol. Microbiol.* **23:**1089–1097.

36. **Harkey, C. W., K. D. Everiss, and K. M. Peterson.** 1995. Isolation and characterization of a *Vibrio cholerae* gene (*tagA*) that encodes a ToxR-regulated lipoprotein. *Gene* **153:**81–84.

37. **Häse, C. C., and J. J. Mekalanos.** 1998. TcpP protein is a positive regulator of virulence gene expression in *Vibrio cholerae. Proc. Natl. Acad. Sci. USA* **95:**730–734.

38. **Herrington, D. A., R. H. Hall, G. A. Losonsky, J. J. Mekalanos, R. K. Taylor, and M. M. Levine.** 1988. Toxin, toxin-coregulated pili, and the *toxR* regulon are essential for *Vibrio cholerae* pathogenesis in humans. *J. Exp. Med.* **168:**1487–1492.

39. **Hill, D. F., N. J. Short, R. N. Perham, and G. B. Peterson.** 1991. DNA sequence of the filamentous bacteriophage Pfl. *J. Mol. Biol.* **218:**349–363.

40. **Hobbs, M., and J. S. Mattick.** 1993. Common components in the assembly of type 4 fimbriae, DNA transfer systems, filamentous phage and protein-secretion apparatus: a general system for the formation of surface-associated protein complexes. *Mol. Microbiol.* **10:**233–243.

41. **Hochhut, B., and M. K. Waldor.** 1999. Site-specific integration of the conjugal *Vibrio cholerae* SXT element into *prfC. Mol. Microbiol.* **32:**99–110.

42. **Hughes, K. J., K. D. Everiss, C. W. Harkey, and K. M. Peterson.** 1994. Identification of a *Vibrio cholerae* ToxR-activated gene (*tagD*) that is physically linked to the toxin-coregulated pilus (*tcp*) gene cluster. *Gene* **148:**97–100.

43. **Hughes, K. J., K. D. Everiss, M. E. Kovach, and K. M. Peterson.** 1994. Sequence analysis of the *Vibrio cholerae acfD* gene reveals the presence of an overlapping reading frame, *orfZ*, which encodes a protein that shares sequence similarity to the FliA and FliC products of *Salmonella. Gene* **146:**79–82.

44. **Iredell, J. R., U. H. Stroeher, H. M. Ward, and P. A. Manning.** 1998. Lipopolysaccharide O-antigen expression and the effect of its absence on virulence in *rfb* mutants of *Vibrio cholerae* O1. *FEMS Immunol. Med. Microbiol.* **20:**45–54.

45. **Jouravleva, E. A., G. A. McDonald, C. F. Garon, M. Boesman-Finkelstein, and R. A. Finkelstein.** 1998. Characterization and possible functions of a new filamentous bacteriophage from *Vibrio cholerae* O139. *Microbiology* **144:**315–324.

46. **Jouravleva, E. A., G. A. McDonald, J. W. Marsh, R. K. Taylor, M. Boesman-Finkelstein, and R. A. Finkelstein.** 1998. The *Vibrio cholerae* mannose-sensitive hemagglutinin is the receptor for a filamentous bacteriophage from *V. cholerae* O139. *Infect. Immun.* **66:**2535–2539.

47. **Kamal, A. M.** 1974. The seventh pandemic of cholera, p. 1–14. *In* D. Barua and W. Burrows (ed.), *Cholera.* The W. B. Saunders Co., Philadelphia, Pa.

48. **Kaper, J. B., and M. M. Baldini.** 1992. Genetics, p. 69–94. *In* D. Barua and W. B. Greenough III (ed.), *Cholera.* Plenum Medical Book Co., New York, N.Y.

49. **Kaper, J. B., J. Michalski, J. M. Ketley, and M. M. Levine.** 1994. Potential for reacquisition of cholera enterotoxin genes by attenuated *Vibrio cholerae* vaccine strain CVD103-HgR. *Infect. Immun.* **62:** 1480–1483.

50. **Kaper, J. B., J. G. Morris, Jr., and M. M. Levine.** 1995. Cholera. *Clin. Microbiol. Rev.* **8:**48–86.

51. **Kar, S., R. K. Ghosh, A. N. Ghosh, and A. Ghosh.** 1996. Integration of the DNA of a novel filamentous bacteriophage VSK from *Vibrio cholerae* O139 into the host chromosomal DNA. *FEMS Microbiol. Lett.* **145:**17–22.

52. **Karaolis, D. K. R., J. A. Johnson, C. C. Bailey, E. C. Boedeker, J. B. Kaper, and P. R. Reeves.** 1998. A *Vibrio cholerae* pathogenicity island associated with epidemic and pandemic strains. *Proc. Natl. Acad. Sci. USA* **95:**3134–3139.

53. **Karaolis, D. K. R., R. Lan, and P. R. Reeves.** 1994. Molecular evolution of the 7th pandemic clone of *Vibrio cholerae* and its relationship to other pandemic and epidemic *V. cholerae* strains. *J. Bacteriol.* **176:** 6199–6206.

54. **Karaolis, D. K. R., R. Lan, and P. R. Reeves.** 1995. The sixth and seventh cholera pandemics are due to independent clones separately derived from environmental, nontoxigenic, non-O1 *Vibrio cholerae. J. Bacteriol.* **177:**3191–3198.

55. **Karaolis, D. K. R., S. Somara, D. R. Maneval, Jr., J. A. Johnson, and J. B. Kaper.** A bacteriophage encoding a pathogenicity island, type IV pilus, and phage receptor in cholera bacteria. *Nature*, in press.

56. **Koblavi, S., F. Grimont, and P. A. D. Grimont.** 1990. Clonal diversity of *Vibrio cholerae* O1 evidenced by rRNA gene restriction patterns. *Res. Microbiol.* **141:**645–657.

57. **Koonin, E. V.** 1992. The second cholera toxin, Zot, and its plasmid-encoded and phage encoded homologues constitute a group of putative ATP-ases with an altered purine NTP-binding motif. *FEBS Lett.* **312:**3–6.

58. **Kovach, M. E., K. J. Hughes, K. D. Everiss, and K. M. Peterson.** 1994. Identification of a ToxR-activated gene, *tagE,* that lies within the accessory colonization factor gene cluster of *Vibrio cholerae* O395. *Gene* **148:**91–95.

59. **Kovach, M. E., M. D. Shaffer, and K. M. Peterson.** 1996. A putative integrase gene defines the distal end of a large cluster of ToxR-regulated colonization genes in *Vibrio cholerae. Microbiology* **142:**2165–2174.

60. **Levine, M. M., J. B. Kaper, D. Herrington, G. Losonsky, J. G. Morris, M. Clements, R. E. Black, B. Tall, and R. Hall.** 1988. Volunteer studies of deletion mutants of *Vibrio cholerae* O1 prepared by recombinant techniques. *Infect. Immun.* **56:**161–167.

61. **Lin, W., K. J. Fullner, R. Clayton, J. A. Sexton, M. B. Rogers, K. E. Calia, S. B. Calderwood, C. Frasier, and J. J. Mekalanos.** 1999. Identification of a *Vibrio cholerae* RTX toxin gene cluster that is tightly linked to the cholera toxin prophage. *Proc. Natl. Acad. Sci. USA* **96:**1071–1076.

62. **Lindsay, J. A., A. Ruzin, H. F. Ross, N. Kurepina, and R. P. Novick.** 1998. The gene for toxic shock toxin is carried by a family of mobile pathogenicity islands in *Staphylococcus aureus. Mol. Microbiol.* **29:** 527–543.

63. **Manning, P. A.** 1997. The *tcp* gene cluster of *Vibrio cholerae. Gene* **192:**63–70.

64. **Manning, P. A., U. W. Stroeher, and R. Morona.** 1994. Molecular basis for O-antigen biosynthesis in *Vibrio cholerae* O1: Ogawa-Inaba switching, p. 77–94. *In* I. K. Wachsmuth, P. A. Blake, and Ø. Olsvik (ed.), Vibrio cholerae *and Cholera.* American Society for Microbiology, Washington, D.C.

65. **Mazel, D., B. Dychinco, V. A. Webb, and J. Davies.** 1998. A distinctive class of integron in the *Vibrio cholerae* genome. *Science* **280:**605–608.

66. **Mekalanos, J. J.** 1985. Cholera toxin: genetic analysis, regulation, and role in pathogenesis. *Curr. Top. Microbiol. Immunol.* **118:**97–118.

67. **Mekalanos, J. J.** 1983. Duplication and amplification of toxin genes in *Vibrio cholerae. Cell* **35:**253–263.

68. **Michalski, J., J. E. Galen, A. Fasano, and J. B. Kaper.** 1993. CVD110, an attenuated *Vibrio cholerae* O1 El Tor live oral vaccine strain. *Infect. Immun.* **61:**4462–4468.

69. **Miller, V. L., R. K. Taylor, and J. J. Mekalanos.** 1987. Cholera toxin transcriptional activator ToxR is a transmembrane DNA binding protein. *Cell* **48:**271–279.

70. **Model, P., and M. Russel.** 1988. Filamentous bacteriophage, p. 375–456. *In* R. Calender (ed.), *The Bacteriophages.* Plenum Publishing Corp., New York, N.Y.

71. **Morris, J. G., Jr.** 1994. Non-O1 group 1 *Vibrio cholerae* strains not associated with epidemic disease, p. 103–115. *In* I. K. Wachsmuth, P. A. Blake, and Ø Olsvik (ed.), Vibrio cholerae *and Cholera: Molecular to Global Perspectives.* American Society for Microbiology, Washington, D.C.

72. **Mukhopadhyay, A. K., A. Basu, P. Garg, P. K. Bag, A. Ghosh, S. K. Bhattacharya, Y. Takeda, and G. B. Nair.** 1998. Molecular epidemiology of reemergent *Vibrio cholerae* O139 Bengal in India. *J. Clin. Microbiol.* **36:**2149–2152.

73. **Nesper, J., J. Blass, M. Fountoulakis, and J. Reidl.** 1999. Characterization of the major control region of *Vibrio cholerae* bacteriophage K139: immunity, exclusion, and integration. *J. Bacteriol.* **181:**2902–2913.

74. **Ogawa, A., and T. Takeda.** 1993. The gene encoding the heat-stable enterotoxin of *Vibrio cholerae* is flanked by 123-base pair direct repeats. *Microbiol. Immunol.* **37:**607–616.

75. **Ogierman, M. A., A. Fallarino, T. Riess, S. G. Williams, S. R. Attridge, and P. A. Manning.** 1997. Characterization of the *Vibrio cholerae* El Tor lipase operon *lipAB* and a protease gene downstream of the *hly* region. *J. Bacteriol.* **179:**7072–7080.

76. **Olsvik, Ø., J. Wahlberg, B. Petterson, M. Uhlen, T. Popovic, I. K. Wachsmuth, and P. I. Fields.** 1993. Use of automated sequencing of polymerase chain reaction-generated amplicons to identify three types of cholera toxin subunit B in *Vibrio cholerae* O1 strains. *J. Clin. Microbiol.* **31:**22–25.

77. **Parsot, C., and J. J. Mekalanos.** 1991. Expression of the *Vibrio cholerae* gene encoding aldehyde dehydrogenase is under control of ToxR, the cholera toxin transcriptional activator. *J. Bacteriol.* **173:**2842–2851.

78. **Pearson, G. D. N., A. Woods, S. L. Chiang, and J. J. Mekalanos.** 1993. CTX genetic element encodes a site-specific recombinase system and an intestinal colonization factor. *Proc. Natl. Acad. Sci. USA* **90:** 3750–3754.

79. **Peterson, K. M., and J. J. Mekalanos.** 1988. Characterization of the *Vibrio cholerae* ToxR regulon: identification of novel genes involved in intestinal colonization. *Infect. Immun.* **56:**2822–2829.

80. **Pollitzer, R.** 1959. *Cholera.* World Health Organization, Geneva, Switzerland.

81. **Popovic, T., C. A. Bopp, Ø. Olsvik, and K. Wachsmuth.** 1993. Epidemiologic application of a standardized ribotype scheme for *V. cholerae* O1. *J. Clin. Microbiol.* **31:**2474–2482.

82. **Rader, A. E., and J. R. Murphy.** 1988. Nucleotide sequences and comparison of the hemolysin determinants of *Vibrio cholerae* El Tor RV79(Hly$^+$) and RV79(Hly$^-$) and classical 569B(Hly$^-$). *Infect. Immun.* **56:**1414–1419.

83. **Ramamurthy, T., S. Garg, R. Sharma, S. K. Bhattacharya, G. B. Nair, T. Shimada, T. Takeda, T. Karasawa, H. Kurazano, A. Pal, and Y. Takeda.** 1993. Emergence of a novel strain of *Vibrio cholerae* with epidemic potential in southern and eastern India. *Lancet* **341:**703–704.

84. **Reidl, J., and J. J. Mekalanos.** 1995. Characterization of *Vibrio cholerae* bacteriophage K139 and use of a novel mini-transposon to identify a phage-encoded virulence factor. *Mol. Microbiol.* **18:**685–701.

85. **Rhine, J. A., and R. K. Taylor.** 1994. TcpA pilin sequences and colonization requirements for O1 and O139 *Vibrio cholerae. Mol. Microbiol.* **13:**1013–1020.

86. **Rowe, B., and J. A. Frost.** 1992. Vibrio phages and phage-typing, p. 95–105. *In* D. Barua and W. B. Greenough III (ed.), *Cholera.* Plenum Publishing Corp., New York, N.Y.

87. **Rubin, E. J., W. Lin, J. J. Mekalanos, and M. K. Waldor.** 1998. Replication and integration of a *Vibrio cholerae* cryptic plasmid linked to the CTX prophage. *Mol. Microbiol.* **28:**1247–1254.

88. **Rubin, E. J., M. K. Waldor, and J. J. Mekalanos.** 1998. Mobile genetic elements and the evolution of new epidemic strains of *Vibrio cholerae,* p. 147–161. *In* R. M. Krause (ed.), *Emerging Infections.* Academic Press, Inc., New York, N.Y.

89. **Russel, M.** 1995. Moving through the membrane with filamentous phages. *Trends Microbiol.* **3:**223–228.

90. **Salles, C. A., and H. Momen.** 1991. Identification of *Vibrio cholerae* by enzyme electrophoresis. *Trans. R. Soc. Trop. Med. Hyg.* **85:**544–547.

91. **Samadi, A. R., N. Shahid, A. Eusof, M. Yunus, M. I. Huq, M. U. Khan, A. S. M. M. Rahman, and A. S. G. Faruque.** 1983. Classical *Vibrio cholerae* biotype displaces El Tor in Bangladesh. *Lancet* **i:** 805–807.

92. **Sears, C. L., and J. B. Kaper.** 1996. Enteric bacterial toxins: mechanisms of action and linkage to intestinal secretion. *Microbiol. Rev.* **60:**167–215.

93. **Sharma, D. P., C. Thomas, R. H. Hall, M. M. Levine, and S. R. Attridge.** 1989. Significance of toxin-coregulated pilus as protective antigens of *Vibrio cholerae* on the infant mouse model. *Vaccine* **7:**451–456.

94. **Shaw, C. E., and R. K. Taylor.** 1990. *Vibrio cholerae* O395 *tcpA* pilin gene sequence and comparison of predicted protein structural features to those of type 4 pilins. *Infect. Immun.* **58:**3042–3049.

95. **Shimada, T., G. B. Nair, B. C. Deb, M. J. Albert, R. B. Sack, and Y. Takeda.** 1993. Outbreak of *Vibrio cholerae* non-O1 in India and Bangladesh. *Lancet* **341:**1346.

96. **Shimodori, S., K. Iida, F. Kojima, A. Takade, M. Ehara, and K. Amako.** 1997. Morphological features of a filamentous phage from *Vibrio cholerae* O139 Bengal. *Microbiol. Immunol.* **41:**757–763.

97. **Shousha, A. T.** 1947. Cholera epidemic in Egypt: a preliminary report. *Bull. W. H. O.* **1:**353–381.

98. **Stroeher, U. H., K. E. Jedani, B. K. Dredge, R. Morona, M. H. Brown, L. E. Karageorgos, M. J. Albert, and P. A. Manning.** 1995. Genetic rearrangements in the *rfb* regions of *Vibrio cholerae* O1 and O139. *Proc. Natl. Acad. Sci. USA* **92:**10374–10378.

99. **Stroeher, U. H., K. E. Jedani, and P. A. Manning.** 1998. Genetic organization of the genes associated with surface polysaccharide synthesis in *Vibrio cholerae* O1, O139 and *Vibrio anguillarum* O1 and O2: a review. *Gene* **223:**269–282.

100. **Stroeher, U. H., L. E. Karageorgos, R. Morona, and P. A. Manning.** 1992. Serotype conversion in *Vibrio cholerae* O1. *Proc. Natl. Acad. Sci. USA* **89:**2566–2570.

101. **Stroeher, U. H., G. Parasivam, B. K. Dredge, and P. A. Manning.** 1997. Novel *Vibrio cholerae* O139 genes involved in lipopolysaccharide biosynthesis. *J. Bacteriol.* **179:**2740–2747.

102. **Sun, D., J. J. Mekalanos, and R. K. Taylor.** 1990. Antibodies directed against the toxin-coregulated pilus isolated from *Vibrio cholerae* provide protection in the infant mouse experimental cholera model. *J. Infect. Dis.* **161:**1231–1236.

103. **Tacket, C. O., R. K. Taylor, G. Losonsky, Y. Lim, J. P. Nataro, J. B. Kaper, and M. M. Levine.** 1998. Investigation of the roles of toxin-coregulated pili and mannose sensitive hemagglutinin pili in the pathogenesis of *Vibrio cholerae* O139 infection. *Infect. Immun.* **66:**692–695.

104. **Taylor, R. K., V. L. Miller, D. B. Furlong, and J. J. Mekalanos.** 1987. The use of *phoA* gene fusions to identify a pilus colonization factor coordinately regulated with cholera toxin. *Proc. Natl. Acad. Sci. USA* **84:**2833–2837.

105. **Taylor, R. K., C. E. Shaw, K. M. Peterson, P. Spears, and J. J. Mekalanos.** 1988. Safe, live *Vibrio cholerae* vaccines? *Vaccine* **6:**151–154.

106. **Trucksis, M., J. E. Galen, J. Michalski, A. Fasano, and J. B. Kaper.** 1993. Accessory cholera enterotoxin (Ace), the third toxin of a *Vibrio cholerae* virulence cassette. *Proc. Natl. Acad. Sci. USA* **90:**5267–5271.

107. **Trucksis, M., J. Michalski, Y. K. Deng, and J. B. Kaper.** 1998. The *Vibrio cholerae* genome contains two unique circular chromosomes. *Proc. Natl. Acad. Sci. USA* **95:**14464–14469.

108. **Waldor, M. K., and J. J. Mekalanos.** 1996. Lysogenic conversion by a filamentous phage encoding cholera toxin. *Science* **272:**1910–1914.

109. **Waldor, M. K., E. J. Rubin, G. D. N. Pearson, H. Kimsey, and J. J. Mekalanos.** 1997. Regulation, replication, and integration functions of the *Vibrio cholerae* CTXΦ are encoded by region RS2. *Mol. Microbiol.* **24:**917–926.

110. **Waldor, M. K., H. Tschape, and J. J. Mekalanos.** 1996. A new type of conjugative transposon encodes resistance to sulfamethoxazole, trimethoprim, and streptomycin in *Vibrio cholerae* O139. *J. Bacteriol.* **178:**4157–4167.

Chapter 10

cag, the Pathogenicity Island of *Helicobacter pylori*, Triggers Host Responses

Antonello Covacci and Rino Rappuoli

H. PYLORI AND ASSOCIATED DISEASES

During the last 100 years of microscopic examination of human pathological samples, we have become aware that the number of bacterial species living as saprophytes or infecting different areas of the body is larger than expected. Most of them are not culturable and cannot be propagated in vitro (55). Some of them, like *Treponema pallidum* and *Mycobacterium leprae,* can be propagated only in vivo by using surrogate animal systems.

Helicobacter pylori was isolated by accidental extended incubation. It is a spiral-shaped, gram-negative, microaerophilic microorganism that colonizes and survives in the hostile environment of the human stomach, in an equilibrium that permanently links the parasite to the host (25). The infection is strongly associated with an increased risk of chronic active gastritis, peptic ulcer disease (PUD), and atrophic gastritis and with a high incidence of antral adenocarcinoma and mucosa-associated lymphoid tissue lymphoma (8). Approximately half of the world's human population is infected for life by *H. pylori,* but only 10% of infections progress to clinical diseases (53). Strains isolated from patients with PUD contain the *cagA* gene (cytotoxin-associated gene A) and express the immunodominant CagA antigen (18, 68).

cagA AND vacA ARE FREQUENTLY COEXPRESSED

Strains isolated from patients with PUD also produce vacuolating toxin VacA (encoded by *vacA* [vacuolating toxin gene A]), which is responsible for the cytopathic effects seen in vitro and in vivo (21, 54, 61, 65). CagA and VacA are frequently coexpressed; however, their genes are 300 kb apart and VacA expression does not require the presence of the *cagA* gene, since null *cagA* mutants still produce the VacA protein (23, 69, 75). The vacuolating toxin was identified as a multimeric complex that interferes with the traffic of late endosomes (expressing the Rab 7 marker) toward the Golgi apparatus and the lysosomal pathway in HeLa and HEp-2 cells (49, 52). Hybrid vesicles that have both late endosomal and lysosomal features accumulate and fuse into acidic vacuoles generated by

Antonello Covacci and Rino Rappuoli • Department of Molecular Biology, Immunobiological Research Institute of Siena, Chiron Vaccines, Via Fiorentina 1, 53100 Siena, Italy.

the vacuolar ATPase proton pump, causing cytoplasmic swelling (5, 22). *vacA* alleles with a selective vacuolating activity have recently been described, and they could be linked to a toxin receptor present in various allelomorphic forms in the human population (51). In most industrialized countries, 70 to 80% of the clinical isolates express CagA (75). Other virulence factors, such as urease or flagellin, which are required for infection and long-term colonization, are produced by all *H. pylori* strains (25). Clinical isolates have been grouped into two broad families, type I and type II, in which type I strains possess the *cag* pathogenicity island (PAI). Interestingly, only type I strains are correlated with severe gastroduodenal diseases and have a predominant antral localization (75).

cag STRUCTURE, STRUCTURAL FRAGMENTATION, AND PHENOTYPIC SWITCHES

Data accumulated in the last 20 years suggest that pathogenic bacteria evolved from nonpathogenic commensal progenitors after rapid acquisition of new genetic traits inherited from unknown microorganisms by horizontal transfer, reminiscent of a phage or a plasmid integrated into the main chromosome or into a large plasmid (34, 35, 43, 51). These genetic traits represent regions of instability that are sometimes flanked by direct repeats. A type III or type IV secretory apparatus is frequently resident (in *Salmonella typhimurium* and *H. pylori*) (44). Evidence for the emergence of new pathogenic variants is very strong and may account for differences in the clinical outcomes of a disease and host range specificity.

Integration

The nucleotide sequence of the *cag* PAI of *H. pylori* CCUG 17874 (identical to NCTC 11638) was released in 1996; this was probably the first full-length PAI accessible to computer analyses (2, 12, 67). The genomic sequence from strain 26695 confirmed the genetic organization of the *cag* PAI, with minor differences emerging as a consequence of different criteria for prediction of open reading frames (66). The 40-kb locus has a G+C content significantly different from the genomic G+C content (35 and 39% of the genome, respectively). The presence of two 31-bp direct repeats at the ends of *cag* indicates that it was originally acquired as a single unit inserted into the chromosomal glutamate racemase gene (*glr*) (12, 56) (Fig. 1a). *glr* mutations are lethal, suggesting that the precise excision of *cag* may depend on a physiological requirement of an intact *glr* gene. *cag* integration does not disrupt the coding sequence of the *glr* gene: the 31-bp module, corresponding to the last nucleotides of the gene surrounding the stop codon, is simply duplicated at the 5'- end of *cag* (12). Within this sequence, a 6-nucleotide region, which also forms the core of the left and right ends of the IS*605* element (an insertion sequence of *Helicobacter*), may serve as a site of recombination (12).

Fragmentation

In reference strain CCUG 17874, the *cag* region is split into *cag*I and *cag*II domains by an intervening sequence flanked on both sides by an IS*605* element (2, 12) (Fig. 1b). The IS*605* element has ends with internal dyad symmetry (centered on the hexanucleotide also present in the *glr* gene) and encodes two putative transposases, TnpA and TnpB; it

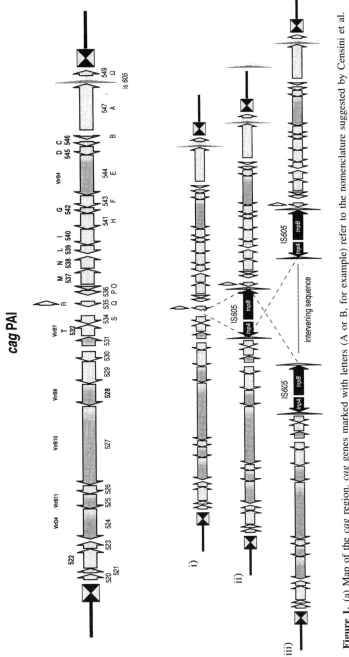

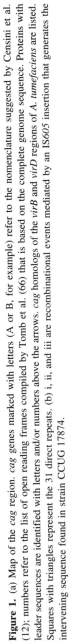

Figure 1. (a) Map of the *cag* region. *cag* genes marked with letters (A or B, for example) refer to the nomenclature suggested by Censini et al. (12); numbers refer to the list of open reading frames compiled by Tomb et al. (66) that is based on the complete genome sequence. Proteins with leader sequences are identified with letters and/or numbers above the arrows. *cag* homologs of the *virB* and *virD* regions of *A. tumefaciens* are listed. Squares with triangles represent the 31 direct repeats. (b) i, ii, and iii are recombinational events mediated by an IS*605* insertion that generates the intervening sequence found in strain CCUG 17874.

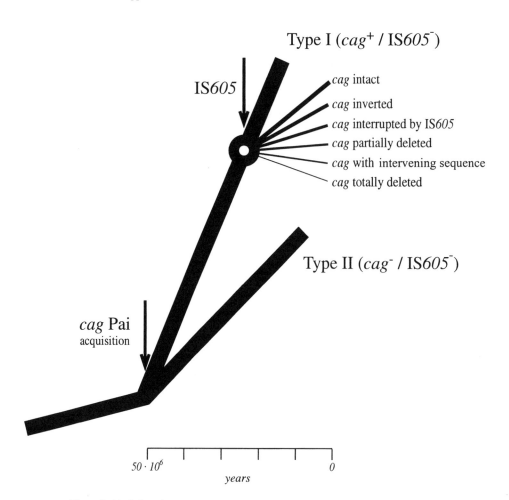

Type I (cag^+ / IS605⁻)

IS605

cag intact
cag inverted
cag interrupted by IS605
cag partially deleted
cag with intervening sequence
cag totally deleted

Type II (cag^- / IS605⁻)

cag Pai
acquisition

50 · 10⁶   0
years

Figure 2. Evolution of type I, intermediate, and type II strains. *cag* acquisition is indicated by an arrow. The white circle indicates the IS605 insertion. The type I and type II lineages show little divergence. Intermediate strains branch from type I, and the level of *cag* fragmentation is progressively increasing (top to bottom). All intermediate strains are positive for IS605. A tentative bar scale is indicated and was obtained by computer simulation calculated on the basis of DNA amelioration rates.

resembles analogous genes found in IS*200* from gram-negative bacteria and IS*1341* from thermophilic bacterium PS3 (12). Intermediate strains, ideally represented as branches from the type I lineage, presumably emerged following IS605 insertion and homologous recombination (12) (Fig. 2).

Excision

Southern analysis shows that the structure of the *cag* locus varies. For example, although 10 of 40 different strains from a set of clinical isolates contained *cag*I and *cag*II fused

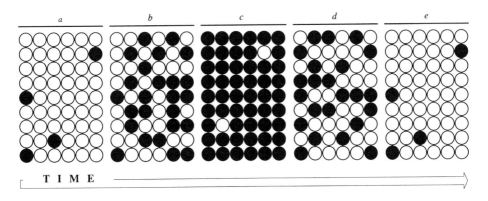

Figure 3. Model illustrating cycles of contraction and expansion of the *H. pylori* population during a chronic infection. Open circles represent *cag*⁺ bacteria, and solid circles represent *cag* bacteria. Loss of the *cag* PAI is the most frequent event in vivo. (a) After infection with a type I strain, the acute phase is dominated by *cag*⁺ bacteria. (b and c) During the remission phase, *cag*⁻ clones, originated by selective pressure, expanded. (d and e) After remission, another wave of clonal expansion of *cag*⁺ bacteria starts. This model was originally proposed by J. Hacker to explain chronic urinary infections by *E. coli* 536.

without IS*605,* other strains with multiple copies of IS*605* exhibited partial or total deletion of *cag*I or total deletion of *cag*I and *cag*II. Type II strains lack both *cag* and IS*605* sequences (12). In summary, the *cag* locus is unstable, simply inverted, or mutilated by partial or total deletions and functionally impaired so that the mutants resemble type II strains. Deletion of *cag* by an inductive signal or selective forces may promote the readaptation of the pathogen at different stages of infection and might explain chronic persistence as a result of continual fluctuations in the proportion of *cag*⁺ and *cag*⁻ bacteria (6, 9, 19, 28) (Fig. 3).

cag-DEPENDENT HOST RESPONSES

Pathogens activate host signal transduction pathways through ligand-receptor interactions with secreted virulence factors that differ among species but with secretion apparatuses that in some cases are interchangeable. Mechanisms involved include enzymatic tyrosine kinase activity, bacterial tyrosine phosphatase activity, local cytoskeletal rearrangements of actin and actin-binding proteins with sustained polymerization, and alterations in intracellular traffic (29, 30, 46). Secreted products are responsible for the activation of the cellular program of apoptosis (programmed cellular death) for host cell responses to *Helicobacter* and also for responses to *Shigella flexneri, Salmonella typhimurium, Staphylococcus aureus, Pseudomonas aeruginosa,* and *Yersinia pestis* (76). The release of molecules which are targeted outside the bacterial cell or transferred between cells depends on secretion pathways. Proteins encoded by genes located in *cag* are involved in *H. pylori*-host cell interaction as part of a type IV secretion apparatus that reroutes molecules synthesized in the bacterial cytoplasm to the cytoplasm of the eukaryotic cells (29, 30). Isogenic *cag* mutants negatively affect interleukin-8 (IL-8) production (23), which suggests that *cag* plays a role in chronic inflammation, inducing epithelial cell secretion of IL-8 after increased transcription of responsive promoters by activated NF-κB molecules (32, 50). Activation of NF-κB is accompanied by drastic changes in the recipient cells. Production of long protrusions of the apical pole, forming pedestals that cup bacteria, follows remodelling of the cell surface by an intense cytoskeletal activity, with actin and actin-associated proteins polymerization (62). Tyrosine phosphorylation of a 145-kDa host protein becomes evident (63); by analogy to anteropathogenic *Escherichia coli* (EPEC) strains, this molecule can be either a protein encoded by the host, phosphorylated as a consequence of the intimate adhesion, or a bacterial product, encoded by a putative gene located within *cag*, phosphorylated by a bacterial tyrosine kinase and later injected into the host (24, 26, 38, 57). The cytoskeletal remodelling after contact with type I *H. pylori* is drastically reduced when cells are exposed to type II strains and *cag* mutants (63). It has proposed that bacterial secretion systems were constitutive elements of primitive bacteria and were used for cell communication and that they later evolved into specialized machines for virulence and other forms of bacterial specialization (29).

cag AS TYPE IV SECRETION APPARATUS AND PUTATIVE *cag* SUBSTRATES

Type IV systems are present in the genome of *Bordetella pertussis* (pertussis toxin liberation genes) (17, 73), *Agrobacterium tumefaciens* (*virBDE* regions of the Ti plasmid) (7, 31), *E. coli* (*tra* genes) (13, 74), *Legionella pneumophila* (39, 64), *Rickettsia prowazekii* (4), and *H. pylori* (*cag* PAI) (2, 12, 66, 67). Secretion of autotransporting proteins such as immunoglobulin A protease has also been referred to as type IV secretion. This secretion process involves a mechanism completely different from what we refer to as type IV secretion as exhibited by *H. pylori*.

Recently it has become clear that a plant pathogen and at least five human pathogens have adapted a version of a conjugative transfer machinery to secrete macromolecules that are targeted during bacterial contact with epithelia or plant cells (13, 74). The channel serves as a transenvelope conduit through which unfolded molecules pass, while the pilus is proposed to mediate the physical contact between the bacterium and a recipient cell. The genes coding for related proteins are colinear in the various operons, providing further evidence of common ancestry (13).

Members of a Family

B. pertussis, the causative agent of whooping cough, uses the Ptl transporter to export the six-subunit pertussis toxin across the bacterial envelope (17, 73). Very recently, another member of the type IV family was shown to be important for the virulence of *L. pneumophila,* the causative agent of Legionnaires' disease and Pontiac fever (39, 64). Mutational studies aimed at identifying genes involved in intracellular growth and in macrophage killing resulted in the identification of the *icm/dot* genes. Products of two of these genes, *dotG* and *dotB,* are related to VirB proteins, and products of several other *icm/dot* genes have homologs in bacterial conjugation systems (39, 64). As with the related Cag proteins of *H. pylori,* the Icm/Dot proteins act as an exporters for the virulence factor(s) targeted to the intracellular environment to enhance survival and to kill host macrophages (39, 64).

Two homologs of VirB4 and one homolog each of VirB8, VirB9, VirB10, VirB11, and VirD4 were detected in the complete nucleotide sequence of *R. prowazekii*, suggesting that this microorganism contains another type IV transport system similar to the *H. pylori* and *Legionella* system (4).

System Architecture

VirB2 is the major pilin subunit recruited to the outer membrane for pilus polymerization (41). The VirB proteins are required for pilus assembly, but it is not known whether the VirB proteins participate directly in pilus morphogenesis or simply provide an anchor at the membrane for pilus attachment. VirB4 and VirB11 hydrolyze ATP in vitro. These proteins utilize the energy of ATP hydrolysis to drive transporter assembly or substrate translocation (7, 13). Both ATPases are tightly associated with the inner membrane. Each forms a homodimer early during assembly with other transporter components, although the final oligomeric structure of these proteins in the fully assembled transporter is unknown. VirB4 is an integral membrane protein with two domains embedded either into or through the membrane into the periplasm (13). VirB11 is tightly bound to the membrane and probably is localized exclusively on the cytoplasmic face of the membrane (13). VirB7 and VirB9 are likely candidates for components of an outer membrane pore. The functions of the remaining transporter components have not been defined, but structural predictions indicate that most of the *cag*-encoded proteins are composed of membrane-associated domains and suggest that the PAI may actually arise from combinations of different primitive PAIs until an optimum was reached. The recent discovery of the inflammatory PAI of *Shigella* unveiled the presence of a distant homolog of CagO that has no counterpart in other type IV systems and is associated with an inflammatory reaction (77).

Assisted Folding

The remaining VirB proteins may be structural subunits of the putative transenvelope channel or may transiently assist in the assembly of this structure. Studies of *cag* mutants revealed that some of the proteins, most notably the lipoprotein CagT (a VirB7 homolog) and the VirB9 homolog, provide important stabilizing functions for other VirB proteins (42).

The existence of 30 different proteins all encoded within *cag* underscores the functional importance of specialized chaperones in macromolecular export. The dependence of CagT stability on CagM may be functionally related to periplasmic chaperons (42). Recent data suggest that VirB4, VirB7, VirB9, VirB10, and VirB11 assemble as a complex and form the core of the transporter (4, 12, 14, 67) (Fig. 4). Therefore, all the components of a simplified type IV system are present, and an intriguing feature is the presence of the VirD4 homolog, which is associated with type IV secretion systems to couple conjugative DNA transfer. We can broaden the scope of this section speculating that the *cag* region can export proteins and nucleoproteins across kingdom boundaries (14).

Substrates

Conjugal DNA transfer intermediates are thought to be delivered across the donor cell envelope in a single step through a proteinaceous channel or mating pore. In striking

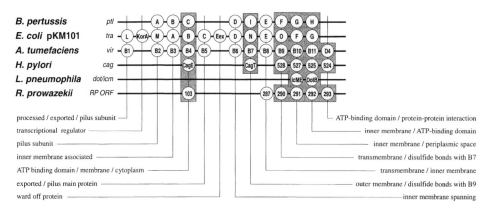

Figure 4. Evolutionary relationships between members of the type IV secretion apparatuses. Boxes indicate individual gene products, and the order reflects their relative position within the operons. Functions and localization are provided for each member. The shaded areas refer to the minimal set of Vir homologs present within *cag*.

contrast, the highly related Ptl exporter is proposed to function quite differently. *B. pertussis* excretes functional pertussis toxin into the extracellular milieu, which has led to the hypothesis that the Ptl proteins do not elaborate a pilus. However, it is notable that PtlA is related to the VirB2 pilin subunit (14, 17, 73, 74). This could mean that the Ptl system does in fact assemble at least a vestige of a pilus or that VirB2-type proteins supply a function which is critical to transporter assembly but unrelated to pilus assembly. The proposed toxin substrates exported by the *H. pylori cag* and *L. pneumophila icm/dot* systems have not yet been identified. However, the *L. pneumophila icm/dot* system directs the interbacterial movement of plasmid RSF1010 (39, 64). Cells carrying RSF1010 display a reduction in intracellular multiplication and human macrophage killing. Both these features of the infection process are thought to result from export of a toxin effector via the *icm/dot* system (39, 64). These observations suggest that the *icm/dot* system has retained a functional vestige of the ancestral DNA conjugation system from which it evolved (39, 64). Whether other type IV toxin export systems, including the *B. pertussis* Ptl system and the *H. pylori* Cag system, also are capable of directing conjugative DNA transfer to recipient bacteria or even to eukaryotic cells remains to be tested.

Together, these findings raise the intriguing possibility that this subset of proteins corresponds to a minimal ancestral protein subassembly upon which bacteria have built construct transporters designed for novel purposes including intercellular DNA transfer, toxin export, and, possibly, direct injection of virulence factors into eukaryotic cells.

cag MOLECULAR CELL BIOLOGY

The flagellar apparatus, or a simplified version of it, was proposed as a common ancestor of the type III secretion machines (40, 45). These systems eventually specialized as extracellular tubular protrusions or as an intracellular gated complex involved in substrate transfer between different subcellular compartments (16, 71). This analogy can be extended to the type IV family, which is thought to originate from a conjugative apparatus that later associated with other classes of genes, providing an entirely new range of functions over an evolutionary time scale. Type III and IV systems have a progenitor in the filamentous phage assembly/secretion processes (58–60). These systems deliver toxins and nucleoprotein particles that interact with discrete receptors and, for all of the known systems, are internalized, where they mediate a variety of intracellular responses. Within the eukaryotic cell, the effector molecules may perturb cellular functions through direct structural interactions. Alternatively, the transferred molecule may be DNA, in which case gene expression alters the cellular physiology. In type IV secretion systems, the variety of effects is extremely great, even though the exported substrate and its precise mode of action are not defined. In *Helicobacter*, the *cag* system induces the epithelial secretion of IL-8, which depends on the NF-κB activation (12, 32, 50, 67). In addition, the 145-kDa protein is tyrosine phosphorylated and pedestals are formed after actin rearrangements and vasodilator-stimulated phosphoprotein (VASP) accumulation (62, 63) (Fig. 5). Interestingly, all these events are controlled by a type III secretion system in EPEC strains (26, 57). The *Legionella icm/dot* system transfers DNA to other bacterial cells, although DNA is not thought to be the substrate involved in *Legionella* virulence (39, 64). Rather, in mammalian hosts, the *dot/icm* gene products are thought to export a toxin that promotes intracellular multiplication, killing of human macrophages, and prevention of phagosome-lysosome fusion. This latter response suggests that both types III and IV play a direct role in altering communication processes between cells but also within distinct subcellular compartments (15, 70).

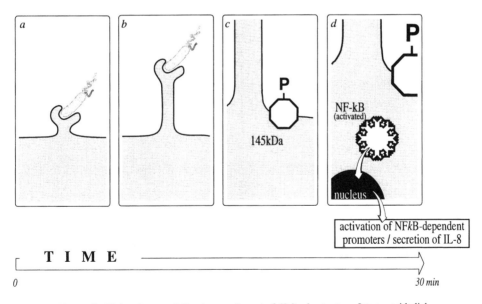

Figure 5. Chain of events following attachment of *Helicobacter* type I to an epithelial cell in culture. (a) Pedestal induction. (b) Growth of the pseudopodium and triggering of intracellular reactions. (c) Resulting tyrosine phosphorylation of the 145-kDa protein localized in the membrane fraction. (d) Resulting activation of NF-κB and IL-8 secretion.

COEVOLUTION WITH THE HOST

Helicobacter is a nonclonal pathogen with a pronounced interstrain variability (1, 37). Most of the differences between sequenced genomes (two at the time of this review [3]) are chromosomal inversions with silent mutations accumulated in the third position at a rate of 1 every 21 bp. More than 30% of the genome is essentially made up of duplication products. Strains isolated in clinical practice tend to cultural coevolution: they are genetically more homogeneous within the ethnic group of the patient when measured by random amplification of polymorphic DNA (10, 33, 36, 47, 72). Anatomically modern humans originated in Africa, and they migrated toward New Guinea and Australia 60,000 years ago and to Europe probably 40,000 years ago, and they reached the Americas around 15,000 years ago. Geographic expansions of populations spread their genes. In turn, technological innovations that favor transport sparked new expansions (27). During the major radiations, descendants of African ancestors almost exterminated the great mammals (and did exterminate the mammoth and the giant marsupials) and giant birds, limiting the number of domesticable species. Agriculture and breeding spread quite recently, between 10,500 years ago (Middle East) and 4,500 years ago (Atlantic coast of North America) and reached a peak in southern Europe. As a result of exposure to domestic animals, Europeans were targeted by transmissible diseases such as smallpox, mumps, typhoid fever, influenza, tuberculosis, plague, cholera, and syphilis, and so they developed a relative immunity (27).

It is now clear that most of the infectious diseases have an animal origin, require an intermediate host, and occasionally infect humans. Epidemics originated only after groups merged into a complex sociocultural structure, i.e., a population (27). The diffusion of *H. pylori* entails the spread of a population's culture. This was influenced by the history of parasitic association of the bacterium with the human species and the migratory expansion (20). *Helicobacter,* like ''cultural traits transmitted vertically, and therefore in a way similar to that of our genes,'' shares the same evolutionary history of humans and reflects the stratification of cultures, genes, and pathogens (11).

Acknowledgments. We thank S. Falkow, J. Hacker, and J. Kaper for helpful suggestions. The work of L. L. Cavalli-Sforza was a major source of inspiration. We acknowledge P. Christie and A. Zychlinsky for their unpublished observations and N. Lange, S. Censini, S. Guidotti, M. Marchetti, M. Stein, E. Segal, and H. Pahl for granting access to experimental data. We gratefully acknowledge G. Corsi for the illustrations and C. Mallia for editorial assistance. R. Beltrami generously assisted in the computer analyses.

REFERENCES

1. **Akopyanz, N., N. O. Bukanov, T. U. Westblom, and D. E. Berg.** 1992. PCR-based RFLP analysis of DNA sequence diversity in the gastric pathogen *Helicobacter pylori. Nucleic Acids Res.* **20:**6221–6225.
2. **Akopyanz, N. S., S. W. Clifton, D. Kersulyte, J. E. Crabtree, B. E. Youree, C. A. Reece, N. O. Bukanov, E. S. Drazek, B. A. Roe, and D. E. Berg.** 1998. Analyses of the *cag* pathogenicity island of *Helicobacter pylori. Mol. Microbiol.* **28:**37–53.
3. **Alm, R. A., L. L. Lo-See, D. T. Moir, B. L. King, E. D. Brown, P. C. Doig, D. R. Smith, B. Noonan, B. C. Guild, B. L. Dejonge, C. Carmel, P. J. Tummino, A. Caruso, M. Uria-Nickelsen, D. M. Mills, C. Ives, R. Gibson, D. Merberg, S. D. Mills, Q. Jiang, D. E. Taylor, G. F. Vovis, and T. J. Trust.** 1999. Genomic-sequence comparison of two unrelated isolates of the human gastric pathogen *Helicobacter pylori. Nature* **397:**176–180.
4. **Andersson, S. G., A. Zomorodipour, J. O. Andersson, T. Sicheritz-Ponten, U. C. Alsmark, R. M.**

Podowski, A. K. Naslund, A. S. Ericksson, H. H. Winkler, and C. G. Kurland. 1998. The genome sequence of *Rickettsia prowazekii* and the origin of mitochondria. *Nature* **396:**133–140.

5. **Atherton, J. C., P. Cao, R. M. Peek, Jr., M. K. Tummuru, M. J. Blaser, and T. L. Cover.** 1995. Mosaicism in vacuolating cytotoxin alleles of *Helicobacter pylori.* Association of specific *vacA* types with cytotoxin production and peptic ulceration. *J. Biol. Chem.* **270:**17771–17777.

6. **Atherton, J. C., K. T. Tham, R. M. Peek, Jr., T. L. Cover, and M. J. Blaser.** 1996. Density of *Helicobacter pylori* infection in vivo as assessed by quantitative culture and histology. *J. Infect. Dis.* **174:**552–556.

7. **Baker, B., P. Zambryski, B. Staskawicz, and S. P. Dinesh-Kumar.** 1997. Signaling in plant-microbe interactions. *Science* **276:**726–733.

8. **Blaser, M. J.** 1998. *Helicobacter pylori* and gastric diseases. *Br. Med. J.* **316:**1507–1510.

9. **Blum, G., M. Ott, A. Lischewski, A. Ritter, H. Imrich, H. Tschape, and J. Hacker.** 1994. Excision of large DNA regions termed pathogenicity islands from tRNA-specific loci in the chromosome of an *Escherichia coli* wild-type pathogen. *Infect. Immun.* **62:**606–614.

10. **Campbell, S., A. Fraser, B. Holliss, J. Schmid, and P. W. O'Toole.** 1997. Evidence for ethnic tropism of *Helicobacter pylori. Infect. Immun.* **65:**3708–3712.

11. **Cavalli-Sforza, L. L., P. Menozzi, and A. Piazza.** 1993. Demic expansions and human evolution. *Science* **259:**639–646.

12. **Censini, S., C. Lange, Z. Xiang, J. E. Crabtree, P. Ghiara, M. Borodovsky, R. Rappuoli, and A. Covacci.** 1996. *cag,* a pathogenicity island of *Helicobacter pylori,* encodes type I-specific and disease-associated virulence factors. *Proc. Natl. Acad. Sci. USA* **93:**14648–14653.

13. **Christie, P.** 1997. *Agrobacterium tumefaciens* T-complex transport apparatus: a paradigm for a new family of multifunctional transporters in eubacteria. *J. Bacteriol.* **179:**3085–3094.

14. **Christie, P. J.** 1997. The *cag* pathogenicity island: mechanistic insights. *Trends Microbiol.* **5:**264–265.

15. **Cirillo, D. M., R. H. Valdivia, D. M. Monack, and S. Falkow.** 1998. Macrophage-dependent induction of the *Salmonella* pathogenicity island 2 type III secretion system and its role in intracellular survival. *Mol. Microbiol.* **30:**175–188.

16. **Cormack, B. P., R. H. Valdivia, and S. Falkow.** 1996. FACS-optimized mutants of the green fluorescent protein (GFP). *Gene* **173:**33–38.

17. **Covacci, A., and R. Rappuoli.** 1993. Pertussis toxin export requires accessory genes located downstream from the pertussis toxin operon. *Mol. Microbiol.* **8:**429–434.

18. **Covacci, A., S. Censini, M. Bugnoli, R. Petracca, D. Burroni, G. Macchia, A. Massone, E. Papini, Z. Xiang, N. Figura, and R. Rappuoli.** 1993. Molecular characterization of the 128-kDa immunodominant antigen of *Helicobacter pylori* associated with cytotoxicity and duodenal ulcer. *Proc. Natl. Acad. Sci. USA* **90:**5791–5795.

19. **Covacci, A., S. Falkow, D. E. Berg, and R. Rappuoli.** 1997. Did the inheritance of a pathogenicity island modify the virulence of *Helicobacter pylori? Trends Microbiol.* **5:**205–208.

20. **Covacci, A., and R. Rappuoli.** 1998. *Helicobacter pylori:* molecular evolution of a bacterial quasi-species. *Curr. Opin. Microbiol.* **1:**96–102.

21. **Cover, T. L., P. Cao, C. D. Lin, K. T. Tham, and M. J. Blaser.** 1993. Correlation between vacuolating cytotoxin production by *Helicobacter pylori* isolates in vitro and in vivo. *Infect. Immun.* **61:**5008–5012.

22. **Cover, T. L.** 1996. The vacuolating cytotoxin of *Helicobacter pylori. Mol. Microbiol.* **20:**241–246.

23. **Crabtree, J. E., Z. Xiang, I. J. Lindley, D. S. Tompkins, R. Rappuoli, and A. Covacci.** 1995. Induction of interleukin-8 secretion from gastric epithelial cells by a *cagA* negative isogenic mutant of *Helicobacter pylori. J. Clin. Pathol.* **48:**967–969.

24. **Deibel, C., S. Kramer, T. Chakraborty, and F. Ebel.** 1998. EspE, a novel secreted protein of attaching and effacing bacteria, is directly translocated into infected host cells, where it appears as a tyrosine-phosphorylated 90 kDa protein. *Mol. Microbiol.* **30:**147–161.

25. **Dundon, W. G., S. M. Beesley, and C. J. Smyth.** 1998. *Helicobacter pylori*—a conundrum of genetic diversity. *Microbiology* **144:**2925–2939.

26. **Ebel, F., T. Podzadel, M. Rohde, A. U. Kresse, S. Kramer, C. Deibel, C. A. Guzman, and T. Chakraborty.** 1998. Initial binding of Shiga toxin-producing *Escherichia coli* to host cells and subsequent induction of actin rearrangements depend on filamentous EspA-containing surface appendages. *Mol. Microbiol.* **30:** 147–161.

27. **Falkow, S.** 1998. Who speaks for the microbes? *Emerg. Infect. Dis.* **4:**495–497.

28. **Figura, N., C. Vindigni, A. Covacci, L. Presenti, D. Burroni, R. Vernillo, T. Banducci, F. Roviello, D.**

Marrelli, M. Biscontri, S. Kristodhullu, C. Gennari, and D. Vaira. 1998. *cagA* positive and negative *Helicobacter pylori* strains are simultaneously present in the stomach of most patients with non-ulcer dyspepsia: relevance to histological damage. *Gut* **42**:772–778.

29. **Finlay, B. B., and S. Falkow.** 1997. Common themes in microbial pathogenicity revisited. *Microbiol. Mol. Biol. Rev.* **61**:136–169.

30. **Finlay, B. B., and P. Cossart.** 1997. Exploitation of mammalian host cell functions by bacterial pathogens. *Science* **276**:718–725.

31. **Fullner, K. J., J. C. Lara, and E. W. Nester.** 1996. Pilus assembly by *Agrobacterium* T-DNA transfer genes. *Science* **273**:1107–1109.

32. **Glocker, E., C. Lange, A. Covacci, S. Bereswill, M. Kist, and H. L. Pahl.** 1998. Proteins encoded by the *cag* pathogenicity island of *Helicobacter pylori* are required for NF-*κ*B activation. *Infect. Immun.* **66**: 2346–2348.

33. **Go, M. F., V. Kapur, D. Y. Graham, and J. M. Musser.** 1996. Population genetic analysis of *Helicobacter pylori* by multilocus enzyme electrophoresis: extensive allelic diversity and recombinational population structure. *J. Bacteriol.* **178**:3934–3938.

34. **Groisman, E. A., and H. Ochman.** 1996. Pathogenicity islands: bacterial evolution in quantum leaps. *Cell* **87**:791–794.

35. **Hacker, J., G. Blum-Oehler, I. Muhldorfer, and H. Tschape.** 1997. Pathogenicity islands of virulent bacteria: structure, function and impact on microbial evolution. *Mol. Microbiol.* **23**:1089–1097.

36. **Hazell, S. L., R. H. Andrews, H. M. Mitchell, and G. Daskalopoulous.** 1997. Genetic relationship among isolates of *Helicobacter pylori:* evidence for the existence of a *Helicobacter pylori* species-complex. *FEMS Microbiol. Lett.* **150**:27–32.

37. **Jiang, Q., K. Hiratsuka, and D. E. Taylor.** 1996. Variability of gene order in different *Helicobacter pylori* strains contributes to genome diversity. *Mol. Microbiol.* **20**:833–842.

38. **Kenny, B., R. DeVinney, M. Stein, D. J. Reinscheid, E. A. Frey, and B. B. Finlay.** 1997. Enteropathogenic *E. coli* (EPEC) transfers its receptor for intimate adherence into mammalian cells. *Cell* **91**:511–520.

39. **Kirby, J. E., and R. R. Isberg.** 1998. Legionnaires' disease: the pore macrophage and the legion of terror within. *Trends Microbiol.* **6**:256–258.

40. **Kubori, T., Y. Matsushima, D. Nakamura, J. Uralil, M. Lara-Tejero, A. Sukhan, J. E. Galan, and S. I. Aizawa.** 1998. Supramolecular structure of the *Salmonella typhimurium* type III protein secretion system. *Science* **280**:602–605.

41. **Lai, E. M., and C. I. Kado.** 1998. Processed VirB2 is the major subunit of the promiscuous pilus of *Agrobacterium tumefaciens. J. Bacteriol.* **180**:2711–2717.

42. **Lange, C., A. Covacci, and R. Rappuoli.** The CagT of *cag,* the pathogenicity island of *Helicobacter pylori,* is a lipoprotein that assembles into a core system and requires CagM for stabilization. Submitted for publication.

43. **Lee, C. A.** 1996. Pathogenicity islands and the evolution of bacterial pathogens. *Infect. Agents Dis.* **5**:1–7.

44. **Lee, C. A.** 1997. Type III secretion systems: machines to deliver bacterial proteins into eukaryotic cells? *Trends Microbiol.* **5**:148–156.

45. **Macnab, R. M.** 1992. Genetics and biogenesis of bacterial flagella. *Annu. Rev. Genet.* **26**:131–158.

46. **Menard, R., C. Dehio, and P. J. Sansonetti.** 1996. Bacterial entry into epithelial cells: the paradigm of *Shigella. Trends Microbiol.* **4**:220–226.

47. **Mitchell, H. M., T. Bohane, R. A. Hawkes, and A. Lee.** 1993. *Helicobacter pylori* infection within families. *Int. J. Med. Microbiol. Virol. Parasitol. Infect. Dis.* **280**:128–136.

48. **Mitchell, H. M., S. L. Hazell, T. Kolesnikow, J. Mitchell, and D. Frommer.** 1996. Antigen recognition during progression from acute to chronic infection with a *cagA*-positive strain of *Helicobacter pylori. Infect. Immun.* **4**:1166–1172.

49. **Molinari, M., C. Galli, N. Norais, J. L. Telford, R. Rappuoli, J. P. Luzio, and C. Montecucco.** 1997. Vacuoles induced by *Helicobacter pylori* toxin contain both late endosomal and lysosomal markers. *J. Biol. Chem.* **272**:25339–25344.

50. **Munzenmaier, A., C. Lange, E. Glocker, A. Covacci, A. Moran, S. Bereswill, P. A. Baeuerle, M. Kist, and H. L. Pahl.** 1997. A secreted/shed product of *Helicobacter pylori* activates transcription factor nuclear factor-kappa B. *J. Immunol.* **159**:6140–6147.

51. **Pagliaccia, C., M. de Bernard, P. Lupetti, X. Ji, D. Burroni, T. L. Cover, E. Papini, R. Rappuoli, J.**

L. Telford, and J. M. Reyrat. 1998. The m2 form of the *Helicobacter pylori* cytotoxin has cell type-specific vacuolating activity. *Proc. Natl. Acad. Sci. USA* **95:**10212–10217.

52. **Papini, E., B. Satin, C. Bucci, M. de Bernard, J. L. Telford, R. Manetti, R. Rappuoli, M. Zerial, and C. Montecucco.** 1997. The small GTP binding protein rab7 is essential for cellular vacuolation induced by *Helicobacter pylori* cytotoxin. *EMBO J.* **16:**15–24.

53. **Parsonnet, J., G. D. Friedman, N. Orentreich, and H. Vogelman.** 1997. Risk for gastric cancer in people with CagA positive or CagA negative *Helicobacter pylori* infection. *Gut* **40:**297–301.

54. **Phadnis, S. H., D. Ilver, L. Janzon, S. Normark, and T. U. Westblom.** 1994. Pathological significance and molecular characterization of the vacuolating toxin gene of *Helicobacter pylori. Infect. Immun.* **62:** 1557–1565.

55. **Relman, D. A., and S. Falkow.** 1992. Identification of uncultured microorganisms: expanding the spectrum of characterized microbial pathogens. *Infect. Agents Dis.* **1:**245–253.

56. **Ritter, A., G. Blum, L. Emody, M. Kerenyi, A. Bock, B. Neuhierl, W. Rabsch, F. Scheutz, and J. Hacker.** 1995. tRNA genes and pathogenicity islands: influence on virulence and metabolic properties of uropathogenic *Escherichia coli. Mol. Microbiol.* **17:**109–121.

57. **Rosenshine, I., S. Ruschkowski, M. Stein, D. J. Reinscheid, S. D. Mills, and B. B. Finlay.** 1996. A pathogenic bacterium triggers epithelial signals to form a functional bacterial receptor that mediates actin pseudopod formation. *EMBO J.* **15:**2613–2624.

58. **Russel, M.** 1995. Moving through the membrane with filamentous phages. *Trends Microbiol.* **3:**223–228.

59. **Russel, M.** 1998. Macromolecular assembly and secretion across the bacterial cell envelope: type II protein secretion systems. *J. Mol. Biol.* **279:**485–499.

60. **Salmond, G. P., B. W. Bycroft, G. S. Stewart, and P. Williams.** 1995. The bacterial 'enigma': cracking the code of cell-cell communication. *Mol. Microbiol.* **16:**615–624.

61. **Schmitt, W., and R. Haas.** 1994. Genetic analysis of the *Helicobacter pylori* vacuolating cytotoxin: structural similarities with the IgA protease type of exported protein. *Mol. Microbiol.* **12:**307–319.

62. **Segal, E. D., S. Falkow, and L. S. Tompkins.** 1996. *Helicobacter pylori* attachment to gastric cells induces cytoskeletal rearrangements and tyrosine phosphorylation of host cell proteins. *Proc. Natl. Acad. Sci. USA* **93:**1259–1264.

63. **Segal, E. D., C. Lange, A. Covacci, L. S. Tompkins, and S. Falkow.** 1997. Induction of host signal transduction pathways by *Helicobacter pylori. Proc. Natl. Acad. Sci. USA* **94:**7595–7599.

64. **Segal, G., and H. A. Shuman.** 1998. How is the intracellular fate of the *Legionella pneumophila* phagosome determined? *Trends Microbiol.* **6:**253–255.

65. **Telford, J. L., P. Ghiara, M. Dell'Orco, M. Comanducci, D. Burroni, M. Bugnoli, M. F. Tecce, S. Censini, A. Covacci, Z. Xiang, and R. Rappuoli.** 1994. Gene structure of the *Helicobacter pylori* cytotoxin and evidence of its key role in gastric disease. *J. Exp. Med.* **179:**1653–1658.

66. **Tomb, J. F., O. Whith, A. R. Kerlavage, R. A. Clayton, G. G. Sutton, R. D. Fleischmann, K. A. Ketchum, H. P. Klenk, S. Gill, B. A. Dougherty, K. Nelson, J. Quackenbush, L. Zhou, E. F. Kirkness, S. Peterson, B. Loftus, D. Richardson, R. Dodson, H. G. Khalak, A. Glodek, K. McKenney, L. M. Fitzegerald, N. Lee, M. D. Adams, and J. C. Venter.** 1997. The complete genome sequence of the gastric pathogen *Helicobacter pylori. Nature* **388:**539–547.

67. **Tummuru, M., S. A. Sharma, and M. J. Blaser.** 1995. *Helicobacter pylori picB*, a homolog of the *Bordetella pertussis* toxin secretion protein, is required for induction of IL-8 in gastric epithelial cells. *Mol. Microbiol.* **18:**867–876.

68. **Tummuru, M. K., T. L. Cover, and M. J. Blaser.** 1993. Cloning and expression of a high-molecular-mass major antigen of *Helicobacter pylori:* evidence of linkage to cytotoxin production. *Infect. Immun.* **61:** 1799–1809.

69. **Tummuru, M. K., T. L. Cover, and M. J. Blaser.** 1994. Mutation of the cytotoxin-associated *cagA* gene does not affect the vacuolating cytotoxin activity of *Helicobacter pylori. Infect. Immun.* **62:**2609–2613.

70. **Valdivia, R. H., and S. Falkow.** 1997. Fluorescence-based isolation of bacterial genes expressed within host cells. *Science* **277:**2007–2011.

71. **Valdivia, R. H., and S. Falkow.** 1997. Probing bacterial gene expression within host cells. *Trends Microbiol.* **5:**360–363.

72. **van der Ende, A., E. A. Rauws, M. Feller, C. J. Mulder, G. N. Tytgat, and J. Dankert.** 1996. Heterogeneous *Helicobacter pylori* isolates from members of a family with a history of peptic ulcer disease. *Gastroenterology* **111:**638–647.

73. **Weiss, A. A., F. D. Johnson, and D. L. Burns.** 1993. Molecular characterization of an operon required for pertussis toxin secretion. *Proc. Natl. Acad. Sci. USA* **90:**2970–2974.

74. **Winans, S. C., D. L. Burns, and P. J. Christie.** 1996. Adaptation of a conjugal transfer system for the export of pathogenic macromolecules. *Trends Microbiol.* **4:**64–68.

75. **Xiang, Z., S. Censini, P. F. Bayeli, J. L. Telford, N. Figura, R. Rappuoli, and A. Covacci.** 1995. Analysis of expression of CagA and VacA virulence factors in 43 strains of *Helicobacter pylori* reveals that clinical isolates can be divided into two major types and that CagA is not necessary for expression of the vacuolating cytotoxin. *Infect. Immun.* **63:**94–98.

76. **Zychlinsky, A., and P. J. Sansonetti.** 1997. Apoptosis as a proinflammatory event: what can we learn from bacteria-induced cell death? *Trends Microbiol.* **5:**201–204.

77. **Zychlinsky, A.** 1999. Personal communication.

Pathogenicity Islands and Other Mobile Virulence Elements
Edited by J. B. Kaper and J. Hacker
© 1999 American Society for Microbiology, Washington, D.C.

Chapter 11

Are the *vap* Regions of *Dichelobacter nodosus* Pathogenicity Islands?

Brian F. Cheetham, Gabrielle Whittle, and Margaret E. Katz

Foot rot is a mixed bacterial infection of the hoof and affects sheep, goats, cattle, and deer. The gram-negative anaerobic bacterium *Dichelobacter nodosus* is the principal causative agent, since only *D. nodosus* can initiate the infection when applied to the hoof as a pure culture (1). Benign foot rot begins as interdigital dermatitis, which then extends into the avascular epidermal tissue of the hoof. This results in mild lameness, which usually heals spontaneously when dry environmental conditions return. In virulent foot rot, which is highly contagious, the underlying epidermal tissue is progressively eroded, which eventually leads to separation of the hoof from the epidermis and severe lameness. Although environmental conditions contribute to the development of foot rot, the difference in severity of disease is due to innate genetic differences in *D. nodosus* strains, which are classified as benign, intermediate, or virulent. Sheep affected by foot rot show decreased wool production and quality and lower fertility. The treatment of foot rot is labor-intensive and costly. As a result of the reduced wool production and the high costs of treatment, virulent foot rot is one of the most economically important endemic diseases of sheep and is responsible for considerable economic loss to the Australian wool industry.

TAXONOMIC STATUS OF *D. NODOSUS*

D. nodosus is a strictly anaerobic, non-spore-forming, nonflagellated gram-negative rod (15). The cells have knob-like swellings at their termini and polar type 4 *N*-methylphenylalanine fimbriae (11). *D. nodosus* (formerly *Bacteroides nodosus*) has recently been assigned to a new family, *Cardiobacteriaceae,* in the gamma subdivision of the *Proteobacteria* (14). Based on the K-agglutination reaction, isolates of *D. nodosus* can be divided into nine serogroups, A to I (9). The serogroups have been divided into two classes, I and II, according to the organization of the fimbrial genes (34). There is no correlation between the serogroup and the relative virulence of the strain. The extracellular proteases produced by virulent strains are more thermostable than those produced by benign strains (13). In addition, virulent strains exhibit significantly greater elastolytic activity (44) and show greater fimbria-mediated twitching motility (12) than do benign strains.

Brian F. Cheetham, Gabrielle Whittle, and Margaret E. Katz • Division of Molecular and Cellular Biology, School of Biological Sciences, University of New England, Armidale, New South Wales 2351, Australia.

THE *vap* REGIONS OF THE *D. NODOSUS* GENOME

Isolation of the *vap* Regions and Preferential Distribution in Virulent Strains

The *vap* (virulence-associated protein) regions of the *D. nodosus* chromosome were isolated as DNA sequences which were present in the virulent strain A198 but absent from the benign strain C305 (28). This study also resulted in the isolation of a different segment of the *D. nodosus* genome associated with virulence, the *vrl* (virulence-related locus) region, which is discussed below. The G+C content of the *vap* regions (40.6%) is lower than that reported for the *D. nodosus* genome (45% [25]), suggesting that the *vap* regions may have been acquired by horizontal transfer. The *vap* regions are found in almost all virulent strains which have been studied (28, 42) but are absent from about two-thirds of benign strains. Hence, there is a preferential distribution of the *vap* regions in virulent strains. There is one report (42) of a small number of virulent strains which appear to lack at least part of the *vap* regions, but we have been unable to obtain these strains for analysis due to inviability of the stored stocks.

Multiple Copies of the *vap* Regions

Multiple copies of the *vap* regions are found in many strains; for example, there are three copies of the *vap* regions in virulent strain A198. These are designated *vap* regions 1, 2, and 3. There is no correlation between the number of copies of the *vap* regions and the degree of virulence, since some virulent strains have only one copy, while some benign strains have multiple copies (28).

Functions of the Genes Found in the *vap* Regions

Based on similarities to known genes, functions have been assigned to most of the genes of the *vap* regions. There is at present no transformation system for *D. nodosus,* which precludes the direct testing of the role of these genes in virulence. Attempts by others to develop a transformation system with plasmids derived from other bacteria or with the one *D. nodosus* plasmid which has been reported previously have been unsuccessful (2). We have recently identified and characterized a new native plasmid, pDN1 (49), that has a high degree of similarity to plasmids belonging to *Escherichia coli* incompatibility group Q. We have constructed derivatives of pDN1 for use in transformation experiments, which are in progress. Development of a transformation system would provide a means by which the role of the *vap* and other virulence-associated genes in the pathogenesis of ovine foot rot could be determined directly.

The major genes which have been identified in *vap* region 1 (Fig. 1) of the virulent strain A198 include an integrase gene, *intA*; a gene encoding a putative toxin, *toxA*; and genes designated *vapA* to *vapH*. None of the genes found in the *vap* regions encode known virulence factors of *D. nodosus,* such as thermostable proteases or proteins required for fimbrial function, nor do they encode proteins with similarity to virulence factors from other organisms. The proteins to which the predicted *vap* gene products show homology are summarized in Table 1.

The *toxA-vapA* operon is similar to the *higB-higA* operon (45) from the killer plasmid Rts1 of *E. coli.* The *higB-higA* operon encodes a stable toxin molecule, HigB, and an unstable antidote molecule, HigA. *E. coli* cells which lose plasmid Rts1 are killed by

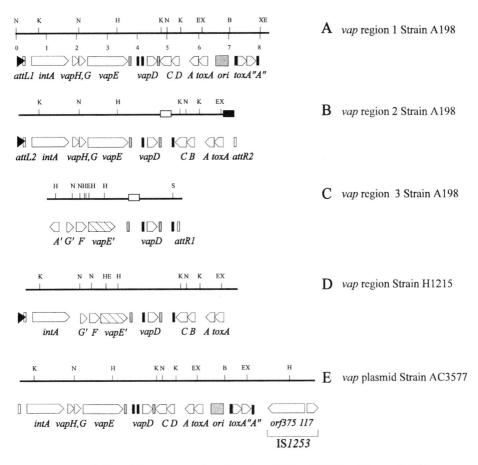

Figure 1. Map of the *vap* regions from *D. nodosus* A198 and H1215 and the *vap* plasmid from strain AC3577. The numbers show the distance (in kilobases) from the leftmost *Nru*I site in *vap* region 1, strain A198. The restriction sites shown are *Bam*HI (B), *Eco*RI (E), *Hind*III (H), *Kpn*I (K), *Nru*I (N), *Sac*I (S), and *Xho*I (X). The major potential genes are indicated by open arrows. Repeated sequences (8) are indicated as follows: 19-bp *att* sites are indicated by small open boxes, 103-bp repeats or partial copies are indicated by small shaded boxes, 102-bp repeats or partial copies are indicated by small solid boxes, and the putative origin of replication is indicated by a large shaded box. The tRNA-*ser* genes are indicated by solid triangles. DNA sequences found in *vap* region 2 but not in *vap* region 1 are indicated by boxes on the scale line for *vap* region 2. The complete DNA sequence of *vap* regions 1 and 3 (8, 29) and part of the DNA sequences of *vap* region 2 (30) and the *vap* plasmid (2) have been determined. The map of the *vap* region of strain H1215 is based on the results of Southern blotting and PCR experiments (4).

Table 1. Sequence analysis of *vap* regions 1 and 3[a] of *D. nodosus* A198

Gene	Coordinates (5′–3′)	Size (aa)[b]	% Identity to nucleotide or putative protein[b]	Homolog (integration site)[c]	Accession no.	P[d]
intA	418–1623	402	41.5/400 aa[e]	*E. coli* retronphage φR73 integrase (*selC*tRNA)	M64113	1.5×10^{-61}
			34.6/405 aa	*V. cholerae* 0395 integrase from CTXfPAI (*ssr*A)	U02372	4.4×10^{-51}
			39.4/393 aa	*E. coli* K-12 cryptic prophage P4-57 integrase (*ssr*A)	U03737	1.9×10^{-50}
			37.6/394 aa	*M. loti* symbiosis island integrase (tRNA-*phe*)	AF049242	4.1×10^{-50}
			34.3/397 aa	*S. flexneri* fSF6 integrase	X59553	3.9×10^{-40}
			34.0/396 aa	*E. coli* K-12 integrase (tRNA-*argW*)	U11296	3.8×10^{-39}
			32.2/273 aa	*E. coli* K-12 integrase (tRNA-*leuX*)	AE00323	1.3×10^{-38}
			35.6/135 aa	*R. capsulatus* putative prophage integrase	U57682	1.4×10^{-32}
			44.7/123 aa	*E. aerogenes* putative integrase	AF039582	9×10^{-19}
			45.2/124 aa	Bacteriophage P4 integrase	X05947	1.7×10^{-18}
			23.3/408 aa	*S. typhimurium* LT2 integrase of Gif sy-1 prophage (*lepA*)	AF001386	2.9×10^{-16}
			47.2/117 aa	*P. putida* integrase from clc element (tRNA-*gly*)	PPAJ4950	1×10^{-15}
			22.0/239 aa	Lambda bacteriophage φ80 integrase	X04051	1.2×10^{-12}
			40.1/167 aa	*D. nodosus* integrase, IntB (tRNA-*ser*$_{GCU}$ or tRNA-*ser*$_{GCA}$)	X98547	1.6×10^{-10}
vapA	5936–5628	103	50.0/60 aa	Putative ORF from *Synechococcus* sp.	U04356	2.4×10^{-9}
			38.4/73 aa	ORF from *Acetobacter europaeus* plasmid	AEY17109	2.5×10^{-8}
			39.7/78 aa	Putative ORF from *E. coli* K-12	AE000154	1.1×10^{-6}
			22.0/70 aa	HigA antidote protein from killer plasmid Rts1	U43847	2.5×10^{-6}
			30.0/78 aa	Putative ORF from *E. coli* K-12	AE000244	2.6×10^{-6}
			41.4/70 aa	VapA (HI1251) from *H. influenzae*	U32805	6.1×10^{-5}
toxA	6305–5949	92	45.6/92 aa	HigB killer protein from killer plasmid Rts1	U43847	6.8×10^{-20}
			33.7/89 aa	HI1250 from *H. influenzae*	U32805	1.6×10^{-5}
vapB	5292–5062	77	38.7/75 aa	Encoded within ORF *patA* from *Synechocystis* sp.	D90902	2.7×10^{-10}
			36.0/75 aa	VapB (HI0321) from *H. influenzae*	U32776	8.5×10^{-7}
			34.8/66 aa	VagC from *S. dublin* virulence plasmid	X66934	9.7×10^{-7}
			42.4/59 aa	HI0953 from *H. influenzae* within ORF	U32717	1.3×10^{-5}
			34.7/72 aa	Encoded by an unidentified ORF from *A. tumefaciens*	M59852	1.3×10^{-5}
			34.7/72 aa	Encoded from within ORF *traD* of *E. coli* F plasmid	M29254	4×10^{-4}
			34.7/72 aa	Encoded from within ORF *traI* of *E. coli* F plasmid	M54796	7×10^{-4}
			33.3/72 aa	Stborf1 from *S. flexneri* virulence plasmid pMYSH6000	U82621	2.3×10^{-3}
vapC	5065–4658	136	40.6/133 aa	Stborf2 from *S. flexneri* virulence plasmid pMYSH6000	U82621	1×10^{-12}
			35.7/132 aa	VapC (HI0322) from *H. influenzae*	U32776	6.3×10^{-9}
			40.9/132 aa	VagD from *H. influenzae*	U32776	7×10^{-7}
			40.9/129 aa	HI0953 from *H. influenzae* within ORF	U32717	1.2×10^{-21}
			47.1/128 aa	Encoded from within ORF *patA* from *Synechocystis* sp.	D90902	1.4×10^{-21}
			38.2/85 aa	Putative protein from *Synechocystis* sp.	D90902	2.2×10^{-18}
			42.7/82 aa	VagD from *S. dublin* virulence plasmid	X66934	4×10^{-16}
			39.9/133 aa	Encoded from within ORF *traD* of *E. coli* F plasmid	X57431	2.2×10^{-13}

Table 1. *Continued*

Gene	Coordinates 5'–3'	Size (aa)[b]	% Identity to nucleotide or putative protein[b]	Homolog (integration site)[c]	Accession no.	P[d]
vapD	4255–4536	281	80.6/93 aa[e]	Orf2 from *A. actinomycetemcomitans* plasmid pVT736-1	L24000	7.2×10^{-40}
			68.8/93 aa	HP0309 from *H. pylori*	AE000549	1×10^{-31}
			66.7/91 aa	VapD from *H. pylori*	U94318	2.8×10^{-29}
			70.3/74 aa	Protein encoded within ORFA-ORFB of *Treponema denticola* plasmid pTD1	M87856	2.5×10^{-26}
			46.0/91 aa	Orf5 from cryptic plasmid pJD1 of *N. gonorrhoeae*	M10316	2.4×10^{-21}
			40.7/91 aa	VapD from *H. influenzae*	U32728	5.5×10^{-21}
			33.3/93 aa	HP0969 from *H. pylori*	AE000605	4.3×10^{-7}
			29.0/93 aa	VapD from *A. actinomycetemcomitans* chromosome	D88189	7.6×10^{-3}
vapE	2304–3617	438	37.9/353 aa	Potential protein from *S. aureus* bacteriophage-like Tn*557*	U93688	2.2×10^{-53}
			30.0/307 aa	Orf1 of cryptic plasmid pMA1 of cyanobacterium *M. aeruginosa*	Z28337	9.4×10^{-21}
vapG	2002–2208	69		NSH[f]		
vapH	1718–2023	102	62.8/145 nt	*S. flexneri* IS2 *orf179* putative bacteriophage immunity region	Z23101	8×10^{-2}

[a] *intA* element from *D. nodosus* strain A198 (GenBank accession number L31763).
[b] aa, amino acids; nt, nucleotides.
[c] Where the site of integration is known for an integrase gene, it is indicated in parentheses following the description of the Int homolog. ORF, open reading frame.
[d] The number of sequences with this level of similarity which would be expected in a database of this size by chance alone.
[e] The length over which the putative proteins (aa) or genes (nt) from the *vap* regions have identity to homologous proteins or genes.
[f] NSH, no significant homology to sequences in databases.

HigB, and hence these gene products act to prevent plasmid loss. We have experimental evidence to suggest that ToxA (the toxin) and VapA (the antidote) perform a similar function (4).

The *vapB-vapC* operon of *D. nodosus* is similar to the *vagC-vagD* operon on the virulence plasmid of *Salmonella dublin* (37) and to the *stborf1-stborf2* operon from the plasmid stability locus of the *Shigella flexneri* virulence plasmid pMYSH6000 (38). The gene products from these *Salmonella* and *Shigella* operons coordinate plasmid replication with cell division. The mechanism by which this occurs is unknown (38).

The only protein of known function to which VapD is similar is the product of *orf2* from the rolling circle replicating plasmid pVT736-1 of *Actinobacillus actinomycetemcomitans* (18), which has a function in plasmid maintenance and incompatibility (19). VapE is similar at the amino acid level to two proteins of unknown function. The first is the product of *orf1* of the cryptic plasmid pMA1 from the cyanobacterium *Microcystis aeruginosa* (46), and the second is a potential protein from the bacteriophage-like transposon Tn*557* of *Staphylococcus aureus,* which carries a gene encoding toxic shock toxin (33).

The *vapG-vapH* region has DNA sequence similarity to *orf179* of *S. flexneri*, which is a homolog of the *E. coli dicF* gene (16). This gene encodes DicF RNA, an antisense inhibitor of the cell division gene *ftsZ*, and thus the *dicF* gene product inhibits cell division in *E. coli* (16). The arrangement of *vapG-vapH* is very similar to that of *orf199* and *kil* from the immunity region of bacteriophage P4 (20), and *kil* is also a homolog of *dicF* (16).

It is of interest that on the basis of similarity to genes of known function, the *toxA*, *vapA*, *vapB*, *vapC*, *vapD*, *vapG*, and *vapH* genes are likely to be involved with plasmid maintenance, control of cell division, or both. The only gene to which no function can yet be assigned is *vapE*. It is possible that the *vap* genes constitute an integrated plasmid carrying genes involved in plasmid maintenance and that this integrated plasmid cannot be lost easily from the *D. nodosus* genome due to the presence of the *vapA-toxA* system. If this is correct, the *vap* genes would play no role in virulence, and their preferential distribution in virulent strains would be coincidental. However, an alternative explanation is that the *vap* gene products interact with the cell division machinery in *D. nodosus* and that this interaction plays a role in virulence.

The determination of the complete DNA sequence of several bacterial genomes has allowed us to search for homologs of the *vap* genes and to examine their arrangement. For example, in the *Haemophilus influenzae* genome (17), there are homologs of *toxA*, *vapA*, *vapB*, *vapC*, and *vapD*. *vapA* and *toxA* are adjacent, as are *vapB* and *vapC*. However, the *vapA-toxA*, *vapB-vapC*, and *vapD* genes are widely separated in the *H. influenzae* chromosome. A similar situation exists in other bacterial genomes which contain homologs of *vap* genes. Thus, although the *vap* genes are clustered in *D. nodosus*, *vap*-related genes from other organisms are not contiguous.

MOBILITY FUNCTIONS ASSOCIATED WITH THE *vap* REGIONS

Integrase Gene and Origin of Replication

The *vap* regions contain a gene, *intA*, encoding an integrase which has 35 to 40% amino identity to the integrases of coliphages φR73 and P4 and bacteriophage Sf6 from *S. flexneri* (8). We have also identified within the *vap* regions a putative origin of replication, consisting of a series of repeats of two related 21-bp sequences flanked by two AT-rich sequences, with a DnaA box located nearby (8). This resembles the origins of replication of several plasmids and bacteriophages.

IntA is most similar to integrases carried by bacteriophages of the P4 family, and the arrangement of *vapG* and *vapH* is very similar to that of *orf199* and *kil* from the immunity region of bacteriophage P4 (20). However, most of the genes which show similarity to *toxA* and *vapA* to *vapD* are carried by plasmids. Thus, the *vap* regions show some characteristics of both these types of mobile elements, plasmids and bacteriophages. The *vap* region is relatively small for a functional bacteriophage or conjugative plasmid but is similar in size to the genome of defective bacteriophage P4 (23).

vap Plasmid pJIR896 and Insertion Sequence IS*1253*

A native plasmid, designated pJIR896, was isolated from *D. nodosus* AC3577 and found to consist of the genes from *vap* region 1 of strain A198, together with a putative insertion sequence, IS*1253* (Fig. 1) (2). Since this plasmid is capable of replication as a circular molecule, it must contain a functional origin of replication, which may be the putative origin identified on the basis of sequence analysis. Plasmid pJIR896 (*vap* plasmid) is probably the circular progenitor of the *vap* regions found in the chromosome of many

D. nodosus strains. However, this plasmid does not encode functions associated with conjugation and is therefore not self-transmissible in its present form. The *vap* plasmid may have been transferred into *D. nodosus* strains by a coresident conjugative plasmid or conjugative transposon or by a transducing bacteriophage. Alternatively, the present *vap* plasmid may have been derived from a larger, conjugative plasmid, from which the conjugation functions were lost. The low copy number of the *vap* plasmid (2) and the presence of several plasmid maintenance systems, which are usually found on low-copy-number conjugative plasmids, support this view (19). IS*1253* may have played a role in the deletion of the genes required for conjugation. Strains which now carry the *vap* regions may have evolved from a common ancestor carrying the *vap* plasmid.

IS*1253* is not located next to the *vap* regions of strain A198, but a copy is found elsewhere in the genome (2), near the outer membrane protein genes (35). It is of interest that insertion elements (IS elements) with high similarity to IS*1253* are located close to virulence-associated genes in many other pathogenic bacteria. These include the *cag* pathogenicity island (PAI) of *Helicobacter pylori* (7), the *Salmonella typhimurium* virulence plasmid (21), the *Yersinia pestis* invasin genes (43), the flagellin genes of *Vibrio cholerae* (31), the hemolysin gene of a *Synechocystis* sp. (26), and the invasin and enterotoxin genes of *Clostridium perfringens* (6, 27).

THE *vap* REGIONS ARE INTEGRATED INTO tRNA GENES

Many bacteriophages, plasmids, and PAIs are found integrated into tRNA genes (22, 39). A tRNA-*ser*$_{GCU}$ gene is located about 200 bp upstream from the start codon of the *intA* gene from *vap* region 1 in *D. nodosus* A198 (Fig. 2), suggesting that *vap* region 1 arose by the integration of a genetic element into this tRNA gene (8). A different tRNA gene, tRNA-*ser*$_{GGA}$, is found next to *vap* region 2 in strain A198. These tRNA genes appear to be the two predominant integration sites for the *vap* element in *D. nodosus*. In strain A198, *vap* region 3, which lacks many of the genes from the *vap* regions (Fig. 1), is adjacent to *vap* region 1 (Fig. 2). A 19-bp sequence, the attachment (*attL1*) site, from the 3′ end of tRNA-*ser*$_{GCU}$ is almost perfectly conserved at the end of *vap* region 3 (*attR1*). This sequence is also found at the 3′ end of tRNA-*ser*$_{GGA}$, at the left-hand end of *vap* region 2 (*attL2*), and at the right-hand junction of *vap* region 2 (*attR2*). These results are compatible with the integration of a circular form of the *vap* element by site-specific recombination between the 3′ end of tRNA-*ser* (*attB*) and an *att* site (*attP*) on the circular DNA molecule. A single copy of the *att* site is found on the *vap* plasmid (2), which supports this hypothesis. We have evidence suggesting that *vap* regions 1, 2, and 3 arose by independent integration into the *D. nodosus* genome (4).

FLUIDITY OF THE *vap* REGIONS

Differences in *vap* Regions within and between Strains

There are considerable differences between the three *vap* regions in strain A198 and between *vap* regions found in different *D. nodosus* strains (Fig. 1). These differences include the insertion or deletion of short sequences, the loss of *vap* genes, and the presence of related but distinct copies of some *vap* genes. In strain A198, *vap* regions 1 and 2 are

Virulent strain A198

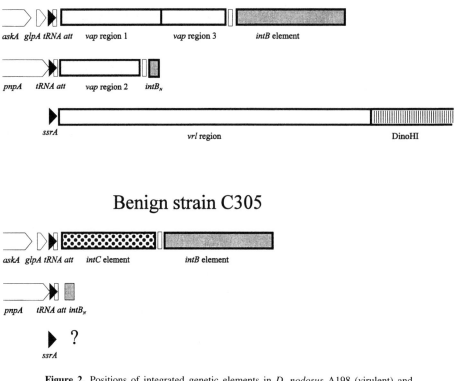

Benign strain C305

Figure 2. Positions of integrated genetic elements in *D. nodosus* A198 (virulent) and C305 (benign). The tRNA genes are shown as black triangles. The figure is not drawn to scale.

almost identical up to the end of *toxA* (Fig. 1A and B). However, there is a 600-bp insertion between *vapC* and *vapD* in *vap* region 2 (Fig. 1B), and a short sequence at the end of *vap* region 2 (Fig. 1B) is not found in *vap* region 1. The genes *toxA″* and *vapA″* found in *vap* region 1 are absent from *vap* region 2. ToxA″ and VapA″ have about 30% amino acid identity to ToxA and VapA, respectively. These genes may have evolved by duplication of *toxA* and *vapA* followed by divergence or may have been acquired separately. The absence of these genes from *vap* region 2 may be explained by failure to acquire the genes, or by loss at a later time.

In strain A198, *vap* region 3 is immediately adjacent to vap region 1. However, region 3 lacks most of the genes from the *vap* region, including *intA, toxA, vapA, vapB,* and *vapC* (Fig. 1C). There is a copy of *vapD* in *vap* region 3, and this is identical to *vapD* in *vap* regions 1 and 2. There is no copy of *vapE,* but a related gene, *vapE′*, is found in the same position (8). VapE′, which is 293 amino acids, has 67% amino acid identity over the first 246 amino acids to VapE, which is 437 amino acids. The amino acid sequences diverge due to a frameshift mutation, but the DNA sequences are still closely related. It is tempting to speculate that *vapE′* has evolved from *vapE.* However, the divergence between *vapE'* and *vapE* is puzzling, since the adjacent gene, *vapD,* is identical in *vap* regions 1 and 3. In region 3, there is also a gene, *vapA',* whose predicted protein product has 38% identity to VapA. This gene may have been acquired separately. The DNA segment immediately upstream from *vapE* in region 1, which contains *vapG* and *vapH,* is related to the segment immediately upstream from *vapE'.* However, there has been a small insertion between *vapG'* and *vapE',* and the *vapH* coding region has been disrupted.

The *vap* regions of most strains which have been studied contain *vapE* (4). However, the genome of strain H1215 (Fig. 1D) lacks *vapE* but contains *vapE'* at the position where *vapE* is usually found (Fig. 1). DNA sequence analysis of the *vap* regions in this strain has not been carried out, but the results of Southern blot analysis and PCR experiments suggest that the region immediately upstream from *vapE'* in strain H1215 is more similar to the region immediately upstream from *vapE'* in strain A198 than to the region upstream from *vapE.* Hence, the *vap* region in strain H1215 is more similar to *vap* region 3 of strain A198 than to *vap* region 1. This suggests that *vap* region 3 arose by integration of a *vap* element similar to the *vap* element in strain H1215, rather than by partial duplication of *vap* region 1.

The *vap* plasmid is almost identical to *vap* region 1 up to the end of *vapA''* (Fig. 1E). However, unlike other *vap* regions, the *vap* plasmid has a copy of IS*1253* following *vapA''.* After the IS element, there is a segment of about 500 bp, which is found at the right-hand end of *vap* region 3 in strain A198.

Repeated Sequences within the *vap* Regions

Two families of repeated sequences have been identified within *vap* regions 1 and 3 of strain A198 (8). There are three complete copies and one partial copy of a 103-bp sequence, which flank *vapD* in both *vap* region 1 and *vap* region 3. In addition, copies or partial copies of an unrelated 102-bp repeat are found at five positions within *vap* regions 1 and 3 (Fig. 1). These repeated sequences may play a role in DNA rearrangements within the *vap* regions. The *vapD* gene from *vap* region 3 is identical to *vapD* from *vap* region 2. Sequence identity begins within the 102-bp repeat upstream from *vapD* in each case and ends within the 103-bp repeat. The sequence between *vapD* and *vapC* in *vap* region 2, which is not found in *vap* region 1, is found upstream from *vapD* in *vap* region 3. This sequence is also bounded by a 103-bp repeat and a 102-bp repeat (8). Similarly, the identity between the *vap* plasmid and the end of *vap* region 3 begins with a 102-bp repeat. *toxA''* and *vapA'',* which are absent from *vap* region 2, are also closely bounded by 102-bp repeats. We have not identified a mechanism by which these repeats could be used for the movement of sequences.

INTEGRATION SITES FOR THE *vap* REGIONS

Analysis of the integration sites for the *vap* regions in a number of strains of *D. nodosus* (4, 48) has identified two predominant integration sites for the *vap* regions (Fig. 2). Most *vap* regions are integrated into the 3' end of tRNA-*ser*$_{GGA}$, which is the site of integration for *vap* region 2 in strain A198. This tRNA gene is immediately downstream from the gene encoding polynucleotide phosphorylase (Pnp), *pnpA* (4). In other bacteria, Pnp is one of the two principal enzymes involved in the degradation of bacterial mRNA to nucleotides and also plays a role in tRNA processing (32). In *D. nodosus,* the *pnpA* gene is very close to tRNA-*ser*$_{GGA}$, with the stop codon located just 1 nucleotide before the start of the tRNA gene.

The other integration site which has been identified for the *vap* regions in *D. nodosus* is tRNA-*ser*$_{GCU}$, which is the site of integration for *vap* region 1 in strain A198 (8). Upstream from this tRNA gene is a gene designated *glpA* (48), which is highly related to *rsmA* from *Erwinia carotovora*. RsmA acts as a global repressor of virulence in *E. carotovora* by repressing extracellular enzyme production. This is mediated by a reduction in the stability of the transcript from *hslI*, which is required for the production of the signalling molecule *N*-(3-oxohexanoyl)-L-homoserine lactone (OhHSL) (10). GlpA may play a similar role as a repressor of virulence in *D. nodosus*.

In *Pseudomonas aeruginosa*, elastase activity is controlled by *N*-(3-oxodecanoyl)-L-homoserine lactone (36). This is of particular interest since extracellular proteases are virulence factors in *D. nodosus* and since virulent strains of *D. nodosus* also have greater elastase activity than benign strains do (44). Given the similarity between GlpA and RsmA of *E. carotovora,* which is involved in the OhHSL-mediated secretion of virulence-associated exoenzymes, it is likely that the production of virulence-associated extracellular enzymes in *D. nodosus* is also controlled by acylated HSL derviatives.

POSSIBLE ROLES FOR THE *vap* REGIONS IN VIRULENCE

Altering the Expression of Adjacent Genes

The integration of the *vap* element into tRNA-*ser*$_{GCU}$ or tRNA-*ser*$_{GGA}$ could alter the expression of these tRNA genes, since this integration event would alter the sequences downstream from the 3′ end of the tRNAs. A direct regulatory role for tRNA molecules in virulence has been proposed by others (40). For example, the deletion of two PAIs from uropathogenic *E. coli* 536 disrupts *selC,* which encodes the selenocysteine-tRNA, and *leuX,* which encodes a leucine-specific tRNA (5). This results in loss of in vivo virulence, which can be restored by introduction of the intact *selC* and *leuX* genes. There is no direct evidence for a role for tRNA-*ser*$_{GCU}$ or tRNA-*ser*$_{GGA}$ in virulence in *D. nodosus,* primarily due to the lack of a transformation system which could be used to investigate such a possibility.

Integration of the *vap* element downstream from *glpA* or *pnpA* may alter the expression of these genes, since both genes are located very close to these tRNA genes. If GlpA does play a role in virulence similar to that proposed for the highly related RsmA from *E. carotovora,* modulation of the expression of *glpA* by integration of the *vap* element could play a key role in virulence. PnpA may also be important in virulence, since Pnp in other bacteria affects mRNA stability. We are currently investigating transcripts from *glpA* and *pnpA* in virulent and benign strains of *D. nodosus.*

Inhibition of Cell Division—a Role in Virulence?

The *glpA* gene, which is adjacent to *vap* region 1 (Fig. 2), is highly related to *rsmA* from *E. carotovora,* a global repressor of virulence, and to *csrA* from *E. coli.* CsrA acts as a global repressor of the starvation response in *E. coli.* When *E. coli* cells enter the stationary phase due to nutrient limitation, cell division is inhibited, cell size increases, and glycogen biosynthesis is activated (41). We hypothesize that the secretion of extracellular enzymes, which differs between virulent and benign strains in both *E. carotovora* and *D. nodosus,* is an adaptation of the starvation response, whereby increased nutrients are made available by the action of the extracellular enzymes upon plant tissue in *E. carotovora* or hoof tissue in *D. nodosus.* All of the *vap* genes except *vapE* show similarity to genes whose products are involved in interaction with the cell division machinery. In this situation, the inhibition of cell division in *D. nodosus* by the products of the *vap* genes may be functionally connected to the expression of extracellular proteases and may thus contribute to virulence. We have noted that virulent strains of *D. nodosus,* in general, grow more slowly than benign strains and often have very elongated cells. Thus, there may be a direct role for the *vap* gene products in virulence, involving inhibition of cell division.

Acquisition of Other Virulence Determinants

The *vap* regions may influence virulence by altering the expression of neighboring genes or by direct action of the *vap* gene products, such as inhibition of cell division. In addition, a further potential role has been proposed, which is the acquisition or maintenance of other virulence determinants. In two extensive studies in which 872 isolates of *D. nodosus* were examined, it was found that all strains which carried the 27-kb virulence-related locus (*vrl* region) also carried the *vap* region (28, 42). However, there are strains which carry the *vap* region but not the *vrl* region. The *vap* region may therefore play a role in the acquisition or maintenance of other virulence determinants, such as the *vrl* region.

OTHER INTEGRATED GENETIC ELEMENTS IN *D. NODOSUS*

The Virulence-Related Locus (*vrl*)

The 27-kb *vrl* region is found in most virulent strains of *D. nodosus* and is absent from most benign strains, suggesting that it may play a role in virulence (24, 28). In the reports published so far, no genes from the region have been identified which have similarity to known virulence determinants in either *D. nodosus* or other pathogenic bacteria (24). The *vrl* region appears to have arisen by the integration of a plasmid or a bacteriophage into the *D. nodosus* genome, although no integrase gene has been identified and the right-hand *att* site has not been identified. The integration site of the *vrl* region is the gene *ssrA,* which encodes a small, stable RNA molecule, designated 10Sa RNA. This integration site is different from the two integration sites which have been identified so far for the *vap* regions.

Since no integrase gene has been identified so far in the *vrl* region, it is possible that the integrase from the *vap* region, IntA, is required for integration of the *vrl* region. The *vrl* region is integrated into *ssrA* (24), part of which shows strong similarity to the pseudouridine arm of tRNA genes from other organisms (47). IntA may recognize *ssrA,* as well as tRNA-*ser*$_{GCU}$ and tRNA-*ser*$_{GGA}$, as an integration site. This hypothesis is supported by the observation that two of the integrases to which IntA is most highly related, the integrases of the CTXφ PAI from *V. cholerae* and cryptic prophage P4-57 from *E. coli* (Table 1), integrate into *ssrA* genes.

The *intB* Element

In the virulent *D. nodosus* strain A198, there is an integrase gene, *intB,* located 200 bp past the end of *vap* region 3. We have determined the DNA sequence of a further 4.8 kb of DNA past the attachment site for *vap* region 3 and identified a genetic element, designated the *intB* element, which may be an integrated prophage or conjugative transposon (4). IntB is most closely related to the same integrases as IntA—the integrases from phages φR73 and Sf6 and from a *V. cholerae* PAI, and the symbiosis island of *Mesorhizobium loti.* The degree of similarity between IntB and IntA is almost the same as that between IntB and the integrase from φR73. Next to *intB* is a gene, *regA,* encoding a putative DNA-binding regulatory protein, followed by three genes of unknown function, *gepA, gepB,* and *gepC.* None of these genes show any similarity to known virulence determinants.

There is a partial copy of *intB,* designated *intB$_N$*, at the end of *vap* region 2 in strain A198; in other strains we have found the *intB* gene, or a partial copy thereof, next to tRNA-*ser*$_{GCU}$ and tRNA-*ser*$_{GGA}$ (48). These results suggest that the *intB* element integrates at the same two sites as the *vap* element and that expression of *pnpA, glpA,* and the tRNA-*ser* genes may differ according to whether *intA* or *intB* is adjacent to them. A copy of at least part of the *intB* element has been found in all strains studied so far, both benign and virulent, and so there is no association between the presence of the *intB* gene and virulence. We are using chromosome walking to further characterize the *intB* element, since we have not yet found the expected attachment site at the other end of the element. Deletions of at least part of the *intB* element have occurred in some strains; therefore, it is possible that the *intB* element does carry genes involved in virulence and that the virulence-associated part of the *intB* element is missing from benign strains.

Bacteriophage DinoHI

Our work on the *vap* and *intB* elements suggested that these may be integrated bacteriophages, which led us to attempt to induce bacteriophages from *D. nodosus* strains. We have induced a bacteriophage, DinoHI, from one strain of *D. nodosus* but found that it did not carry *intA* or *intB* and hence is a separate integrated genetic element (3). DNA from DinoHI also failed to hybridize to two probes from the *vrl* region. At least part of the DinoHI genome is integrated into the bacterial chromosome in several strains of *D. nodosus.* We are currently characterizing the integrase gene from DinoHI, and preliminary results suggest that the integrase is different from the integrases which have so far been isolated from *D. nodosus.* The site of integration of DinoHI in strain H1215 is unknown, but in strain A198 part of the DinoHI genome is located next to the *vrl* region (3). This suggests that DinoHI and the *vrl* region share the same integration site.

The *intC* Element

We have identified another genetic element, the *intC* element (48), which integrates into tRNA-*ser*$_{GCU}$, next to *glpA.* The integrase, IntC, from this element, is most closely related to IntA, with 55% amino acid identity. This is considerably higher than the amino acid identity to the next most closely related integrase from the databases, the integrase from phage φR73, to which it has 40% amino acid identity. The *intC* element contains genes related to *vapG-vapH,* but the rest of the genes from the *intC* element are unrelated to genes from the *vap* element. However, there is a copy of the insertion sequence IS*1253* at the end of the *intC* element. It is of interest that a copy of this IS element is found on the *vap* plasmid and on the *intC* element.

In addition, we have preliminary evidence for the presence of another genetic element which integrates into tRNA-*ser*GGA. This new element has been detected in only six strains, and characterization is in progress.

EVOLUTIONARY IMPLICATIONS

At least six different genetic elements can integrate into the genome of *D. nodosus*, using at least three different genomic integration sites—tRNA-*ser*GCU, tRNA-*ser*GGA, and *ssrA*. A plasmid form of the *vap* element has been identified but appears not to be self-transmissible. The bacteriophage DinoHI should be capable of infecting other strains of *D. nodosus*, although we have so far been unable to achieve this in the laboratory. This may be due to the presence of at least part of the DinoHI genome in other strains, which may confer immunity to superinfection. At present, a nonintegrated form of the *intB*, *intC*, or *vrl* element has not been identified. The roles in virulence of these elements have not been defined, but some of them may carry genes with a defined role in virulence or may alter the expression of adjacent cellular genes upon integration. It is possible that virulence in *D. nodosus* is modulated by the integration and excision of one or more of these elements.

SUMMARY

The *vap* regions of *D. nodosus* satisfy most of the criteria for classification of PAIs (22). They are found much more frequently in virulent strains than in benign strains, have a different G+C content from the DNA of the host, occupy large chromosomal regions, and are distinct genetic units, flanked by direct repeats. They are integrated into tRNA genes and contain an integrase gene and a putative origin of replication. However, unlike most PAIs, they are stably inherited, since loss of the *vap* regions has not been seen to occur during passage in the laboratory. The presence of the *vapA-toxA* maintenance system in the *vap* regions may prevent their loss. The major reason for disputing the classification of the *vap* regions of *D. nodosus* as PAIs is that there is at present no evidence for a direct role of the *vap* gene products in virulence. However, we propose that the *vap* regions may influence virulence by altering the expression of neighboring genes, and, since many of the *vap* genes are similar to genes which affect the bacterial cell division process, we speculate that the *vap* genes may play a direct role in virulence.

Integrated genetic elements in *D. nodosus* and other pathogenic bacteria may affect virulence by carrying genes encoding virulence determinants, such as toxins, invasins, or proteins involved in resistance to host defense mechanisms or acquisition of iron. In addition, they may affect virulence either by carrying regulatory genes which affect the expression of existing virulence determinants or by integrating into chromosomal positions such that the expression of virulence determinants or their regulators is altered. A broader definition of PAIs may be needed to encompass these possibilities.

In addition to the *vap* regions, five other genetic elements that are integrated into the

D. nodosus genome have been identified. Some of these may also be classified as PAIs when their role in virulence has been determined.

Acknowledgment. This work was supported by a grant from the Australian Research Council.

REFERENCES

1. **Beveridge, W. I. B.** 1941. Footrot in sheep: a transmissible disease due to infection with *Fusiformis nodosus*. *C. S. I. R. O. Bull.* **140:**1–40.
2. **Billington, S. J., M. Sinistaj, B. F. Cheetham, A. Ayres, E. K. Moses, M. E. Katz, and J. I. Rood.** 1996. Identification of a native *Dichelobacter nodosus* plasmid and implications for the evolution of the *vap* regions. *Gene* **172:**111–116.
3. **Bloomfield, G. A., M. E. Katz, and B. F. Cheetham.** Unpublished data.
4. **Bloomfield, G. A., G. Whittle, M. B. McDonagh, M. E. Katz, and B. F. Cheetham.** 1997. Analysis of sequences flanking the *vap* regions of *Dichelobacter nodosus:* evidence for multiple integration events, a killer system, and a new genetic element. *Microbiology* **143:**553–562.
5. **Blum, G., M. Ott, A. Lischewski, A. Ritter, H. Imrich, H. Tschaepe, and J. Hacker.** 1994. Excision of large DNA regions termed pathogenicity islands from tRNA-specific loci in the chromosome of an *Escherichia coli* wild-type pathogen. *Infect. Immun.* **62:**606–614.
6. **Brynestad, S., L. A. Iwanejiko, G. S. A. B. Stewart, and P. E. Granum.** 1994. A complex array of Hpr consensus DNA recognition sequences proximal to the enterotoxin gene in *Clostridium perfringens* type A. *Microbiology* **140:**97–104.
7. **Censini, S., C. Lange, Z. Xiang, J. E. Crabtree, P. Ghiara, M. Borodovsky, R. Rappuoli, and A. Covacci.** 1996. *cag,* a pathogenicity island of *Helicobacter pylori,* encodes type I-specific and disease-associated virulence factors. *Proc. Natl. Acad. Sci. USA* **93:**14648–14653.
8. **Cheetham, B. F., D. B. Tattersall, G. A. Bloomfield, J. I. Rood, and M. E. Katz.** 1995. Identification of a bacteriophage-related integrase gene in a *vap* region of the *Dichelobacter nodosus* genome. *Gene* **162:** 53–58.
9. **Claxton, P. D., L. A. Ribeiro, and J. R. Egerton.** 1983. Classification of *Bacteroides nodosus* by agglutination tests. *Aust. Vet. J.* **60:**331–334.
10. **Cui, Y., A. Chatterjee, Y. Liu, C. K. Dumenyo, and A. K. Chatterjee.** 1995. Identification of a global repressor gene, *rsmA,* of *Erwinia carotovora* subsp. *carotovora* that controls extracellular enzymes, *N*-(3-oxohexanoyl)-L-homoserine lactone, and pathogenicity in soft-rotting *Erwinia* spp. *J. Bacteriol.* **177:** 5108–5115.
11. **Dalrymple, B., and J. S. Mattick.** 1987. An analysis of the organization and evolution of type 4 fimbrial (MePhe) subunit proteins. *J. Mol. Evol.* **25:**261–269.
12. **Depiazzi, L. J., and R. B. Richards.** 1985. Motility in relation to virulence of *Bacteroides nodosus*. *Vet. Microbiol.* **10:**107–116.
13. **Depiazzi, L. J., and J. I. Rood.** 1984. The thermostability of proteases from virulent and benign strains of *Bacteroides nodosus*. *Vet. Microbiol.* **9:**227–236.
14. **Dewhirst, F. E., B. J. Paster, S. La Fontaine, and J. I. Rood.** 1990. Transfer of *Kingella indologenes* (Snell and Lapage 1976) to the genus *Suttonella* gen. nov. as *Suttonella indologenes* comb. nov.; transfer of *Bacteroides nodosus* (Beveridge 1941) to the genus *Dichelobacter* gen. nov. as *Dichelobacter nodosus* comb. nov.; and assignment of the genera *Cardiobacterium, Dichelobacter,* and *Suttonella* to *Cardiobacteriaceae* fam. nov. in the gamma division of *Proteobacteria* on the basis of 16S rRNA sequence comparisons. *Int. J. Syst. Bacteriol.* **40:**426–433.
15. **Egerton, J. R.** 1989. Footrot of cattle, goats and deer, p. 47–56. *In* J. R. Egerton, W. K. Yong, and G. G. Riffkin (ed.), *Footrot and Foot Abscess of Ruminants.* CRC Press, Inc., Boca Raton, Fla.
16. **Faubladier, M., and J.-P. Bouche.** 1994. Division inhibitor gene *dicF* of *Escherichia coli* reveals a widespread group of prophage sequences in bacterial genomes. *J. Bacteriol.* **176:**1150–1156.
17. **Fleischmann, R. D.** 1995. Whole-genome random sequencing and assembly of *Haemophilus influenzae* Rd. *Science* **269:**496–512.
18. **Galli, D. M., and D. J. LeBlanc.** 1994. Characterization of pVT736-1, a rolling circle plasmid from the gram-negative bacterium *Actinobacillus actinomycetemcomitans*. *Plasmid* **31:**31–39.

19. **Galli, D. M., and D. J. LeBlanc.** 1997. Identification of a maintenance system on rolling circle replicating plasmid pVT736-1. *Mol. Microbiol.* **25:**649–659.

20. **Ghisotti, D., R. Chiaramonte, F. Forti, S. Zangrossi, G. Sironi, and G. Deho.** 1992. Genetic analysis of the immunity region of phage-plasmid P4. *Mol. Microbiol.* **6:**3405–3413.

21. **Gulig, P. A., A. I., Caldwell, and V. A. Chiodo.** 1992. Identification, genetic analysis and DNA sequence of a 7.8-kb virulence region of the *Salmonella typhimurium* virulence plasmid. *Mol. Microbiol.* **6:**1395–1411.

22. **Hacker, J., G. Blum-Oehler, I. Muhldorfer, and H. Tschape.** 1997. Pathogenicity islands of virulent bacteria: structure, function and impact on microbial evolution. *Mol. Microbiol.* **23:**1089–1097.

23. **Halling, C., R. Calendar, G. E. Christie, E. C. Dale, G. Deho, S. Finkel, J. Flensburg, D. Ghisotti, M. L. Kahn, K. B. Lane, B. H. Lindqvist, L. S. Pierson III, E. W. Six, M. G. Sunshine, and R. Ziermann.** 1990. DNA sequence of satellite bacteriophage P4. *Nucleic Acids Res.* **18:**1649.

24. **Haring, V., S. J. Billington, C. L. Wright, A. S. Huggins, M. E. Katz, and J. I. Rood.** 1995. Delineation of the virulence-related locus (*vrl*) of *Dichelobacter nodosus. Microbiology* **149:**2081–2086.

25. **Holdeman, L. V., R. W. Kelley, and W. E. C. Moore.** 1984. Genus I. *Bacteroides,* p. 604–631. *In* N. G. Krieg and J. G. Holt (ed.), *Bergey's Manual of Systematic Bacteriology,* vol. 1. The Williams & Wilkins Co., Baltimore, Md.

26. **Kaneko, T.** 1996. Sequence analysis of the genome of the unicellular cyanobacterium *Synechocystis sp.* strain PCC6803II. Sequence determination of the entire genome and assignation of potential protein-coding regions. *DNA Res.* **3:**109–136.

27. **Katayama, S., B. Dupuy, T. Garnier, and S. T. Cole.** 1995. Rapid expansion of the physical and genetic map of the chromosome of *Clostridium perfringens* CPN50. *J. Bacteriol.* **177:**5680–5686.

28. **Katz, M. E., P. M. Howarth, W. K. Yong, G. G. Riffkin, L. J. Depiazzi, and J. I. Rood.** 1991. Identification of three gene regions associated with virulence in *Dichelobacter nodosus,* the causative agent of ovine footrot. *J. Gen. Microbiol.* **137:**2117–2124.

29. **Katz, M. E., R. A. Strugnell, and J. I. Rood.** 1992. Molecular characterization of a genomic region associated with virulence in *Dichelobacter nodosus. Infect. Immun.* **60:**4586–4592.

30. **Katz, M. E., C. L. Wright, T. S. Gartside, B. F. Cheetham, C. V. Doidge, E. K. Moses, and J. I. Rood.** 1994. Genetic organization of the duplicated *vap* region of the *Dichelobacter nodosus* genome. *J. Bacteriol.* **176:**2663–2669.

31. **Klose, K. E., and J. J. Mekalanos.** 1998. Differential regulation of multiple flagellins in *Vibrio cholerae. J. Bacteriol.* **180:**303–316.

32. **Li, Z., and M. P. Deutscher.** 1994. The role of individual exoribonucleases in processing at the 3' end of *Escherichia coli* tRNA precursors. *J. Biol. Chem.* **269:**6064–6071.

33. **Lindsay, J. A., A. Ruzin, H. F. Ross, N. Kurepina, and R. P. Novick.** 1998. The gene for toxic shock toxin is carried by a family of mobile pathogenicity islands in *Staphylococcus aureus. Mol. Microbiol.* **29:**527–543.

34. **Mattick, J. S., B. J. Anderson, P. T. Cox, B. P. Dalrymple, M. M. Bills, M. Hobbs, and J. R. Egerton.** 1991. Gene sequences and comparison of the fimbrial subunits representative of *Bacteroides nodosus* serotypes A to I: class I and class II strains. *Mol. Microbiol.* **5:**561–573.

35. **Moses, E. K., R. T. Good, M. Sinistaj, S. J. Billington, C. J. Langford, and J. I. Rood.** 1995. A multiple site-specific inversion model for the control of Omp1 phase and antigenic variation in *Dichelobacter nodosus. Mol. Microbiol.* **17:**183–196.

36. **Pearson, J. P., E. C. Pesci, and B. H. Iglewski.** 1997. Roles of *Pseudomonas aeruginosa las* and *rhl* quorum-sensing systems in control of elastase and rhamnolipid biosynthesis genes. *J. Bacteriol.* **179:**5756–5767.

37. **Pullinger, G. D., and A. J. Lax.** 1992. A *Salmonella dublin* virulence plasmid locus that affects bacterial growth under nutrient-limited conditions. *Mol. Microbiol.* **6:**1631–1643.

38. **Radnedge, L., M. A. Davis, B. Youngren, and S. J. Austin.** 1997. Plasmid maintenance functions of the large virulence plasmid of *Shigella flexneri. J. Bacteriol.* **179:**3670–3675.

39. **Reiter, W.-D., P. Palm, and S. Yeats.** 1989. Transfer RNA genes frequently serve as integration sites for prokaryotic genetic elements. *Nucleic Acids Res.* **17:**1907–1914.

40. **Ritter, A., G. Blum, L. Emody, M. Kerenyi, A. Bock, B. Neuhier, W. Rabsch, F. Scheutz, and J. Hacker.** 1995. tRNA genes and pathogenicity islands: influence on virulence and metabolic properties of uropathogenic *Escherichia coli. Mol. Microbiol.* **17:**109–121.

41. **Romeo, T., M. Gong, M. Y. Liu, and A.-M. Brun-Zinkernagel.** 1993. Identification and molecular charac-

terization of *csrA*, a pleiotropic gene from *Escherichia coli* that affects glycogen biosynthesis, gluconeogenesis, cell size and surface properties. *J. Bacteriol.* **175:**4744–4755.

42. **Rood, J. I., P. A. Howart, V. Haring, W. K. Yong, D. Liu, M. A. Palmer, D. R. Pitman, I. Links, D. J. Stewart, and J. A. Vaughan.** 1996. Comparison of gene probe and conventional methods for the diagnosis of ovine footrot. *Vet. Microbiol.* **52:**127–142.

43. **Simonet, M., and S. Falkow.** 1992. Invasin expression in *Yersinia pseudotuberculosis. Infect. Immun.* **60:** 4414–4417.

44. **Stewart, D. J.** 1979. The role of elastase in the differentiation of *Bacteroides nodosus* infections in sheep and cattle. *Res. Vet. Sci.* **27:**99–105.

45. **Tian, Q. B., M. Ohnishi, A. Tabuchi, and Y. Terawaki.** 1996. A new plasmid-encoded killer gene system: cloning, sequencing, and analyzing *hig* locus of plasmid Rts1. *Biochem. Biophys. Res. Commun.* **220:** 280–284.

46. **Tominaga, H., S. Kawagishi, H. Ashida, Y. Sawa, and H. Ochiai.** 1995. Structure and replication of cryptic plasmids, pMA1 and pMA2, from a unicellular cyanobacterium, *Microcystis aeruginosa. Biosci. Biotechnol. Biochem.* **59:**1217–1220.

47. **Tyagi, J. S., and A. K. Klinger.** 1992. Identification of the 10Sa RNA structural gene of *Mycobacterium tuberculosis. Nucleic Acids Res.* **20:**138.

48. **Whittle, G., G. A. Bloomfield, M. E. Katz, and B. F. Cheetham.** Modulation of virulence by the integration of genetic elements into the genome of *Dichelobacter nodosus,* the causative agent of ovine footrot. Submitted for publication.

49. **Whittle, G., M. E. Katz, E. H. Clayton, and B. F. Cheetham.** Unpublished data.

Pathogenicity Islands and Other Mobile Virulence Elements
Edited by J. B. Kaper and J. Hacker
© 1999 American Society for Microbiology, Washington, D.C.

Chapter 12

Virulence Gene Clusters and Putative Pathogenicity Islands in Listeriae

Jürgen Kreft, José-Antonio Vázquez-Boland, Eva Ng, and Werner Goebel

The genus *Listeria* comprises six characterized species, *Listeria monocytogenes, L. ivanovii, L. seeligeri, L. innocua, L. welshimeri,* and *L. grayi.* Members of this genus are gram-positive, rod-shaped, nonsporulating, heterotrophic bacteria that are commonly found in soil, water, sewage, and decaying vegetation. In addition, several species of *Listeria* have been isolated from many wild and domestic animals (32, 57). Classical taxonomy places *Listeria* next to *Lactobacillus,* while more recent 16S rRNA sequence analysis indicates that its closest relationship is to *Streptococcus* (5) and 23S rRNA analysis groups it next to *Staphylococcus* and *Bacillus* (56). Not surprisingly, homology searches carried out with the deduced amino acid sequences of the known genes (see below) of *Listeria* species yielded significant similarities to gene products of many gram-positive bacteria, e.g., *Lactobacillus, Streptococcus, Staphylococcus,* and particularly to different members of the genus *Bacillus.* The listerial genome, as has been found for many other bacteria, is likely to be a genetic mosaic, containing DNA which has been acquired by horizontal gene transfer from other, mostly gram-positive bacteria. The ongoing *Listeria* genome sequencing project might shed more light on this complex genome arrangement.

Two species of *Listeria* possess pathogenic potential: *L. monocytogenes* can cause disease in humans and animals with clinical manifestations such as septicemia, meningitis and/or encephalitis, abortion, granulomatosis, and gastroenteritis (22, 32, 44), and *L. ivanovii* infects predominantly sheep and cattle, without causing the central nervous system symptoms typical of infections by *L. monocytogenes.* Human infections by *L. ivanovii* are extremely rare (8). *L. seeligeri,* although weakly hemolytic, is nonpathogenic, but it has occasionally been isolated from patients (55). The other three species are typical heterotrophic saprophytes, living exclusively in different natural environments (32, 57). Recent phylogenetic studies based on sequence analysis of the listerial 16S rRNA and the *iap* gene (64) suggest a phylogenetic tree for *Listeria* where *L. grayi* has a clear phylogenetic

Jürgen Kreft, Eva Ng, and Werner Goebel • Lehrstuhl für Mikrobiologie, Biozentrum Universität Würzburg, D-97074 Würzburg, Germany. *José-Antonio Vázquez-Boland* • Grupo de Patogénesis Molecular Bacteriana, Microbiologia e Inmunologia, Facultad de Veterinaria, Universidad Complutense de Madrid, E-28040 Madrid, Spain.

distance from the other five *Listeria* species, which are again phylogenetically separated into the *L. ivanovii/L. seeligeri/L. welshimeri* and *L. monocytogenes/L. innocua* groups.

The two pathogenic species, *L. monocytogenes* and *L. ivanovii,* are facultatively intracellular bacteria capable of infecting a broad spectrum of normally nonphagocytic mammalian cell types in vitro (7, 11, 13, 18, 28, 29, 42). After infection of these host cells as well as of professional phagocytic cells, predominantly monocytes and macrophages, these bacteria are released from the primary phagosome into the host cell cytosol, where they replicate efficiently. They are also able to spread from the originally infected cell into neighboring homologous and heterologous host cells, a phenomenon commonly called cell-to-cell spread.

Several specific genes which are apparently involved in these steps and hence in virulence of *L. monocytogenes* and *L. ivanovii* were identified in the last decade. The ability to undergo intracellular (cytosolic) replication and cell-to-cell spread is conferred by a cluster of genes which are coordinately regulated by the transcription activator PrfA, whose locus is within this cluster (7, 38, 49, 58). This set of genes is therefore often referred to as the *prfA* virulence gene cluster. The products of these genes are necessary and apparently sufficient for survival and replication in mammalian host cell cytosol.

Several *L. monocytogenes* genes have been implicated in adhesion and internalization of *L. monocytogenes* and possibly also *L. ivanovii* (7). Among these, the best-studied factors are the internalin (*inl*) genes *inlA* and *inlB,* both of which are members of the rather large group of cell-associated large internalins (7, 19). Genes for this internalin group have been identified only in *L. monocytogenes* to date.

There is another class of internalins, termed small internalins or internalin-related-protein (irp) (43). These proteins, in contrast to the large internalins, represent secreted proteins with unknown functions. It should be stressed at this point that the term ''internalin'' in this context does not necessarily imply that the specific protein is really involved in the process of internalization. Such a function has been shown only for InlA and InlB, as discussed below. Both large and small internalins share the leucine-rich repeat (LRR) domain and are thus paralogous members of a growing family of LRR proteins (33). Genes encoding the small internalins have been found in *L. monocytogenes* and *L. ivanovii,* but there seem to be more of these genes in *L. ivanovii* than in *L. monocytogenes* (see below).

THE *prfA* VIRULENCE GENE CLUSTER—FINAL OUTCOME OF AN ANCIENT PATHOGENICITY ISLAND?

The *prfA* gene cluster, which was first characterized in *L. monocytogenes* and shown to control intracellular (cytosolic) replication and cell-to-cell spread, comprises six genes in the order *prfA, plcA, hly, mpl, actA,* and *plcB.* These genes encode two phospholipases of the C type (PlcA and PlcB), the pore-forming protein listeriolysin O (LLO or Hly), the ActA protein, and a Zn-dependent metalloprotease (Mpl). The first three gene products participate in the opening of the phagosomal compartments (24, 38, 49, 58), while ActA is responsible for the widely studied bacterium-induced polymerization of host cell actin (6, 7, 38, 49, 59). The function of Mpl is unknown. PlcA and PlcB show high similiarity to corresponding enzymes from *Staphylococcus aureus* and *Bacillus cereus,* respectively, and Mpl highly resembles metalloproteases from bacilli. However, no extended sequence similarity has been observed for the ActA protein.

The 8.8-kbp gene cluster is not only found in all *L. monocytogenes* isolates tested but is also located at a defined position on the listerial chromosome between the two house-keeping genes *ldh* (encoding lactate dehydrogenase) and *prs* (encoding phosphoribosyl-pyrophosphate synthetase). While the intergenic region between the first gene of this virulence gene cluster, *prfA,* and the flanking *prs* is only 47 bp long, the distance between the last gene *plcB,* and *ldh* is 2.2 kb. This intergenic region contains five small open reading frames (ORFs), termed ORFX, ORFY, ORFZ, ORFB, and ORFA (63). *prfA* encodes a transcription activator of the Crp/Fnr family (31, 39), which recognizes a specific palindromic sequence of 14 bp located at bp -41 with respect to the transcriptional start site of each PrfA-dependent gene or operon (37). The virulence gene cluster is subdivided into four PrfA-dependent transcription units, rendering the expression of all the genes in this cluster fully dependent on PrfA. The entire PrfA regulon, however, also comprises genes outside of this gene cluster including some of the *inl* genes, e.g., *inlA, inlB,* and *inlC,* as well as a yet undefined gene(s) involved in uptake and/or metabolism of phosphor-ylated sugars (53), stress response (54), and possibly events that are as yet unidentified.

A similar *prfA* gene cluster is also present on the chromosome of *L. ivanovii* (26, 36, 39). Not only are the number and the arrangement of the six genes identical to those of *L. monocytogenes,* but so is their localization between the housekeeping genes *prs* and *ldh.* The sequence homology between the corresponding genes, including *prfA,* of *L. ivanovii* and *L. monocytogenes* is high with the exception of *actA.* The *actA* equivalent of *L. ivanovii,* termed *Li-actA,* is considerably larger (3,069 bp) than its *L. monocytogenes* counterpart (1,920 bp), and the Li-ActA protein has only 46% sequence similarity to ActA (36). Recent studies demonstrate, however, that ActA and Li-ActA function in a similar mode due to two highly conserved, major functional domains involved in actin polymeriza-tion (23).

Expression of all the genes within the *L. ivanovii* virulence gene cluster is likewise strictly dependent on PrfA, and PrfA regulation seems to function in a fashion similar to that in *L. monocytogenes.* Interestingly, the known PrfA regulon of *L. ivanovii* is larger than that of *L. monocytogenes* and includes all genes encoding small internalins (see below).

In contrast to *L. monocytogenes* and *L. ivanovii, L. seeligeri,* albeit being weakly hemo-lytic on blood agar plates, is avirulent in the murine animal model. Consistent with this observation is the inability of this species to trigger its uptake in nonphagocytic mammalian host cells and to be released into the cytosol when internalized by phagocytic cells. It was therefore surprising to find in *L. seeligeri* a gene cluster highly reminiscent of the *prfA* virulence gene cluster of the two pathogenic *Listeria* species. This gene cluster is also located at the same position on the chromosome of *L. seeligeri* as the virulence gene clusters of *L. monocytogenes* and *L. ivanovii.* It contains all six genes identified in the latter *prfA* gene clusters, including a functional equivalent of the *prfA* gene (40).

The *L. seeligeri* gene cluster is, however, substantially larger than those of the patho-genic *Listeria* species and contains three additional ORFs, which, based on their flanking regulatory features (putative promoters, ribosome binding sites, and transcription termina-tors), represent potentially transcribed genes. In addition, there is an apparently deleted second copy of *plcB* downstream of *actA,* which may have been generated by the duplica-tion of *plcB* followed by a subsequent deletion within one of the *plcB* copies. The localiza-

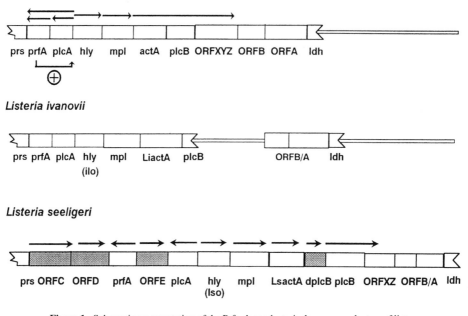

Figure 1. Schematic representation of the Prfa-dependent virulence gene clusters of listeriae. The direction of transcription is indicated by arrows; in *L. ivanovii* it is identical to that in *L. monocytogenes.* Note that in *L. monocytogenes* and *L. ivanovii,* the product of *prfA* stimulates the transcription of the bicistronic *plcA-prfA* mRNA; in *L. seeligeri* this autoregulatory loop is interrupted by the divergently transcribed ORFE. The sequences for *L. ivanovii mpl* and *plcB* have not yet been completely determined. For *L. ivanovii* and *L. seeligeri,* the presence of sequences homologous to ORFB and ORFA has been shown by DNA hybridization (63); the sequence has not yet been determined. For further details and references, see the text.

tion of the three additional genes, called ORFC to ORFE, within the *prfA* gene cluster of *L. seeligeri* is depicted in Fig. 1.

The deduced amino acid sequences suggest that ORFC is a cell surface-associated protein of 96 kDa, containing five highly conserved repeat units of 78 to 80 amino acids. These repeats show a significant similarity (59%) to the C-protein alpha antigen of *Streptococcus agalactiae.* ORFD encodes a putative protein which is homologous (63% similarity) to the *araD* gene product of *Escherichia coli* and *Salmonella typhimurium; araD* codes for an L-ribulose-5-phosphate epimerase. ORFE may encode a cytoplasmic protein (50 kDa) with no known homologs. ORFX to ORFZ, located at the *ldh*-proximal end of the virulence gene cluster of *L. monocytogenes,* appear in *L. seeligeri* as a fusion of these reading frames (ORFXZ). Most interestingly, there are well-conserved and possibly functionally operative PrfA boxes in the upstream sequences of ORFD, ORFE, and ORFXZ, suggesting that these genes are also under PrfA control. The location of ORFE between *prfA* and *plcA* leads to a different regulation of *prfA* expression in *L. seeligeri* from that in *L. monocytogenes* and *L. ivanovii.* The autoregulation of *prfA* transcription by the PrfA-dependent promoter in front of *plcA,* observed in *L. monocytogenes* and *L. ivanovii,* can no longer function in *L. seeligeri;* instead, the PrfA-dependent promoter of ORFE drives transcription in the opposite direction relative to the *prfA* gene (Fig. 1). Thus, in *L. seeligeri, prfA* expression may depend solely on the two promoters directly in front of *prfA,* which resemble their counterparts in *L. monocytogenes* and *L. ivanovii.* Transcription of *prfA* from these promoters is not very efficient (40) and may even be negatively influenced by PrfA, as has been shown for *L. monocytogenes* (17). This may explain the low expression of the PrfA-dependent genes in *L. seeligeri* under conditions which are favorable for PrfA-dependent expression in *L. monocytogenes* and *L. ivanovii.*

Although *Listeria innocua* is phylogenetically more closely related to *L. monocytogenes* than to *L. ivanovii* and *L. seeligeri* (see above), it does not possess the *prfA* gene cluster between the *ldh* and *prs* genes or at any other position on the chromosome. This fact suggests that *L. innocua* may have deleted the *prfA* gene cluster, since *L. monocytogenes, L. ivanovii,* and *L. seeligeri* all contain this cluster; otherwise, one would have to invoke three independent insertion events into the same site or to question the accuracy of the 16S rRNA/*iap*-derived phylogenetic tree. Furthermore, this finding suggests that this set of genes was acquired by *Listeria* after the divergence of *L. grayi* and possibly *L. welshimeri* but before the divergence of the progenitor of *L. monocytogenes* and *L. innocua* from the progenitor of *L. ivanovii* and *L. seeligeri.*

Functionally speaking, the *prfA* gene cluster seems to act in two ways. The nonpathogenic *L. innocua, L. welshimeri,* and *L. grayi* possess no *prfA* gene cluster, whereas the nonpathogenic *L. seeligeri* has an extended one, which expresses lower levels of PrfA and all the PrfA-dependent gene products compared to *L. monocytogenes* and *L. ivanovii* under the same conditions. The two pathogenic species, *L. monocytogenes* and *L. ivanovii,* share a very similar *prfA* gene cluster in which all six genes encode the same functions and seem to be identically regulated. Expression of all the genes of this gene cluster is low when *L. monocytogenes* grows in rich culture media but becomes highly induced under certain conditions, particularly when the bacteria grow within mammalian cells (3). In the laboratory, growth of *L. monocytogenes* has also been demonstrated in acanthamoebae and other protists. In contrast to the situation in mammalian cells, listerial replication in these lower eukaryotes is not very efficient (45), suggesting that the arrangement and regulation of the genes in the virulence gene cluster of *L. monocytogenes* and *L. ivanovii* may be best adapted for the intracellular life of these bacteria in mammalian cells.

The additional genes in the *prfA* gene cluster of *L. seeligeri* do not appear to be randomly inserted in a cluster of the *L. monocytogenes* (*ivanovii*) type. Instead, the arrangement of these additional genes and their potential expression from PrfA-dependent promoters suggests an adaptation to another environment. This does not seem to be the mammalian host cell, since *L. seeligeri* is unable to invade and/or replicate within phagocytic or nonphagocytic mammalian cell lines (18, 34). Although speculative, it is intriguing to entertain the idea that this *prfA* gene cluster may be better adapted for life in lower eukaryotes. It is interesting in this context that the isoelectric point of ActA (pH 9.85) from *L. seeligeri* is high compared to those of the *L. monocytogenes* and *L. ivanovii* ActA proteins, which are pH 4.8 and 4.6, respectively. Possibly the ActA protein of *L. seeligeri* functions in an environment which requires this particular physical property for triggering actin polymerization; interestingly, no actin tails are induced by *L. seeligeri* in mammalian cells even under experimental conditions which allow the release of *L. seeligeri* into the host cell cytosol by the enhanced expression of its *hly* and *plcA* genes (34).

A possible scenario for the evolution of the different *prfA* gene clusters in the *Listeria* species is as follows. The ancestral members of *Listeria* were heterotrophic bacteria which in their natural environments might have frequently encountered protozoa, like acantha-moebae and other environmental bacterivores. The interaction between these professional phagocytic protists and *Listeria* selected for variants which had acquired functions (possi-bly by horizontal gene transfer) enabling them to survive and replicate in these eukaryotic hosts. Today's *L. seeligeri prfA* gene cluster may still represent a set of genes more adapted to such an intracellular environment. The functions which have allowed these progenitor "environmental pathogens" to survive and to replicate in the intracellular compartment of protists might be preadaptations for the lifestyle of *Listeria* in phagocytes of higher animals. The conversion of the *L. seeligeri*-type *prfA* gene cluster to the *prfA* virulence gene clusters of *L. monocytogenes* and *L. ivanovii* probably would have involved the removal of all unnecessary genes and the optimization of the expression of these genes in a mammalian cell. Based on the sequence information available to date (ca. 38 kbp in addition to the virulence gene cluster and the internalin genes), we calculated the G+C content, relative dinucleotide abundance, and codon frequency and could not find a signifi-cant difference between the genes of the *prfA* gene cluster and genes of the residual listerial chromosome in any of the listerial species carrying the *prfA* gene cluster. All deviations from the mean could be attributed to the particular amino acid composition of the respective protein. This apparently extensive adaptation of the genetic composition of the *prfA* gene cluster to the listerial chromosome suggests an ancient origin of this "genetic cassette for intracellular survival." The generation of such a "lean" virulence gene cluster, stably anchored in the bacterial chromosome, may thus represent the ultimate outcome in the evolution of what is called today a pathogenicity island (PAI) (30). The probable loss of this gene cluster by *L. innocua* has converted this species again into a saprophytically living microorganism similar to the other two environmental *Listeria* species, *L. welshimeri* and *L. grayi*.

PATHOGENICITY ISLANDS AND ISLETS—THE INTERNALIN MULTIGENE FAMILY

During a systemic infection, *L. monocytogenes* has to cross several tissue barriers which consist of different cell types. After being ingested, the bacteria first encounter the intestinal epithelium, where they are probably internalized by enterocytes and the specialized M cells (50). In the underlying mucosa-associated lymphoid tissue, they are phagocytosed primarily by macrophages and possibly also by dendritic cells and are transported into the liver and spleen. It has been demonstrated that *L. monocytogenes* enters and replicates in hepatocytes (11, 38, 58). Normally the *L. monocytogenes* cells will be cleared from these organs, but occasionally they enter the peripheral bloodstream and eventually cross the blood-brain barrier, causing meningitis or encephalomeningitis. In pregnant women or animals, *Listeria* cells can cross the placental barrier, causing stillbirth or abortion. In the latter cases, they have to overcome either micro- or macrovascular endothelia, and there is evidence that *L. monocytogenes* is internalized by both types of endothelial cells (13, 28, 29, 48). There is ample evidence that *L. monocytogenes* and *L. ivanovii* are capable of invading these and other cell types at least in established cell cultures. Host cell invasion by *Listeria* is not accompanied by drastic morphological changes in the host cell membrane, and the invasion process is comparable to the zipper mechanism observed with *Yersinia enterocolitica* (7, 61).

Several listerial proteins seem to be able to trigger the internalization of *L. monocytogenes* and *L. ivanovii* in some host cell types (1, 2, 7), suggesting that more than one receptor on the host cell surface may be engaged in receptor-mediated phagocytosis.

Here we will concentrate on the best-studied *L. monocytogenes* invasins, which belong to the large family of internalins. There is unambiguous evidence for the involvement of the products of *inlA* and *inlB* in internalization into epithelial cells, hepatocytes, and endothelial cells (11, 13, 18–21, 27–29). The only host cell receptor known is E-cadherin, which is associated with InlA (46). *inlA* and *inlB* form an operon whose expression is under partial control of PrfA (10, 42) (Fig. 2A). This operon has been mapped in the vicinity of the *prfA* virulence gene cluster but is not directly linked to it (58). These genes have not been detected in *L. ivanovii*; the faint bands which are observed by hybridization of *L. ivanovii* chromosomal DNA with an *inlA* probe may well be attributed to other internalin genes (see below) due to the LRR and other common sequences (19). *L. innocua* does not seem to carry these genes, and there is also no evidence for the occurrence of *inlA-inlB* in *L. seeligeri* and the more distantly related species *L. welshimeri* and *L. grayi*.

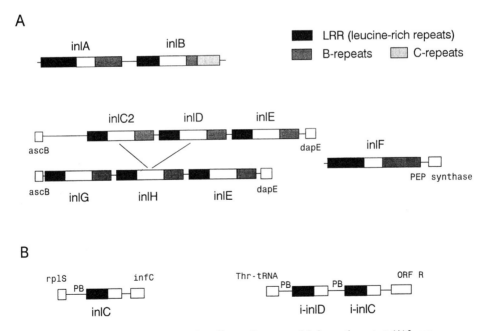

Figure 2. Schematic representation of internalin genes and their genetic context. (A) Large internalins of *L. monocytogenes*. *inlH* was generated by a deletion of the C terminus of *inlC2* and the N terminus of *inlD*. (B) Small internalins: *inlC* of *L. monocytogenes* and *i-inlCD* of *L. ivanovii*. PB, PrfA-box. For further details see the text. Additional small internalins of *L. ivanovii* are shown in Fig. 3.

There is more sequence information available on the recently described *inlC2DE* genes of *L. monocytogenes* (12), which form a gene cluster flanked by the metabolic genes *ascB* (encoding 6-phospho-β-glucosidase) and *dapE* (encoding succinyl-diaminopimelate-desuccinylase). Interestingly, a similar but not identical gene cluster (*inlGHE*), framed by the same metabolic genes, has been identified in another *L. monocytogenes* strain (51). Sequence comparison between the two gene clusters revealed that *inlH* apparently was generated by a recombination of the 5′-terminal part of *inlC2* and the 3′-terminal part of *inlD*. The *inlG* gene is probably also present in the *inlC2DE* gene cluster (12, 51) and presumably went undetected by the first investigators, suggesting that this strain may contain a cluster of four *inl* genes (Fig. 2). Expression studies suggest that all three (or four) *inl* genes are arranged in an operon which is transcribed independently of PrfA (12, 51). These genes encode large, cell-associated internalins with substantial homology to InlA and InlB, but the functions of these internalins are unknown. Our preliminary data suggest, however, that they may not be directly involved in the internalization of *L. mono-cytogenes* by host cells. The chromosomal regions of *L. ivanovii* and *L. innocua* corre-sponding to the *inlGHE* cluster have been determined (47) and show the complete absence of this *inl* gene cluster; the two flanking genes, *ascB* and *dapE,* are next to each other on the chromosome of both *Listeria* species. This gene cluster also seems to be absent in *L. seeligeri*. These data suggest that the *inlGHE* (*inlC2DE*) gene cluster is highly specific for *L. monocytogenes*. *L. monocytogenes* contains another *inl* gene, termed *inlF*, encoding a large internalin. The map position of *inlF* has not been reported, but an ORF with homology to PEP synthase has been identified downstream of this gene (12) (Fig. 2A).

The other class of internalins are the small, secreted internalins, all of which are strictly under the control of PrfA (14–16). In *L. monocytogenes,* only a single gene, *inlC* (or *irpA*), has been identified (14, 43) (Fig. 2B). This gene is embedded on the *L. monocytogenes* chromosome between the housekeeping genes *rplS,* encoding the ribosomal protein L19, and *infC,* encoding the translation initiation factor IF3 (15). In *L. innocua,* two ORFs have been detected in the region between *rplS* and *infC,* one showing homology to NAD(P)H oxidoreductases and the other being homologous to a conserved protein of unknown func-tion (47). Both of these genes are present in multiple copies in *Bacillus subtilis*; in *L. monocytogenes,* even though the insertion of the *inlC* gene may have coincided with the deletion of these two genes, it did so without causing large deleterious effects. Most interestingly, in *L. ivanovii* the *inlC* gene is also present, but its genomic insertion site is entirely different from that of *L. monocytogenes inlC*. First, a tandem duplication of *inlC* has occurred, giving rise to two very similar but differently expressed genes, named *i-inlC* and *i-inlD* (15) (Fig. 2B). Second, these genes may be part of a much larger chromo-somal insert which has not yet been fully unravelled. The 5′-flanking sequence is a Thr-tRNA gene whose integrity is destroyed by the insertion. Upstream of the Thr-tRNA gene are additional tRNA genes in an arrangement similar to that observed in a ribosomal gene cluster of *B. subtilis*. If this operon is similar in *Listeria,* one would expect another tRNA gene as the 3′-flanking gene of this insert. The sequence immediately downstream of *i-inlC, i-inlD,* instead represents an ORF with homology to a transcription regulator of the transposonborne TetR family (Fig. 2). The intergenic region between *rplS* and *infC,* where *inlC* is located in *L. monocytogenes,* is more closely related to that of *L. innocua* (47). It is therefore likely that *i-inlC* and *i-inlD* reside on the *L. ivanovii* chromosome within a structure related to a PAI.

AN UNSTABLE, VIRULENCE-ASSOCIATED CHROMOSOMAL REGION OF *L. IVANOVII* WHICH CONTAINS SEVERAL GENES FOR SECRETED INTERNALINS AND A SPHINGOMYELINASE GENE

At least three additional small, secreted internalin genes are present on the *L. ivanovii* chromosome. The *i-inlE* gene was identified by using degenerate oligonucleotide primers derived from the N-terminal sequence of one of the major secreted proteins of *L. ivanovii* (16). An in-frame *i-inlE* deletion mutant turned out to be significantly impaired in virulence in the mouse infection model, indicating that i-InlE is involved in virulence (16). Upstream from *i-inlE,* there is another gene for a small internalin, *i-inlF,* and further upstream an ORF encoding yet another secreted internalin, provisionally termed *i-inlG,* has recently been identified (9) (Fig. 3). Expression of all these internalin genes is PrfA dependent, and they may have arisen from gene duplication events, similar to *i-inlCD.* No counterparts of these members of the internalin multigene family have been detected in *L. monocytogenes* or other *Listeria* species, indicating they are probably *L. ivanovii* specific.

Interestingly, the gene coding for the *L. ivanovii* sphingomyelinase C (*smcL*) is located between *i-inlF* and *i-inlG* but is transcribed in the opposite orientation (25) (Fig. 3). This sphingomyelinase is also *L. ivanovii* specific and is responsible for the strong, bizonal hemolysis that distinguishes this pathogenic *Listeria* species from *L. monocytogenes* (which is weakly hemolytic) (35, 52, 62). The deduced amino acid sequence of the *L. ivanovii* sphingomyelinase, SmcL, is highly similar to that of the sphingomyelinases C of *S. aureus* (beta-toxin) and *B. cereus* (52.4 and 46.8% identity, respectively). Mutational inactivation of this fourth (see below) membrane-damaging, cytolytic determinant of *L. ivanovii* revealed that it is required for full virulence in mice. Preliminary results indicate that SmcL may play a role in intracellular survival of the bacteria, probably by contributing, together with listeriolysin O, PlcA, and PlcB, to phagosomal membrane disruption (25). In contrast to the surrounding internalin genes, the monocistronically transcribed *smcL* is totally PrfA independent (25). This fact and its opposite orientation with respect to the encompassing *i-inl* genes suggest that *smcL* may have been acquired by horizontal gene transfer and inserted in a preexisting PrfA-dependent internalin locus.

Most interestingly, spontaneous mutants have been isolated in which this newly identified *L. ivanovii*-specific virulence gene cluster is deleted (9). The frequency of this excision is very low; by pulsed-field gel electrophoresis and Southern hybridization analyses, the size of the deleted region was estimated to be at least 23 kb, showing that it contains much more than the four genes characterized to date. The deletion mutants are severely impaired in virulence in the murine model and are less pathogenic for sheep (9). These observations support the notion that *smcL* and the secreted internalin genes *i-inlE, i-inlF,* and *i-inlG* form part of a PAI. Together with the recently described 15.2-kb *tst* element

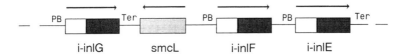

Figure 3. Schematic representation of the known genes of the *L. ivanovii*-specific virulence locus. The direction of transcription is indicated by arrows. PB, PrfA box; Ter, transcriptional terminator. The sphingomyelinase gene (*smcL*) is PrfA independent.

of *S. aureus,* which carries the gene for toxic shock syndrome toxin 1 (41), this is the second example of an unstable, virulence-associated chromosomal locus in a gram-positive bacterium. This may indicate that the acquisition of foreign genetic material carrying information related to virulence functions does not occur only in gram-negative pathogens but, rather, is a universal phenomenon of utmost importance in the evolution of bacterial virulence. The observation that at least three genes of this *L. ivanovii* element, i.e., *i-inlE, i-inlF,* and *i-inlG,* are PrfA dependent suggests that it arose in *L. ivanovii* at later stages of listerial virulence evolution. This is in line with the fact that most of the known LRR proteins have been found in eukaryotes (33), supporting the idea that the few bacterial proteins found in this family, e.g., the internalins, are a rather recent development in the prokaryotic world. With respect to this chromosomal region, *L. ivanovii* is clearly distinct from *L. monocytogenes* and *L. seeligeri.* In this context, it is interesting that, in contrast to *L. monocytogenes,* which has a wide host range (it infects many species of mammals [including humans], birds, and other vertebrates), *L. ivanovii* is specifically pathogenic for ruminants. The cell membranes of these animals are by far the richest in sphingomyelin (51%, versus, for example, 27% in humans or 13.5% in horses), and so it is tempting to speculate that *smcL* and, possibly, the other virulence genes carried by this *L. ivanovii*-specific locus are involved in host tropism.

CONCLUSION

Today's knowledge of the genetics of the pathogenic *Listeria* species, *L. monocytogenes* and *L. ivanovii,* and its comparison with that of the nonpathogenic *Listeria* species *L. innocua* and *L. seeligeri,* suggests a stepwise acquisition of virulence genes which may have occurred by common as well as species-specific mechanisms. The *prfA* virulence gene cluster is common to both pathogenic species, with virtually no difference in the genomic arrangement, the number of genes, and their regulation. While most of the corresponding genes in the two gene clusters show high similarity, there is a significant divergence in the *actA* genes in spite of the functional conservation of the two gene products; furthermore, the *actA* gene of *L. monocytogenes* exhibits a striking polymorphism (4, 60, 65), suggesting a low selective pressure on several domains of the ActA protein. Interestingly, a similar but larger *prfA* gene cluster is also present on the chromosome of the nonpathogenic *L. seeligeri.* The additional genes and the mode of their regulation by PrfA suggest that the *L. seeligeri* gene cluster is not adapted to support intracellular survival in mammalian host cells as do those of *L. monocytogenes* and *L. ivanovii.* In the light of the phylogenetic relationship of the *Listeria* species, the occurrence of this virulence gene cluster in *L. monocytogenes, L. ivanovii,* and *L. seeligeri* suggests that it may have been first acquired as an intracellular survival cassette for *Listeria* inside phagocytic protists and was only later adapted for supporting life in mammalian cells. It is likely that the genes were acquired through horizontal gene transfer, since the other phylogenetic branch of *Listeria,* including *L. welshimeri* and *L. grayi,* does not possess these clustered virulence genes. Today's *prfA* virulence gene clusters of *L. monocytogenes* and *L. ivanovii* may therefore represent a trimmed version of a very old PAI.

L. innocua is an interesting member of the genus *Listeria.* While showing the closest phylogenetic relationship to *L. monocytogenes,* it is nonpathogenic and lacks the *prfA* gene cluster. This leads one to conclude that *L. innocua* must have deleted the *prfA* gene cluster, thus becoming a normal heterotrophic soil saprophyte.

As for the genes for the other families of presumed virulence factors, the large cell-associated internalins and the small secreted internalin most probably were generated in *L. monocytogenes* and *L. ivanovii* at a later stage, i.e. (except for *inlC*), probably after the bifurcation of their progenitor species. In *L. monocytogenes,* the known *inl* genes are all inserted in clusters (*inlA-inlB, inlC2DE,* and *inlGHE*) or as single genes (*inlC* and *inlF*) between housekeeping genes. To date, no large internalins have been found in *L. ivanovii,* but this species carries a large number of small internalin genes; of these, only *inlC* is shared between *L. monocytogenes* and *L. ivanovii.* Interestingly, in *L. ivanovii,* all these genes are located on large inserts in the genome which possess properties reminiscent of today's PAIs.

At present, the available genomic data on the *inl* genes do not permit any conclusion on how or when any internalin first materialized in *Listeria.* However, one can safely conclude that the proliferation by gene duplication and the very frequent and apparently random insertion into different chromosomal sites among the members of the recently divergent branches of *L. monocytogenes-L. innocua* and *L. ivanovii-L. seeligeri* are marks of later events than the acquisition and fixation of the *prfA* gene cluster. Although limited, our present knowledge of the function of internalins suggests that they specifically interact with mammalian cells. This also could argue that these genes arose after incorporation of the *prfA* gene cluster.

Acknowledgments. We are grateful to A. Bubert, F. Engelbrecht, G. Dominguez-Bernal, B. Gonzalez-Zorn, D. Raffelsbauer, and M. Wagner for communicating unpublished results. Our work has been supported by grants from the Dirección General de Enseñanza Superior (PB97-0327), the Deutsche Forschungsgemeinschaft (Kr 1206/3-1 and SFB 165-B4), the Fonds der Chemischen Industrie, the European Commission (BMH4-CT96-0659), and the Spanish-German Integrated Actions Program (HA94-141B and HA95-114B).

REFERENCES

1. **Alvarez-Dominguez, C., J.-A. Vazquez-Boland, E. Carrasco-Marin, P. Lopez-Mato, and F. Leyva-Cobian.** 1997. Host cell heparan sulfate proteoglycans mediate attachment and entry of *Listeria monocytogenes,* and the listerial surface protein ActA is involved in heparan sulfate receptor recognition. *Infect. Immun.* **65:**78–88.

2. **Bubert, A., M. Kuhn, W. Goebel, and S. Köhler.** 1992. Structural and functional properties of the p60 proteins from different *Listeria* species. *J. Bacteriol.* **174:**8166–8171.

3. **Bubert, A., S.-K. Chun, L. Papatheodorou, A. Simm, W. Goebel, and Z. Sokolovic.** 1999. Differential virulence gene expression by *Listeria monocytogenes* growing within host cells. *Mol. Gen. Genet.* **261:**323–326.

4. **Chakraborty, T., F. Ebel, J. Wehland, J. Dufrenne, and S. Notermans.** 1994. Naturally occurring virulence-attenuated isolates of *Listeria monocytogenes* capable of inducing long term protection against infection by virulent strains of homologous and heterologous serotypes. *FEMS Immunol. Med. Microbiol.* **10:**1–10.

5. **Collins, M. D., S. Wallbanks, D. J. Lane, J. Shah, R. Nietupski, J. Smida, M. Dorsch, and E. Stackebrandt.** 1991. Phylogenetic analysis of the genus *Listeria* based on reverse transcriptase sequencing of 16S rRNA. *Int. J. Syst. Bacteriol.* **41:**240–246.

6. **Cossart, P., P. Bouquet, S. Normark, and R. Rappuoli.** 1996. Cellular microbiology emerging. *Science* **271:**315–316.

7. **Cossart, P., and M. Lecuit.** 1998. Interaction of *Listeria monocytogenes* with mammalian cells during entry and actin-based movement: bacterial factors, cellular ligands and signaling. *EMBO J.* **17:**3797–3806.

8. **Cummins, A. J., A. K. Fielding, and J. McLauchlin.** 1994. *Listeria ivanovii* infection in a patient with AIDS. *J. Infect.* **28:**89–91.

9. **Domínguez-Bernal, G., B. González-Zorn, and J. A. Vázquez-Boland.** Unpublished data.

10. **Dramsi, S., C. Kocks, C. Forestier, and P. Cossart.** 1993. Internalin-mediated invasion of epithelial cells by *Listeria monocytogenes* is regulated by the bacterial growth state, temperature and the pleiotropic activator PrfA. *Mol. Microbiol.* **9:**931–941.

11. **Dramsi, S., I. Biswas, E. Maguin, L. Braun, P. Mastroeni, and P. Cossart.** 1995. Entry of *Listeria monocytogenes* into hepatocytes requires expression of InlB, a surface protein of the internalin multigene family. *Mol. Microbiol.* **16:**251–261.

12. **Dramsi, S., P. Dehoux, M. Lebrun, P. L. Goossens, and P. Cossart.** 1997. Identification of four new members of the internalin multigene family of *Listeria monocytogenes* EGD. *Infect. Immun.* **65:**1615–1625.

13. **Drevets, D. A., R. T. Sawyer, T. A. Potter, and P. A. Campbell.** 1995. *Listeria monocytogenes* infects human endothelial cells by two distinct mechanisms. *Infect. Immun.* **63:**4268–4276.

14. **Engelbrecht, F., S.-K. Chun, C. Ochs, J. Hess, F. Lottspeich, W. Goebel, and Z. Sokolovic.** 1996. A new PrfA-regulated gene of *Listeria monocytogenes* encoding a small, secreted protein which belongs to the family of internalins. *Mol. Microbiol.* **21:**823–837.

15. **Engelbrecht, F., C. Dickneite, R. Lampidis, M. Götz, U. DasGupta, and W. Goebel.** 1998. Sequence comparison of the chromosomal regions encompassing the internalin C genes (*inlC*) of *Listeria monocytogenes* and *Listeria ivanovii. Mol. Gen. Genet.* **257:**186–197.

16. **Engelbrecht, F., G. Dominguez-Bernal, C. Dickneite, J. Hess, L. Greiffenberg, R. Lampidis, D. Raffelsbauer, S. H. E. Kaufmann, J. Kreft, J.-A. Vazquez-Boland, and W. Goebel.** 1998. A novel PrfA-regulated chromosomal locus of *Listeria ivanovii* encoding two small, secreted internalins is essential for virulence in mice. *Mol. Microbiol.* **30:**405–417.

17. **Freitag, N. E., L. Rong, and D. A. Portnoy.** 1993. Regulation of the *prfA* transcriptional activator of *Listeria monocytogenes*: multiple promoter elements contribute to intracellular growth and cell-to-cell spread. *Infect. Immun.* **61:**2537–2544.

18. **Gaillard, J. L., P. Berche, J. Mounier, S. Richard, and P. J. Sansonetti.** 1987. In vitro model of penetration and intracellular growth of *Listeria monocytogenes* in the human enterocyte-like cell line Caco-2. *Infect. Immun.* **55:**2822–2829.

19. **Gaillard, J.-L., P. Berche, C. Frehel, E. Gouin, and P. Cossart.** 1991. Entry of *Listeria monocytogenes* into cells is mediated by internalin, a repeat protein reminiscent of surface antigens from gram-positive cocci. *Cell* **65:**1127–1141.

20. **Gaillard, J. L., F. Jaubert, and P. Berche.** 1996. The *inlAB* locus mediates the entry of *Listeria monocytogenes* into hepatocytes *in vivo. J. Exp. Med.* **183:**359–369.

21. **Gaillard, J. L., and B. B. Finlay.** 1996. Effect of cell polarization and differentiation on entry of *Listeria monocytogenes* into the enterocyte-like Caco-2 cell line. *Infect. Immun.* **64:**1299–1308.

22. **Gellin, B. G., and C. V. Broome.** 1989. Listeriosis. *JAMA* **261:**1313–1320.

23. **Gerstel, B., L. Gröbe, S. Pistor, T. Chakraborty, and J. Wehland.** 1996. The ActA polypeptides of *Listeria ivanovii* and *Listeria monocytogenes* harbor related binding sites for host microfilament proteins. *Infect. Immun.* **64:**1929–1936.

24. **Goebel, W., and J. Kreft.** 1997. Cytolysins and the intracellular life of bacteria. *Trends Microbiol.* **5:** 86–88.

25. **González-Zorn, B., G. Domínguez-Bernal, and J. A. Vázquez-Boland.** Unpublished data.

26. **Gouin, E., J. Mengaud, and P. Cossart.** 1994. The virulence gene cluster of *Listeria monocytogenes* is also present in *Listeria ivanovii,* an animal pathogen, and *Listeria seeligeri,* a nonpathogenic species. *Infect. Immun.* **62:**3550–3553.

27. **Gregory, S. H., A. J. Sagnimeni, and E. J. Wing.** 1996. Expression of the *inlAB* operon by *Listeria monocytogenes* is not required for entry into hepatic cells in vivo. *Infect. Immun.* **64:**3983–3986.

28. **Greiffenberg, L., Z. Sokolovic, H.-J. Schnittler, A. Spory, R. Böckmann, W. Goebel, and M. Kuhn.** 1997. *Listeria monocytogenes*-infected human umbilical vein endothelial cells: internalin-independent invasion, intracellular growth, movement, and host cell responses. *FEMS Microbiol. Lett.* **157:**163–170.

29. **Greiffenberg, L., W. Goebel, K. S. Kim, I. Weiglein, A. Bubert, F. Engelbrecht, M. Stins, and M. Kuhn.** 1998. Interaction of *Listeria monocytogenes* with human brain microvascular endothelial cells: InlB-dependent invasion, long-term intracellular growth and spread from macrophages to endothelial cells. *Infect. Immun.* **66:**5260–5267.

30. **Hacker, J., G. Blum-Oehler, I. Mühldorfer, and H. Tschäpe.** 1997. Pathogenicity islands of virulent bacteria: structure, function and impact on microbial evolution. *Mol. Microbiol.* **23:**1089–1097.

31. **Irvine, A. S., and J. R. Guest.** 1993. *Lactobacillus casei* contains a member of the CRP-FNR family. *Nucleic Acids Res.* **21:**753.

32. **Jones, D.** 1990. Foodborne listeriosis. *Lancet* **336:**1171–1174.

33. **Kajava, A. V.** 1998. Structural diversity of leucine-rich repeat proteins. *J. Mol. Biol.* **277:**519–527.

34. **Karunasagar, I., R. Lampidis, W. Goebel, and J. Kreft.** 1997. Complementation of *Listeria seeligeri* with the *plcA-prfA* genes from *L. monocytogenes* activates transcription of seeligerolysin and leads to bacterial escape from the phagosome of infected mammalian cells. *FEMS Microbiol. Lett.* **146:**303–310.

35. **Kreft, J., D. Funke, A. Haas, F. Lottspeich, and W. Goebel.** 1989. Production, purification and characterization of hemolysins from *Listeria ivanovii* and *Listeria monocytogenes* Sv4b. *FEMS Microbiol. Lett.* **57:** 197–202.

36. **Kreft, J., M. Dumbsky, and S. Theiss.** 1995. The actin-polymerization protein from *Listeria ivanovii* is a large repeat protein which shows only limited amino acid sequence homology to ActA from *Listeria monocytogenes*. *FEMS Microbiol. Lett.* **126:**113–122.

37. **Kreft, J., J. Bohne, R. Gross, H. Kestler, Z. Sokolovic, and W. Goebel.** 1995. Control of *Listeria monocytogenes* virulence by the transcriptional regulator PrfA, p. 129–142. *In* R. Rappuoli, V. Scarlato, and B. Aricó (ed.), *Signal Tranduction and Bacterial Virulence.* R. G. Landes Co., Austin, Tex.

38. **Kuhn, M., and W. Goebel.** 1995. Molecular studies on the virulence of *Listeria monocytogenes*. *Genet. Eng.* **17:**31–51.

39. **Lampidis, R., R. Gross, Z. Sokolovic, W. Goebel, and J. Kreft.** 1994. The virulence regulator protein of *Listeria ivanovii* is highly homologous to PrfA from *Listeria monocytogenes* and both belong to the Crp-Fnr family of transcription regulators. *Mol. Microbiol.* **13:**141–151.

40. **Lampidis, R., M. Emmerth, I. Karunasagar, and J. Kreft.** The virulence gene cluster from *Listeria seeligeri* contains large insertions and a partial gene duplication. Unpublished data.

41. **Lindsay, J. A., A. Ruzin, H. F. Ross, N. Kurepina, and R. P. Novick.** 1998. The gene for toxic shock toxin is carried by a family of mobile pathogenicity islands in *Staphylococcus aureus*. *Mol. Microbiol.* **29:** 527–543.

42. **Lingnau, A., E. Domann, M. Hudel, M. Bock, T. Nichterlein, J. Wehland, and T. Chakraborty.** 1995. Expression of *Listeria monocytogenes* EGD *inlA* and *inlB* genes, whose products mediate bacterial entry into tissue culture cell lines, by PrfA-dependent and -independent mechanisms. *Infect. Immun.* **64:**1002–1006.

43. **Lingnau, A., T. Chakraborty, K. Niebuhr, E. Domann, and J. Wehland.** 1996. Identification and purification of novel internalin-related proteins in *Listeria monocytogenes* and *Listeria ivanovii*. *Infect. Immun.* **64:** 1002–1006.

44. **Lorber, B.** 1997. Listeriosis. *Clin. Infect. Dis.* **24:**1–11.

45. **Ly, T. M., and H. E. Müller.** 1990. Ingested *Listeria monocytogenes* survive and multiply in protozoa. *J. Med. Microbiol.* **33:**51–54.

46. **Mengaud, J., H. Ohayon, P. Gounon, R.-M. Mege, and P. Cossart.** 1996. E-cadherin is the receptor for internalin, a surface protein required for entry of *Listeria monocytogenes* into epithelial cells. *Cell* **84:** 923–932.

47. **Ng, E., and W. Goebel.** Unpublished data.

48. **Parida, S. K., E. Domann, M. Rohde, S. Müller, A. Darji, T. Hain, J. Wehland, and T. Chakraborty.** 1998. Internalin B is essential for adhesion and mediates the invasion of *Listeria monocytogenes* into human endothelial cells. *Mol. Microbiol.* **28:**81–93.

49. **Portnoy, D. A., T. Chakraborty, W. Goebel, and P. Cossart.** 1992. Molecular determinants of *Listeria monocytogenes* pathogenesis. *Infect. Immun.* **60:**1263–1267.

50. **Pron, B., C. Boumaila, F. Jaubert, S. Sarnacki, J. P. Monnet, P. Berche, and J. L. Gaillard.** 1998. Comprehensive study of the intestinal stage of listeriosis in a rat ligated ileal loop system. *Infect. Immun.* **66:**747–755.

51. **Raffelsbauer, D., A. Bubert, F. Engelbrecht, J. Scheinpflug, A. Simm, J. Hess, S. H. E. Kaufmann, and W. Goebel.** 1998. The gene cluster *inlC2DE* of *Listeria monocytogenes* contains additional new internalin genes and is important for virulence in mice. *Mol. Gen. Genet.,* **260:**144–158.

52. **Ripio, M.-T., C. Geoffroy, G. Domínguez-Bernal, J. E. Alouf, and J. A. Vázquez-Boland.** 1995. The sulphydryl-activated cytolysin and a sphingomyelinase C are the major membrane-damaging factors involved in cooperative (CAMP-like) haemolysis of *Listeria* spp. *Res. Microbiol.* **146:**303–313.

53. **Ripio, M.-T., K. Brehm, M. Lara, M. Suárez, and J.-A. Vázquez-Boland.** 1997. Glucose-1-phosphate utilization by *Listeria monocytogenes* is PrfA dependent and coordinately expressed with virulence factors. *J. Bacteriol.* **197:**7174–7180.

54. **Ripio, M.-T., J.-A. Vázquez-Boland, Y. Vega, S. Nair, and P. Berche.** 1998. Evidence for expressional crosstalk between the central virulence regulator PrfA and the stress response mediator ClpC in *Listeria monocytogenes. FEMS Microbiol. Lett.* **158:**45–50.

55. **Roucourt, J., H. Hof, A. Schrettenbrunner, R. Malinverni, and J. Bille.** 1986. Méningite purulente aigue à *Listeria seeligeri* chez un adulte immuno-compétent. *Schweiz. Med. Wochenschr.* **116:**248–251.

56. **Sallen, B., A. Rajoharison, S. Desvarenne, F. Quinn, and C. Mabilat.** 1996. Comparative analysis of 16S and 23S rRNA sequences of *Listeria* species. *Int. J. Syst. Bacteriol.* **46:**669–674.

57. **Schuchat, A., B. Swaminathan, and C. V. Broome.** 1991. Epidemiology of human listeriosis. *Clin. Microbiol. Rev.* **4:**169–183.

58. **Sheehan, B., C. Kocks, S. Dramsi, E. Gouin, A. D. Klarsfeld, J. Mengaud, and P. Cossart.** 1994. Molecular and genetic determinants of the *Listeria monocytogenes* infectious process. *Curr. Top. Microbiol. Immunol.* **192:**187–216.

59. **Smith, G. A., and D. A. Portnoy.** 1997. How the *Listeria monocytogenes* ActA protein converts actin polymerization into a motile force. *Trends Microbiol.* **5:**272–276.

60. **Sokolovic, Z., S. Schüller, J. Bohne, A. Baur, U. Rdest, C. Dickneite, T. Nichterlein, and W. Goebel.** 1996. Differences in virulence and in expression of PrfA and PrfA-regulated virulence genes of *Listeria monocytogenes* strains belonging to serogroup 4. *Infect. Immun.* **64:**4008–4019.

61. **Swanson, J. A., and S. C. Baer.** 1995. Phagocytosis by zippers and triggers. *Trends Cell Biol.* **5:**89–93.

62. **Vázquez-Boland, J. A., L. Domínguez, E. F. Rodríguez-Ferri, and G. Suárez.** 1989. Purification and characterization of two *Listeria ivanovii* cytolysins, a sphingomyelinase C and a thiol-activated toxin (ivanolysin O). *Infect. Immun.* **57:**3928–3935.

63. **Vazquez-Boland, J.-A., C. Kocks, S. Dramsi, H. Ohayon, C. Geoffroy, J. Mengaud, and P. Cossart.** 1992. Nucleotide sequence of the lecithinase operon of *Listeria monocytogenes* and possible role of lecithinase in cell-to-cell spread. *Infect. Immun.* **60:**219–230.

64. **Wagner, M.** Personal communication.

65. **Wiedmann, M., J. L. Bruce, C. Keating, A. E. Johnson, P. L. McDonough, and C. A. Batt.** 1997. Ribotypes and virulence gene polymorphisms suggest three distinct *Listeria monocytogenes* lineages with differences in pathogenic potential. *Infect. Immun.* **65:**2707–2716.

Pathogenicity Islands and Other Mobile Virulence Elements
Edited by J. B. Kaper and J. Hacker
© 1999 American Society for Microbiology, Washington, D.C.

Chapter 13

Virulence-Associated Mobile Elements in Bacilli and Clostridia

Veit Braun and Christoph von Eichel-Streiber

Bacilli and clostridia are prominent examples of bacteria whose lifestyle is determined by their growth properties and survival strategies. Since these two genera have the capacity to form spores, their members may even kill the hosts in the process of infection without committing suicide. Bacilli grow aerobically and in the presence of CO_2, whereas clostridia prefer an anaerobic atmosphere and grow poorly or not at all under CO_2.

The genus *Bacillus* consists of approximately 40 species arranged in eight groups (144). Often found as a laboratory contaminant, they inhabit soil and the environment in general. *Bacillus anthracis* and *B. cereus* are most frequently encountered in clinical specimens, causing anthrax (a disease in cattle, sheep, and sometimes humans) and acute intestinal intoxication, respectively (192). Clostridia are isolated from severe acute or chronic infections; some are highly pathogenic or toxinogenic, while others are rare pathogens. Approximately 300 species have been described; in clinical samples the spectrum is restricted to a mere 13 species (147).

Due to space limitations, this chapter focuses on (i) species that induce human diseases, (ii) species that are able to produce toxins, and (iii) the association of appropriate virulence factors with possible mobile elements (Table 1). With reference to bacilli, we discuss mainly *B. anthracis* and *B. cereus*. The main topics in the section on clostridia are *Clostridium perfringens,* neurotoxin-producing clostridia, and species capable of producing large clostridial cytotoxins. Finally, we discuss the contribution of the genetic mobility of virulence genes to the evolution of pathogenic bacilli and clostridia.

BACILLI

B. anthracis, B. cereus, B. thuringiensis, and *B. cereus* subsp. *mycoides* belong to group I of the genus *Bacillus*. Their G+C content varies between 32 and 37% (96, 145). One anticipates that the sequences of these species are very similar, so that it is extremely difficult to differentiate between them, and it has been suggested that they be reorganized into one species with four subspecies (191). Only two differences could be found, for

Veit Braun and Christoph von Eichel-Streiber • Institut für Medizinische Mikrobiologie und Hygiene, Johannes Gutenberg-Universität Mainz, 55101 Mainz, Germany.

Table 1. Important toxins produced by bacilli and clostridia

Toxin	Source	Localization
Bacilli		
PA (protective antigen)	*B. anthracis*	Toxin plasmid pXO1
EF (edema factor)	*B. anthracis*	Toxin plasmid pXO1
LF (lethal factor)	*B. anthracis*	Toxin plasmid pXO1
Poly-γ-D-glutamic acid capsule	*B. anthracis*	Capsule plasmid pXO2
Emetic toxin	*B. cereus*	Unknown
Enterotoxin (hemolysin)	*B. cereus*	Chromosome
δ-Endotoxins (crystal proteins)	*B. thuringiensis*	Conjugative plasmids
Clostridia		
α-Toxin	*C. perfringens*	Chromosome
β-Toxin	*C. perfringens*	Plasmid
ι-Toxin	*C. perfringens*	Plasmid
ε-Toxin	*C. perfringens*	Plasmid
θ-Toxin	*C. perfringens*	Chromosome
κ-Toxin	*C. perfringens*	Chromosome
μ-Toxin	*C. perfringens*	Chromosome
λ-Toxin	*C. perfringens*	Plasmid
Enterotoxin	*C. perfringens*	Chromosome or plasmid
TeNT	*C. tetani*	Plasmid
BoNT/A	*C. botulinum*	Chromosome
BoNT/B	*C. botulinum*	Chromosome
BoNT/C	*C. botulinum*	Lysogenic phage
BoNT/D	*C. botulinum*	Lysogenic phage
BoNT/E	*C. botulinum*	Chromosome
BoNT/F	*C. botulinum*	Chromosome
BoNT/G	*C. botulinum*	Plasmid
BuNT/E	*C. butyricum*	Plasmid and defective phage
BaNT	*C. barati*	Unknown
C2-toxin	*C. botulinum*	Chromosome
C3-toxin	*C. botulinum*	Lysogenic phage
TcdA (enterotoxin)	*C. difficile*	Chromosome
TcdB (cytotoxin)	*C. difficile*	Chromosome
TcsL (lethal toxin)	*C. sordellii*	Chromosome
TcsH (hemorrhagic toxin)	*C. sordellii*	Unknown
Tcnα	*C. novyi*	Lysogenic phage

example, in the 23S ribosomal DNAs (rDNAs) of *B. anthracis* and *B. cereus* (3, 4). A series of modern methods has been used in an attempt to distinguish between *B. anthracis*, *B. cereus*, and *B. thuringiensis* (3, 4, 100, 111). Regions of DNA diversity, such as *vrrA*, are used for epidemiological differentiation. *vrrA* varies between individual isolates (2, 90); it is associated with a 12-bp tandem array sequence that expands and contracts during the period of evolution.

Bacillus anthracis

Brief Introduction to the Disease

B. anthracis is the only member of the *Bacillus* genus which is capable of causing epidemic disease in humans and other mammals. It is the etiological agent of anthrax, a disease transmitted from animals to humans. Anthrax was a serious disease among farm animals in many parts of the world before a vaccine for domestic animals became available. Apparent human infection with *B. anthracis* is directly or indirectly traceable to contact with infected animals.

The development of efficient antibiotic treatment and an effective veterinary vaccine has reduced the frequency of cases of anthrax in both animals and humans. Anthrax is, however, still endemic in various regions of the globe. Recent reviews on the epidemiology and the clinical characteristics of anthrax have been published elsewhere (73, 109).

Pathogenicity Factors

B. anthracis strains produce a tripartite protein toxin, comprising PA (protective antigen), EF (edema factor) and LF (lethal factor) (116, 118). PA builds two different A-B toxins through the interaction of PA and EF, referred to as edema toxin, and of PA and LF, called lethal toxin (61, 118). In these composite toxins, PA is the ligand domain which binds to the cell receptors. It forms a membrane channel that mediates the entry of EF and LF into the cell (61, 140). EF is a calmodulin-dependent adenyl cyclase catalyzing the modification of ATP into cyclic AMP (115, 117). Lethal toxin is the dominant virulence factor and one of the principal causes of death in infected animals (73, 150). The time to death after intravenous injection of lethal toxin in rats is 38 min (49). For mice treated in vivo with LF, the massive release of cytokines by macrophages has been suggested as a reason for the onset of the shock symptoms seen in anthrax (54). LF is a Zn-metalloprotease (102) whose proteolytic activity on mitogen-activated protein kinase kinase 1 (MAPKK1) and MAPKK2 has been recently reported on (40). The possible role of this protease activity with respect to anthrax is currently the subject of controversial discussion (40, 74, 177).

Genetic Localization of Virulence Genes

Genes on chromosomes and phages. The main scientific interest is focused on the toxin plasmid (pXO1) and the capsule plasmid (pXO2), since they were recognized at an early stage as carrying the major virulence factors of *B. anthracis* (64, 139). Only a few chromosomal loci have been implicated in the virulence of *B. anthracis* strains (150, 202). Two proteins, Sap (137) and EA1 (48), encoded on the chromosome form a paracrystalline surface layer. Their function as major antigens is largely accepted; whether this surface layer also serves as a virulence factor has not yet been clarified (136). However, the surface layer and capsule may be expressed at the same time (136).

Phages have been found in several *B. anthracis* strains (19, 22, 31, 88, 131). Others originate from *B. cereus* (183). Phages CP-51, CP-2, and CP-20 infect both pXO1-cured and uncured strains; phage yields produced on cured strains, however, are considerably higher than those on the uncured parent strain (183). A temperate phage, φ20, was induced by mitomycin C treatment or UV light in some *B. anthracis* strains [such as *B. anthracis* Sterne(pXO1$^+$ pXO2$^-$), a veterinary vaccine strain]. φ20 exists as a plasmid but is not located on pXO1, the toxin plasmid, or on the chromosome. Taken together, the phages known to us seem not to encode virulence factors, yet all phages may be used as vehicles for mobilization of virulence genes, such as those found on pXO1 and pXO2 (see below), between *B. anthracis, B. cereus,* and *B. thuringiensis.*

pXO1- and pXO2-encoded extrachromosomal virulence genes. The pXO1 plasmid, of approximately 174 kb (97, 139), carries the major virulence genes of *B. an-*

thracis (*pag* [201], *lef* [15], and *cya* [160, 187]), encoding PA, LF, and EF, respectively. The main *B. anthracis* regulatory gene, *atxA* (1.5 kb), maps between the *cya* and *pag* genes (33, 103, 193) and is thus an integral component of toxin plasmid pXO1. The three toxin genes (*cya, lef,* and *pag*) can be seen as a regulon, in which transcription of the genes is activated by *atxA* in response to temperature and CO_2 (32, 81). *atxA* is the only *B. anthracis* gene known to play a role in toxin gene expression. It acts at the transcriptional level on the toxins (pXO1) and the capsule (pXO2) (7, 103, 173, 196). The four genes *capB, capC, capA,* and *dep,* on the 90-kb plasmid pXO2, encode the poly-γ-D-glutamic acid capsule (127, 194), and it has been suggested that they form an operon (194). pXO2 also contains a regulatory gene, *acpA,* that influences capsule expression triggered by CO_2 (196).

To display its full virulence, *B. anthracis* needs to be encapsulated and toxinogenic, i.e., to carry both pXO1 and pXO2. Accordingly, vaccine strains contain only one plasmid (the Sterne strain is pXO1$^+$ pXO2$^-$, and the Pasteur strain is pXO1$^-$ pOX2$^+$) (71, 151). Strains cured of a single plasmid (pXO1 or pXO2), however, are not completely attenuated in virulence for mice. Avirulent strains without plasmids have been isolated from the field (190) or have been created in the laboratory (200).

The effect of the two plasmids on the regulation of *B. anthracis* virulence factor expression is differential (52). AtxA is currently under discussion as the molecule mediating most of this unilateral cross talk between pXO1 and pXO2 (67). pXO1-encoded AtxA strongly enhances capsule formation, whereas pXO2-encoded AcpA does not have a similar effect on the production of the toxins (33, 103, 193). AtxA null mutants are avirulent in vivo and show a decreased immunological response to the toxin proteins (33). Despite their sequence homology (196), AtxA and AcpA respond differentially to the presence of bicarbonate/CO_2 (173, 196) and temperature (52, 173). An increase in toxin and capsule production was measured when *B. anthracis* was grown in minimal media under elevated CO_2 pressure (7, 33, 52, 118, 138, 183, 196). Toxin gene transcription is increased at higher temperatures (173); *capB* transcription seems to be temperature independent (52). Regulation by CO_2 seems logical for an organism which invades mammalian cell tissues and even kills its host. Differential expression of virulence factors as a result of environmentally programmed shifts in temperature is a phenomenon known for a variety of pathogenic bacteria (114, 129, 154).

Mobility of Virulence Plasmids

Horizontal gene transfer is fairly feasible among natural populations of *Bacillus* species. Under laboratory conditions, gene transfer has been achieved by transduction, conjugation, or conduction and has been reported to occur between *B. anthracis, B. cereus,* and *B. thuringiensis* strains (183).

Gene exchange via phages. In experiments in which *B. cereus* was used as the host organism, bacteriophages CP-51 and CP-54, originally isolated from bacilli taken from soil, were found to transduce DNA to *B. anthracis* and *B. thuringiensis* as well as to *B. cereus* (185, 186, 207). The two phages are serologically related but not identical. Since both are cold labile and fairly lytic for all three species, problems evolve because potential transductants are in danger of becoming lysed. Inactivating phage infectivity with UV light or plating transduction mixtures on media containing phage antisera increased the number of transductants obtained (183). Using a temperature-sensitive mutant of CP-51 could reduce the loss of potential transductants through phage-induced lysis (183).

CP-51 not only transduces chromosomal markers (185); it also has been used for trans-duction of plasmids (164) between *B. anthracis, B. cereus,* and *B. thuringiensis.* The phage can package and transduce even larger plasmids (206). Although CP-51 and pXO2 have similar DNA sizes, there was no problem in obtaining CAP⁺ transductants of *B. cereus* and *B. anthracis* previously cured of pXO2 when the phage was grown on a donor carrying pXO2 (64, 65).

Other phages capable of transducing plasmids between bacilli are CP-52 (176) and TP-21 (183). TP-21, isolated from *B. thuringiensis* subsp. *kurstaki,* has a fairly wide range of hosts among *B. thuringiensis, B. cereus,* and *B. anthracis* strains.

Transfer of plasmids through mating. Conjugative plasmids pXO11 through pXO16, isolated from various *B. thuringiensis* strains, function efficiently in *B. anthracis* (8, 159). With their use, DNA was effectively transferred. Cell-to-cell contact and a period during which the donor and recipients grow together is necessary before plasmid transfer can occur, indicating a process similar to conjugation (8). Further analysis has shown that transfer is mediated by conduction involving the formation of cointegrate structures be-tween these self-conjugative plasmids and chromosomal DNA or nonconjugative plasmids (65). The frequency of pXO12-mediated transfer of the 4.2-kb tetracycline resistance plasmid pBC16 (183) was approximately 8×10^{-1} transcipient per donor. With larger plasmids, such as pXO2, tagged with Tn*917,* transfer occurred at a frequency 200 to 1,000 times lower than the transfer of pBC16 (183). Molecular analysis has indicated that pBC16 is transferred by donation whereas the larger *B. anthracis* plasmids pXO1 and pXO2 are mobilized by conduction as described above (65). In the transferred pBC16 plasmid, no alterations were observed. In the majority of transcipients acquiring pXO1 or pXO2 in pXO12-mediated matings, the mobilized plasmid inherited a copy of Tn*4430* from pXO12 (119). Several transcipients even contained cointegrates from pXO12 and pXO1 or pXO2, suggesting that Tn*4430* functions as a mediator in cointegrate formation between the conjugative plasmid pXO12 and the conducted plasmids. Tn*4430* is not unique in this function; in matings with donor pXO12::Tn*917* and pXO2, many CAP⁺ transcipients inherited a pXO2 plasmid containing a copy of Tn*917* (not of Tn*4430*) (65).

Transfer of pXO1 and pXO2 not only to the homologous environment of *B. anthracis* but also to the *B. cereus* or *B. thuringiensis* background has led to the successful expression of plasmid-encoded virulence factors (8). Inversely, *B. anthracis* transcipients have effi-ciently expressed parasporal crystals—the *B. thuringiensis* virulence factors—after acqui-sition of pXO12 (184). These experiments indicate that the virulence factors of *B. an-thracis, B. cereus,* and *B. thuringiensis* seem to be widely interchangeable between the species. Thus, a major adaptive function of conjugative plasmids and their transposable elements may involve the horizontal dissemination of genetic material, including virulence factors, within group I bacilli (171).

Bacillus cereus

Opportunistic *B. cereus* infections are rare and because of this are often the subject of case reports (39). In the majority of cases, *B. cereus* infections are linked to food-borne outbreaks (62). Few patients seek medical help during the active phase. The infection is self-limiting and does not normally pose a severe problem to patients and physicians, meaning that quite often the diagnosis is not properly set and that symptoms are not correlated with *B. cereus.*

Two groups of toxins have been detected (63). The emetic toxin consists of a ring structure of four amino acids repeated three times (105). It is not known whether the toxin is genetically encoded or enzymatically produced through modification of the components of the growth medium. The three-component enterotoxin proved to be identical to hemolysin BL and seems to be produced during growth in the gut (1, 9, 124). Two of the genes encoding this toxin (*hblC* and *hblD*) have been cloned and sequenced from genomic DNA (165). The course of the disease is characterized by acute vomiting, provoked by the small emetic toxin, and acute diarrhea, induced by the enterotoxins.

Genome analysis of *B. cereus* uncovered two genome sizes, 2.4 and 5.3 Mb (27). While the smaller genome component seems to be conserved, the additional component is observed only in the large genomes, where it might even be located on extrachromosomal DNA (27). Detailed information on the genetic organization of the enterotoxin region, in particular the possible variations of it, has not yet been provided. However, the fact that the *hbl* enterotoxin genes are localized within the variable section of the genome (26, 63) can be taken as an indication that, again, a dynamic component of the genetic information—here of *B. cereus*—may be the target site of insertions and deletions. This section obviously carries the variability of the genome and is probably responsible for the adaptation of the genome to the demands exerted by the environment on the bacterium.

Bacillus thuringiensis

At this point we shall briefly mention *B. thuringiensis* infections. We do not intend to give a detailed summary of what is known about *B. thuringiensis,* since it is principally not a human pathogen. However, the genetics of *B. thuringiensis*—especially with reference to its crystal protein δ-endotoxins—has been investigated in detail, and there are clear indications that its virulence genes are genetically mobile (171). There are a few very recent and comprehensive reviews to which the interested reader is referred to for more detailed information (123, 125, 126, 171).

B. thuringiensis is an insect pathogen. Its crystal δ-endotoxins are processed in the insect midgut to form the active toxin. Their toxicity is achieved when they bind to epithelial cells in the midgut, causing osmotic lysis of these cells through pore formation in the membrane. This process disintegrates the regular structure of the gut barrier, leading to the death of the infected insects. This property is today used to eradicate mosquitoes, especially in areas where malaria is endemic (34). *B. cereus* and *B. thuringiensis* are highly homologous, and it remains to be clarified if they should be defined as subspecies within one species (4, 100, 157). The differences between the two species are due mainly to additional plasmids found in *B. thuringiensis.* The *cry* genes are generally associated with these large and often conjugative plasmids (59, 60). The frequent association of the *cry* genes with conjugative plasmids suggests that new *cry* genes can be transferred and acquired among *B. thuringiensis* and *B. cereus.* Further analysis of the genetic environment of the crystal genes uncovered a plethora of insertion (IS) and transposon (Tn) elements, suggesting their involvement in the inter- and intramolecular mobility of the *cry* genes (14, 106, 120, 121). Similar experimental genetic exchange has even been used to alter the host range of certain Cry endotoxins (122). Insertion elements and transposons have been extensively reviewed by Mahillon et al. (126) and Mahillon and Chandler (125). The sequences of *B. thuringiensis* have been associated with the IS4, IS21, IS3, and Tn4430 families. More than 20 different IS- or Tn-like structures have been identified in *B. thuringiensis* to date. At least four elements, IS231A, IS232, Tn4430, and Tn5401, are active not only in *B. thuringiensis* but also in *B. subtilis* and even in *Escherichia coli* (126).

These four elements are located close to the *cry* genes, and there are serious presumptions that they are involved in the translocation of these genes. Two possible roles of the transposable elements are currently under discussion (171). These are (i) that the amplification or even accumulation of the *cry* genes within a single host may result from the association of the IS and Tn elements with the *cry* genes, and (ii) that the dissemination of the *cry* genes by gene transfer processes may arise from their association with conjugative transposons (plasmids). The extensive arsenal of crystal toxins may have been generated by processes similar to conduction (65). Phylogenetic analysis of the Cry toxin family and its great variability in biocidal activity has been discussed with regard to two fundamental evolutionary processes: (i) the independent evolution of its three functional domains and (ii) the exchange of domains among different toxins (18).

Such short-term adaptive and long-term evolutionary processes seem to be greatly needed, since insects—i.e., the hosts of the soil bacterium *B. thuringiensis*—have a short generation time and eventually develop toxin resistance (134). The survival of *B. thuringiensis* through adaptation is surely facilitated by the association of *cry* genes with the movable IS and Tn elements and conjugative plasmids mentioned above. Thus, genetic mobility and, through this, genetic variation seem to be a prerequisite for *B. thuringiensis* with its particular living space and lifestyle.

Mobility of Virulence Factors

Group I bacilli are closely related and differ primarily in their content of extrachromosomal DNA, which encodes the major virulence factors. Analysis of *B. cereus* indicates that the amount of extrachromosomal DNA could even equal that of chromosomal DNA. The transfer of genetic information between "close relatives" seems to be very possible; that of virulence factors often also encompasses the transfer of their own regulatory genes, as can be seen for pXO1 and pXO2 of *B. anthracis*. Mechanisms of horizontal gene transfer, such as conjugation, transduction, or conduction, have been observed under laboratory conditions but probably also occur in the wild. With regard to the virulence plasmids of *B. anthracis*, pXO1 and pXO2 are obviously not mobile by themselves but require additional elements, such as phages or plasmids, to be mobilized. In general, pathogenic bacillus isolates contain mobile virulence elements; their cured derivatives even serve as vaccine strains. Under field conditions, strains may accidentally lose or acquire virulence factors by virtue of the horizontal transfer of the mobile elements, thereby modulating (or adopting) their virulence potential.

CLOSTRIDIA

C. perfringens

Brief Introduction to the Disease

The pathogenic bacterium *C. perfringens* is found in soil but is also frequently discovered in the gastrointestinal tract of humans and animals. *C. perfringens* causes various serious human diseases such as gas gangrene, clostridial myonecrosis, food poisoning, necrotizing enterocolitis in infants, and pigbel. *C. perfringens* is also the etiologic agent of animal diseases such as lamb dysentery, ovine enterotoxemia (struck), and pulpy kidney disease in sheep, as well as further enterotoxemia diseases in lambs and calves (163). Whereas the diseases mentioned above are caused by extracellular enzymes or toxins, the major pathogenicity factor in food poisoning in humans is a sporulation-specific entero-toxin (CPE). As recently shown, enterotoxigenic *C. perfringens* isolates also contribute to CPE-associated human non-food-borne diseases, such as antibiotic-associated diarrhea and sporadic non-food-borne diarrhea (130).

Toxins

The enterotoxin is found in only ca. 2 to 6% of all *C. perfringens* isolates (37, 104, 195), yet in such cases is not limited to one particular type of *C. perfringens* (163). *C. perfringens* isolates are classified into five types (A to E) based on their ability to produce a certain combination of the four major lethal toxins, α-toxin, β-toxin, ϵ-toxin, and ι-toxin, which are also called typing toxins. The *C. perfringens* α-toxin has phospholipase C and sphingomyelinase activity (188, 189); the ι-toxin is a binary toxin with ADP-ribosyltransferase activity (149). The exact mechanisms of action of the β- and ϵ-toxins have not yet been described. β-Toxin is a lethal necrotizing toxin which causes hemor-rhagic necrosis and destruction of the intestinal villi; ϵ-toxin is classified as a potent neurotoxin which causes brain edema and influences vascular permeability (148).

Besides these four major toxins, *C. perfringens* can produce at least nine further extra-cellular toxins and enzymes (133, 163). These include, for example, the θ-toxin, a thiol-activated hemolysin; the κ-toxin, a collagenase; the λ-toxin, a metalloprotease; the μ-toxin, a hyaluronidase; and the sialidases NanH and NanI (162). However, an individual *C. perfringens* cell can produce only a defined subset of these 13 toxins.

Organization of the Toxin Genes

The genes of the four major toxins (α, β, ϵ, and ι), the enterotoxin gene, and most of the other known virulence factors in *C. perfringens* have been identified and sequenced (162). Virulence genes in *C. perfringens* can be localized both on chromosomes and on episomes. In both instances, there is often an association of virulence genes with mobile genetic elements.

Chromosomal localization. The circular chromosome of the *C. perfringens* refer-ence strain CPN50 is ca. 3.6 Mbp (24). An analysis of the chromosome has shown that many of the virulence genes localized on chromosomes are within a 250-kb region around the origin of replication (*oriC*) (99). These genes include *plc* (α-toxin), *pfoA* (θ-toxin), *colA* (κ-toxin), and *nagH* (μ-toxin). A comparison of the genomic organization of eight different isolates has demonstrated that the overall chromosomal organization of *C. per-fringens* types A, B, D, and E is relatively constant. However, the same analysis also uncovered the existence in the chromosome of three hypervariable regions (a to c) which are flanked by rRNA operons. It is noticeable that the virulence genes clustered around *oriC* always lie within the defined hypervariable regions (25). Hypervariable region a contains the *plc* gene, and region b contains *pfoA, colA,* and *nagH* (25). Region c can contain the enterotoxin gene (*cpe*), which is discussed later in this chapter. Why many of the virulence genes localized on chromosomes are associated with hypervariable and thus potentially unstable regions is not clear. Canard et al. (25) reported that many of the minor size variations of chromosomal segments were found near the rRNA operon. The authors pointed out that horizontal transfer of DNA, coupled with homologous recombination between the *rrn* genes, could be one cause of genomic diversification in *C. perfringens*. Such a process would correspond to a segmental exchange of DNA, as described for *E. coli* and *Salmonella typhimurium* (25).

Two further virulence genes, encoding the sialidases NanH and NanI, lie in conserved and not hypervariable regions of the chromosome. Their positions in strain CPN50 are ca. 1.0 Mb (*nanI*) and 1.2 Mb (*nanH*) away from *oriC* (25, 99). There are indications that the sialidases first evolved in animals of deuterostomate lineage and were then acquired by bacteria (161). A series of data (reviewed by Roggentin and Schauer [161]) suggests that the sialidase genes in the kingdom *Bacteria* are spread by horizontal gene transfer (83). The fact that *nanH* is located close to a phage attachment site on the chromosome is seen as an indication for a possible involvement of bacteriophages in the sialidase gene transfer (25, 161).

Extrachromosomal localization. Most of the remaining extracellular virulence factors known to us are encoded on extrachromosomal elements in *C. perfringens*. The λ-toxin gene (*lam*) has been found on plasmids of 120 and 140 kb in two type D strains. The three major toxins β-toxin (*cpb*), ι-toxin (*iap/ibp*), and ε-toxin (*etx*), are also plasmid encoded. Here it is of note that all three plasmid-encoded major toxins (β, ε, and ι) are associated with the insertion sequence IS*1151*, which is significantly similar to IS*231* from *B. thuringiensis*. Deeper investigation of the large plasmids, which contain *cpb* and *iap/ibp*, has not yet been undertaken; this is not the case, however, with the genetic vicinity of the *etx* gene (36, 85, 162).

In the proximity of the plasmid-encoded ε-toxin gene (*etx*) are three structures reminiscent of mobile elements. The insertion sequence IS*1151* is located 96 bp upstream from the *etx* gene (36). Immediately upstream from IS*1151* is an open reading frame (ORF) coding for a protein which bears significant similarity to TnpA, a transposase of the Tn*3* family (162). According to Rood (162), the DNA upstream from *etx* is reminiscent of the relations in transposon Tn*4430* from *B. thuringiensis*. Downstream from the *etx* gene are sequences which have certain similarities to transposon Tn*4001* from *Staphylococcus aureus*. In this region are two overlapping ORFs which appear to encode a fusion protein resembling transposases of the insertion sequences IS*1201* and IS*905* from *Lactococcus helveticus* and *Lactococcus lactis*, respectively (85, 162). Indications for a mobilizing function of the sequences flanking the *etx* gene, however, have not yet been proved through experiment.

The association of all of the plasmid-encoded main toxins (β, ε, and ι) with the insertion sequence IS*1151* is a priori a situation which suggests gene transfer processes. The similarity between IS*1151* and the insertion sequence IS*231* from *B. thuringiensis* also supports such a process (the latter sequence is allegedly involved in the gene transfer or mobility of virulence genes [36]). The toxin genes associated with IS*1151* can be localized on plasmids of different size, as described for the *etx* gene (25). This, too, can be interpreted as the result of a mobilization of genetic elements. The exchange of toxin genes between various plasmids could enlarge the selection of potential hosts for the toxins and thus contribute decisively to the pathogenicity of the host.

Enterotoxin gene. A localization on both the chromosome and plasmids in *C. perfringens* has to date been described only for the enterotoxin gene (*cpe*). Similar to the toxin genes *plc*, *pfoA*, *colA*, and *nagH* (see above), the chromosomal *cpe* gene is in a

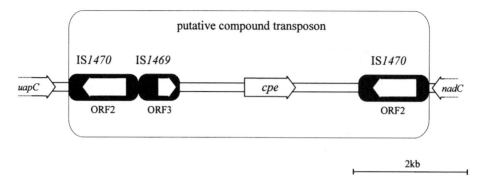

Figure 1. Genetic organization of the chromosomal enterotoxin gene (*cpe*). ORFs are shown as arrows, and IS elements are indicated by solid boxes. *uapC* encodes the putative purine permease; *nadC* encodes the putative quinolinate phosphoribosyltransferase. The figure is based on data from references 20 and 21.

hypervariable area, region c of the *C. perfringens* genome (25). The chromosomal *cpe* gene is associated with several insertion sequences up- and downstream (Fig. 1) (20, 21). The next elements upstream, at a distance of 1.2 kb, are the 789-bp insertion sequence IS*1469*, similar to IS*200*, and (in strain NCTC 8239), directly adjacent to IS*1469*, an IS*1470* element attributed to the IS*30* family. A second copy of this IS*1470* is on the other side, approximately 1.1 kb downstream from the *cpe*. Directly up- and downstream from the two "flanking" IS*1470* copies are direct repeats of 14 bp, which were obviously created at the integration of a DNA fragment in the chromosome (21). Organized in this way, the toxin locus around the *cpe* gene can be understood to be a ca. 6.3-kb compound transposon which contains both the toxin gene itself and an internal insertion sequence, IS*1469* (Fig. 1). Again, experimental data which would prove the ability of this structure to transpose is not available.

With plasmid localization of the *cpe* gene, IS*1469* is found at the same position as for enterotoxin genes localized on chromosomes, whereas the two flanking IS*1470* elements, typical for chromosomal localization, are lacking (30). Thus, when the *cpe* gene is localized on a plasmid, there is no organization in a structure similar to a transposon. However, IS*1151* elements have been found on the host plasmids of the *cpe* gene. In strain F3686, IS*1151* is ca. 260 bp downstream and directly associated with the enterotoxin. In strain 945P, however, IS*1151* does not appear to be coupled with the *cpe* gene but with the *etx* toxin gene localized on the same plasmid (see above).

The obligatory association of the *cpe* with insertion sequences with simultaneous, alternative localization either on a potential transposon or on a plasmid speaks in favor of mobility, i.e., the spreading of the enterotoxin genes by gene transfer. This could also explain the observation that *C. perfringens* strains can spontaneously lose or gain the ability to produce enterotoxin (20, 21, 29).

Significance of Mobile Elements for Virulence

The association of the various toxin genes with mobile genetic elements is a clear indication of the possible transfer of toxin genes between *C. perfringens* strains. A mobilization of important virulence factors such as this has far-reaching effects on the pathogenic potential of *C. perfringens*. This applies in particular to the plasmid-encoded lethal main toxins (β, ε, and ι) and the enterotoxin, since a distinct correlation between the induced disease and (i) localization or (ii) the existence of toxin genes can be shown for these toxins.

(i) A correlation between disease and localization—chromosomally or plasmid located—of the enterotoxin gene can be deduced from two studies. Cornillot et al. (30) showed that *C. perfringens* isolates with chromosomal localization of the *cpe* gene were involved in cases of food poisoning in humans. In contrast, the enterotoxin in strains significant to veterinary medicine appears to be plasmid encoded. Recently, Collie and McClane (29) reported that isolates from human non-food-borne gastrointestinal diseases also contain a plasmid-encoded enterotoxin. Isolates from cases of human non-food-borne gastrointestinal diseases as well as animal isolates are not subjected to the heat treatment prior to infection that is typical for isolates which are ingested from heat-preserved foodstuffs. It is in this heat treatment that Brynestad et al. (21) see the main difference in the environments between strains from animals and those isolated from patients with food poisoning. Heat treatment could affect the movement and in consequence the localization of the *cpe* gene. The fact that enterotoxin-positive strains can lose the enterotoxin gene in the course of repeated subcultivation without heat shock treatment would fit in with this theory (21). Whether heat treatment really has an effect on the mobilization of the enterotoxin gene between the chromosome and plasmids remains to be proven. Only when scientists are successful in mobilizing *cpe* from the chromosome to the episome (and vice versa) can one investigate if the localization of *cpe* really is the decisive factor for the type of disease. Such experiments could substantiate the theory that the mobility of the *cpe* gene can be allotted a significant role for the virulence of enterotoxigenic *C. perfringens* strains.

(ii) Each of the five *C. perfringens* types (A to E) is responsible for specific disease syndromes (163). Type A strains, for example, cause gas gangrene, food poisoning, or necrotizing enteritis of infants, whereas type C strains cause necrotizing enteritis in animals and human enteritis necroticans (pigbel). Biochemically and genetically, strains of *C. perfringens* types B to E are distinguished from those of type A by being able to produce, in addition to the α-toxin, a certain combination of the plasmid-encoded β-, ε-, and ι-toxins. Through PCR typing, it has been shown that the presence or absence of the β-, ε-, and ι-toxin genes and not differences in gene expression is of prime importance for the biotype of *C. perfringens* isolates (35). Therefore, according to Katayama et al. (98), the localization of the three typing toxins (β-, ε-, and ι-toxins) on plasmids provides a logical explanation for the "biotype drift" with *C. perfringens* strains, discussed some time ago (133). The unequal distribution of these toxinogenic plasmids and their ability to be lost or acquired are held responsible as the actual cause of differences in the toxinotype of individual *C. perfringens* isolates (98). The association of major toxin genes with mobile genetic elements thus generally appears to exert a decisive influence on the pathogenic potential of *C. perfringens*.

Neurotoxin-Producing Clostridia

Brief Introduction to the Disease

The group of neurotoxin-producing, pathogenic clostridia includes relatively unknown pathogens, such as *C. barati* and *C. butyricum,* but also more important pathogens, such as *C. tetani* and *C. botulinum*. In humans, the major diseases caused by these pathogenic bacteria are tetanus, food-borne botulism, infant botulism, and wound botulism. Whereas the tetanus toxin is produced by one species exclusively (*C. tetani*), a whole range of *Clostridium* species produce botulinus toxin (BoNT). BoNT-producing clostridia are split into four physiological groups (I to IV). *Clostridium* species seldom counted among the neurotoxin producers (*C. butyricum* and *C. barati*) make up a fifth group (75).

Toxins

In total, at least eight different neurotoxins (TeNT, BoNT/A to BoNT/G) and the two toxins C2 and C3 are produced by neurotoxin-forming clostridia. Toxins C2 and C3 both show ADP-ribosylating activity. The A-B toxin C2 was first discovered in *C. botulinum* type C and type D. C2 modifies intracellular actin, whereas C3, also produced by type C and type D strains, modifies the GTP-binding protein Rho from the Ras superfamily (28). The role that toxins C2 and C3 might play in the formation of botulism has not yet been clearly defined.

BoNTs are categorized in seven types (types A to G) according to their specific antigen characteristics. BoNTs are related to the tetanus toxin (TeNT) in both structure and function. All neurotoxins are synthesized as single-chain proteins (ca. 150 kDa) which are proteolytically activated in a light chain (L chain; ca. 50 kDa) and a heavy chain (H chain; ca. 100 kDa). L and H chains remain linked covalently to each other via a disulfide bridge. The clostridial neurotoxins are zinc-dependent metalloproteases which inhibit the exocytosis of neurotransmitters on interneuron synapses in the central nervous system (TeNT) and neuromuscular junctions (BoNT). The specific substrates of the neurotoxins are proteins which are involved in synaptic vesicle docking and fusion (synaptobrevin/VAMP, SNAP25, and syntaxin) (12, 13, 169, 170).

A typical characteristic of BoNT is their association with nontoxic-nonhemagglutinin components (NTNH) and hemagglutinins (HA), which are composed of several subcomponents to form complexes varying in size from 230 to about 900 kDa. Several of the toxin complexes show HA activity (166). The function of these ''neurotoxin complexes'' is not precisely known. It is assumed, however, that the formation of a complex could represent a form of protection against acid pH and protease degradation, especially with the passage of toxins through the stomach. This assumption is based on the fact that the toxicity of the neurotoxins increases with the size of the complex following peroral application (70, 180). Also, for TeNT, no formation of a complex is found with nontoxic proteins, and TeNT is inactive in laboratory animals after oral application.

Organization of the Toxin Genes

The toxin locus in *C. botulinum*. The BoNT genes, the NTNH genes, and their genetic vicinity were sequenced from a series of *C. botulinum* strains of toxin types A to G (41–43, 55–57, 86, 101, 107, 108, 143, 146, 155, 181, 204). The 3′ region of the BoNT locus contains the genes for the BoNT and NTNH proteins, forming an operon. In all *C. botulinum* strains which have been examined to date, this area is organized in a similar manner (Fig. 2) (42). The toxin clusters in the 5′ region, on the other hand, differ greatly from one another. Here, various combinations of *ha33*, *ha35*, *ha17*, *ha70*, *orf22*, *p47*, *orfX*$_1$, and *orfX*$_2$ are found in the individual strains (108). The proteins encoded by the *ha* genes are held responsible for the HA activity of the neurotoxin complex (174); ORF22 (BotR) has been identified as the positive regulator of the neurotoxin expression (128).

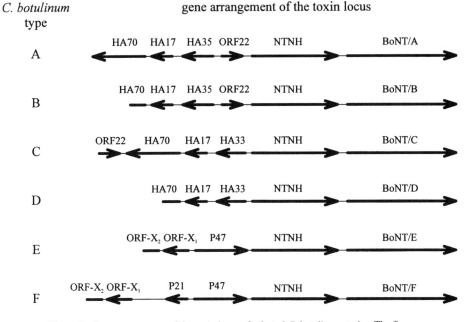

Figure 2. Gene arrangement of the toxin locus of selected *C. botulinum* strains. The figure is based on data summarized by Kubota et al. (108).

The functions of genes *p47, orfX$_1$,* and *orfX$_2$* are not known; however, it is worth noting that these genes occur only in strains without a *ha* gene (Fig. 2).

Whether all genes which constitute the toxin locus in the individual *C. botulinum* strains have been identified and which of the genes already characterized can be allotted to the respective toxin loci has not yet been finally clarified. However, a sequence comparison of two type A strains (62A and NCTC 2916) could define the 3' border of the toxin loci in these strains. Here it has been shown that the DNA sequences downstream from the *bont/A* gene correspond in an additional 97 bp but that further downstream they differ totally (11, 78, 181). It is not yet possible to precisely define the 5' border of the respective toxin loci. However, due to the functions of the NTNH, HA, and BotR proteins and their relation to the neurotoxins (see above), one can assume that these affiliated genes belong to the toxin locus directly. If one were then to suppose that the toxin loci are distinct genetic elements, then gene *p47* must also be attributable to the toxin locus, since it is localized between the putative regulator of the toxin expression and the *ntnh/bont* operon in type F strains (Fig. 2). Questions about assigning *orfX$_1$* and *orfX$_2$* found in type E, type F, and type A (infant botulism) strains upstream from *p47* and *orf22,* respectively (108), to a toxin locus cannot yet be answered. A conclusive definition of the extension of the botulinus toxin locus at a genetic level is currently not possible.

The C2 and C3 toxins have been found in addition to the neurotoxins in some strains of *C. botulinum* types C and D. In all strains examined to date, the C3 toxin gene is genetically coupled with the BoNT gene. The experimentally induced loss of neurotoxicity (phage curing) always results in the loss of the C3 toxin. An equivalent coupling has been ruled out for the C2 toxin (44).

Neurotoxin loci in *C. butyricum* and *C. barati*. Botulinus toxins are produced not just by *C. botulinum* but also by certain toxinogenic *C. butyricum* and *C. barati* strains. These strains have been isolated in connection with infant botulism (5, 69, 132) and food-borne botulism (135). In *C. barati* ATCC 43756, a neurotoxin gene (*bant*) coding for a protein with high homology to BoNT/F has been identified (182). Directly upstream from this *bant* gene is the gene encoding an NTNH protein, typical for the BoNT locus. Butyricum neurotoxins are almost identical to BoNT/E (155, 203). In addition to this, the toxin loci of *C. botulinum* type E and the toxinogenic strains of *C. butyricum* examined to date also show an equivalent organization; the genes which encode proteins with homology to ORFX$_2$, ORFX$_1$, P47, NTNH, and the neurotoxin are in the same order (108).

Toxin locus in *C. tetani*. If one examines the situation for TeNT, it is apparent that apart from the TeNT gene, only one other gene (*tetR*) which displays homologies to a gene (*botR*) from the BoNT locus exists in *C. tetani*. Like *botR, tetR* is localized upstream from the neurotoxin gene (50). It has been shown that TetR and BotR (ORF22) both exercise functions as positive regulators for the expression of the toxin (128). Furthermore, to date no other genes have been characterized in *C. tetani* which have an equivalent in the BoNT gene cluster. The TeNT locus thus probably consists of just the two genes for TeNT and its regulator, TetR.

Toxin Loci and Mobile Genetic Elements

The toxin clusters in the various strains of neurotoxin-producing clostridia were found in association with various potentially mobile genetic elements, such as phages, plasmids, and transposons.

Plasmid-encoded neurotoxins. In *C. tetani* and in *C. botulinum* type G, the neurotoxin genes have been localized together with their associated genes on large plasmids of 75 and 114 kb (46, 51, 110, 209). However, no indications of a transfer of the toxin genes by way of mobilization of the corresponding plasmids have been found.

Association of the *bunt*/E toxin locus with a defect prophage. On the basis of PCR experiments, Hauser et al. (76) assumed that the neurotoxin complex around BuNT/E in *C. butyricum* was plasmid encoded. In contrast, Zhou et al. (208) found through DNA-DNA hybridization that in *C. butyricum* the BuNT/E complex is encoded on the chromosome. Interestingly, the toxin complex on the chromosome appears to be linked to a defect prophage. While no direct proof of the localization of the BuNT/E complex on the isolated phage DNA could be derived from hybridization experiments, phage DNA could serve as templates to detect the *bunt*/E gene by PCR. Furthermore, successful transfer of the *bunt*/E gene from the toxinogenic *C. butyricum* strain 5839 to the nontoxinogenic *C. botulinum* type E-like strain S-5 (208) favors localization on a phage. However, transfer was successful only when phage particles from strain 5839 were cultivated with the recipient strain S-5 in the culture filtrate of a nontoxinogenic helper strain (*C. butyricum* ATCC 19398) (208).

Phage-encoded neurotoxins. The toxin gene clusters around *bont*/C and *bont*/D are localized on bacteriophages in *C. botulinum*. Through experiment, these can be used to effect an interconversion of type C to type D strains and vice versa. If type C and D *C. botulinum* strains are cured of their neurotoxigenic phages, no more neurotoxin is formed.

Through reinfection of cured strains with phages from toxinogenic type C and D strains, these can be converted back into neurotoxin-producing bacteria. The specific phage with which the bacteria are infected determines the toxinotype of the strain (44).

A pseudolysogenic relationship exists between the phages and the host; i.e., bacteriophages are found free in the bacterial cytoplasm. A certain number of bacteria are lysed under laboratory conditions, depending on the strain and conditions of growth, and phages are released. Cells which have lost their phages can be reinfected by the released phages. These cycles of lysogeny and reinfection can also occur in natural habitats and can be responsible for the creation of nontoxinogenic or low-producing variants of *C. botulinum* types C and D (153).

A mosaic gene which is made up of parts of the genes encoding neurotoxin types C1 and D was recently characterized in *C. botulinum* C6813 (142). The results of this study show that in nature the genetic information of the neurotoxins is altered, probably through homologous recombination. The localization of this chimeric gene on a mobile genetic element, a bacteriophage, could propagate a rapid dissemination of the new variant neurotoxin.

In type C and D strains, the phages contain genes encoding both the neurotoxins and the C3 toxin. The C3 toxin gene was localized on an element of ca. 21.5 kb with a number of different type C and type D phages (C-468, C-St, and D-1873). This distinct genetic element is flanked by a 6-bp core motif (AAGGAG) and displays several of the characteristics common to the site-specific transposon family Tn*1554*. These include (i) asymmetrical ends, (ii) the absence of inverse or terminal repeats, and (iii) the existence of a 6-bp core motif at both ends of the element and at the insertion site (77). In the three phages examined (C-468, C-St, and D-1873), the C3 toxin gene and the ends of the 21.5-kb element almost exactly match in the sequences. The existence of the same DNA fragment in differing *C. botulinum* phages provides grounds for the assumption that this 21.5-kb fragment constitutes an independent, mobile genetic element which is responsible for the dissemination of the C3 toxin in *C. botulinum* type C and D strains (78).

ADP-ribosyltransferases, related to the C3 toxin, are produced not only by *C. botulinum* but also by other species of bacteria, such as *Clostridium limosum, Staphylococcus aureus, B. cereus,* and *Legionella pneumophila* (10, 89, 91, 92, 179). The striking homology between the known C3-like gene sequences suggests that the C3 genes have a common origin and that they are spread by horizontal gene transfer. Structures typical for the 21.5-kb element have to date been found only in phages C-468, C-St, and D-1873; however, there are probably other modes of transfer which promote the dissemination of the C3 gene (77).

Chromosomally encoded neurotoxins. Although plasmids and bacteriophages have been found in *C. botulinum* types A, B, E, and F, it has not been possible to directly link the toxicity of the strains to these genetic elements (178, 199). The fact that the neurotoxins of these toxinotypes are cloned from chromosomal DNA supports the theory that the corresponding toxin genes are localized on chromosomes. Remarkably, and again pointing to a phage as the source of these particular toxins, a gene (*lyc*) was identified ca. 1 kb downstream from the *bont* genes in *C. botulinum* type A and F strains, whose predicted protein shows similarity to various lysozyme types (79). These include the lytic enzymes of the bacteriophages φMV-1 from *Lactobacillus bulgaricus* and φCP-1 from *Streptococcus pneumoniae* (79). Enzymes such as these are involved in the lytic cycle of bacteriophages.

The existence of *lyc* genes in the vicinity of *bont/A* and *bont/F* genes could, according to Henderson et al. (79), indicate that the neurotoxin genes constitute parts of an integrated prophage. It is also interesting that in this context the toxin loci around *bont/A* in *C. botulinum* 62A and NCTC 2916 are localized on different regions of the chromosome (11, 78, 181). This would also point to possible mobility of the BoNT toxin locus, derived here for a type A strain.

Mobility of the Toxin Loci

Neurotoxin genes are transferred as parts of toxin gene loci. As discussed above, mobility and horizontal gene transfer obviously play a significant role in neurotoxin-producing clostridia. One precondition for this is undoubtedly the association of the neurotoxin genes with mobile genetic elements. The organization of the neurotoxin gene loci themselves is also important. As a sign of the organization on a distinct genetic element, the neurotoxin genes in the various strains are always localized in the direct vicinity of several of their associated genes (*ha, ntnh, botR, tetR,* etc.). When mobilized, many of the genes can be transferred to the recipient organism in one step, with their proteins being important for the regulation (BotR and TetR) and function (HA and NTNH) of the neurotoxins. This increases the probability that successful expression of functional neurotoxin complexes occurs in the recipient organism.

It is thus hardly surprising that besides the classic neurotoxin producers *C. botulinum* and *C. tetani,* toxin loci have been described in neurotoxin-producing strains of *C. butyricum* and *C. barati* which are similarly or identically organized to those in *C. botulinum* (see above). With an identity of almost 97%, BuNT/E and BoNT/E are the most closely related neurotoxins which have been described to date, although they are produced by different species of clostridia (78). Nontoxinogenic *C. butyricum* strains do not contain the *bunt/E* gene (76). It thus seems obvious that toxinogenic *C. butyricum* strains can be generated from nontoxinogenic *C. butyricum* strains by the horizontal gene transfer of the entire BoNT/E toxin locus, transferred from the donor *C. botulinum* type E via mobile genetic elements (78). It can also be assumed that horizontal gene transfer takes place in the generation of neurotoxin-producing *C. barati* strains. However, the lower homology of the type F neurotoxin from *C. barati* to BoNT indicates that *C. barati* gained its neurotoxin earlier in the process of evolution than did *C. butyricum* (182).

In all neurotoxinogenic *C. barati* and *C. butyricum* strains isolated thus far (5, 69, 132, 135), the toxin genes are actually expressed and functional neurotoxins are produced. The integration of the acquired genes into the normal physiological processes of the recipient bacteria seems to have been successful. Nonproteolytic *C. botulinum* type E and F strains are clustered with *C. barati* and *C. butyricum* on a shared branch of the phylogenetic clostridial family tree (87). The phylogenetic proximity of *C. barati* and *C. butyricum* to the potential donor strains of their neurotoxin genes *bant/F* and *bunt/E* could have encouraged the successful integration of the genes.

Is the horizontal gene transfer of neurotoxins limited to certain species? Very close relationships have been described between *C. botulinum* strains from groups I, III, and IV and special, nonneurotoxinogenic species of clostridia. Thus, distinct phylogenetic lineages are formed from (i) *C. botulinum* types C and D and *C. novyi* type A, (ii) *C. botulinum* types A, B, and F and *C. sporogenes,* and (iii) *C. botulinum* type G and *C. subterminale* (87). Specific isolates of *C. novyi* type A, *C. sporogenes,* and *C. subterminale* could thus be the nonneurotoxinogenic counterparts of the corresponding neurotoxinogenic *C. botulinum* strains. Systematic molecular biological examinations have shown that many nonneurotoxinogenic strains are genotypically authentic *C. botulinum* (87). It seems reasonable to speculate that *C. novyi* type A provides a suitable genetic background for the production of BoNT/C and BoNT/D whereas *C. sporogenes* strains have a suitable genetic background for the production of functional BoNT/A, BoNT/F, and BoNT/B and *C. subterminale* has a suitable genetic background for the production of BoNT/G. The identification of a silent BoNT/B gene in two *C. subterminale* strains is worth particular mention in the context of this discussion (53). The existence of a *bont/B* gene in the genome of *C. subterminale* strains could be understood as an example of "accidental" horizontal gene transfer into a genetic environment which seems unsuitable for the functional production of BoNT/B. This would clearly show that besides the actual transfer of the genetic element, additional factors are necessary if the horizontal gene transfer of clostridial neurotoxins is to be successful, such as the fitting of the transferred genes into suitable regulation networks in the host organism or the stabilization of the integrated DNA. The successful dissemination of neurotoxin genes by horizontal gene transfer (without further evolutionary adaptation) could be limited to certain combinations of neurotoxin genes and *Clostridium* spp. Nevertheless, the possibility should not be ruled out that the missing BoTN/B expression in *C. subterminale* is not a matter of principle but is caused by coincidence, such as a point mutation within the BoTN/B gene which leads to the termination of translation.

Clostridia Which Produce Large Clostridial Cytotoxins

Brief Introduction to the Disease

Large clostridial cytotoxins (LCTs) are produced by toxinogenic strains of *C. sordellii*, *C. novyi* and *C. difficile* and by one *C. barati* strain. *C. sordellii* is responsible for a number of illnesses in animals and humans. Diseases in animals include fatal myositis, liver disease, and sudden death in cows, sheep, and horses (175). The most serious *C. sordellii* diseases found among humans are gas gangrene-like infections (75). The more common gas gangrene pathogen is, however, *C. novyi,* the cause of ca. one-third of the infections of this kind in humans. Disease caused by *C. novyi* has also been described in conjunction with diseases of animals, such as infection of wounds or infectious necrotic hepatitis in sheep and cattle (75). *C. difficile* is associated primarily with illness in humans. The bacterium is regarded as the etiologic agent of antibiotic-associated diarrhea and pseudomembranous colitis. *C. difficile* infections have also been observed in many animals, such as cats, dogs, and horses (175).

The Family of Large Clostridial Cytotoxins

To date, five toxins which belong to the LCTs have been identified as being produced by *C. difficile, C. sordellii,* or *C. novyi.* These are the two *C. difficile* toxins TcdA and TcdB, the *C. novyi* α-toxin (Tcnα), and the *C. sordellii* lethal (TcsL) and hemorrhagic (TcsH) toxins. Typical characteristics of LCTs are their cytotoxicity toward cultivated cells, a high molecular mass (250 to 308 kDa), and a modular structure consisting of three functional domains. The C-terminal domain is responsible for binding toxins to cell receptors; computer analysis assigns potential functions to the central domain during the translocation of the toxins; and the N-terminal one-third carries the enzymatic activity (197). All LCTs are glycosyltransferases, which in cytosol glycosylate small GTP-binding proteins (GTPases) with activated sugars as a cosubstrate (58, 93, 94, 152, 172). The relationship of LCTs at a structural and functional level is also reflected in the sequences of the individual toxins. With reference to the amino acid sequence of TcdB, TcdA has 63%, TcsL has 90%, and Tcnα has 48% homology (197). The sequence of the TcsH gene has not yet been determined.

Organization of the Toxin Genes

At the molecular level, *C. difficile* is the most thoroughly researched of the LCT-producing *Clostridium* species. As early as at the end of the 1980s, overlapping, recombinant clones representing both toxin genes were isolated from genomic libraries in *E. coli* (156, 198). The sequences of both toxins were published at the beginning of the 1990s (6, 38, 167). By comparing toxinogenic and nontoxinogenic isolates, we and others were later able to define the toxin locus and its integration site in the *C. difficile* genome (17, 72). The toxin locus is referred to below as the pathogenicity locus (PaLoc). The PaLoc is a distinct genetic element of 19.6 kb which includes the five genes *tcdA* to *tcdE* (Fig. 3). *tcdA* encodes the enterotoxin (TcdA), and *tcdB* encodes the cytotoxin (TcdB). Following a reporter gene analysis with *E. coli* and the transcription analysis of the *tcd* genes from *C. difficile,* it has been postulated that TcdD functions as a positive regulator (84, 141). Transcription analyses also suggest that TcdC is involved in the negative regulation of toxin expression (Fig. 3) (16, 84). The function of TcdE is unknown.

The five PaLoc genes in *C. difficile* are organized in two transcription units. One unit comprises only the *tcdC* gene, and the other contains the four genes *tcdDBEA* (84). The two units are obviously coupled, as can be deduced from the organization of the genes and their mode of transcription (16). By reading through the transcription terminator be-

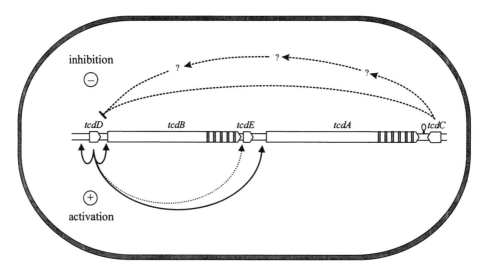

Figure 3. Model for the regulation of the toxin expression in *C. difficile*. The model is based on work in our laboratory (16, 84) and a reporter gene analysis by Moncrief et al. (141). The antagonistic functions of the two putative regulatory molecules, TcdC and TcdD, for the expression of the *C. difficile* toxins are indicated. The model is described in detail by Braun (16).

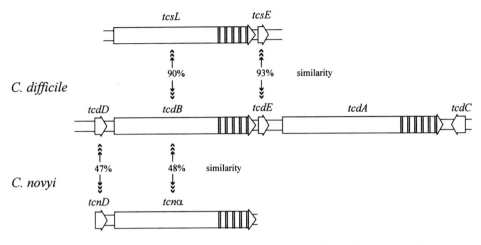

Figure 4. Genetic organization of the pathogenicity locus of *C. difficile*, *C. sordellii* (partial), and *C. novyi* (partial). The figure is based on data from references 16, 17, 66, and 82.

tween *tcdA* and *tcdC,* transcription unit *tcdDBEA* generates antisense RNA for the *tcdC* gene and thus directly influences the production of TcdC. In the model developed in our laboratory, PaLoc is seen as a complex unit of regulation equipped with its own positive (TcdD) and negative (TcdC) regulators for toxin expression (Fig. 3). An "autologous" regulation such as this would be highly significant for the successful dissemination of the toxin genes via horizontal gene transfer (see below).

Sequence data available for the *C. sordellii* and *C. novyi* toxins is distinctly more limited. Data collected to date, however, indicates that also these two species have a structure similar in principle to that of the *C. difficile* PaLoc. In *C. novyi,* an ORF (*tcnD*) was identified directly upstream from the *tcnα* gene (Fig. 4). The relative position and orientation of *tcnD* are comparable to those of *tcdD* in the PaLoc of *C. difficile. tcnD* encodes a protein with homology to TcdD (196a). Similarly to TcdD, TcnD also displays structures such as helix-turn-helix motifs, which are typically found in DNA-binding proteins with regulatory functions.

The sequence upstream from the *tcsL* gene is still unknown in *C. sordellii.* However, here a gene has been found downstream from *tcsL* which encodes a protein with 93% homology to TcdE from *C. difficile* (Fig. 4) (66). This gene is also at the site typical for *tcdE* in the *C. difficile* pathogenicity locus. All data collected to date strongly implies that the PaLoc of *C. difficile* could be the paradigm for the genetic organization of all other LCTs (Fig. 4).

Toxin Loci and Mobile Genetic Elements

C. novyi **α-toxin.** The first indication that the α-toxin gene is localized on a phage (i.e., on a mobile genetic element) in *C. novyi* came from results reported by Eklund et al. (47). The authors established that *C. novyi* type A isolates which no longer produce α-toxin are sensitive to phages from toxinogenic derivatives of the same strain. Isolates which continue to produce α-toxin are, on the other hand, immune to these phages (NA1). Nontoxinogenic isolates infected with the NA1 phage again begin to produce the α-toxin. Schallehn et al. (168) reported that nontoxinogenic derivatives of originally toxinogenic strains not only are sensitive to the toxinogenic phages of the parent strain but in some cases also are sensitive to toxinogenic phages from other *C. novyi* strains. The strict correlation between the existence of a toxinogenic phage and the production of the α-toxin was also confirmed in this study.

Eklund et al. (45) proved that the *C. novyi* α-toxin can also be successfully transferred to other species. In this investigation, the phage-cured *C. botulinum* type C isolate HS37 was changed into a bacterium which produces α-toxin by being infected with the NA1 phage. The structure of the actual locus of the α-toxin gene, and especially that of the adjacent phage sequences, in *C. novyi* is not yet known. Thus, with the information currently available, it is not impossible that the PaLoc in *C. novyi* is an independent mobile element on the phage, as found with specific *C. botulinum* type C and D phages for the C3 toxin (see above). This theory is currently being investigated in our laboratory. Localization on an independent mobile element could facilitate the transfer of the α-toxin from its original phage to other mobile elements (phages, conjugative plasmids, etc.) and thus expand its host spectrum.

C. difficile PaLoc. In contrast to *C. novyi*, the *C. difficile* PaLoc has been fully characterized and clearly defined (17, 72). The *C. difficile* PaLoc is reminiscent of genetic elements which are described as pathogenicity islands (PAIs) (see chapter 1). The PaLoc fulfills the definition of a PAI (68) in many respects (17). It encodes the major pathogenicity factors of *C. difficile,* there are nonpathogenic strains which do not contain the PaLoc, and the G+C content of the PaLoc differs from that of the host DNA (16). At ca. 20 kb, the PaLoc is somewhat small for a PAI—which are often larger than 30 kb—yet there are even smaller genetic elements which have been defined as PAIs (68), such as the 11.9-kb Vap region of *Dichelobacter nodosus*. A further characteristic of PAIs is that the PaLoc is a compact, distinct genetic element. However, it does not contain any direct repeats at the borders, a situation which has also been observed for other PAIs, such as the locus of enterocyte effacement from enteropathogenic *E. coli* or SP-II from *S. typhimurium* (68, 113). This lack of direct repeats at PAI borders is often connected with stability of the respective genetic element, otherwise atypical for PAIs (68, 113). This also applies to the PaLoc of *C. difficile*. Another feature, also atypical for PAIs, is that at the borders of the *C. difficile* PaLoc there are neither IS elements nor tRNA genes, structures which often serve as integration sites for mobile genetic elements (68). It is interesting that in nontoxinogenic *C. difficile* strains there is a DNA stretch of 115 bp which must have been lost (or replaced) during the assumed integration of the PaLoc into toxinogenic strains. Within this 115-bp stretch in nontoxinogenic strains is an inverted repeat which can form a stable hairpin loop of 20 bp (17). This hairpin loop could serve as the target structure of the PaLoc during integration. A further important point in relation to PAIs is the existence of "mobility genes," such as IS elements, integrases, or transposases. For the reference strain *C. difficile* VPI 10463, as in most of the other isolates, proof of the existence of elements such as these has not yet been established. However, we have known for a short time now that in specific *C. difficile* isolates, sequences similar to IS elements occur in the PaLoc (196a). The function of these IS elements in the mobility and evolution of the PaLoc in *C. difficile* is currently being investigated in our laboratory.

To conclude, it can be ascertained that the PaLoc in *C. difficile* has most but not all of the characteristics common to PAIs. The instances where there are differences from the classic definition of a PAI concentrate on aspects directly linked to the stability of the PaLoc, such as terminal repetitive structures or the existence of mobility genes. One can assume that the PaLoc in *C. difficile* is not an autonomous mobile element. This has led to the hypothesis that it could be an independent, pathogenic part of a larger, virulence-associated element (17). This hypothetical larger genetic element would then be the actual PAI of *C. difficile*. This situation resembles that described above for C3 in *C. botulinum* type C and D strains.

Significance of the PaLoc in Evolution of LCT-Producing Clostridia

Recently, information was published on a *C. barati* strain that had been isolated from a patient with diarrhea and that produced exotoxins similar to *C. difficile* (158). Proof that TcdA- and TcdB-homologous toxins are produced in this specific *C. barati* strain was established by various methods (158). This constitutes the first report on an LCT-producing clostridium besides the three species mentioned above, namely, *C. difficile*, *C. sordellii*, and *C. novyi*. Since there has thus far been no indication of genes in *C. barati* homologous to *tcdA* and *tcdB* of *C. difficile*, we assume that the toxin genes were transferred to the isolated *C. barati* bacterium via horizontal transfer and that the transfer must have encompassed the entire, functional PaLoc. Detailed molecular biological characterization of the *C. barati* strain will thus also help us to resolve unanswered questions about the *C. difficile* PaLoc. We could clarify, for example, whether only the PaLoc as currently defined (17, 72) or, indeed, a larger DNA element was transferred by the horizontal gene transfer supported here and whether an integration site, similar to that described in *C. difficile*, also exists in *C. barati*.

The neurotoxin-producing *C. barati* isolates are distantly related to the potential donor strains of the transferred DNA, namely, *C. botulinum* types C and D. There is no close relationship, however, between *C. difficile* and *C. barati* (87, 112). Nevertheless, the fact that toxins homologous to those of *C. difficile* were detected in *C. barati*, assuming that the toxin genes were acquired from *C. difficile*, suggests that *C. barati* is obviously capable of functionally expressing *C. difficile* genes. It is interesting to speculate on the reasons for this successful production of toxins in *C. barati*.

The close genetic coupling of the five *tcd* genes on a distinct genetic element allows us to assume that the entire PaLoc, either on its own or as part of a larger PAI, was transferred to the toxinogenic *C. barati* strain. The transfer of the PaLoc as a complete element could be partly responsible for the successful expression of the toxins in *C. barati*. As discussed above, the PaLoc contains an internal regulation mechanism for toxin expression, comprising the *tcdC* and *tcdD* genes. If this internal regulation mechanism can be successfully integrated in the physiological processes of this recipient bacterium, a completely regulated production of toxins should be ensured. In *C. difficile*, the expression of the toxins is associated with processes of the stationary phase of growth, probably even with the sporulation process itself (95). All clostridia are capable of sporulation. If the internal PaLoc regulation can indeed be embedded in regulating networks of sporulation, this would provide one optimum condition for the successful dissemination of *C.*

difficile toxins between clostridia. An integration process such as this could explain the expression of the toxin genes acquired by *C. barati.*

Comments on the Mobility of Clostridial Toxins

The gene transfer of virulence factors within and between the species is obviously an important factor in the evolution of pathogenic clostridia. The question why the clostridial toxin genes were able to spread to such an extent then arises.

The basis of this is most probably that the toxin genes are organized in compact gene clusters and obviously that they are also associated with mobile genetic elements. Another prerequisite for the transfer of genes is that the contact between the donor and recipient organism should be as close and frequent as possible. For clostridia, the intestinal tract could be the communal habitat where gene transfer occurs within or between the species. Potential donor (e.g., *C. botulinum, C. difficile, C. perfringens,* toxinogenic *C. barati,* and *C. butyricum* strains) and recipient (nontoxinogenic *C. barati* and *C. butyricum* strains, *C. subterminale, C. sporogenes,* etc.) organisms of the toxin genes can, at least on a temporary basis, colonize the intestinal area of humans and animals (147). With a bacterial concentration of sometimes over 10^{11} organisms/g of intestinal content, the colon is the most densely colonized habitat in humans, and the number of anaerobes exceeds that of aerobes by a factor of 10^2 to 10^3 (80). Thus, the number and density of bacteria from the individual *Clostridium* spp. are probably also much higher in the human colon than in other natural habitats such as soil. In the human colon, the number of clostridia is probably even temporarily increased following treatment with antibiotics, since clostridia form spores and can withstand the effects of antibiotics by sporulation as well as by antibiotic resistance. Once the patient terminates his or her course of antibiotics, the spores germinate and overgrow the intestine before the normal intestinal flora has a chance to reestablish itself. This overgrowth of *C. difficile* following suppression of the normal intestinal flora during the course of treatment with antibiotics is currently being discussed for *C. difficile* as an important feature in the pathogenesis of the disease (205). A considerable accumulation of clostridia was also observed under specific conditions in the gastrointestinal tract of animals. In the ileum in sheep, for example, up to 10^9 living *C. perfringens* cells per g of intestinal content in the ileum was found following a radical change of diet (23). The large number of bacteria in the gastrointestinal tract, combined with the side-by-side existence of potential donor and recipient organisms, could support the transfer of genes or even enable transfer at all.

CONCLUDING REMARKS

Mobile virulence-associated genetic elements have been observed in clostridia and in bacilli. If one studies the frequency of such elements, it can be established that an association of mobility and virulence factors in both species of bacteria described not only is apparent but also is the rule rather than the exception. This conclusion can be reached despite the limited amount of genetic information currently available in many cases. As research on the genetics of virulence factors progresses, more examples of virulence factor mobility in *Clostridium* and *Bacillus* species will surely be found in the near future.

With virulence factors we know to be mobile, the significance of the association of mobile genetic elements with virulence genes for the evolution of the pathogenic clostridia and bacilli becomes clear. This applies to evolution, through gene transfer, of a specific isolate (chromosomal or extrachromosomal localization of *cpe*), of a single species (biotype drift with *C. perfringens*), or even of a genus (generation of neurotoxinogenic *C. butyricum* and *C. barati* strains through horizontal gene transfer). However, among pathogenic bacilli and clostridia, the principle of genetic variation is obviously based not just on the acquisition of virulence factors through exchange of their vehicles (plasmids and phages, for example) but also on their loss, as reflected, for example, by the differences between fully virulent *B. anthracis* strains (carrying both virulence plasmids) and vaccine strains (which have lost at least one of the two). The ecological sense behind this phenomenon could be to keep individual isolates in a population receptive to new, mobile genetic elements, such as plasmids, phages (bypassing plasmid and phage incompatibility), and PAIs (free integration sites). Often it is not until virulence factors are lost that conditions are provided which enable other virulence-associated genes to be acquired. The extreme flexibility of the bacteria toward the loss and acquisition of virulence factors could help pathogenic bacteria adapt to the excessive pressure of selection to which they are subjected during the complex interactions between pathogens and their hosts.

Acknowledgments. We thank Michel Popoff (Institut Pasteur, Paris, France) and Julian Rood (Monash University, Clayton, Australia) for supplying preprints of in-press reviews. C.V.E.-S. thanks his laboratory crew for their spirit, encouragement, and enthusiasm through the years. Special gratitude goes to the University of Mainz and the Naturwissenschaftlich-Medizinischem Forschungszentrum Mainz, which supplied the group with laboratory space in the Verfügungsgebäude für Forschung und Entwicklung. A true personal thanks is directed to the former head of the department, Paul Klein, who died on 20 March 1998.

REFERENCES

1. **Agata, N., M. Ohta, Y. Arakawa, and M. Mori.** 1995. The *bceT* gene of *Bacillus cereus* encodes an enterotoxic protein. *Microbiology* **141:**983–988.
2. **Andersen, G. L., J. M. Simchock, and K. H. Wilson.** 1996. Identification of a region of genetic variability among *Bacillus anthracis* strains and related species. *J. Bacteriol.* **178:**377–384.
3. **Ash, C., and M. D. Collins.** 1992. Comparative analysis of 23S ribosomal RNA gene sequences of *Bacillus anthracis* and emetic *Bacillus cereus* determined by PCR-direct sequencing. *FEMS Microbiol. Lett.* **73:** 75–80.
4. **Ash, C., J. A. Farrow, M. Dorsch, E. Stackebrandt, and M. D. Collins.** 1991. Comparative analysis of *Bacillus anthracis, Bacillus cereus,* and related species on the basis of reverse transcriptase sequencing of 16S rRNA. *Int. J. Syst. Bacteriol.* **41:**343–346.
5. **Aureli, P., L. Fenicia, B. Pasolini, M. Gianfranceschi, L. M. McCroskey, and C. L. Hatheway.** 1986. Two cases of type E infant botulism caused by neurotoxigenic *Clostridium butyricum* in Italy. *J. Infect. Dis.* **154:**207–211.
6. **Barroso, L. A., S. Z. Wang, C. J. Phelps, J. L. Johnson, and T. D. Wilkins.** 1990. Nucleotide sequence of *Clostridium difficile* toxin B gene. *Nucleic Acids Res.* **18:**4004.
7. **Bartkus, J. M., and S. H. Leppla.** 1989. Transcriptional regulation of the protective antigen gene of *Bacillus anthracis. Infect. Immun.* **57:**2295–2300.
8. **Battisti, L., B. D. Green, and C. B. Thorne.** 1985. Mating system for transfer of plasmids among *Bacillus anthracis, Bacillus cereus,* and *Bacillus thuringiensis. J. Bacteriol.* **162:**543–550.
9. **Beecher, D. J., and A. C. Wong.** 1994. Improved purification and characterization of hemolysin BL, a hemolytic dermonecrotic vascular permeability factor from *Bacillus cereus. Infect. Immun.* **62:**980–986.
10. **Belyi, Y. F., I. S. Tartakovskii, Y. V. Vertiev, and S. V. Prosorovskii.** 1991. Partial purification and characterization of ADP-ribosyltransferase produced by *Legionella pneumophila. Biomed. Sci.* **2:**169–174.
11. **Binz, T., H. Kurazono, M. Wille, J. Frevert, K. Wernars, and H. Niemann.** 1990. The complete

sequence of botulinum neurotoxin type A and comparison with other clostridial neurotoxins. *J. Biol. Chem.* **265:**9153–9158.

12. **Blasi, J., E. R. Chapman, E. Link, T. Binz, S. Yamasaki, P. De Camilli, T. C. Sudhof, H. Niemann, and R. Jahn.** 1993. Botulinum neurotoxin A selectively cleaves the synaptic protein SNAP-25. *Nature* **365:**160–163.

13. **Blasi, J., E. R. Chapman, S. Yamasaki, T. Binz, H. Niemann, and R. Jahn.** 1993. Botulinum neurotoxin C1 blocks neurotransmitter release by means of cleaving HPC-1/syntaxin. *EMBO J.* **12:**4821–4828.

14. **Bourgouin, C., A. Delecluse, J. Ribier, A. Klier, and G. Rapoport.** 1988. A *Bacillus thuringiensis* subsp. *israelensis* gene encoding a 125-kilodalton larvicidal polypeptide is associated with inverted repeat sequences. *J. Bacteriol.* **170:**3575–3583.

15. **Bragg, T. S., and D. L. Robertson.** 1989. Nucleotide sequence and analysis of the lethal factor gene (lef) from *Bacillus anthracis. Gene* **81:**45–54.

16. **Braun, V.** 1997. Ph.D. thesis. Johannes Gutenberg-Universität, Mainz, Germany.

17. **Braun, V., T. Hundsberger, P. Leukel, M. Sauerborn, and C. von Eichel-Streiber.** 1996. Definition of the single integration site of the pathogenicity locus in *Clostridium difficile. Gene* **181:**29–38.

18. **Bravo, A.** 1997. Phylogenetic relationships of *Bacillus thuringiensis* delta-endotoxin family proteins and their functional domains. *J. Bacteriol.* **179:**2793–2801.

19. **Brown, E. R., and W. B. Cherry.** 1955. Specific identification of *Bacillus anthracis* by means of a variant bacteriophage. *J. Infect. Dis.* **96:**34–39.

20. **Brynestad, S., L. A. Iwanejko, G. S. Stewart, and P. E. Granum.** 1994. A complex array of Hpr consensus DNA recognition sequences proximal to the enterotoxin gene in *Clostridium perfringens* type A. *Microbiology* **140:**97–104.

21. **Brynestad, S., B. Synstad, and P. E. Granum.** 1997. The *Clostridium perfringens* enterotoxin gene is on a transposable element in type A human food poisoning strains. *Microbiology* **143:**2109–2115.

22. **Buck, C. A., R. L. Anacker, F. S. Newman, and A. Eisentark.** 1963. Phage isolated from lysogenic *Bacillus anthracis. J. Bacteriol.* **85:**1423–1430.

23. **Bullen, J. J., and R. Scarisbrick.** 1957. Enterotoxaemia of sheep: experimental reproduction of the disease. *J. Pathol. Bacteriol.* **73:**494–509.

24. **Canard, B., and S. T. Cole.** 1989. Genome organization of the anaerobic pathogen *Clostridium perfringens. Proc. Natl. Acad. Sci. USA* **86:**6676–6680.

25. **Canard, B., B. Saint Joanis, and S. T. Cole.** 1992. Genomic diversity and organization of virulence genes in the pathogenic anaerobe *Clostridium perfringens. Mol. Microbiol.* **6:**1421–1429.

26. **Carlson, C. R., T. Johansen, and A. B. Kolsto.** 1996. The chromosome map of *Bacillus thuringiensis* subsp. *canadensis* HD224 is highly similar to that of the *Bacillus cereus* type strain ATCC 14579. *FEMS Microbiol. Lett.* **141:**163–167.

27. **Carlson, C. R., and A. B. Kolsto.** 1994. A small (2.4 Mb) *Bacillus cereus* chromosome corresponds to a conserved region of a larger (5.3 Mb) *Bacillus cereus* chromosome. *Mol. Microbiol.* **13:**161–169.

28. **Chardin, P., P. Boquet, P. Madaule, M. R. Popoff, E. J. Rubin, and D. M. Gill.** 1989. The mammalian G protein rhoC is ADP-ribosylated by *Clostridium botulinum* exoenzyme C3 and affects actin microfilaments in Vero cells. *EMBO J.* **8:**1087–1092.

29. **Collie, R. E., and B. A. McClane.** 1998. Evidence that the enterotoxin gene can be episomal in *Clostridium perfringens* isolates associated with non-food-borne human gastrointestinal diseases. *J. Clin. Microbiol.* **36:**30–36.

30. **Cornillot, E., B. Saint Joanis, G. Daube, S. Katayama, P. E. Granum, B. Canard, and S. T. Cole.** 1995. The enterotoxin gene (*cpe*) of *Clostridium perfringens* can be chromosomal or plasmid-borne. *Mol. Microbiol.* **15:**639–647.

31. **Cowles, P. B.** 1931. A bacteriophage for *Bacillus anthracis. J. Bacteriol.* **21:**161–166.

32. **Dai, Z., and T. M. Koehler.** 1997. Regulation of anthrax toxin activator gene (*atxA*) expression in *Bacillus anthracis*: temperature, not CO_2/bicarbonate, affects AtxA synthesis. *Infect. Immun.* **65:**2576–2582.

33. **Dai, Z., J. C. Sirard, M. Mock, and T. M. Koehler.** 1995. The atxA gene product activates transcription of the anthrax toxin genes and is essential for virulence. *Mol. Microbiol.* **16:**1171–1181.

34. **Das, P. K., and D. D. Amalraj.** 1997. Biological control of malaria vectors. *Indian J. Med. Res.* **106:**174–197.

35. **Daube, G., B. China, P. Simon, K. Hvala, and J. Mainil.** 1994. Typing of *Clostridium perfringens* by in vitro amplification of toxin genes. *J. Appl. Bacteriol.* **77:**650–655.

36. **Daube, G., P. Simon, and A. Kaeckenbeeck.** 1993. IS1151, an IS-like element of *Clostridium perfringens. Nucleic Acids Res.* **21:**352.

37. **Daube, G., P. Simon, B. Limbourg, C. Manteca, J. Mainil, and A. Kaeckenbeeck.** 1996. Hybridization of 2,659 *Clostridium perfringens* isolates with gene probes for seven toxins (alpha, beta, epsilon, iota, theta, mu, and enterotoxin) and for sialidase. *Am. J. Vet. Res.* **57:**496–501.

38. **Dove, C. H., S. Z. Wang, S. B. Price, C. J. Phelps, D. M. Lyerly, T. D. Wilkins, and J. L. Johnson.** 1990. Molecular characterization of the *Clostridium difficile* toxin A gene. *Infect. Immun.* **58:**480–488.

39. **Drobniewski, F. A.** 1993. *Bacillus cereus* and related species. *Clin. Microbiol. Rev.* **6:**324–338.

40. **Duesbery, N. S., C. P. Webb, S. H. Leppla, V. M. Gordon, K. R. Klimpel, T. D. Copeland, N. G. Ahn, M. K. Oskarsson, K. Fukasawa, K. D. Paull, and G. F. Vande Woude.** 1998. Proteolytic inactivation of MAP-kinase-kinase by anthrax lethal factor. *Science* **280:**734–737.

41. **East, A. K., M. Bhandari, J. M. Stacey, K. D. Campbell, and M. D. Collins.** 1996. Organization and phylogenetic interrelationships of genes encoding components of the botulinum toxin complex in proteolytic *Clostridium botulinum* types A, B, and F: evidence of chimeric sequences in the gene encoding the nontoxic nonhemagglutinin component. *Int. J. Syst. Bacteriol.* **46:**1105–1112.

42. **East, A. K., and M. D. Collins.** 1994. Conserved structure of genes encoding components of botulinum neurotoxin complex M and the sequence of the gene coding for the nontoxic component in nonproteolytic *Clostridium botulinum* type F. *Curr. Microbiol.* **29:**69–77.

43. **East, A. K., P. T. Richardson, D. Allaway, M. D. Collins, T. A. Roberts, and D. E. Thompson.** 1992. Sequence of the gene encoding type F neurotoxin of *Clostridium botulinum. FEMS Microbiol. Lett.* **75:** 225–230.

44. **Eklund, M. W.** 1993. The role of bacteriophages and plasmids in the production of toxins and other biologically active substances by *Clostridium botulinum* and *Clostridium novyi*, p. 179–194. *In* M. Sebald (ed.), *Genetics and Molecular Biology of Anaerobic Bacteria.* Springer-Verlag, Heidelberg, Germany.

45. **Eklund, M. W., F. T. Poysky, J. A. Meyers, and G. A. Pelroy.** 1974. Interspecies conversion of *Clostridium botulinum* type C to *Clostridium novyi* type A by bacteriophage. *Science* **186:**456–458.

46. **Eklund, M. W., F. T. Poysky, L. M. Mseitif, and M. S. Strom.** 1988. Evidence for plasmid-mediated toxin and bacteriocin production in *Clostridium botulinum* type G. *Appl. Environ. Microbiol.* **54:**1405–1408.

47. **Eklund, M. W., F. T. Poysky, M. E. Peterson, and J. A. Meyers.** 1976. Relationship of bacteriophages to alpha toxin production in *Clostridium novyi* types A and B. *Infect. Immun.* **14:**793–803.

48. **Etienne Toumelin, I., J. C. Sirard, E. Duflot, M. Mock, and A. Fouet.** 1995. Characterization of the *Bacillus anthracis* S-layer: cloning and sequencing of the structural gene. *J. Bacteriol.* **177:**614–620.

49. **Ezzell, J. W., B. E. Ivins, and S. H. Leppla.** 1984. Immunoelectrophoretic analysis, toxicity, and kinetics of in vitro production of the protective antigen and lethal factor components of *Bacillus anthracis* toxin. *Infect. Immun.* **45:**761–767.

50. **Fairweather, N. F., and V. A. Lyness.** 1986. The complete nucleotide sequence of tetanus toxin. *Nucleic Acids Res.* **14:**7809–7812.

51. **Finn, C. W., Jr., R. P. Silver, W. H. Habig, M. C. Hardegree, G. Zon, and C. F. Garon.** 1984. The structural gene for tetanus neurotoxin is on a plasmid. *Science* **224:**881–884.

52. **Fouet, A., and M. Mock.** 1996. Differential influence of the two *Bacillus anthracis* plasmids on regulation of virulence gene expression. *Infect. Immun.* **64:**4928–4932.

53. **Franciosa, G., J. L. Ferreira, and C. L. Hatheway.** 1994. Detection of type A, B, and E botulism neurotoxin genes in *Clostridium botulinum* and other *Clostridium* species by PCR: evidence of unexpressed type B toxin genes in type A toxigenic organisms. *J. Clin. Microbiol.* **32:**1911–1917.

54. **Friedlander, A. M.** 1986. Macrophages are sensitive to anthrax lethal toxin through an acid-dependent process. *J. Biol. Chem.* **261:**7123–7126.

55. **Fujii, N., K. Kimura, N. Yokosawa, K. Oguma, T. Yashiki, K. Takeshi, T. Ohyama, E. Isogai, and H. Isogai.** 1993. Similarity in nucleotide sequence of the gene encoding nontoxic component of botulinum toxin produced by toxigenic *Clostridium butyricum* strain BL6340 and *Clostridium botulinum* type E strain Mashike. *Microbiol. Immunol.* **37:**395–398.

56. **Fujii, N., K. Kimura, N. Yokosawa, T. Yashiki, K. Tsuzuki, and K. Oguma.** 1993. The complete nucleotide sequence of the gene encoding the nontoxic component of *Clostridium botulinum* type E progenitor toxin. *J. Gen. Microbiol.* **139:**79–86.

57. **Fujinaga, Y., K. Inoue, S. Shimazaki, K. Tomochika, K. Tsuzuki, N. Fujii, T. Watanabe, T. Ohyama,**

K. Takeshi, and K. Inoue. 1994. Molecular construction of *Clostridium botulinum* type C progenitor toxin and its gene organization. *Biochem. Biophys. Res. Commun.* **205**:1291–1298.

58. **Genth, H., F. Hofmann, J. Selzer, G. Rex, K. Aktories, and I. Just.** 1996. Difference in protein substrate specificity between hemorrhagic toxin and lethal toxin from *Clostridium sordellii. Biochem. Biophys. Res. Commun.* **229**:370–374.

59. **Gonzalez, J. M., Jr., B. J. Brown, and B. C. Carlton.** 1982. Transfer of *Bacillus thuringiensis* plasmids coding for delta-endotoxin among strains of *B. thuringiensis* and *B. cereus. Proc. Natl. Acad. Sci. USA* **79**:6951–6955.

60. **Gonzalez, J. M., Jr., H. T. Dulmage, and B. C. Carlton.** 1981. Correlation between specific plasmids and delta-endotoxin production in *Bacillus thuringiensis. Plasmid* **5**:352–365.

61. **Gordon, V. M., S. H. Leppla, and E. L. Hewlett.** 1988. Inhibitors of receptor-mediated endocytosis block the entry of *Bacillus anthracis* adenylate cyclase toxin but not that of *Bordetella pertussis* adenylate cyclase toxin. *Infect. Immun.* **56**:1066–1069.

62. **Granum, P. E.** 1994. *Bacillus cereus* and its toxins. *Soc. Appl. Bacteriol. Symp. Ser.* **23**:61s–66s.

63. **Granum, P. E., and T. Lund.** 1997. *Bacillus cereus* and its food poisoning toxins. *FEMS Microbiol. Lett.* **157**:223–228.

64. **Green, B. D., L. Battisti, T. M. Koehler, C. B. Thorne, and B. E. Ivins.** 1985. Demonstration of a capsule plasmid in *Bacillus anthracis. Infect. Immun.* **49**:291–297.

65. **Green, B. D., L. Battisti, and C. B. Thorne.** 1989. Involvement of Tn*4430* in transfer of *Bacillus anthracis* plasmids mediated by *Bacillus thuringiensis* plasmid pXO12. *J. Bacteriol.* **171**:104–113.

66. **Green, G. A., V. Schue, and H. Monteil.** 1995. Cloning and characterization of the cytotoxin L-encoding gene of *Clostridium sordellii*: homology with *Clostridium difficile* cytotoxin B. *Gene* **161**:57–61.

67. **Guignot, J., M. Mock, and A. Fouet.** 1997. AtxA activates the transcription of genes harbored by both *Bacillus anthracis* virulence plasmids. *FEMS Microbiol. Lett.* **147**:203–207.

68. **Hacker, J., G. Blum Oehler, I. Muhldorfer, and H. Tschape.** 1997. Pathogenicity islands of virulent bacteria: structure, function and impact on microbial evolution. *Mol. Microbiol.* **23**:1089–1097.

69. **Hall, J. D., L. M. McCroskey, B. J. Pincomb, and C. L. Hatheway.** 1985. Isolation of an organism resembling *Clostridium barati* which produces type F botulinal toxin from an infant with botulism. *J. Clin. Microbiol.* **21**:654–655.

70. **Hambleton, P.** 1992. *Clostridium botulinum* toxins: a general review of involvement in disease, structure, mode of action and preparation for clinical use. *J. Neurol.* **239**:16–20.

71. **Hambleton, P., J. A. Carman, and J. Melling.** 1984. Anthrax: the disease in relation to vaccines. *Vaccine* **2**:125–132.

72. **Hammond, G. A., and J. L. Johnson.** 1995. The toxigenic element of *Clostridium difficile* strain VPI 10463. *Microb. Pathog.* **19**:203–213.

73. **Hanna, P.** 1998. Anthrax pathogenesis and host response. *Curr. Top. Microbiol. Immunol.* **225**:13–35.

74. **Hanna, P.** 1998. How anthrax kills. *Science* **280**:1671, 1673–1674.

75. **Hatheway, C. L.** 1990. Toxigenic clostridia. *Clin. Microbiol. Rev.* **3**:66–98.

76. **Hauser, D., M. Gibert, P. Boquet, and M. R. Popoff.** 1992. Plasmid localization of a type E botulinal neurotoxin gene homologue in toxigenic *Clostridium butyricum* strains, and absence of this gene in non-toxigenic *C. butyricum* strains. *FEMS Microbiol. Lett.* **78**:251–255.

77. **Hauser, D., M. Gibert, M. W. Eklund, P. Boquet, and M. R. Popoff.** 1993. Comparative analysis of C3 and botulinal neurotoxin genes and their environment in *Clostridium botulinum* types C and D. *J. Bacteriol.* **175**:7260–7268.

78. **Hauser, D., M. Gibert, J. C. Marvaud, M. W. Eklund, and M. R. Popoff.** 1995. Botulinal neurotoxin C1 complex genes, clostridial neurotoxin homology and genetic transfer in *Clostridium botulinum. Toxicon* **33**:515–526.

79. **Henderson, I., T. Davis, M. Elmore, and N. Minton.** 1997. The genetic basis of toxin production in *Clostridium botulinum* and *Clostridium tetani*, p. 261–294. *In* J. I. Rood, B. A. McClane, J. G. Songer, and R. W. Titball (ed.), *The Clostridia: Molecular Biology and Pathogenesis*. Academic Press, Ltd., London, United Kingdom.

80. **Hentges, D. J.** 1993. The anaerobic microflora of the human body. *Clin. Infect. Dis.* **16**(Suppl. 4): S175–S180.

81. **Hoffmaster, A. R., and T. M. Koehler.** 1997. The anthrax toxin activator gene *atxA* is associated with CO_2-enhanced nontoxin gene expression in *Bacillus anthracis. Infect. Immun.* **65**:3091–3099.

82. **Hofmann, F., A. Herrmann, E. Habermann, and C. von Eichel-Streiber.** 1995. Sequencing and analysis of the gene encoding the alpha-toxin of *Clostridium novyi* proves its homology to toxins A and B of *Clostridium difficile*. *Mol. Gen. Genet.* **247**:670–679.

83. **Hoyer, L. L., A. C. Hamilton, S. M. Steenbergen, and E. R. Vimr.** 1992. Cloning, sequencing and distribution of the *Salmonella typhimurium* LT2 sialidase gene, nanH, provides evidence for interspecies gene transfer. *Mol. Microbiol.* **6**:873–884.

84. **Hundsberger, T., V. Braun, M. Weidmann, P. Leukel, M. Sauerborn, and C. von Eichel-Streiber.** 1997. Transcription analysis of the genes tcdA-E of the pathogenicity locus of *Clostridium difficile*. *Eur. J. Biochem.* **244**:735–742.

85. **Hunter, S. E., I. N. Clarke, D. C. Kelly, and R. W. Titball.** 1992. Cloning and nucleotide sequencing of the *Clostridium perfringens* epsilon-toxin gene and its expression in *Escherichia coli*. *Infect. Immun.* **60**:102–110.

86. **Hutson, R. A., M. D. Collins, A. K. East, and D. E. Thompson.** 1994. Nucleotide sequence of the gene coding for non-proteolytic *Clostridium botulinum* type B neurotoxin: comparison with other clostridial neurotoxins. *Curr. Microbiol.* **28**:101–110.

87. **Hutson, R. A., D. E. Thompson, and M. D. Collins.** 1993. Genetic interrelationships of saccharolytic *Clostridium botulinum* types B, E and F and related clostridia as revealed by small-subunit rRNA gene sequences. *FEMS Microbiol. Lett.* **108**:103–110.

88. **Inal, J. M., and K. V. Karunakaran.** 1996. phi 20, a temperate bacteriophage isolated from *Bacillus anthracis* exists as a plasmidial prophage. *Curr. Microbiol.* **32**:171–175.

89. **Inoue, S., M. Sugai, Y. Murooka, S. Y. Paik, Y. M. Hong, H. Ohgai, and H. Suginaka.** 1991. Molecular cloning and sequencing of the epidermal cell differentiation inhibitor gene from *Staphylococcus aureus*. *Biochem. Biophys. Res. Commun.* **174**:459–464.

90. **Jackson, P. J., E. A. Walthers, A. S. Kalif, K. L. Richmond, D. M. Adair, K. K. Hill, C. R. Kuske, G. L. Andersen, K. H. Wilson, M. Hugh Jones, and P. Keim.** 1997. Characterization of the variable-number tandem repeats in *vrrA* from different *Bacillus anthracis* isolates. *Appl. Environ. Microbiol.* **63**: 1400–1405.

91. **Just, I., C. Mohr, G. Schallehn, L. Menard, J. R. Didsbury, J. Vandekerckhove, J. van Damme, and K. Aktories.** 1992. Purification and characterization of an ADP-ribosyltransferase produced by *Clostridium limosum*. *J. Biol. Chem.* **267**:10274–10280.

92. **Just, I., G. Schallehn, and K. Aktories.** 1992. ADP-ribosylation of small GTP-binding proteins by *Bacillus cereus*. *Biochem. Biophys. Res. Commun.* **183**:931–936.

93. **Just, I., J. Selzer, C. von Eichel-Streiber, and K. Aktories.** 1995. The low molecular mass GTP-binding protein Rho is affected by toxin A from *Clostridium difficile*. *J. Clin. Investig.* **95**:1026–1031.

94. **Just, I., J. Selzer, M. Wilm, C. von Eichel Streiber, M. Mann, and K. Aktories.** 1995. Glucosylation of Rho proteins by *Clostridium difficile* toxin B. *Nature* **375**:500–503.

95. **Kamiya, S., H. Ogura, X. Q. Meng, and S. Nakamura.** 1992. Correlation between cytotoxin production and sporulation in *Clostridium difficile*. *J. Med. Microbiol.* **37**:206–210.

96. **Kaneko, T., R. Nozaki, and K. Aizawa.** 1978. Deoxyribonucleic acid relatedness between *Bacillus anthracis, Bacillus cereus* and *Bacillus thuringiensis*. *Microbiol. Immunol.* **22**:639–641.

97. **Kaspar, R. L., and D. L. Robertson.** 1987. Purification and physical analysis of *Bacillus anthracis* plasmids pXO1 and pXO2. *Biochem. Biophys. Res. Commun.* **149**:362–368.

98. **Katayama, S., B. Dupuy, G. Daube, B. China, and S. T. Cole.** 1996. Genome mapping of *Clostridium perfringens* strains with I-CeuI shows many virulence genes to be plasmid-borne. *Mol. Gen. Genet.* **251**: 720–726.

99. **Katayama, S., B. Dupuy, T. Garnier, and S. T. Cole.** 1995. Rapid expansion of the physical and genetic map of the chromosome of *Clostridium perfringens* CPN50. *J. Bacteriol.* **177**:5680–5685.

100. **Keim, P., A. Kalif, J. Schupp, K. Hill, S. E. Travis, K. Richmond, D. M. Adair, M. Hugh Jones, C. R. Kuske, and P. Jackson.** 1997. Molecular evolution and diversity in *Bacillus anthracis* as detected by amplified fragment length polymorphism markers. *J. Bacteriol.* **179**:818–824.

101. **Kimura, K., N. Fujii, K. Tsuzuki, T. Murakami, T. Indoh, N. Yokosawa, K. Takeshi, B. Syuto, and K. Oguma.** 1990. The complete nucleotide sequence of the gene coding for botulinum type C1 toxin in the C-ST phage genome. *Biochem. Biophys. Res. Commun.* **171**:1304–1311.

102. **Klimpel, K. R., N. Arora, and S. H. Leppla.** 1994. Anthrax toxin lethal factor contains a zinc metalloprotease consensus sequence which is required for lethal toxin activity. *Mol. Microbiol.* **13**:1093–1100.

103. **Koehler, T. M., Z. Dai, and M. Kaufman Yarbray.** 1994. Regulation of the *Bacillus anthracis* protective antigen gene: CO_2 and a *trans*-acting element activate transcription from one of two promoters. *J. Bacteriol.* **176:**586–595.

104. **Kokai Kun, J. F., J. G. Songer, J. R. Czeczulin, F. Chen, and B. A. McClane.** 1994. Comparison of Western immunoblots and gene detection assays for identification of potentially enterotoxigenic isolates of *Clostridium perfringens. J. Clin. Microbiol.* **32:**2533–2539.

105. **Kramer, J. M., and R. J. Gilbert.** 1989. *Bacillus cereus* and other *Bacillus* species, p. 21–70. *In* M. P. Doyle (ed.), *Foodborne Bacterial Pathogens.* Marcel Dekker, New York, N.Y.

106. **Kronstad, J. W., and H. R. Whiteley.** 1984. Inverted repeat sequences flank a *Bacillus thuringiensis* crystal protein gene. *J. Bacteriol.* **160:**95–102.

107. **Kubota, T., S. Shirakawa, S. Kozaki, E. Isogai, H. Isogai, K. Kimura, and N. Fujii.** 1996. Mosaic type of the nontoxic-nonhemagglutinin component gene in *Clostridium botulinum* type A strain isolated from infant botulism in Japan. *Biochem. Biophys. Res. Commun.* **224:**843–848.

108. **Kubota, T., N. Yonekura, Y. Hariya, E. Isogai, H. Isogai, K. Amano, and N. Fujii.** 1998. Gene arrangement in the upstream region of *Clostridium botulinum* type E and *Clostridium butyricum* BL6340 progenitor toxin genes is different from that of other types. *FEMS Microbiol. Lett.* **158:**215–221.

109. **LaForce, F. M.** 1994. Anthrax. *Clin. Infect. Dis.* **19:**1009–1013.

110. **Laird, W. J., W. Aaronson, R. P. Silver, W. H. Habig, and M. C. Hardegree.** 1980. Plasmid-associated toxigenicity in *Clostridium tetani. J. Infect. Dis.* **142:**623.

111. **Lawrence, D., S. Heitefuss, and H. S. Seifert.** 1991. Differentiation of *Bacillus anthracis* from *Bacillus cereus* by gas chromatographic whole-cell fatty acid analysis. *J. Clin. Microbiol.* **29:**1508–1512.

112. **Lawson, P. A., P. Llop Perez, R. A. Hutson, H. Hippe, and M. D. Collins.** 1993. Towards a phylogeny of the clostridia based on 16S rRNA sequences. *FEMS Microbiol. Lett.* **113:**87–92.

113. **Lee, C. A.** 1996. Pathogenicity islands and the evolution of bacterial pathogens. *Infect. Agents Dis.* **5:**1–7.

114. **Leimeister Wachter, M., E. Domann, and T. Chakraborty.** 1992. The expression of virulence genes in *Listeria monocytogenes* is thermoregulated. *J. Bacteriol.* **174:**947–952.

115. **Leppla, S. H.** 1982. Anthrax toxin edema factor: a bacterial adenylate cyclase that increases cyclic AMP concentrations of eukaryotic cells. *Proc. Natl. Acad. Sci. USA* **79:**3162–3166.

116. **Leppla, S. H.** 1995. Anthrax toxins, p. 543–567. *In* J. Moss, B. Iglewski, M. Vaughan, and A. T. Tu (ed.), *Handbook of Natural Toxins,* vol. 8. Marcel Dekker, New York, N.Y.

117. **Leppla, S. H.** 1984. *Bacillus anthracis* calmodulin-dependent adenylate cyclase: chemical and enzymatic properties and interactions with eucaryotic cells. *Adv. Cyclic Nucleotide Protein Phosphorylation Res.* **17:**189–198.

118. **Leppla, S. H.** 1988. Production and purification of anthrax toxin. *Methods Enzymol.* **165:**103–116.

119. **Lereclus, D., J. Mahillon, G. Menou, and M. M. Lecadet.** 1986. Identification of Tn4430, a transposon of *Bacillus thuringiensis* functional in *Escherichia coli. Mol. Gen. Genet.* **204:**52–57.

120. **Lereclus, D., G. Menou, and M. M. Lecadet.** 1983. Isolation of a DNA sequence related to several plasmids from *Bacillus thuringiensis* after a mating involving the *Streptococcus faecalis* plasmid pAM beta 1. *Mol. Gen. Genet.* **191:**307–313.

121. **Lereclus, D., J. Ribier, A. Klier, G. Menou, and M. M. Lecadet.** 1984. A transposon-like structure related to the delta-endotoxin gene of *Bacillus thuringiensis. EMBO J.* **3:**2561–2567.

122. **Lereclus, D., M. Vallade, J. Chaufaux, O. Arantes, and S. Rambaud.** 1992. Expansion of insecticidal host range of *Bacillus thuringiensis* by in vivo genetic recombination. *Bio/Technology* **10:**418–421.

123. **Lesieur, C., B. Vecsey Semjen, L. Abrami, M. Fivaz, and F. Gisou van der Goot.** 1997. Membrane insertion: the strategies of toxins. *Mol. Membr. Biol.* **14:**45–64.

124. **Lund, T., and P. E. Granum.** 1996. Characterisation of a non-haemolytic enterotoxin complex from *Bacillus cereus* isolated after a foodborne outbreak. *FEMS Microbiol. Lett.* **141:**151–156.

125. **Mahillon, J., and M. Chandler.** 1998. Insertion sequences. *Microbiol. Mol. Biol. Rev.* **62:**725–774.

126. **Mahillon, J., R. Rezsohazy, B. Hallet, and J. Delcour.** 1994. IS231 and other *Bacillus thuringiensis* transposable elements: a review. *Genetica* **93:**13–26.

127. **Makino, S., I. Uchida, N. Terakado, C. Sasakawa, and M. Yoshikawa.** 1989. Molecular characterization and protein analysis of the cap region, which is essential for encapsulation in *Bacillus anthracis. J. Bacteriol.* **171:**722–730.

128. **Marvaud, J. C., M. Gibert, K. Inoue, V. Fujinaga, K. Oguma, and M. R. Popoff.** 1998. botR/A is a

positive regulator of botulinum neurotoxin and associated non-toxin protein genes in *Clostridium botulinum* A. *Mol. Microbiol.* **29:**1009–1018.

129. **Maurelli, A. T.** 1989. Temperature regulation of virulence genes in pathogenic bacteria: a general strategy for human pathogens? *Microb. Pathog.* **7:**1–10.

130. **McClane, B. A.** 1998. New insights into the genetics and regulation of expression of *Clostridium perfringens* enterotoxin. *Curr. Top. Microbiol. Immunol.* **225:**37–55.

131. **McCloy, E. W.** 1951. Studies on a lysogenic *Bacillus* strain. I. A bacteriophage specific for *Bacillus anthracis. J. Hyg.* **49:**114–125.

132. **McCroskey, L. M., C. L. Hatheway, L. Fenicia, B. Pasolini, and P. Aureli.** 1986. Characterization of an organism that produces type E botulinal toxin but which resembles *Clostridium butyricum* from the feces of an infant with type E botulism. *J. Clin. Microbiol.* **23:**201–202.

133. **McDonel, J. L.** 1986. Toxins of *Clostridium perfringens* types A, B, C, D and E, p. 477–517. *In* F. Dorner and H. Drews (ed.), *Pharmacology of Bacterial Toxins.* Pergamon, Oxford, United Kingdom.

134. **McGaughey, W. H., F. Gould, and W. Gelernter.** 1998. Bt resistance management. *Nat. Biotechnol.* **16:**144–146.

135. **Meng, X., T. Karasawa, K. Zou, X. Kuang, X. Wang, C. Lu, C. Wang, K. Yamakawa, and S. Nakamura.** 1997. Characterization of a neurotoxigenic *Clostridium butyricum* strain isolated from the food implicated in an outbreak of food-borne type E botulism. *J. Clin. Microbiol.* **35:**2160–2162.

136. **Mesnage, S., E. Tosi Couture, P. Gounon, M. Mock, and A. Fouet.** 1998. The capsule and S-layer: two independent and yet compatible macromolecular structures in *Bacillus anthracis. J. Bacteriol.* **180:** 52–58.

137. **Mesnage, S., E. Tosi Couture, M. Mock, P. Gounon, and A. Fouet.** 1997. Molecular characterization of the *Bacillus anthracis* main S-layer component: evidence that it is the major cell-associated antigen. *Mol. Microbiol.* **23:**1147–1155.

138. **Meynell, E., and G. G. Meynell.** 1964. The roles of serum and carbon dioxide in capsule formation by *Bacillus anthracis. J. Gen. Microbiol.* **34:**153–164.

139. **Mikesell, P., B. E. Ivins, J. D. Ristroph, and T. M. Dreier.** 1983. Evidence for plasmid-mediated toxin production in *Bacillus anthracis. Infect. Immun.* **39:**371–376.

140. **Milne, J. C., D. Furlong, P. C. Hanna, J. S. Wall, and R. J. Collier.** 1994. Anthrax protective antigen forms oligomers during intoxication of mammalian cells. *J. Biol. Chem.* **269:**20607–20612.

141. **Moncrief, J. S., L. A. Barroso, and T. D. Wilkins.** 1997. Positive regulation of *Clostridium difficile* toxins. *Infect. Immun.* **65:**1105–1108.

142. **Moriishi, K., M. Koura, N. Abe, N. Fujii, Y. Fujinaga, K. Inoue, and K. Oguma.** 1996. Mosaic structures of neurotoxins produced from *Clostridium botulinum* types C and D organisms. *Biochim. Biophys. Acta* **1307:**123–126.

143. **Moriishi, K., M. Koura, N. Fujii, Y. Fujinaga, K. Inoue, B. Syuto, and K. Oguma.** 1996. Molecular cloning of the gene encoding the mosaic neurotoxin, composed of parts of botulinum neurotoxin types C1 and D, and PCR detection of this gene from *Clostridium botulinum* type C organisms. *Appl. Environ. Microbiol.* **62:**662–667.

144. **Müller, H. E.** 1992. Bacillaceae, p. 251–257. *In* F. Burkhardt (ed.), *Mikrobiologische Diagnostik.* Thieme Verlag, Stuttgart, Germany.

145. **Normore, W. M.** 1973. Guanine-plus-cytosine composition of the DNA of bacteria, fungi, algae, and protozoa, p. 585–740. *In* A. L. Laskin and H. A. Lechavalier (ed.), *Handbook of Microbiology,* vol. II. The Chemical Rubber Co., Washington, D.C.

146. **Ohyama, T., T. Watanabe, Y. Fujinaga, K. Inoue, H. Sunagawa, N. Fujii, K. Inoue, and K. Oguma.** 1995. Characterization of nontoxic-nonhemagglutinin component of the two types of progenitor toxin (M and L) produced by *Clostridium botulinum* type D CB-16. *Microbiol. Immunol.* **39:**457–465.

147. **Onderdonk, A. B., and S. D. Allen.** 1995. *Clostridium,* p. 574–586. *In* P. R. Murray, E. J. Baron, M. A. Pfaller, F. C. Tenover, and R. H. Yolken (ed.), *Manual of Clinical Microbiology,* 6th ed. ASM Press, Washington, D.C.

148. **Payne, D., and P. Oyston.** 1997. The *Clostridium perfringens* e-toxin, p. 439–447. *In* J. I. Rood, B. A. McClane, J. G. Songer, and R. W. Titball (ed.), *The Clostridia: Molecular Biology and Pathogenesis.* Academic Press, London, United Kingdom.

149. **Perelle, S., M. Gibert, P. Boquet, and M. R. Popoff.** 1993. Characterization of *Clostridium perfringens* iota-toxin genes and expression in *Escherichia coli. Infect. Immun.* **61:**5147–5156.

150. **Pezard, C., P. Berche, and M. Mock.** 1991. Contribution of individual toxin components to virulence of *Bacillus anthracis. Infect. Immun.* **59:**3472–3477.

151. **Pezard, C., M. Weber, J. C. Sirard, P. Berche, and M. Mock.** 1995. Protective immunity induced by *Bacillus anthracis* toxin-deficient strains. *Infect. Immun.* **63:**1369–1372.

152. **Popoff, M. R., E. Chaves Olarte, E. Lemichez, C. von Eichel Streiber, M. Thelestam, P. Chardin, D. Cussac, B. Antonny, P. Chavrier, G. Flatau, M. Giry, J. de Gunzburg, and P. Boquet.** 1996. Ras, Rap, and Rac small GTP-binding proteins are targets for *Clostridium sordellii* lethal toxin glucosylation. *J. Biol. Chem.* **271:**10217–10224.

153. **Popoff, M. R., and J. C. Marvaud.** 1999. Structural and genomic features of clostridial neurotoxins, p. 174–201. *In* J. E. Alouf and J. H. Freer (ed.), *Bacterial Protein Toxins: a Comprehensive Sourcebook.* Academic Press, London, United Kingdom.

154. **Portnoy, D. A., T. Chakraborty, W. Goebel, and P. Cossart.** 1992. Molecular determinants of *Listeria monocytogenes* pathogenesis. *Infect. Immun.* **60:**1263–1267.

155. **Poulet, S., D. Hauser, M. Quanz, H. Niemann, and M. R. Popoff.** 1992. Sequences of the botulinal neurotoxin E derived from *Clostridium botulinum* type E (strain Beluga) and *Clostridium butyricum* (strains ATCC 43181 and ATCC 43755). *Biochem. Biophys. Res. Commun.* **183:**107–113.

156. **Price, S. B., C. J. Phelps, T. D. Wilkins, and J. L. Johnson.** 1987. Cloning of the carbohydrate-binding portion of the toxin A gene of *Clostridium difficile. Curr. Microbiol.* **16:**55–60.

157. **Priest, F. G.** 1993. Systematics and ecology of *Bacillus,* p. 3–16. *In* A. U. Sonenshein, J. Hoch, and R. Losick (ed.), Bacillus subtilis *and Other Gram-Positive Bacteria.* American Society for Microbiology, Washington, D.C.

158. **Ravizzola, G., N. Manca, F. Dima, C. Signorini, E. Garrafa, and A. Turano.** 1998. Isolation of a *Clostridium* exotoxin producer other than *Clostridium difficile* from a patient with diarrhea. *J. Clin. Microbiol.* **36:**2396.

159. **Reddy, A., L. Battisti, and C. B. Thorne.** 1987. Identification of self-transmissible plasmids in four *Bacillus thuringiensis* subspecies. *J. Bacteriol.* **169:**5263–5270.

160. **Robertson, D. L., M. T. Tippetts, and S. H. Leppla.** 1988. Nucleotide sequence of the *Bacillus anthracis* edema factor gene (*cya*): a calmodulin-dependent adenylate cyclase. *Gene* **73:**363–371.

161. **Roggentin, T., and R. Schauer.** 1997. Clostridial sialidases, p. 423–437. *In* J. I. Rood, B. A. McClane, J. G. Songer, and R. W. Titball (ed.), *The Clostridia: Molecular Biology and Pathogenesis.* Academic Press, London, United Kingdom.

162. **Rood, J. I.** 1998. Virulence genes of *Clostridium perfringens. Annu. Rev. Microbiol.* **52:**333–360.

163. **Rood, J. I., and S. T. Cole.** 1991. Molecular genetics and pathogenesis of *Clostridium perfringens. Microbiol. Rev.* **55:**621–648.

164. **Ruhfel, R. E., N. J. Robillard, and C. B. Thorne.** 1984. Interspecies transduction of plasmids among *Bacillus anthracis, B. cereus,* and *B. thuringiensis. J. Bacteriol.* **157:**708–711.

165. **Ryan, P. A., J. D. Macmillan, and B. A. Zilinskas.** 1997. Molecular cloning and characterization of the genes encoding the L1 and L2 components of hemolysin BL from *Bacillus cereus. J. Bacteriol.* **179:** 2551–2556.

166. **Sakaguchi, G., I. Ohishi, and S. Kozaki.** 1988. Botulism—structure and chemistry of botulinum, p. 191–216. *In* M. C. Hardegree and A. T. Tu (ed.), *Handbook of Natural Toxins,* vol. 4. Marcel Dekker, Inc., New York, N.Y.

167. **Sauerborn, M., and C. von Eichel-Streiber.** 1990. Nucleotide sequence of *Clostridium difficile* toxin A. *Nucleic Acids Res.* **18:**1629–1630.

168. **Schallehn, G., M. W. Eklund, and H. Brandis.** 1980. Phage conversion of *Clostridium novyi* type A. *Zentbl. Bakteriol. Microbiol. Hyg. Ser. A.* **247:**95–100.

169. **Schiavo, G., and C. Montecucco.** 1997. The structure and mode of action of botulinum and tetanus toxin, p. 295–322. *In* J. I. Rood, B. A. McClane, J. G. Songer, and R. W. Titball (ed.), *The Clostridia: Molecular Biology and Pathogenesis.* Academic Press, London, United Kingdom.

170. **Schiavo, G., C. C. Shone, O. Rossetto, F. C. Alexander, and C. Montecucco.** 1993. Botulinum neurotoxin serotype F is a zinc endopeptidase specific for VAMP/synaptobrevin. *J. Biol. Chem.* **268:**11516–11519.

171. **Schnepf, E., N. Crickmore, J. Van Rie, D. Lereclus, J. Baum, J. Feitelson, D. R. Zeigler, and D. H. Dean.** 1998. *Bacillus thuringiensis* and its pesticidal crystal proteins. *Microbiol. Mol. Biol. Rev.* **62:** 775–806.

172. **Selzer, J., F. Hofmann, G. Rex, M. Wilm, M. Mann, I. Just, and K. Aktories.** 1996. *Clostridium*

novyi alpha-toxin-catalyzed incorporation of GlcNAc into Rho subfamily proteins. *J. Biol. Chem.* **271:** 25173–25177.

173. **Sirard, J. C., M. Mock, and A. Fouet.** 1994. The three *Bacillus anthracis* toxin genes are coordinately regulated by bicarbonate and temperature. *J. Bacteriol.* **176:**5188–5192.

174. **Somers, E., and B. R. DasGupta.** 1991. *Clostridium botulinum* types A, B, C1, and E produce proteins with or without hemagglutinating activity: do they share common amino acid sequences and genes? *J Protein Chem.* **10:**415–425.

175. **Songer, J. G.** 1997. Clostridial diseases of animals, p. 153–182. *In* J. I. Rood, B. A. McClane, J. G. Songer, and R. W. Titball (ed.), *The Clostridia: Molecular Biology and Pathogenesis.* Academic Press, London, United Kingdom.

176. **Stepanov, A. S., S. V. Gavrilov, O. B. Puzanova, T. M. Grigor'eva, and R. R. Azizbekian.** 1989. Plasmid transduction by *Bacillus anthracis* bacteriophage CP54. *Mol. Gen. Mikrobiol. Virusol.* **1:**14–19.

177. **Strauss, E.** 1998. New clue to how anthrax kills. *Science* **280:**676.

178. **Strom, M. S., M. W. Eklund, and F. T. Poysky.** 1984. Plasmids in *Clostridium botulinum* and related *Clostridium* species. *Appl. Environ. Microbiol.* **48:**956–963.

179. **Sugai, M., K. Hashimoto, A. Kikuchi, S. Inoue, H. Okumura, K. Matsumoto, Y. Goto, H. Ohgai, K. Moriishi, B. Syuto, et al.** 1992. Epidermal cell differentiation inhibitor ADP-ribosylates small GTP-binding proteins and induces hyperplasia of epidermis. *J. Biol. Chem.* **267:**2600–2604.

180. **Sugiyama, H.** 1980. *Clostridium botulinum* neurotoxin. *Microbiol. Rev.* **44:**419–448.

181. **Thompson, D. E., J. K. Brehm, J. D. Oultram, T. J. Swinfield, C. C. Shone, T. Atkinson, J. Melling, and N. P. Minton.** 1990. The complete amino acid sequence of the *Clostridium botulinum* type A neurotoxin, deduced by nucleotide sequence analysis of the encoding gene. *Eur. J. Biochem.* **189:**73–81.

182. **Thompson, D. E., R. A. Hutson, A. K. East, D. Allaway, M. D. Collins, and P. T. Richardson.** 1993. Nucleotide sequence of the gene coding for *Clostridium barati* type F neurotoxin: comparison with other clostridial neurotoxins. *FEMS Microbiol. Lett.* **108:**175–182.

183. **Thorne, C. B.** 1993. *Bacillus anthracis*, p. 113–124. *In* A. L. Sonenshein, J. A. Hoch, and R. Losick (ed.), Bacillus subtilis *and Other Gram-Positive Bacteria.* American Society for Microbiology, Washington, D.C.

184. **Thorne, C. B.** 1985. Genetics of *Bacillus anthracis*, p. 56–62. *In* L. Leive, P. F. Bonventre, J. A. Morello, S. Schlesinger, S. D. Silver, and H. C. Wu (ed.), *Microbiology—1985.* American Society for Microbiology, Washington, D.C.

185. **Thorne, C. B.** 1968. Transduction in *Bacillus cereus* and *Bacillus anthracis. Bacteriol. Rev.* **32:**358–361.

186. **Thorne, C. B.** 1978. Transduction in *Bacillus thuringiensis. Appl. Environ. Microbiol.* **35:**1109–1115.

187. **Tippetts, M. T., and D. L. Robertson.** 1988. Molecular cloning and expression of the *Bacillus anthracis* edema factor toxin gene: a calmodulin-dependent adenylate cyclase. *J. Bacteriol.* **170:**2263–2266.

188. **Titball, R. W.** 1993. Bacterial phospholipases C. *Microbiol. Rev.* **57:**347–366.

189. **Titball, R. W.** 1997. Clostridial phospholipases, p. 223–242. *In* J. I. Rood, B. A. McClane, J. G. Songer, and R. W. Titball (ed.), *The Clostridia: Molecular Biology and Pathogenesis.* Academic Press, London, United Kingdom.

190. **Turnbull, P. C., R. A. Hutson, M. J. Ward, M. N. Jones, C. P. Quinn, N. J. Finnie, C. J. Duggleby, J. M. Kramer, and J. Melling.** 1992. *Bacillus anthracis* but not always anthrax. *J. Appl. Bacteriol.* **72:** 21–28.

191. **Turnbull, P. C., and J. M. Kramer.** 1991. *Bacillus*, p. 296–303. *In* A. Balows, W. J. Hausler, Jr., K. L. Herrmann, H. D. Isenberg, and H. J. Shadomy (ed.), *Manual of Clinical Microbiology*, 5th ed. American Society for Microbiology, Washington, D.C.

192. **Turnbull, P. C. B., and J. M. Kramer.** 1995. *Bacillus*, p. 349–359. *In* P. R. Murray, E. J. Baron, M. A. Pfaller, F. C. Tenover, and R. H. Yolken (ed.), *Manual of Clinical Microbiology,* 6th ed. ASM Press, Washington, D.C.

193. **Uchida, I., J. M. Hornung, C. B. Thorne, K. R. Klimpel, and S. H. Leppla.** 1993. Cloning and characterization of a gene whose product is a trans-activator of anthrax toxin synthesis. *J. Bacteriol.* **175:**5329–5338.

194. **Uchida, I., S. Makino, C. Sasakawa, M. Yoshikawa, C. Sugimoto, and N. Terakado.** 1993. Identification of a novel gene, *dep*, associated with depolymerization of the capsular polymer in *Bacillus anthracis. Mol. Microbiol.* **9:**487–496.

195. **Van Damme Jongsten, M., J. Rodhouse, R. J. Gilbert, and S. Notermans.** 1990. Synthetic DNA probes for detection of enterotoxigenic *Clostridium perfringens* strains isolated from outbreaks of food poisoning. *J. Clin. Microbiol.* **28:**131–133.

196. **Vietri, N. J., R. Marrero, T. A. Hoover, and S. L. Welkos.** 1995. Identification and characterization of a trans-activator involved in the regulation of encapsulation by *Bacillus anthracis*. *Gene* **152:**1–9.

196a.**von Eichel-Streiber, C.** Unpublished data.

197. **von Eichel-Streiber, C., P. Boquet, M. Sauerborn, and M. Thelestam.** 1996. Large clostridial cytotoxins—a family of glycosyltransferases modifying small GTP-binding proteins. *Trends Microbiol.* **4:** 375–382.

198. **von Eichel-Streiber, C., D. Suckau, M. Wachter, and U. Hadding.** 1989. Cloning and characterization of overlapping DNA fragments of the toxin A gene of *Clostridium difficile*. *J. Gen. Microbiol.* **135:**55–64.

199. **Weickert, M. J., G. H. Chambliss, and H. Sugiyama.** 1986. Production of toxin by *Clostridium botulinum* type A strains cured by plasmids. *Appl. Environ. Microbiol.* **51:**52–56.

200. **Welkos, S. L.** 1991. Plasmid-associated virulence factors of non-toxigenic (pX01 −) *Bacillus anthracis*. *Microb. Pathog.* **10:**183–198.

201. **Welkos, S. L., J. R. Lowe, F. Eden McCutchan, M. Vodkin, S. H. Leppla, and J. J. Schmidt.** 1988. Sequence and analysis of the DNA encoding protective antigen of *Bacillus anthracis*. *Gene* **69:**287–300.

202. **Welkos, S. L., N. J. Vietri, and P. H. Gibbs.** 1993. Non-toxigenic derivatives of the Ames strain of *Bacillus anthracis* are fully virulent for mice: role of plasmid pX02 and chromosome in strain-dependent virulence. *Microb. Pathog.* **14:**381–388.

203. **Whelan, S. M., M. J. Elmore, N. J. Bodsworth, T. Atkinson, and N. P. Minton.** 1992. The complete amino acid sequence of the *Clostridium botulinum* type-E neurotoxin, derived by nucleotide-sequence analysis of the encoding gene. *Eur. J. Biochem.* **204:**657–667.

204. **Willems, A., A. K. East, P. A. Lawson, and M. D. Collins.** 1993. Sequence of the gene coding for the neurotoxin of *Clostridium botulinum* type A associated with infant botulism: comparison with other clostridial neurotoxins. *Res. Microbiol.* **144:**547–556.

205. **Wilson, K. H.** 1993. The microecology of *Clostridium difficile*. *Clin. Infect. Dis.* **16**(Suppl. 4)**:**S214–S218.

206. **Yelton, D. B., and C. B. Thorne.** 1971. Comparison of *Bacillus cereus* bacteriophages CP-51 and CP-53. *J. Virol.* **8:**242–253.

207. **Yelton, D. B., and C. B. Thorne.** 1970. Transduction in *Bacillus cereus* by each of two bacteriophages. *J. Bacteriol.* **102:**573–579.

208. **Zhou, Y., H. Sugiyama, and E. A. Johnson.** 1993. Transfer of neurotoxigenicity from *Clostridium butyricum* to a nontoxigenic *Clostridium botulinum* type E-like strain. *Appl. Environ. Microbiol.* **59:**3825–3831.

209. **Zhou, Y., H. Sugiyama, H. Nakano, and E. A. Johnson.** 1995. The genes for the *Clostridium botulinum* type G toxin complex are on a plasmid. *Infect. Immun.* **63:**2087–2091.

Pathogenicity Islands and Other Mobile Virulence Elements
Edited by J. B. Kaper and J. Hacker
© 1999 American Society for Microbiology, Washington, D.C.

Chapter 14

Mobile Elements, Phages, and Genomic Islands of Staphylococci and Streptococci

Knut Ohlsen, Wilma Ziebuhr, Werner Reichardt, Wolfgang Witte, Friedrich Götz, and Jörg Hacker

INTRODUCTION

Staphylococci and streptoccocci are gram-positive bacteria which are widespread in nature. Most species of both genera are harmless saprophytes. However, some species are dreaded pathogens, causing a range of severe infections. The most important pathogenic species of the two genera, *Staphylococcus aureus* and *Streptococcus pyogenes,* have been studied more extensively than most other bacterial pathogens by microbiologists and physicians. Remarkably, they have several features in common, including the production of superantigenic toxins, which cause pyogenic infections, and the production of a great variety of extracellular proteins, many of which are involved in pathogenicity.

Pathogenic Staphylococci

Most staphylococcal species occur as natural inhabitants of the skin and mucosal membranes of mammals, birds, and fish. However, staphylococci are also common human and animal pathogens. The most important pathogenic species is the coagulase-positive species *Staphylococcus aureus.* It causes a number of diseases in humans, including wound infections, superficial and deep infections of the skin, septicemia, pneumonia, osteomyelitis, and other infections of internal organs. In addition, individual strains of *S. aureus* produce a range of biologically highly active toxins which cause severe toxin-mediated diseases including food poisoning, toxic shock, and exfoliative diseases of the skin. The broad spectrum of diseases caused by *S. aureus* is associated with the presence of a number of

Knut Ohlsen, Wilma Ziebuhr, and Jörg Hacker • Institut für Molekulare Infektionsbiologie der Universität Würzburg, Röntgenring 11, 97070 Würzburg, Germany. *Werner Reichardt* • Institut für Experimentelle Mikrobiologie, Friedrich-Schiller-Universität Jena, Winzerlaer Str. 10, 07745 Jena, Germany. *Wolfgang Witte* • Robert-Koch-Institut, Bereich Wernigerode, Burgstr. 37, 38855 Wernigerode, Germany. *Friedrich Götz* • Mikrobielle Genetik, Universität Tübingen, Auf der Morgenstelle 28, 72076 Tübingen, Germany.

Table 1. Extracellular and surface-associated
proteins of *Staphylococcus aureus*

Extracellular proteins
  Membrane-damaging toxins
    α-, β-, γ-, and δ-hemolysins
  Staphylococcal superantigens
    Enterotoxins A–E, G, and H
    Toxic shock syndrome toxin 1
    Exfoliative toxins A and B
  Accessory extracellular proteins
    Coagulase
    Staphylokinase
    Hyaluronidase
    Nuclease
    Lipase

Surface-associated proteins
  Protein A
  Fibrinogen-binding protein (clumping factor)
  Fibronectin-binding protein
  Collagen-binding protein

surface and extracellular proteins (Table 1). Surface-associated proteins interact with host factors and mediate the attachment to matrix proteins, soluble factors, or host cells. They contribute to virulence by acting as adhesins and by evading host defense mechanisms. Extracellular proteins of *S. aureus* comprise a variety of proteins which are associated with the invasion by bacteria of host tissues and cells. Other proteins, including the entero-toxins, the epidermiolytic toxins, and toxic shock syndrome toxin 1 (TSST-1), are powerful T-cell stimulators. They act as bacterial superantigens. Many extracellular and surface-associated proteins involved in pathogenesis are controlled by global regulatory elements such as accessory gene regulator (*agr*) (88) and staphylococcal accessory regulator (*sar*) (19). *agr* encodes a two-component signaling pathway whose activating ligand is an *agr*-encoded autoinducing peptide (53). In addition, environmental factors including tempera-ture, osmolarity, glucose, oxygen, and subinhibitory concentrations of antibiotics modulate the expression of virulence genes (39, 57, 89, 90).

Currently, the heterogeneous group of coagulase-negative staphylococci (CoNS) con-sists of 31 species. Most of these bacteria have a low pathogenic potential and represent a substantial part of the saprophytic microflora of the skin and mucosa. In recent years, however, CoNS have emerged as pathogens, especially in immunocompromised patients with implanted medical devices. The most common species in polymer-associated infec-tions is *Staphylococcus epidermidis*. Individual strains of this species are capable of gener-ating biofilms on smooth surfaces, which is assumed to be a major virulence mechanism. Moreover, *S. epidermidis* exhibits a rapid variation of phenotypic properties including colony morphology, antibiotic susceptibility, biofilm formation, and biochemical profiles (82). Finally, nosocomial isolates of both *S. aureus* and CoNS are characterized by an increasing resistance to antibiotics, which is a challenge for the management of hospital-acquired infections.

Pathogenic Streptococci

Only a few serogroups of the genus *Streptococcus* are known to cause diseases, with the most important pathogens being *Streptococcus pyogenes* (Lancefield group A [GAS]), *Streptococcus agalactiae* (Lancefield group B [GBS]), and *Streptococcus pneumoniae* (pneumococcus).

By far the largest number of streptococcal infections in humans are caused by *S. pyogenes* (GAS). Acute (and recurrent) pharyngitis, impetigo (pyoderma), and more severe manifestations of streptococcal infection such as otitis, retropharyngeal abscess, gangrene, puerperal sepsis, scarlet fever, necrotizing fasciitis, and the streptococcal toxic shock-like syndrome show the broad range of clinical symptoms due to skin and mucus membrane infections and to deep connective-tissue infections and septicemia. Moreover, *S. pyogenes* is responsible for two nonsuppurative sequelae, acute rheumatic fever and acute glomerulonephritis. As with *Staphylococcus aureus,* the broad spectrum of diseases caused by *S. pyogenes* is associated with the presence of a great variety of extracellular and surface proteins (Table 2). Compared to *Staphylococcus aureus, S. pyogenes* has an enhanced capacity to invade connective tissues and survive and even propagate in human blood. In these cases, exotoxins (superantigens) are directly secreted into the bloodstream and thus may overstimulate lymphocytes, which in turn produce severe cytokine-mediated shocks (37).

Another very important virulence factor of group A streptococci is the M protein (36), which is primarily responsible for the resistance of GAS to phagocytosis by polymorphonuclear leukocytes. M protein has a helical structure of the tropomyosin type. It is currently considered to be the main cause of the above-mentioned postinfectious sequelae and possibly of myocarditis resulting from an autoimmune response.

In the past 15 years, the incidence and severity of clinical episodes involving both

Table 2. Extracellular and surface-associated proteins of *Streptococcus pyogenes*

Extracellular proteins
  Membrane-damaging toxins
    Streptolysins O and S
  Streptococcal superantigens (pyrogenic exotoxins)
    Pyrogenic (erythrogenic) exotoxin types A, C, G, H, and J
    Streptococcal mitogenic exotoxin Z
    Streptococcal superantigen
  Accessory extracellular proteins
    Streptococcal cysteine proteinase (pyrogenic exotoxin type B)
    C5a peptidase
    Apolipoproteinase (opacity factor)
    Streptokinase
    Hyaluronidase
    DNases

Surface-associated proteins
  M protein and M-related proteins (bind different plasma proteins, IgA, and IgG)
  Proteins H and G
  Fibronectin-binding proteins
  Collagen-binding proteins
  Plasminogen-binding proteins

invasive streptococcal infections and rheumatic fever have changed dramatically. After many decades with only rare association of streptococcal infections with systemic diseases, a ''new'' syndrome—streptococcal toxic shock syndrome—has been described (24). The resurgence of the ''old'' severe group A infections presents new incentives to study the still undetermined molecular epidemiology of this process (60).

S. agalactiae was originally described as a causative agent of bovine mastitis and was later found to be serologically identical to the members of Lancefield group B (GBS). With a growing incidence in neonates since 1960, GBS has emerged as one of the major causes of sepsis and meningitis, with a mortality rate of up to 10% and with a 25 to 50% rate of serious long-term neurologic sequelae among survivors of meningitis (5). The major virulence factor of GBS is the type-specific capsular polysaccharide that confers resistance to phagocytosis on the infecting strains (92).

S. pneumoniae is carried in the nasopharynx of up to 70% or more of healthy individuals. Particularly in young children and in the elderly, this organism can cause life-threatening invasive diseases such as pneumonia, septicemia, and meningitis, but it is also the most frequent causative agent of the less severe episodes of otitis media and sinusitis. As in *S. agalactiae,* the polysaccharide capsule of pneumococci is the major virulence factor, conferring resistance to phagocytosis on the infecting strain. All fresh clinical isolates are encapsulated, with spontaneously nonencapsulated (rough) variants being completely avirulent. The experimental transformation of the smooth colony morphology trait in pneumococci was the first evidence obtained by Avery et al. that DNA is the genetic material (4). In addition to the polysaccharide capsule, several proteins are considered to be virulence factors; these include pneumolysin, autolysin, hyaluronidase, neuraminidase, and pneumococcal surface protein A (93, 100).

A striking feature of pneumococci is their natural competence. The components of the competence system are encoded by the *com* locus and consist of a cell density-dependent peptide pheromone and a two-component regulatory system. Natural competence of pneumococci is involved in the development of penicillin-resistant pneumococci, which are now encountered worldwide and whose spread is a matter of major concern.

ACCESSORY GENETIC ELEMENTS AND RESISTANCE DETERMINANTS

The genome of staphylococci and streptococci is not a rigid structure with stable genetic information but, instead, is rather dynamic. It reflects the ongoing processes of evolution. Mobile genetic elements, including plasmids, insertion elements (IS elements), transposons and phages, are nonessential parts of the genome; however, they play a major role in the plasticity of the genome and in the creation of new variants. In staphylococci, accessory genetic elements contribute to resistance to antibiotics, antiseptics, and disinfectants and are involved in genetic rearrangements and formation of virulence traits.

Insertion Sequence Elements and Transposons in Staphylococci

A number of transposons and insertion sequences have been identified in staphylococci. Most of them are associated with antibiotic resistance determinants. Currently, 12 staphylococcal IS elements have been analyzed and found to be members of three distinct IS

Table 3. Examples of *Staphylococcus* IS elements[a]

IS element	Origin	Family	Length (bp)	Reference
IS*431*/L	*S. aureus*(pI524)	IS6	788	6
IS*431*/R	*S. aureus*(pI524)	IS6	790	6
IS*431*mec	*S. aureus* BB270	IS6	790	111
IS*257*-1	*S. aureus*(pSH6)	IS6	791	108
IS*257*-2	*S. aureus*(pSH6)	IS6	790	108
IS*257*-3	*S. aureus*(pSH6)	IS6	789	108
IS*257*R1	*S. aureus* (Tn*4003* from pSK1)	IS6	790	107
IS*257*R2	*S. aureus* (Tn*4003* from pSK1)	IS6	789	107
IS*256*	*S. aureus* (Tn*4001* from pSK1)	IS*256*	1,324	15
IS*1181*	*S. aureus* BM3121	ISL*3*	1,512	27
IS*1182*	*S. aureus* BM3121	Not classified	1,864	28
IS*1272*	*S. haemolyticus* Y176	Not classified	1,935	3

[a] Data from reference 73.

families (Table 3) (73). They can form composite transposons or can be inserted into resistance-mediating plasmids. However, these elements also occur independently at multiple sites of the host genome.

The staphylococcal members of the IS6 family can be regarded as isoforms of the IS257R1 element. They are associated with either the methicillin resistance determinant or the trimethoprim resistance-mediating gene in Tn4003. Also, in other bacteria, many IS6-related elements form composite transposons. Transposition of these elements proceeds by a replicative mechanism involving the formation and resolution of cointegrates (73).

IS256 was originally identified in the aminoglycoside resistance transposon Tn4001, where two copies of the element flank the central resistance-mediating gene as inverted repeats (15, 68–70). The element is widespread in gentamicin-resistant clinical *Staphylococcus* and *Enterococcus* isolates (31, 106). In these isolates it also occurs in multiple copies independently of Tn4001 or related transposons. Based on structural similarities of the putative transposase, IS256 has been grouped with some other bacterial insertion elements in the *Mutator* family of maize (32). However, the mode of action of IS256 has not been elucidated. Recently, it was shown that IS256 can be involved in the phase variation of the polysaccharide intercellular adhesin expression in biofilm-forming strains of *Staphylococcus epidermidis* (131).

The transposons identified in staphylococci represent a heterogeneous group of elements (Table 4). For some of them, transposition has been demonstrated (Tn4001 and Tn552). For others, mobility is indicated by the presence of terminal inverted repeats and the presence of an open reading frame which is homologous to a transposase (Tn4003). For Tn4291, mobility has been demonstrated with regard to integration into plasmids along with transduction (120).

Plasmids in Staphylococci

Most naturally occurring staphylococcal strains contain plasmids. These plasmids can be grouped into three major classes (Table 5). Class I consists of small (1- to 1.5-kb)

Table 4. Antibiotic resistance transposons in *Staphylococcus aureus*

Transposon	Size (kb)	Resistance gene(s)[a]	Terminal repeat	Target specificity	Reference(s)
Tn*551*	5.3	*ermB*	40 bp	None	58
Tn*552* [Tn*4002*, Tn*4201*][b]	6.5	*blaZ*	116/121 bp	ND[c]	109
Tn*554*	6.7	*ermA, spc*	None	High	8
Tn*4001* [Tn*3851*, Tn*4031*]	4.7	*aacA-aphD*	IS*256*	ND	69
Tn*4003*	4.7	*dfrA*	IS*257*	ND	107
Tn*4291*	7.5	*mecA*	IS*257*	ND	41, 120
Tn*5405*	12	*aphA-3, aadE*	IS*1182*	ND	28
Tn*916* [Tn*918*, Tn*1545*]	18	*tetM*	28 bp	Low	25, 56

[a] Resistance genes confer resistance to antibiotics as follows: *aacA-aphD*, gentamicin, tobramycin, kanamycin; *aadE*, streptomycin; *aphA*, neomycin, kanamycin; *blaZ*, penicillin; *dfrA*, trimethoprim; *ermA, ermB*, MLS; *spc*, spectinomycin; *tetM*, tetracycline.

[b] Related transposons are shown in brackets.

[c] ND, not determined.

multicopy plasmids that either are cryptic or carry a single resistance determinant (87). Plasmids of this class mainly contribute to the development of resistance against oxytetracycline, chloramphenicol, and macrolides-lincosamides-streptogramins (MLS) (87, 122).

Plasmids of class II are 15 to 30 kb, have low copy numbers (4 to 6/cell), and mostly carry several resistance determinants: for β-lactam resistance on transposon Tn*552*, for mercury resistance on an element flanked by IS*431*, and for resistance to cadmium and lead and (in pI258) for MLS resistance of the *ermB* type on Tn*551* (68, 87, 112). Plasmids

Table 5. Examples of *Staphylococcus* resistance plasmids

Class	Plasmid	Resistance determinant(s)[a]	Size (kb)
I	pT181	*tetA*	4.4
	pC221	*cat*	4.6
	pS194	*str*	4.5
	pC194	*cat*	2.9
	pSK89	*smr*	2.4
	pUB110	*aadD, ble*	4.5
	pE194	*ermC*	3.7
II	pI258	*blaZ, arsB, arsC, cadA, merAB, ermB*	29.2
	pII147	*blaZ, arsB, arsC, cadA, cadB, merAB*	32.6
	pSK57	*blaZ, cadA, merAB, qacA*	28.8
III	pCRG1600	*blaZ, aacA-aphD, aadD, smr*	52.9
	pJE1	*aacA-aphD, aadD, dfrA, smr*	50.0
	pSK1	*aacA-aphD, dfrA, qacA*	28.4
	pSK41	*aacA-aphD, aadD, smr*	46.4

[a] Resistance genes confer resistance to the following antibiotics: *aacA-aphD*, gentamicin, tobramycin, kanamycin; *aadD*, neomycin, kanamycin, tobramycin, amikacin; *arsB, arsC*, arsenate, arsenite, antimony(III); *blaZ*, penicillin; *ble*, bleomycin; *cadA, cadB*, cadmium, zinc; *cat*, chloramphenicol; *dfrA*, trimethoprim; *ermB, ermC*, MLS; *merAB*, mercury; *qacA*, quaternary ammonium compounds, ethidium bromide, acriflavine, diamidines; *smr*, quaternary ammonium compounds, ethidium bromide; *str*, streptomycin; *tetA*, tetracycline.

of the pI258 type are nearly exclusively associated with an old epidemic hospital strain (strain 80/81) (123).

Class III plasmids are conjugative multiresistance plasmids and are therefore of special epidemiological interest. They are comparatively large (30 to 60 kb), and besides carrying determinants for conjugative transfer, they carry a number of different resistance determinants: for aminoglycoside resistance on Tn*4001*, for trimethoprim resistance on Tn*4003*, and for resistance to quaternary ammonium compounds and (in some cases) also for resistance to β-lactams on a transposon related to Tn*552* (68, 114). Plasmids carrying Tn*4001* emerged rather recently (9, 69). The association of resistance determinants in *S. aureus* with transposable elements has led to a clustering of resistance determinants on plasmids.

There is evidence that certain multiresistance plasmids have evolved by sequential acquisition of resistance determinants based on cointegration of target molecules (chromosomal stretches or small plasmids) (114). This process is mediated by IS*257*, which can already exist on the captured DNA sequence (e.g., plasmid pSK1, *drfA* [66]; plasmid pIP1156, *vat3, dfrA, blaZ, linA* [34]; plasmid pJ3358, *tetA, mupA* [84]; plasmid pSK41, *aacA-aphD, aadD, smr* [9]). Also, the insertion of plasmid pT181 into the *mec*-associated DNA of *S. aureus* ANS46 is most probably mediated by IS*257* (118).

Some staphylococcal plasmids carry bacteriocin-like genes. The approximately 40-kb plasmid pACK1 of *Staphylococcus simulans* bv. staphylolyticus ATCC 1362 carries the lysostaphin gene (*lss*), which codes for an extracellular glycylglycine endopeptidase, and the lysostaphin immunity factor gene (*lif*), which codes for products leading to an increase of the serine/glycine ratio of the interpeptide bridges of peptidoglycan (119). Interestingly, *lss* and *lif* are flanked by insertion sequences such as IS*257* and IS*1293*, suggesting that *S. simulans* bv. staphylolyticus received *lif* and *lss* by horizontal gene transfer.

The Staphylococcal *mecA* Region: a Resistance Island?

Methicillin-resistant *Staphylococcus aureus* (MRSA) and methicillin-resistant CoNS are major causes of nosocomial infections (17). High-level methicillin resistance in the pathogenic staphylococci has evolved by acquisition of the *mecA* gene, which encodes the additional penicillin binding protein 2a (PBP2a, also termed PBP2′). This protein has a low binding affinity for β-lactam antibiotics and is not present in susceptible staphylococci (2). PBP2a can perform the essential functions of β-lactam-susceptible PBPs in cross-linking the peptidoglycan of the bacterial cell wall. The *mecA* determinant is part of a 30- to 50-kb DNA element (*mec*) that is unique to methicillin-resistant staphylococci (2, 17). There is no equivalent region in methicillin-susceptible staphylococcal strains, suggesting that the *mec* fragment was acquired by horizontal gene transfer. The core sequence of *mec* DNA consists of *mecA*, 1 to 2 kb of downstream DNA followed by a copy of the insertion sequence element IS*431mec* (an IS*257*-like element), and the regulatory sequences *mecR1* and *mecI* (Fig. 1). In the upstream region of *mecI*, the transposon Tn*554* is often detectable. Finally, genes encoding resistance or entire integrated plasmids (pUB110 or pT181) are found in the 3′ region of *mecA*, indicating that recombination events between IS elements on the plasmids and a chromosomal copy of the element have occurred (2).

A number of possibilities have been proposed for the origin of *mec* (2, 33, 49, 116,

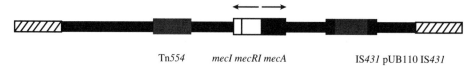

Figure 1. Molecular organization of the *mec* region in *S. aureus* R155. Chromosomal sequences flanking this region are shown as hatched boxes. The *mecA* gene encodes the additional PBP2a. The *mecA* regulatory genes are designated *mecRI* and *mecI*. Tn554 is a transposon carrying *ermA*, encoding inducible MLS resistance. IS431 (the same as IS257) elements flank the kanamycin-tobramycin resistance plasmid pUB110. The directions of transcription for the *mec* genes are indicated by arrows.

124). The evolutionary origin of the precursor *mecA* is probably a CoNS species, and the regulatory sequences, *mecI* and *mecR1,* are probably derived from the staphylococcal β-lactamase regulatory sequences, *blaI* and *blaR1.*

Recently, a *mecA*-like gene with 88% amino acid similarity and 80% DNA sequence identity to *mecA* has been identified in the animal species *Staphylococcus sciuri* (124). The *mecA* homolog is ubiquitous in this species, but its phenotype is methicillin susceptible (26). Interestingly, the 3′ region of *mecA* in *S. sciuri* also has a high homology (85% DNA identity) to the corresponding region of *S. aureus* (125). These and other data support the hypothesis that *S. sciuri* harbors an evolutionary precursor of the structural gene of PBP2a of methicillin-resistant strains of staphylococci.

In the evolution of the *mec* region, a series of events has occurred. Possibly, the *mecA* gene of *S. sciuri* or a related species was mobilized by IS elements or transposons and was fused to the β-lactamase regulatory genes. Additional DNA was acquired by integration of plasmids and plasmid-encoded resistance genes, by insertion of Tn554, and by integration of DNA and gene fragments of unknown origin. Specifically, the IS431 elements, which are derivatives of IS257, are known to have the capacity to capture and cluster resistance genes by homologous recombination and cointegrate formation. This could explain the multiple-drug-resistance phenotype of many methicillin-resistant staphylococcal strains.

In summary, the presence of one or more copies of IS431 within *mec* and directed repeats at the ends of *mecA,* as well as open reading frames within *mec* that may encode recombinases, suggests that *mecA* and its associated DNA are mobile elements. Moreover, identical *mec* sequences found in *S. aureus* and in CoNS imply that horizontal transfer of *mec* DNA has occurred (7, 111). Therefore, by analogy to the "pathogenicity island (PAI)" paradigm, the *mecA* region can be considered a "resistance island."

Mosaic Genes in *Streptococcus pneumoniae*: Penicillin Resistance and Competence

Since the late 1980s, the emergence and global spread of highly penicillin-resistant (and multidrug-resistant) strains of *Streptococcus pneumoniae* have caused severe clinical problems. Clinical isolates generate an enormous variability of PBPs, thus lowering or preventing β-lactam binding while preserving an intact enzymatic activity for murein biosynthesis. Six distinct PBPs have been identified in *S. pneumoniae*: PBP1a, PBP1b, PBP2x, PBP2a, PBP2b, and PBP3. Sequence alignment of PBP genes analyzed from resistant pneumococci reveals a mosaic structure in that cassettes with about 20% divergence have replaced the homologous sequences of genes analyzed in sensitive strains (29, 30, 78). In laboratory strains, the accumulation of point mutations and the subsequent exchange of cassette sequences can be monitored after incrementally increasing the selective pressure (63). In contrast, resistance in clinical isolates is the result of an evolutionary process that most probably involves different rounds of accumulation of point mutations and intraspecies and/or interspecies gene transfer enabled by the natural transformability of pneumococci (44, 113).

Another example of the generation of mosaic genes in pneumococci concerns genes of the competence operon (*com*). Pneumococci are naturally competent and therefore capable of taking up free DNA from the environment. The DNA taken up can in turn replace homologous regions of the recipient chromosome, leading to a new phenotype. This system for competence is highly regulated by an extracellular competence factor of 17 amino acids, the pneumococcal competence-stimulating peptide (CSP), which is produced by the pneumococci themselves with a pheromone-like (hormone) function depending on the cell density in batch cultures and most probably also in vivo (45). CSP is encoded by the *comC* gene of the competence operon. Two further genes, *comD* and *comE*, encode homologs of the histidine kinase sensor (receptor) and the response-regulating (RR) component of a characteristic procaryotic two-component regulatory system that can activate an intracellular phosphorylation cascade (95). The phosphorylated RR component in turn upregulates genes not directly linked to the competence operon (such as *recA*, *dinF*, *cinA*, and *oppA* to *oppC*).

The mosaic structure of *comC* and *comD* provides strong evidence that horizontal gene transfer events have occurred in the evolution of these genes. Similar alleles of the 3′ sequences of *comC* and the 5′ sequences of *comD* imply that they could have been transferred between strains and even species as functional cassettes (46). At least six allelic variants were detected in *Streptococcus mitis,* and four were found in *S. oralis.* This variability could overcome the restriction of one CSP-histidine kinase sensor system by changing the pherotype and rendering different cells inducible to competence by one and the same CSP. (Bacteria belong to a specific pherotype if they respond to a particular pheromone.) Phenotype switching, in turn, then may accelerate the variability of other mosaic genes like those coding for PBPs. Interestingly, the *agr* system of *Staphylococcus aureus,* which is responsible for the coordinate growth-phase-dependent regulation of unlinked virulence genes in this organism, shows a high homology to the competence induction system in *Streptococcus pneumoniae.* The *agr* regulon is also based on a cell density-triggered two-component system with a peptide pheromone as the signal molecule. Recently, different phenotypes were identified in *Staphylococcus aureus* as well (52), suggesting that similar evolutionary mechanisms to that for the *comCDE* system have occurred in the coevolution of pheromone and receptor in the *agr* system. However, whether interspecies recombinational exchanges of sequence blocks or even naturally competent *S. aureus* (110) are involved in the evolution of *agr* phenotypes remains a matter of speculation.

In summary, the mechanism of maintenance of genetic diversity by natural transformation of *S. pneumoniae* which enables intraspecies and interspecies horizontal gene transfer differs fundamentally from that described for the *mecA* region in staphylococci. In contrast to the *mecA* region, neither the mosaic gene structures of the *pbp* genes nor the mosaic structures of the *comC* and *comD* genes of the competence system resemble the features required to consider them part of a PAI. However, it is interesting that the *comCDE* operon is flanked by two tRNA loci and that the G+C content of the region differs from that of the adjoining chromosomal region (46). Since tRNA loci are the preferred integration sites for PAIs and the G+C content of a PAI normally differs from that of the overall chromosome (43), it is tempting to consider the *com* region of *S. pneumoniae* a "competence islet."

MOBILE GENETIC ELEMENTS AND VIRULENCE DETERMINANTS

Phages of Staphylococci

Most of the naturally occurring *Staphylococcus aureus* strains are polylysogenic. On the basis of virus morphology, staphylococcal bacteriophages are members of two groups of tailed phages: the families *Myoviridae* and *Siphoviridae*. Bacteriophages of *S. aureus* belong to seven serological groups, named A, B, C, D, F, G, and L. This phenotypic grouping correlates well with DNA sequence analyses (14, 51).

Various polyvalent staphylococcal phages, such as phage φ812 and phage φSK311, have been described in more detail (42, 91). These phages have an extremely broad host range. Ninety-five percent of a large *S. aureus* collection and 43% of CoNS strains were sensitive to these phages. The phages belong to morphological group A, consisting of the capsid, the isometric head, a rigid tail, a contractile sheath, and a base plate. The approximately 140-kb DNA genome is double stranded and is resistant to digestion by a large number of restriction enzymes.

The best-characterized staphylococcal phage is φ11, which has a 45-kb genome that is circularly permuted, terminally redundant, and flush ended (10). φ11 possesses *int* and *xis* genes, as does φL54a (127). Also, *rinA* and *rinB* functions, required for *int* expression, have been analyzed (126). For phages φ13 and φ42D, no *xis* function has been identified (16).

Staphylococcal phages are also involved in the expression of virulence determinants by mediating both positive and negative lysogenic conversion. The gene for staphylococcal enterotoxin A (*sea*) is carried by a polymorphic family of related temperate bacteriophages which mediate positive lysogenic conversion (13). Staphylococcal enterotoxins are a major cause of food poisoning. Moreover, enterotoxin A is a superantigen belonging to the class of pyrogenic toxins causing toxic shock syndrome. The second example of positive lysogenic conversion involves the gene for the staphylokinase (*sak*) of *S. aureus,* which is also carried by a bacteriophage (61). The *sak* determinant is preferentially associated with prophages of serogroup F.

On the other hand, staphylococcal phages can also mediate negative lysogenic conversion. The determinant encoding the β-toxin (*hlb*) is inactivated by insertion of a converting bacteriophage into the coding sequence (23). By a similar mechanism, the structural gene of the lipase (*geh*) is inactivated by bacteriophage L54a, the *att* site of which is composed of an 18-bp core sequence within the reading frame for lipase (64, 65). Moreover, double- or triple-converting bacteriophages have been described. One type negatively affects the expression of β-toxin but simultaneously confers the ability to produce staphylokinase (61), and a serotype F bacteriophage of *S. aureus* has been found to mediate the simultaneous triple-lysogenic conversion of enterotoxin A, staphylokinase, and β-toxin (22, 115).

Phages of Streptococci

Temperate phages of *Streptococcus pyogenes* are of particular interest because one class of major virulence factors, the streptococcal pyrogenic toxins, reside on their genomes. Based on the streptococcal genome data (for *S. pyogenes* SF370), at least three complete and several nearly complete bacteriophage genomes could be detected (35). So far, virtually all of the known pyrogenic exotoxin genes, except *speB,* which is not a superantigen, are located on phages or defective prophages. Mitomycin induces only one fully functional phage in the M1 *S. pyogenes* strain SF370, and this phage carries the *speC* gene (35). The classical pyrogenic (erythrogenic) exotoxins SpeA (erythrogenic toxin type A) and SpeC (erythrogenic toxin type C) of GAS are encoded by phage T12 (54, 121) and phage CS112 (55), respectively; both could be used for lysogenic conversion of nontoxigenic GAS strains (54, 55, 85). Interestingly, the *speA* gene was also found on two other group A phages involved in lysogenic conversion (128). This is of particular epidemiological importance since *speA* could be detected with significantly enhanced probability in clinical isolates from patients with toxic shock (83, 104, 117).

The association of *speA* with lysogenic phages is a strong indication of horizontal gene transfer; taking into account the very high degree of sequence similarity of SpeA to the staphylococcal enterotoxins B (SEB) and C1 (SEC1) (77), probable interspecies transfer via phage transduction has to be assumed. Consistent with this view is the location of the streptococcal exotoxin genes adjacent to the *attP* site on phage genomes (81), indicating that the exotoxin genes are of chromosomal origin and are picked up during abnormal excision. Genes of recently described new exotoxins (101) are also located on a cryptic phage genome (35). The high content of different prophages and defective phages offers an extremely rich source for the generation of new phages by homologous recombination with a potentially broadened host range. Thus, polylysogeny (with the possibility of phenotypic mixing and transfer induction) may be considered one of the main mechanisms used by streptococci for the intraspecies and interspecies gene transfer of virulence genes. Experimental evidence for all the mentioned phenomena associated with polylysogeny and their potential impact on clinical epidmiology (including the transduction of resistance plasmids) was published before the advent of molecular genetics (74–76).

Staphylococcal Pathogenicity Islands

Toxinogenic variants of *S. aureus* may produce TSST-1, which is a potent superantigen. The genetic origin of the gene encoding TSST-1 has been studied for many years. As already shown in 1983, toxin genes, termed *tst,* are present in toxinogenic *S. aureus* strains and are absent in TSST-1-negative variants (62). These data and the finding that *tst* undergoes phage-mediated transfer have stimulated speculations that the *tst* genes may be located on a distinct genetic element. Indeed, very recently, Lindsay et al. (67) were able to show that the *tst* gene is part of a 15.2-kb element which shares several features with PAIs of gram-negative bacteria (Fig. 2). The element was therefore termed the staphylococcal pathogenicity island (SaPI) (67). The island is flanked by 17-bp directly repeated sequences, and in addition to *tst* it carries other genes whose products are presumably involved in virulence. One gene termed *ent* has sequence homologies to genes encoding superantigens in staphylococci and streptococci; thus, it may encode a second superantigen in TSST-1 strains. Another open reading frame is homologous to the *vapE* gene, which

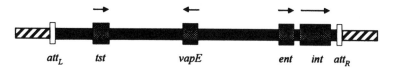

Figure 2. Physical map of the 15.2-kb SaPI1 region. Chromosomal sequences flanking this region are shown as hatched boxes, and the 17-bp direct repeats at left and right are shown as open boxes labelled *att*. The open reading frames encoding TSST-1 (*tst*), a homolog to VapE of *Dichelobacter nodosus* (*vapE*), a putative superantigen (*ent*), and an integrase (*int*) are shown as grey boxes. The directions of transcription for the genes are indicated by arrows.

is part of a putative PAI of *Dichelobacter nodosus*. Like other PAIs, the SaPI also carries a locus which is homologous to loci encoding members of the integrase family of recombinases of bacteriophages. Interestingly, the staphylococcal islands have the capacity to integrate into target sites which are identical to the directly repeated sequences at the ends of SaPIs in different *tst*-negative strains. While SaPI1 of strain RN4282 is integrated near the *tyrB* locus, SaPI2 of strain RN3984 was found to be located near the *trp* gene cluster. It is also obvious from the study of Lindsay et al. (67) that SaPIs represent mobile genetic elements which have the capacity to be excised and circulated by bacteriophages such as φ13 and 80α. Following excision, the islands are transduced to other strains with high frequencies. Since phage 80α has the capacity to transfer SaPI1 with a frequency of 10^{-1}, it is conceivable that the phage and the island represent genetically related elements. The integration of SaPI into the recipient genome is *recA* independent. Thus, the SaPIs belong to mobile genetic elements, and it is tempting to speculate that they may have been derived from bacteriophages. It is also very likely that other chromosomally encoded virulence and resistance gene clusters of staphylococci, including *mec* (see above), are parts of genomic islands similar to the *tst*-carrying SaPIs.

ica Operon of *Staphylococcus epidermidis*

Staphylococcus epidermidis infections are often associated with the use of medical devices. This is because certain strains of *S. epidermidis* are able to generate multilayered biofilms on smooth polymer surfaces. This process involves an extracellular polysaccharide substance (polysaccharide intercellular adhesin [PIA]), which is a major component of staphylococcal biofilms. The PIA is a β-1,6-linked *N*-acetylglucosaminyl polymer and mediates the intercellular adherence of the bacteria and the accumulation of a multilayered biofilm (47, 48, 71, 72). The production of PIA is associated with the expression of the *ica* gene cluster. This cluster comprises four genes (*icaA, icaD, icaB,* and *icaC*), which are organized in an operon structure (Fig. 3). *icaA* encodes an *N*-acetylglucosaminyl transferase, which is the key enzyme for the PIA synthesis. The gene product of *icaB* contains a typical signal sequence and consequently is secreted into the medium. Both the *icaC*- and *icaD*-encoded proteins exhibit properties of membrane proteins. The precise functions of IcaB, IcaC, and IcaD are just beginning to be understood. However, recent data suggest that coexpression of *icaA, icaD,* and *icaC* is absolutely required for the production of the PIA (40). The *ica* operon can be strongly induced by environmental influences (e.g., osmolarity, temperature, carbon sources, and subinhibitory antibiotic concentrations)

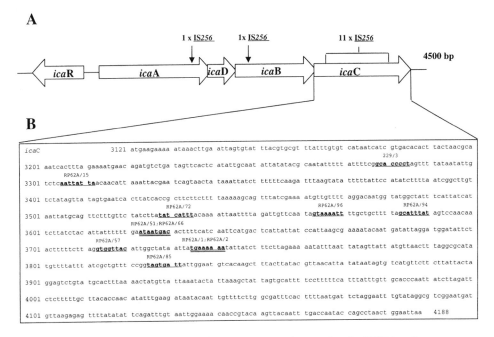

Figure 3. Genetic organization of the *ica* operon and target sites for IS*256* insertions. (A) Overview of the *ica* operon and the adjacent *icaR* gene. The number and positions of IS*256* insertions are marked by arrows. (B) Detailed representation of IS*256* insertions detected in the *icaC* nucleotide sequence of *S. epidermidis* RPG2A and *S. epidermidis* 229 (131). IS*256* target sites are underlined. Double lines mark identical target sequences identified in different insertional mutants. The designations above the targets indicate the individual names of the variants. Numbering of the nucleotide sequence corresponds to that of the published *ica* sequence (accession no. U43366).

(102). However, the components involved in *ica* regulation have not been analyzed in detail.

The evolutionary origin of the *ica* genes is not known, but this genetic information seems to be widespread in clinical *S. epidermidis* isolates (129). Most of these *ica*-positive isolates are multidrug-resistant strains. They carry a range of mobile genetic elements including IS elements, transposons, and plasmids. Recently, it was shown that *ica* expression can be influenced by a naturally occurring insertion sequence element. The PIA expression undergoes a phase variation process which, in a substantial number of variants, is caused by the alternating insertion and excision of IS*256* into different sites of the *ica* gene cluster. Specifically, the *icaC* gene seems to represent a preferred target for IS*256* insertions (Fig. 3B) (131).

At this stage of experimental work, initial conclusions may be drawn about how biofilm-forming *S. epidermidis* strains have evolved. There is a correlation between the occurrence of the *ica* genes and the presence of IS and other mobile genetic elements in *S. epidermidis*. Moreover, in these isolates, large IS-mediated rearrangements of the chromosome which also involve the *ica* gene cluster can be observed (130). It is tempting to speculate that this plasticity of the staphylococcal genome might have contributed to the evolution of biofilm formation in *S. epidermidis*.

mga Virulence Locus of *Streptococcus pyogenes*

In GAS, several important virulence factors are coordinately regulated in the so-called *vir* regulon, thereby responding to the changing conditions during the infectious process (21). Expression of the genes for these factors is positively regulated at the level of transcription by the regulator protein Mga (formerly *virR* or Mry) (94). Besides Mga, two other virulence regulator proteins of GAS have been described: the positively acting regulator protein RofA (38) and the negative regulator Nra (98). Virulence genes upregulated by Mga involve bacterial adhesion, invasion, and evasion of human host defenses. The *vir* regulon (Fig. 4) contains the M protein-encoding *emm* genes; the M-related genes *mrp* (alternative designation, *fcr*) and *enn* (which contributes to phagocytosis resistance by binding of immunoglobulin A [IgA]); the fibronectin-binding protein gene, *sof* (serum

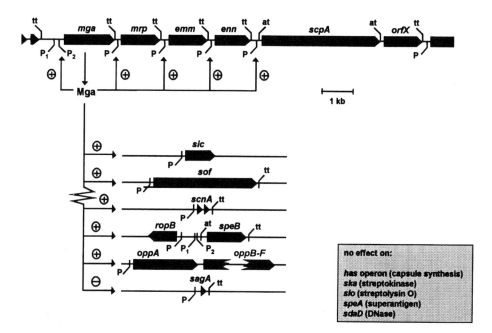

Figure 4. *mga* virulence locus of *S. pyogenes*. Genes controlled by the Mga regulator (*vir* regulon) are indicated by arrows. The genes *mga*, *mrp* (M-related), *emm*, *enn*, *scpA*, and *orfX* form the core *vir* regulon. Genes are transcribed monocistronically from promoters P positively regulated by Mga. The interrupted line indicates unknown direct or indirect regulation of the genes by the Mga regulator. tt indicates transcriptional terminators, and at indicates attenuator sites. The genes encode the following products: *mga*, virulence gene regulator; *mrp*, M-related protein; *emm*, M protein; *enn*, IgA-binding protein; *scpA*, streptococcal C5a peptidase; *sic*, streptococcal inhibitor of complement; *sof*, serum opacity factor; *scnA*, streptococcin; *ropB*, regulator of proteinase; *speA*, cysteine proteinase; *oppA* and *oppB–F*, oligopeptide peptidase; *sagA*, streptolysin S-associated gene (for details, see the text). Genes unaffected by Mga are indicated in the box.

opacity factor); the streptococcal inhibitor of complement gene, *sic* (1); and the complement-inactivating C5a peptidase gene, *scpA* (18). Furthermore, Mga exerts an autoregulation of its own gene, *mga*. The genes encoding the Mga regulator itself (*mga*), M protein (*emm*), M-related proteins (*mrp* and *enn*) and C5a peptidase (*scpA*) are clustered (Fig. 4), thus forming the core *vir* regulon. However, transcription occurs monocistronically except for the *orfX* gene in the downstream region of the cluster, which encodes a 385-amino-acid protein of unknown function. In the so-called SOF-positive strains, which produce apolipoproteinase (serum opacity factor), the encoding gene, *sof,* is located at least 15 kb from the core *vir* regulon (103). In some GAS strains, the gene encoding the streptococcal inhibitor of complement (SIC) belongs to the core *vir* regulon (1, 59). Genes for streptococcin (*scnA*), cysteine proteinase (*speB*), oligopeptide permease (*opp*), and others are positively affected by Mga by an as yet unknown direct or indirect mechanism (99). Interestingly, Nra downregulates transcription of the global regulator Mga, whereas Mga, as a positive regulator, enhances Nra transcription, thus forming a regulatory network within virulence genes (98).

Of the virulence regulators, only the *vir* regulon occurs in all *S. pyogenes* strains (96), which highlights its exceptional role in pathogenicity. In addition to the functions in the infectious process mentioned above, Mga is involved in sensing the iron level, pH, CO_2 level, temperature, and cell density (79, 80). Two major structural types of the *vir* regulon (small and large with a conserved order of core genes) are strongly correlated with the antigenic M protein class (I or II) (12) and the occurrence of the *sof* gene. The reason for this binary evolution within GAS is not understood. However, detailed molecular analysis, mainly of *emm* and *emm*-related genes within the *vir* regulons, revealed evidence of two lineages for generating antigenic variability by horizontal gene transfer events: intergenic exchanges of immunologically relevant portions between *emm* (-related) genes as well as intergenomic exchanges of complete *emm* (-related) genes or at least functional cassettes (11, 50, 97).

IMPLICATIONS FOR THE EVOLUTION OF GRAM-POSITIVE PATHOGENS

Staphylococci represent a heterogeneous group of microorganisms. The strong phenotypic variability of the genus is reflected by the occurrence of numerous IS elements, transposons, plasmids, and bacteriophages. Selective pressure, e.g., treatment of patients with antibiotics, directs the development of resistant subgroups and clones. The evolution of the recently emerged MRSA strains is an example of such an evolutionary process. The *mecA* gene cluster, whose expression forms the basis of methicillin resistance, was probably transferred from the nonpathogenic species *S. sciuri* to pathogenic species, e.g., *S. aureus*. The presence of IS elements, such as IS*257,* and transposase-specific genes on a 30- to 50-kb chromosomal DNA region comprising the *mecA* cluster argues for horizontal gene transfer of the *mecA* determinant. It will be interesting to find whether the *mec* region will encompass additional genetic features often found associated with PAIs; if it does, it may be considered a "resistance island." In contrast to the *mecA* determinant, other resistance genes of staphylococci are parts of transposons or plasmids. Some of these elements have been detected in other species such as enterococci. Gene transfer has been described between staphylococci and enterococci with *Enterococcus faecalis* and *E. faecium* as donors (86).

By analogy to the spread of resistance genes, genes involved in the pathogenesis of staphylococci can also be exchanged by horizontal gene transfer. One example might be the *ica* gene cluster, which converts saprophytic biofilm-negative *S. epidermidis* strains to biofilm-positive variants with the capacity to colonize catheters and other medical devices in immunocompromised patients. In contrast to the *mecA* gene, the origin of the *ica* genes is unknown. They represent a target region for the integration of IS*256* elements, with the consequence that the *ica* expression will be repressed (following IS insertion) or activated (following IS excision). Additionally, the *icaC* gene and the adjacent DNA contain nucleotide sequence regions which show homologies to attachment sites of staphylococcal bacteriophages. However, there is no experimental evidence so far that these sites can indeed be used for the integration of bacteriophages. Nevertheless, the association of the *ica* operon with mobile genetic elements and the occurrence of putative phage attachment sites suggest that gene transfer mechanisms could be involved in the evolution of *ica*-positive *S. epidermidis* strains. Detailed analysis of the factors contributing to this process represents an exciting field of investigation.

Bacteriophages also play an important role in the development of new pathogenic variants of *S. aureus*. While specific virulence-associated genes, such as the *sea* locus encoding the SEA superantigen and the *sak* determinant responsible for staphylokinase expression, are directly transferred by converting bacteriophages, the *tst* gene, encoding TSST-1, is part of a newly described phage-derived PAI. The island, however, can be transferred by generalized transduction between different strains of *S. aureus*. It is tempting to speculate that other gene clusters, such as biofilm-converting genes, other toxin loci, or even resistance determinants such as *mecA,* may be part of distinct staphylococcal islands which may have the capacity to be transferred by bacteriophages. While selective pressures in the evolutionary processes leading to the development of resistant strains are quite obvious, the driving forces in the creation of new pathogenic staphylococcal variants might be an increased capability for surviving in certain ecological niches.

The three pathogenic species of the genus *Streptococcus* considered here, *Streptococcus pyogenes* (Lancefield group A [GAS]), *S. agalactiae* (Lancefield group B [GBS]), and *S. pneumoniae* (pneumococcus), are very heterogeneous in their ecology, morphology, and the types of diseases they cause in humans. One striking example of a surprising and unpredictable evolution in pathogenicity is the reemergence of streptococcal toxic shock and also of acute rheumatic fever caused by *S. pyogenes* since the mid-1980s. Because of a constant decline in the severity of these infections starting from the beginning of this century and later on as a result of effective treatment of streptococci with antibiotics, both diseases were considered rather trivial. Despite growing efforts to explain the observed epidemiological fluctuations in molecular terms, the mechanisms of horizontal intraspecies and interspecies gene transfer are still poorly understood. Some light has been shed on the situation as far as bacteriophages of GAS are concerned. As already discussed in detail, temperate bateriophage genomes harbor genes for one of the most powerful group of virulence factors, the pyrogenic exotoxins (superantigens). Obviously, the strategy of pathogens to destroy human immune defenses by superantigen action was so successful that it has evolved in a variety of bacteria along different phylogenetic lineages (37). Some streptococcal and staphylococcal superantigens were found to be more similar to each other than streptococcal superantigens were among themselves, thus pointing to a possible interspecies transfer. Not surprisingly, all of the streptococcal superantigen genes were found on potentially mobile bacteriophage genomes (35). It has been shown that polylyso-geny offers two advantages to the pathogens: (i) to mobilize virulence genes and (ii) to enable phenotypic mixing by recombination between temperate and cryptic phages (76). So far, bacteriophages may be considered the most likely vehicles for horizontal gene transfer in the natural environment. Whether the streptococcal exotoxin genes are also part of a phage-borne PAI like the *tst* gene of *Staphylococcus aureus* remains to be resolved.

Further evidence for intergenic and intergenomic gene transfer in GAS concerns the M and M-related protein-encoding genes residing on the *vir* regulon. Especially in the so-called large *vir* regulons, which contain the *emm*-related gens *mrp* and *enn* (Fig. 4), the possible generation of surface proteins with new functions could be shown by gene transfer between different serotypes. Since GAS does not develop competence for genetic transfor-mation, conjugative plasmids or bacteriophages might be candidates for mediating genetic exchange that leads to interspecies recombination events.

In contrast to *S. pyogenes, S. pneumoniae* does develop natural competence, and it has become known as the first microorganism with the capacity to take up free DNA experimentally from the environment. In *S. pneumoniae,* transformation is an extremely effective tool for spreading antibiotic resistance and probably also for transferring the *comC* and *comD* genes of the competence operon as functional units between different strains and species. In both cases, the occurrence of mosaic structures in the genes encoding PBPs and the competence-signaling protein (ComC) and its corresponding histidine kinase sensor (ComD) most probably resulted from transformation events. One mosaic structure of *pbp2x,* encoding the primary target PBP2x protein of β-lactams, appeared to be geo-graphically widespread in *S. pneumoniae* as well as in resistant *S. mitis* and *S. oralis* strains from all over Europe (105).

Together with the intriguing suggestion (based mainly on *S. pyogenes* genome data) that a set of competence-regulating genes might also be activated in GAS (20), horizontal interspecies gene transfer involving the two most important pathogens of the genus *Strepto-coccus* would open up the possibility for new approaches to studies of the epidemiology of streptococcal virulence genes.

Acknowledgments. We thank Andreas Podbielski (Ulm, Germany) for providing Fig. 4, Horst Malke (Jena, Germany) and Werner Köhler (Jena, Germany) for valuable discussions of the streptococcal sections, and Ute Hentschel (Würzburg, Germany) for critical reading of the manuscript.

REFERENCES

1. **Akeson, P., A. G. Sjöholm, and L. Björck.** 1996. Protein SIC, a novel extracellular protein of *Streptococcus pyogenes* interfering with complement function. *J. Biol. Chem.* **271:**1081–1088.
2. **Archer, G. L., and D. M. Niemeyer.** 1994. Origin and evolution of DNA associated with resistance to methicillin in staphylococci. *Trends Microbiol.* **2:**343–347.
3. **Archer, G. L., D. M. Niemeyer, and J. A. Thanassi.** 1994. Dissemination among staphylococci of DNA sequences associated with methicillin resistance. *Antimicrob. Agents Chemother.* **38:**447–454.
4. **Avery, O. T., C. M. McLeod, and M. McCarthy.** 1944. Studies on the chemical nature of the substance inducing transformation of pneumococcal phenotypes. Induction of transformation by a deoxyribonucleic acid fraction isolated from pneumococcus type III. *J. Exp Med.* **79:**137–158.
5. **Baker, C. J., and M. S. Edwards.** 1995. Group B streptococcal infections, p. 980–1054. *In* J. S. Remington and J. D. Klein (ed.), *Infectious Diseases of the Fetus and Newborn Infant.* The W. B. Saunders Co., Philadelphia, Pa.

6. **Barberis-Maino, L., B. Berger-Bächi, H. Weber, W. D. Beck, and F. H. Kayser.** 1987. IS*431*, a staphylococcal insertion sequence-like element related to IS*26* from *Proteus mirabilis. Gene* **59:**107–113.

7. **Barberis-Maino, L., C. Ryffel, F. H. Kayser, and B. Berger-Bächi.** 1990. Complete nucleotide sequence of IS*431* mec in *Staphylococcus aureus. Nucleic Acids Res.* **18:**5548.

8. **Bastos, M. C. F., and E. Murphy.** 1988. Transposon *Tn554* encodes three products required for transposition. *EMBO J.* **7:**2935–2941.

9. **Berg, T., N. Firth, S. Apisiridej, A. Hettiaratchi, A. Leelaporn, and R. A. Skurray.** 1998. Complete nucleotide sequence of pSK41: evolution of staphylococcal conjugative multiresistance plasmids. *J. Bacteriol.* **180:**4350–4359.

10. **Berger-Bächi, B.** 1980. Physical mapping of the *Bgl*I, *Bgl*II, *Pst*I and *Eco*RI restriction fragments of staphylococcal phage 11 DNA. *Mol. Gen. Genet.* **180:**391–398.

11. **Bessen, D. E., and S. K. Hollingshead.** 1994. Allelic polymorphism of *emm* loci provides evidence for horizontal gene spread in group A streptococci. *Proc. Natl. Acad. Sci. USA* **91:**3280–3284.

12. **Bessen, D. E., and V. A. Fischetti.** 1990. Differentiation between two distinct classes of group A streptococci by limited substitution of amino acids within the shared region of M protein-like molecules. *J. Exp. Med.* **172:**1757–1764.

13. **Betley, M., and J. J. Mekalanos.** 1985. Staphylococcal enterotoxin A is encoded by phage. *Science* **229:**185–187.

14. **Borecka, P., S. Rosypal, R. Pantucek, and J. Doskar.** 1996. Localization of prophages of serological group B and F on restriction fragments defined in the restriction map of *Staphylococcus aureus* NCTC 8325. *FEMS Microbiol. Lett.* **143:**203–210.

15. **Byrne, M. E., D. A. Rouch, and R. A. Skurray.** 1989. Nucleotide sequence analysis of IS*256* from the *Staphylococcus aureus* gentamicin-tobramycin-kanamycin-resistance transposon Tn*4001. Gene* **81:**361–367.

16. **Carroll, D., M. Kehoe, D. Cavanagh, and D. Coleman.** 1995. Novel organization of the site-specific integration and excision recombination functions of the *Staphylococcus aureus* phi13 and phi42. *Mol. Microbiol.* **16:**877–893.

17. **Chambers, H.** 1997. Methicillin resistance in staphylococci: molecular and biochemical basis and clinical implications. *Clin. Microbiol. Rev.* **10:**781–791.

18. **Chen, C., and P. P. Cleary.** 1990. Complete nucleotide sequence of the streptococcal C5a peptidase gene of *Streptococcus pyogenes. J. Biol. Chem.* **265:**3161–3167.

19. **Cheung, A. L., J. M. Koomey, C. A. Butler, S. J. Projan, and V. A. Fischetti.** 1992. Regulation of exoprotein expression in *Staphylococcus aureus* by a locus (*sar*) distinct from *agr. Proc. Natl. Acad. Sci. USA* **89:**6462–6466.

20. **Claverys, J.-P., and B. Martin.** 1998. Competence regulons, genomics and streptococci. *Mol. Microbiol.* **29:**1125–1127.

21. **Cleary, P. P., D. LaPenta, D. Heath, E. J. Haanes, and C. Chen.** 1991. A virulence regulon in *Streptococcus pyogenes*, p. 147–151. *In* G. M. Dunny, P. P. Cleary, and L. L. McKay (ed.), *Genetics and Molecular Biology of Streptococci, Lactococci, and Enterococci*. American Society for Microbiology, Washington, D.C.

22. **Coleman, D. C., D. J. Sullivan, R. J. Russel, J. P. Arbuthnott, B. F. Carey, and H. M. Pomeroy.** 1989. *Staphylococcus aureus* bacteriophages mediating simultaneous lysogenic conversion of beta-lysin, staphylokinase and enterotoxin A: molecular mechanism of triple conversion. *J. Gen. Microbiol.* **135:**1679–1697.

23. **Coleman, D. C., J. P. Arbuthnott, H. M. Pomeroy, and T. H. Birkbeck.** 1986. Cloning and expression in *Escherichia coli* and *Staphylococcus aureus* of the beta-lysin-determinant from *Staphylococcus aureus:* evidence that bacteriophage conversion of beta-lysin activity is caused by insertional inactivation of the beta-lysin determinant. *Microb. Pathog.* **1:**549–564.

24. **Cone, L. A., D. A. Woodward, P. M. Schlievert, and G. S. Tomory.** 1987. Clinical and bacteriologic observations of a toxic shock-like syndrome due to *Streptococcus pyogenes. N. Engl. J. Med.* **317:**146–149.

25. **Courvalin, P., and C. Carlier.** 1986. Transposable multiple-antibiotic resistance in *Streptococcus pneumoniae. Mol. Gen. Genet.* **205:**291–297.

26. **Couto, L., H. de Lencastre, E. Severina, W. Kloos, J. Webster, I. Santos Sanches, and A. Tomasz.** 1996. Ubiquitous presence of a *mecA* homologue in natural isolates of *Staphylococcus sciuri. Microb. Drug Resist.* **2:**377–391.

27. **Derbise, A., K. G. H. Dyke, and N. El Solh.** 1994. Isolation and characterization of IS*1181*, an insertion sequence from *Staphylococcus aureus. Plasmid* **31:**252–264.

28. **Derbise, A., K. G. H. Dyke, and N. El Solh.** 1996. Characterization of a *Staphylococcus aureus* transposon, Tn*5405*, located within Tn*5404* and carrying the aminoglycoside resistance genes, *aphA-3* and *aadE. Plasmid* **35:**174–188.

29. **Dowson, C. G., A. Hutchison, and B. G. Spratt.** 1989. Extensive re-modelling of the transpeptidase domain of penicillin binding protein 2B of a penicillin-resistant South African isolate of *Streptococcus pneumoniae. Mol. Microbiol.* **3:**95–102.

30. **Dowson, C. G., T. J. Coffey, and B. G. Spratt.** 1994. Origin and molecular epidemiology of penicillin-binding-protein-mediated resistance to β-lactam antibiotics. *Trends Microbiol.* **10:**361–366.

31. **Dyke, K. G. H., S. Aubert, and N. El Solh.** 1992. Multiple copies of IS*256* in staphylococci. *Plasmid* **28:**235–246.

32. **Eisen, J. A., M. J. Benito, and V. Walbot.** 1994. Sequence similarity of putative transposases links the *Mutator* autonomous element and a group of bacterial insertion sequences. *Nucleic Acids Res.* **22:** 2634–2636.

33. **El Kharrhoubi, A., P. Jaques, G. Piras, J. Van Breumen, J. Coyette, and J. M. Ghuysen.** 1991. The *Enterococcus hirae* R40 penicillin-binding protein 5 and the methicillin-resistant *Staphylococcus aureus* penicillin-binding protein 2′ are similar. *Biochem. J.* **280:**463–469.

34. **El Solh, N., J. Allignet, V. Loncle, and P. Mazodier.** 1990. Nucleotide sequence of a staphylococcal plasmid gene *vgb* encoding a hydrolase that inactivates the B components of virginiamycin-like antibiotics, p. 617–622. *In* R. P. Novick (ed.), *Molecular Biology of the Staphylococci.* VCH, New York, N.Y.

35. **Ferretti, J. J., S. Clifton, B. Roe, and W. M. McShan.** 1998. Temperate bacteriophages of *Streptococcus pyogenes:* comparative studies, p. 47. *In ASM Conference on Streptococcal Genetics. Genetics of the Streptococci, Enterococci, and Lactococci.* American Society for Microbiology, Washington, D.C.

36. **Fischetti, V. A.** 1989. Streptococcal M protein: molecular design and biological behavior. *Clin. Microbiol. Rev.* **2:**285–314.

37. **Fleischer, B.** 1994. Superantigens produced by infectious pathogens: molecular mechanism of action and biological significance. *Int. J. Clin. Lab. Res.* **24:**193–197.

38. **Fogg, G. C., C. M. Gibson, and M. G. Caparon.** 1994. The identification of *rofA,* a positive-acting regulatory component of *prtF* expression: *mgd*-based shuttle mutagenesis strategy in *Streptococcus pyogenes. Mol. Microbiol.* **11:**671–684.

39. **Gemmel, C. G.** 1995. Antibiotics and the expression of staphylococcal virulence. *J. Antimicrob. Chemother.* **36:**283–291.

40. **Gerke, C., A. Kraft, R. Süssmuth, O. Schweitzer, and F. Götz.** 1998. Characterization of the N-acetylglucosaminyltransferase activity involved in the biosynthesis of the *Staphylococcus epidermidis* polysaccharide intercellular adhesin. *J. Biol. Chem.* **273:**18586–18593.

41. **Gillespie, M. T., B. R. Lyon, L. S. L. Loo, P. R. Matthews, P. R. Stewart, and R. A. Skurray.** 1987. Homologous direct repeat sequences associated with mercury, methicillin, tetracycline and trimethoprim resistance determinants in *Staphylococcus aureus. FEMS Microbiol. Lett.* **43:**165–171.

42. **Götz, F., F. Popp, and K.-H. Schleifer.** 1984. Isolation and characterization of a virulent bacteriophage from *Staphylococcus carnosus. FEMS Microbiol. Lett.* **23:**303–307.

43. **Hacker, J., G. Blum-Oehler, I. Mühldorfer, and H. Tschäpe.** 1997. Pathogenicity islands of virulent bacteria: structure, function and impact on microbial evolution. *Mol. Microbiol.* **23:**1089–1097.

44. **Hakenbeck, R., T. Briese, L. Chalkley, H. Ellerbrok, R. Kalliakosi, R. Latorre, C. Leimonen, and C. Martin.** 1991. Antigenic variation of penicillin binding proteins from penicillin-resistant clinical strains of *Streptococcus pneumoniae. J. Infect. Dis.* **164:**313–319.

45. **Havarstein, L. S., P. Gaustad, and I. F. Nes.** 1996. Identification of the streptococcal competence pheromone receptor. *Mol. Microbiol.* **21:**863–869.

46. **Havarstein, L. S., R. Hakenbeck, and P. Gaustad.** 1997. Natural competence in the genus *Streptococcus:* evidence that streptococci can change pherotype by interspecies recombinational events. *J. Bacteriol.* **179:** 6589–6594.

47. **Heilmann, C., C. Gerke, F. Perdreau-Remington, and F. Götz.** 1996. Characterization of Tn*917* insertion mutants of *Staphylococcus epidermidis* affected in biofilm formation. *Infect. Immun.* **64:**277–282.

48. **Heilmann, C., O. Schweitzer, C. Gerke, N. Vanittanakom, D. Mack, and F. Götz.** 1996. Molecular

basis of intercellular adhesion in the biofilm-forming *Staphylococcus epidermidis*. *Mol. Microbiol.* **20:** 1083–1091.

49. **Hiramatsu, K.** 1995. Molecular evolution of MRSA. *Microbiol. Immunol.* **39:**531–543.

50. **Hollingshead, S. K., J. Arnold, T. L. Readdy, and D. E. Bessen.** 1994. Molecular evolution of a multigene family in group A streptococci. *Mol. Biol. Evol.* **11:**208–219.

51. **Inglis, B., H. Waldron, and R. P. Stewart.** 1987. Molecular relatedness of *Staphylococcus aureus* typing phages measured by DNA hybridization and high resolution thermal denaturation analysis. *Arch. Virol.* **93:**69–80.

52. **Ji, G., R. Beavis, and R. Novick.** 1997. Bacterial interference caused by autoinducing peptide variants. *Science* **276:**2027–2030.

53. **Ji, G., R. C. Beavis, and R. P. Novick.** 1995. Cell density control of staphylococcal virulence mediated by an octapeptide pheromone. *Proc. Natl. Acad. Sci. USA* **92:**12055–12059.

54. **Johnson, L. P., and P. M. Schlievert.** 1984. Group A streptococcal phage T12 carries the structural gene for pyrogenic exotoxin type A. *Mol. Gen. Genet.* **194:**52–56.

55. **Johnson, L. P., P. M. Schlievert, and D. W. Watson.** 1980. Transfer of group A streptococcal pyrogenic exotoxin production to nontoxigenic strains by lysogenic conversion. *Infect. Immun.* **28:**254–257.

56. **Jones, J., S. Yost, and P. A. Pattee.** 1987. Transfer of the conjugative tetracycline resistance transposon Tn916 from *Streptococcus faecalis* to *Staphylococcus aureus* and identification of some insertion sites in the staphylococcal chromosome. *J. Bacteriol.* **169:**2121–2131.

57. **Kass, E. H., M. I. Kendrick, Y.-C. Tsai, and J. Parsonnet.** 1987. Interaction of magnesium ion, oxygen tension, and temperature in the production of toxic shock syndrome toxin-1 by *Staphylococcus aureus*. *J. Infect. Dis.* **155:**812–814.

58. **Khan, S., and R. P. Novick.** 1980. Terminal nucleotide sequence of Tn551, a transposon specifying erythromycin resistance in *Staphylococcus aureus:* homology with Tn3. *Plasmid* **4:**148–154.

59. **Kihlberg, B. M., J. Cooney, M. G. Caparon, A. Olsen, and L. Björck.** 1995. Biological properties of a *Streptococcus pyogenes* mutant generated by Tn916 insertion in *mga*. *Microb. Pathog.* **19:**299–315.

60. **Köhler, W.** 1990. Streptococcal toxic shock syndrome. *Zentbl. Bakteriol.* **272:**257–264.

61. **Kondo, I.** 1985. Genetic study on staphylokinase. *Zentbl. Bakteriol. Suppl.* **14:**11–29.

62. **Kreiswirth, B. N., S. Lofdahl, M. J. Betley, M. O'Reilly, and P. M. Schlievert.** 1983. The toxic shock syndrome exotoxin structural gene is not detectably transmitted by a prophage. *Nature* **305:**709–712.

63. **Laible, G., and R. Hakenbeck.** 1991. Five independent combinations of mutations can result in low affinity penicillin-binding protein 2x of *Streptococcus pneumoniae*. *J. Bacteriol.* **173:**6986–6999.

64. **Lee, C. Y., and J. J. Iandolo.** 1986. Integration of staphylococcal phage L54a occurs by site-specific recombination: structural analysis of the attachment sites. *Proc. Natl. Acad. Sci. USA* **83:**5474–5478.

65. **Lee, C. Y., and J. J. Iandolo.** 1986. Lysogenic conversion of staphylococcal lipase is caused by insertion of bacteriophage L54a genome into the lipase structural genes. *J. Bacteriol.* **166:**385–391.

66. **Leelaporn, A., N. Firth, I. T. Paulsen, and R. A. Skurray.** 1996. IS257-mediated cointegration in the evolution of a family of staphylococcal trimethoprim resistance plasmids. *J. Bacteriol.* **178:**5070–5073.

67. **Lindsay, J. A., A. Ruzin, H. F. Ross, N. Kurepina, and R. Novick.** 1998. The gene for toxic shock toxin is carried by a family of mobile pathogenicity islands in *Staphylococcus aureus*. *Mol. Microbiol.* **29:** 527–543.

68. **Lyon, B. R., and R. A. Skurray.** 1987. Antimicrobial resistance of *Staphylococcus aureus:* genetic basis. *Microbiol. Rev.* **31:**2281–2285.

69. **Lyon, B. R., J. W. May, and R. A. Skurray.** 1984. Tn4001: a gentamicin and kanamycin resistance transposon in *Staphylococcus aureus*. *Mol. Gen. Genet.* **193:**554–556.

70. **Lyon, B. R., M. T. Gillespie, and R. A. Skurray.** 1987. Detection and characterization of IS256, an insertion sequence in *Staphylococcus aureus*. *J. Gen. Microbiol.* **133:**3031–3038.

71. **Mack, D., M. Nedelmann, A. Krokotsch, A. Schwarzkopf, J. Heesemann, and R. Laufs.** 1994. Characterization of transposon mutants of biofilm-producing *Staphylococcus epidermidis* impaired in the accumulative phase of biofilm production: genetic identification of a hexosamine-containing polysaccharide intercellular adhesin. *Infect. Immun.* **62:**3244–3253.

72. **Mack, D., W. Fischer, A. Krokotsch, K. Leopold, R. Hartmann, H. Egge, and R. Laufs.** 1996. The intercellular adhesin involved in biofilm accumulation of *Staphylococcus epidermidis* is a linear beta-1,6-linked glucosaminoglycan: purification and structural analysis. *J. Bacteriol.* **178:**175–183.

73. **Mahillon, J., and M. Chandler.** 1998. Insertion sequences. *Microbiol. Mol. Biol. Rev.* **62:**725–774.

74. **Malke, H.** 1974. Genetics of resistance to macrolide antibiotics and lincomycine in natural isolates of *Streptococcus pyogenes. Mol. Gen. Genet.* **135:**349–367.

75. **Malke, H., and W. Köhler.** 1973. Transduction among group A streptococci: transducibility of strains representative of thirty different M types. *Zentbl. Bakteriol. Mikrobiol. Hyg. I Abt. Orig. A* **224:**194–201.

76. **Malke, H., R. Starke, W. Köhler, T. K. Kolesnichenko, and A. A. Totolian.** 1975. Bacteriophage P12334mo-mediated intra- and intergroup transduction of antibiotic resistance among streptococci. *Zentbl. Bakteriol. Mikrobiol. Hyg. I Abt. Orig. A* **233:**24–34.

77. **Marrack, P., and J. Kappler.** 1990. The staphylococcal enterotoxins and their relatives. *Science* **248:** 705–711.

78. **Martin, C., C. Sibold, and R. Hakenbeck.** 1992. Relatedness of penicillin binding protein 1a genes from different clones of penicillin-resistant *Streptococcus pneumoniae* isolated in South Africa and Spain. *EMBO J.* **11:**3831–3836.

79. **McIver, K. S., A. S. Heath, and J. R. Scott.** 1995. Regulation of virulence by environmental signals in group A streptococci: influence of osmolarity, temperature, gas exchange, and iron limitation in *emm* transcription. *Infect. Immun.* **63:**4540–4542.

80. **McIver, K., and J. R. Scott.** 1997. Role of *mga* in growth phase regulation of virulence genes of the group A streptococcus. *J. Bacteriol.* **179:**5178–5187.

81. **McShan, W. M., Y.-F. Tang, and J. J. Ferretti.** 1997. Bacteriophage T12 of *Streptococcus pyogenes* integrates into the gene encoding a serine tRNA. *Mol. Microbiol.* **23:**719–728.

82. **Mempel, M., H. Feucht, W. Ziebuhr, M. Endres, R. Laufs, and L. Grüter.** 1994. Lack of *mecA* transcription in slime-negative phase variants of methicillin-resistant *Staphylococcus epidermidis. Antimicrob. Agents Chemother.* **38:**1251–1255.

83. **Musser, J. M., A. R. Hauser, M. H. Kim, P. M. Schlievert, K. Nelson, and R. K. Selander.** 1991. *Streptococcus pyogenes* causing toxic shock-like syndrome and other invasive diseases: clonal diversity and pyrogenic exotoxin expression. *Proc. Natl. Acad. Sci. USA* **89:**2668–2672.

84. **Needham, C., M. Rahman, K. G. H. Dyke, and W. C. Noble.** 1994. An investigation of plasmids from *Staphylococcus aureus* that mediate resistance to mupirocin and tetracycline. *Microbiology* **140:**2577–2583.

85. **Nida, S. K., and J. J. Ferretti.** 1982. Phage influence on the synthesis of extracellular toxins in group A streptococci. *Infect. Immun.* **36:**745–750.

86. **Noble, W. C., M. Rahman, T. Karadec, and S. Schwarz.** 1996. Gentamicin resistance gene transfer from *Enterococcus faecalis* and *E. faecium* to *Staphylococcus aureus, S. intermedius* and *S. hyicus. Vet. Microbiol.* **52:**143–152.

87. **Novick, R. P.** 1989. Staphylococcal plasmids and their replication. *Annu. Rev. Microbiol.* **43:**537–565.

88. **Novick, R. P., H. F. Ross, S. J. Projan, J. Kornblum, B. Kreiswirth, and S. Moghazeh.** 1993. Synthesis of staphylococcal virulence factors is controlled by a regulatory RNA molecule. *EMBO J.* **12:**3967–3975.

89. **Ohlsen, K., K.-P. Koller, and J. Hacker.** 1997. Analysis of expression of the alpha-toxin gene (*hla*) of *Staphylococcus aureus* by using a chromosomally encoded *hla::lacZ* gene fusion. *Infect. Immun.* **65:** 3606–3614.

90. **Ohlsen, K., W. Ziebuhr, K.-P. Koller, W. Hell, T. A. Wichelhaus, and J. Hacker.** 1998. Effects of subinhibitory concentrations of antibiotics on alpha-toxin (*hla*) gene expression of methicillin-sensitive and methicillin-resistant *Staphylococcus aureus* isolates. *Antimicrob. Agents Chemother.* **42:**2817–2823.

91. **Pantucek, R., A. Rosypalova, J. Doskar, J. Kallerova, V. Ruzickova, P. Borecka, S. Snopkova, R. Horvath, F. Götz, and S. Rosypal.** 1998. The polyvalent staphylococcal phage phi812: its host-range mutants and related phages. *Virology* **246:**241–252.

92. **Paoletti, L. C., M. R. Wessels, A. K. Rodewald, A. A. Shroff, H. J. Jennings, and D. L. Kasper.** 1994. Neonatal mouse protection against infection with multiple group B streptococcal (GBS) serotypes by maternal immunization with tetravalent GBS polysaccharide-tetanus toxoid conjugate vaccine. *Infect. Immun.* **62:**3236–3243.

93. **Paton, J. C., P. W. Andrew, G. J. Boulnois, and T. J. Mitchell.** 1993. Molecular analysis of the pathogenicity of *Streptococcus pneumoniae*: the role of pneumococcal proteins. *Annu. Rev. Microbiol.* **47:**89–115.

94. **Perez-Casal, J., M. G. Caparon, and J. R. Scott.** 1991. Mry, a *trans*-acting positive regulator of the M protein gene of *Streptococcus pyogenes* with similarity to the receptor proteins of two-component regulatory systems. *J. Bacteriol.* **173:**2617–2624.

95. **Pestova, E. V., L. S. Havarstein, and D. A. Morrison.** 1996. Regulation of competence for genetic

transformation in *Streptococcus pneumoniae* by an auto-induced peptide and two component regulatory system. *Mol. Microbiol.* **21**:1087–1099.

96. **Podbielski, A.** 1993. Three different types of organization of the *vir* regulon in group A streptococci. *Mol. Gen. Genet.* **237**:287–300.

97. **Podbielski, A., B. Krebs, and A. Kaufhold.** 1994. Genetic variability of the *emm*-related genes of the large *vir* regulon of group A streptococci: potential intra- and intergenomic recombination events. *Mol. Gen. Genet.* **243**:691–698.

98. **Podbielski, A., M. Woischnik, B. A. B. Leonard, and K. H. Schmidt.** 1999. Characterization of *nra*, a global negative regulator gene in group A streptococci. *Mol. Microbiol.* **31**:1051–1064.

99. **Podbielski, A., M. Woischnik, B. Pohl, and K. H. Schmidt.** 1996. What is the size of the group A streptococcal *vir* regulon? The Mga regulator affects expression of secreted and surface virulence factors. *Med. Microbiol. Immunol.* **185**:171–181.

100. **Polissi, A., A. Pontiggia, G. Feger, M. Altieri, H. Mottl, L. Ferrari, and D. Simon.** 1998. Large-scale identification of virulence genes from *Streptococcus pneumoniae*. *Infect. Immun.* **66**:5620–5629.

101. **Proft, T., S. L. Moffatt, C. J. Berkahn, and J. D. Frazer.** 1999. Identification and characterization of novel superantigens from *Streptococcus pyogenes*. *J. Exp. Med.* **189**:89–101.

102. **Rachid, S., K. Ohlsen, J. Hacker, and W. Ziebuhr.** Unpublished data.

103. **Rakonjak, J. V., J. C. Robbins, and V. A. Fischetti.** 1995. DNA sequence of the serum opacity factor of group A streptococci: identification of a fibronectin-binding repeat domain. *Infect. Immun.* **63**:622–631.

104. **Reichardt, W., H. Müller-Alouf, J. E. Alouf, and W. Köhler.** 1992. Erythrogenic toxins A, B, and C: occurrence of the genes and exotoxin formation from clinical *Streptococcus pyogenes* strains associated with streptococcal toxic shock-like syndrome. *FEMS Microbiol. Lett.* **100**:313–322.

105. **Reichmann, P., A. König, J. Linares, F. Alcaide, F. C. Tenover, L. McDougal, S. Swidsinski, and R. Hakenbeck.** 1997. A global gene pool for high level cephalosporin resistance in commensal *Streptococcus* species and *Streptococcus pneumoniae*. *J. Infect. Dis.* **176**:1001–1012.

106. **Rice, L. B., and A. S. Thorisdottir.** 1994. The prevalence of sequences homologous to IS256 in clinical enterococcal isolates. *Plasmid* **32**:344–349.

107. **Rouch, D. A., L. J. Messerotti, L. S. Loo, C. A. Jackson, and R. A. Skurray.** 1989. Trimethoprim resistance transposon Tn4003 from *Staphylococcus aureus* encodes genes for a dihydrofolate reductase and thymidylate synthetase flanked by three copies of IS257. *Mol. Microbiol.* **3**:161–175.

108. **Rouch, D. A., M. E. Byrne, Y. C. Kong, and R. A. Skurray.** 1987. The *aacA-aphD* gentamicin and kanamycin resistance determinant of Tn4001 from *Staphylococcus aureus:* expression and nucleotide sequence analysis. *J. Gen. Microbiol.* **133**:3039–3052.

109. **Rowland, S.-J., D. J. Sherratt, W. M. Stark, and H. R. Boocock.** 1995. Tn552 transposase purification and in vitro activities. *EMBO J.* **14**:196–205.

110. **Rudin, L., J. E. Sjöström, M. Lindberg, and L. Philipson.** 1974. Factors affecting competence for transformation in *Staphylococcus aureus*. *J. Bacteriol.* **118**:155–164.

111. **Ryffel, C., R. Bucher, F. H. Kayser, and B. Berger-Bächi.** 1991. The *Staphylococcus aureus mec* determinant comprises an unusual cluster of direct repeats and codes for a gene product similar to the *Escherichia coli* sn-glycerophosphoryl diester phosphodiesterase. *J. Bacteriol.* **173**:7416–7422.

112. **Shalita, Z., E. Murphy, and R. P. Novick.** 1980. Penicillinase plasmids of *Staphylococcus aureus:* structural and evolutionary relationships. *Plasmid* **3**:291–311.

113. **Sibold, C., J. Henrichsen, A. König, C. Martin, L. Chalkley, and R. Hakenbeck.** 1994. Mosaic *pbpX* gene of major clones of penicillin resistant *Streptococcus pneumoniae* have evolved from *pbpX* genes of a penicillin sensitive *Streptococcus oralis*. *Mol. Microbiol.* **12**:1013–1023.

114. **Skurray, R. A., and N. Firth.** 1997. Molecular evolution of multiple antibiotic-resistant staphylococci, p. 71–75. *In* S. B. Levy (ed.), *Antibiotic Resistance: Origins, Evolution, Selection and Spread*. John Wiley & Sons, Inc., New York, N.Y.

115. **Smeltzer, M. S., M. E. Hart, and J. J. Iandolo.** 1994. The effect of lysogeny on the genomic organization of *Staphylococcus aureus*. *Gene* **138**:51–57.

116. **Song, M. D., M. Wachi, M. Doi, F. Ishino, and M. Matsuhashi.** 1987. Evolution of an inducible penicillin-target protein in methicillin-resistant *Staphylococcus aureus* by gene fusion. *FEBS Lett.* **221**:167–171.

117. **Stevens, D. L., M. H. Tanner, J. Winship, R. Swarts, K. M. Ries, P. M. Schlievert, and E. Kaplan.** 1989. Severe group A streptococcal infections associated with a toxic shock-like syndrome and scarlet fever toxin A. *N. Engl. J. Med.* **321**:1–7.

118. **Stewart, P. R., D. T. Dubin, S. G. Chikramane, B. Inglis, P. R. Matthews, and S. M. Poston.** 1994. IS*257* and small plasmid insertions in the *mec* region of the chromosome of *Staphylococcus aureus. Plasmid* **31:**12–20.

119. **Thumm, G., and F. Götz.** 1997. Studies on prolysostaphin processing and characterization of the lyso-staphin immunity factor (Lif) of *Staphylococcus simulans* biovar *staphylolyticus. Mol. Microbiol.* **23:** 1251–1265.

120. **Trees, D. J., and J. J. Iandolo.** 1988. Identification of a *Staphylococcus aureus* transposon (Tn*4291*) that carries the methicillin resistance gene(s). *J. Bacteriol.* **170:**149–154.

121. **Weeks, C. R., and J. J. Ferretti.** 1984. The gene for type A streptococcal exotoxin (erythrogenic toxin) is located in bacteriophage T12. *Infect. Immun.* **52:**144–150.

122. **Westh, H., P. M. Hongaard, J. Vunst, and V. Rosdahl.** 1995. Prevalence of *erm* gene classes in erythromy-cin-resistant *Staphylococcus aureus* strains isolated between 1959 and 1988. *Antimicrob. Agents Chemother.* **39:**369–373.

123. **Witte, W., and R. Hummel.** 1986. Antibiotic resistance in *Staphylococcus aureus* isolated from man and animals. *Banbury Rep.* **24:**95–106.

124. **Wu, S., C. Piscitelli, H. de Lencastre, and A. Tomasz.** 1996. Tracking the evolutionary origin of the methicillin resistance gene: cloning and sequencing of a homologue of *mecA* from a methicillin susceptible strain of *Staphylococcus sciuri. Microb. Drug Resist.* **2:**435–441.

125. **Wu, S., H. de Lencastre, and A. Tomasz.** 1998. Genetic organization of the *mecA* region in methicillin-susceptible and methicillin-resistant strains of *Staphylococcus sciuri. J. Bacteriol.* **180:**236–242.

126. **Ye, Z. H., and C. Lee.** 1993. Cloning, sequencing and genetic characterization of regulatory genes *rinA* and *rinB* required for activation of staphylococcal phage phi11 *int* expression. *J. Bacteriol.* **175:**1095–1102.

127. **Ye, Z. H., S. Buranen, and C. Lee.** 1990. Sequence analysis and comparison of *int* and *xis* genes from staphylococcal bacteriophage L54a and phi11. *J. Bacteriol.* **172:**2568–2575.

128. **Yu, C. E., and J. J. Ferretti.** 1991. Molecular characterization of new group A bacteriophages containing the gene for streptococcal erythrogenic toxin A (*speA*). *Mol. Gen. Genet.* **231:**161–168.

129. **Ziebuhr, W., C. Heilmann, F. Götz, P. Meyer, K. Wilms, E. Straube, and J. Hacker.** 1997. Detection of the intercellular adhesin gene cluster (*ica*) and phase variation in *Staphylococcus epidermidis* blood culture strains and mucosal isolates. *Infect. Immun.* **65:**890–896.

130. **Ziebuhr, W., I. Lößner, and J. Hacker.** Unpublished data.

131. **Ziebuhr, W., V. Krimmer, S. Rachid, I. Lößner, F. Götz, and J. Hacker.** 1999. A novel mechanism of phase variation of virulence in *Staphylococcus epidermidis:* evidence for control of the polysaccharide intercellular adhesin synthesis by alternating insertion and excision of the insertion sequence element IS*256. Mol. Microbiol.* **32:**345–356.

Pathogenicity Islands and Other Mobile Virulence Elements
Edited by J. B. Kaper and J. Hacker
© 1999 American Society for Microbiology, Washington, D.C.

Chapter 15

Diverse Roles of *Agrobacterium* Ti Plasmid-Borne Genes in the Formation and Colonization of Plant Tumors

*Stephen C. Winans, Virginia Kalogeraki, Samina Jafri,
Reiko Akakura, and Qi Xia*

Bacteria use highly diverse mechanisms to obtain nutrients from higher plants. One of the most intricate strategies is found among the agrobacteria, which obtain nutrients by genetically transforming their hosts. *Agrobacterium* is a pathogen that has served as an important paradigm for molecular host-microbe interactions and has simultaneously become a cornerstone for plant molecular genetics. At the heart of this pathosystem is a large plasmid called the Ti (tumor-inducing) plasmid. This chapter describes the various steps in plant colonization, including binding of the bacteria to host cells, recognition of diffusible host-released chemical signals, and processing and transfer of oncogenic DNA (T-DNA). It concludes with a discussion of the utilization of tumor-released compounds called opines and of the horizontal transfer of the Ti plasmid.

In 1907, *Agrobacterium tumefaciens* was shown to fulfill Koch's postulates as the causative agent of crown gall tumorigenesis of higher plants (128). Four additional species, *A. vitis, A. rubi, A. rhizogenes,* and *A. radiobacter,* were described subsequently (75, 106). The first two of these cause tumors, *A. rhizogenes* causes hairy root disease, and *A. radiobacter* is nonpathogenic. All are members of the family *Rhizobiaceae* within the alpha subgroup of proteobacteria and are extremely closely related to members of the genus *Rhizobium* (120, 147). Species of *Agrobacterium* have been classified primarily by their phytopathogenic properties, which are largely due to differences in plasmid content. With respect to chromosomally encoded properties, *A. rubi* and *A. vitis* are well-defined separate taxa whereas *A. tumefaciens, A. radiobacter,* and *A. rhizogenes* are not. Isolates of the last three species are often placed into one of two biovars. While it has been proposed that these biovars be elevated to taxonomic status (120, 147), this recommendation has not been widely adopted. Bacterial strains and their Ti plasmids are sometimes referred to by the particular opines that they utilize. The most thoroughly studied *A. tumefaciens* strains contain either octopine-type or nopaline-type Ti plasmids.

Stephen C. Winans, Virginia Kalogeraki, Samina Jafri, Reiko Akakura, and Qi Xia • Section of Microbiology, Cornell University, Ithaca, NY 14853.

Ti PLASMIDS AS PATHOGENICITY ISLANDS

During plant infection, agrobacteria transfer fragments of DNA to the nuclei of host plants by a mechanism that requires cell-cell contact and resembles plasmid conjugation. This T-DNA originates on Ti plasmids, which are generally about 200 kb (142, 155) (Fig. 1). T-DNA, after being covalently integrated into the host genome (27), expresses a dozen or so genes, some of which cause infected plant host cells to proliferate, resulting in crown gall tumors (19). Other transferred genes direct the production and release of nutrients called opines, which are derivatives of amino acids or sugars (43). Virtually all genes found on Ti plasmids play direct or indirect roles in some aspect of crown gall tumorigenesis or

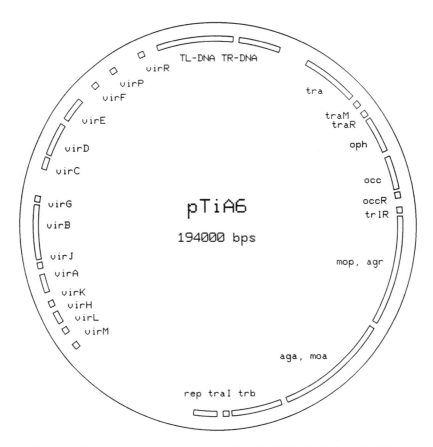

Figure 1. Genetic map of an octopine-type Ti plasmid, pTiΔ6. TL-DNA and TR-DNA, two DNA fragments transferred to plant nuclei; *virA, virB, virC, virD, virE, virF, virG,* and *virJ.* VirG-regulated operons that are essential for efficient plant tumorigenesis; *virH, virK, virL, virM, virP,* and *virR,* VirG-regulated operons that are not required for tumorigenesis; *tra* and *trb,* operons required for Ti plasmid conjugal transfer; *traR, traI, traM,* and *trlR,* regulatory genes that control the expression of the *tra* and *trb* operons; *occ* and *occR,* genes required for catabolism of octopine; *oph,* an ATP-binding cassette-type transporter for an unknown substrate; *mop, agr, aga,* and *moa,* operons required for catabolism of mannopine, agropine, agropinic acid, and mannopinic acid, respectively; *rep,* gene required for vegetative plasmid replication.

tumor colonization. The main features of these plasmids are (i) the T-DNA, (ii) approximately 20 genes that direct the transfer of T-DNA (*vir* genes), (iii) approximately 30 genes that play a role in the uptake or catabolism of opines, and (iv) genes that direct interbacterial Ti plasmid conjugation. These are discussed below.

ATTACHMENT OF *A. TUMEFACIENS* TO PLANT CELLS

One of the earliest steps in most host-pathogen interactions is the binding of the bacterium to host cells. Binding of agrobacteria is thought to be mediated by bacterial polysaccharides and cognate lectins (polysaccharide binding proteins) on the plant cells. Binding to these cells occurs in two steps (86). In the first step, the bacteria bind loosely to an uncharacterized receptor on the plant cell surface. At this stage, the bacteria can be detached by vortexing or by washing wound sites with water. In the second step, an undefined stimulus causes *A. tumefaciens* to produce cellulose fibrils that anchor the bacteria irreversibly to the cell surface. These fibrils also extend into the surrounding medium and entrap additional bacteria, eventually forming a bacterial biofilm (86).

A number of genes have been implicated in attachment, including those found in the *chvAB*, *att*, and *cel* operons. ChvA and ChvB synthesize and export a cyclic β-1,2-glucan, and mutations in these genes cause a 10-fold decrease in binding to leaf mesophyll cells (23, 47, 137). Mutations in the *att* locus also decrease the attachment of bacteria to plant cells, although the role of Att proteins in attachment is not understood (143). *cel* genes are required for cellulose biosynthesis, and mutations in these genes block the second step in attachment (88). Mutations in *chvA*, *chvB*, or *att* abolish tumorigenesis, while mutations in *cel* cause an attenuated tumorigenesis phenotype (87). All these genes are located on the bacterial chromosome, and Ti plasmids are not thought to play central roles in the attachment process.

PROCESSING AND TRANSFER OF T-DNA

Agrobacterium strains harbor a great diversity of Ti plasmids. Some plasmids transfer single DNA fragments to plant nuclei, others transfer two fragments, and at least one transfers three fragments (17, 21, 138). The well-studied nopaline-type Ti plasmid pTiC58 carries a single T-DNA of about 20 kb, while the octopine-type Ti plasmids pTiA6, pTi15955, pTiR10, and pTiAch5 (which are all virtually identical) carry two T-DNAs, one of 13 kb (T_L-DNA) and one of 7 kb (T_R-DNA), separated by 1.5 kb of nontransferred DNA. All T-DNAs are flanked by *cis*-acting, 25-bp direct repeats called border sequences (151, 156). Although the left border is dispensable for T-DNA transfer, the right border is essential and acts in a polar fashion, suggesting that transfer may initiate at the right border repeat and proceed toward the left border (95). Another *cis*-acting element involved in T-DNA transfer is a sequence called *overdrive*, found directly adjacent to the right border (110, 127). Mutations in *overdrive* decrease tumorigenesis approximately 100-fold.

When agrobacteria perceive chemical signals characteristic of wounded plant cells (see below), T-DNA undergoes a series of processing steps. In the first step, each border is cleaved on one DNA strand at a site exactly 4 nucleotides from the left end. By convention, these cleavage sites are designated to lie on the bottom strand. The enzyme that carries out this endonucleolytic attack (VirD2 [see below]) remains covalently bound to the 5′

end of the cleaved DNA strand. In a population of T-DNA molecules, some are not nicked while others are nicked at one or both borders but remain in duplex form. Still other T-DNA bottom strands are found in a single-stranded, linear form (4, 132). These single-stranded, linear molecules are referred to as T-strands and are thought to represent the transferred form of the T-DNA.

T-strands are integrated into the host genome at apparently random sites by a process of illegitimate recombination (139). In one study, the sites of T-DNA integration were studied at the sequence level and compared to the same sites prior to integration (89). In all cases, the chromosomal target sites suffered small deletions. In comparing the left and right ends of the T-strands to the corresponding ends of the integrated T-DNAs, it was evident that small amounts of DNA had often been deleted from either or both ends during integration. In general, the left ends were more prone to these deletions than the right ends were. In several cases, regions of "microhomology" were detected between the T-DNA ends and the target sequence. In three cases, small amounts of "filler" DNA were found at the junctions between T-DNA and host DNA. Integrated T-DNA is stably transmitted to daughter cells upon cell division and is also stably transmitted during meiosis and syngamy.

EXPRESSION OF TRANSFERRED GENES

Each transferred gene possesses many of the features of plant genes, including typical eukaryotic TATA and CAAT boxes, transcriptional enhancers, and poly(A) addition sites (20, 42). No introns have been so far reported for any of the *A. tumefaciens* transferred genes. However, at least one transferred gene in the close relative *A. rhizogenes, rolA,* contains an intron in the 5′ nontranslated portion of the transcript (84).

Most of the transferred genes fall into one of two groups. One group directs the production of plant growth hormones that result in neoplastic growth of the transformed plant cells (98). Two genes on the T-DNA, *iaaM* and *iaaH,* direct the conversion of tryptophan to auxin. *iaaM* encodes tryptophan-2-monooxygenase, while *iaaH* encodes indoleacetamide hydrolase. A third oncogene, *ipt,* codes for an isopentenyl transferase that catalyzes a condensation reaction between isopentenyl pyrophosphate and AMP (38). Plant enzymes are presumed to convert the resulting isopentenyl-AMP into the phytohormone zeatin by removal of the phosphoribose group and hydroxylation of one methyl group of the isopentenyl moiety. Two other T-DNA genes are thought to play roles in tumorigenesis. Gene 5 was found to direct the synthesis of indole-3-lactate, an antagonistic auxin analog (76), while gene 6b increases the sensitivity of plant cells to endogenous or exogenous phytohormones (140).

The second group of genes located on the T-DNA directs the production and release of opines. The *ocs* gene encodes octopine synthase, which reductively condenses pyruvate with either arginine, lysine, histidine, or ornithine to produce octopine, lysopine, histopine, or octopinic acid, respectively (43). The *mas1′* and *mas2′* genes reductively condense glucose with either glutamine or glutamate to produce mannopine or mannopinic acid, respectively. These opines can undergo further rearrangements to form agropine and agropinic acid (43). Octopine-type Ti plasmids therefore direct their hosts to synthesize no fewer than eight opines. The nopaline-type Ti plasmid pTiC58 transfers two opine biosynthetic genes: (i) *nos,* which directs the condensation of α-ketoglutarate with either arginine or lysine, yielding nopaline and nopalinic acid, respectively, and (ii) *ags,* which directs the condensation of sucrose and arabinose, yielding agrocinopine (43). Opines are thought to be released from the plant cells by a protein encoded by the *ons* locus (94).

Ti PLASMID-ENCODED PROTEINS REQUIRED FOR T-DNA PROCESSING, TRANSFER, AND INTEGRATION

Proteins responsible for T-DNA processing and transfer are encoded by the *vir* region of the Ti plasmid. Twenty genes in this region are essential for wild-type levels of pathogenesis and are thought to be expressed in six operons, *virA* to *virG*. The *vir* region of the nopaline-type Ti plasmid was subcloned and shown to be sufficient for tumorigenesis in the absence of a Ti plasmid (116), although such an experiment has never been done for an octopine-type Ti plasmid. Each of these genes is conserved between octopine-type and nopaline-type Ti plasmids (approximately 80% identical at the amino acid level).

The enzymes required for border cleavage are encoded by the *virD1* and *virD2* genes, with the VirD2 protein remaining covalently bound to the 5' end of the T-strands (133, 153, 154). Purified VirD2 efficiently cleaves single-stranded synthetic oligonucleotides containing T-DNA border sequences at the same site as that cleaved in vivo and remains covalently attached to the 5' terminus (108). This reaction is fully reversible, indicating that the DNA-protein bond is a high-energy bond and suggesting that a similar reaction might be required for the integration of T-DNA into the plant genome. Purified VirD2 alone was not able to cleave this sequence in double-stranded form but was able to do so in the presence of VirD1 (121). VirD2 is thought to remain bound to the T-DNA during all stages of transfer and integration.

The T-DNA transfer apparatus is encoded by the *virB* operon, which contains 11 genes (29). All VirB proteins except VirB1 are essential for tumorigenesis (16). Of the 10 essential proteins, 8 either are hydrophobic and could be membrane localized or have signal sequences and could be localized in the periplasm. Two VirB proteins, VirB4 and VirB11, contain mostly hydrophilic residues and are thought to be localized primarily in the cytoplasm (39). VirB4 and VirB11 show ATPase activity and are speculated to provide the energy required for export of other protein subunits or for DNA (30, 126). VirB proteins direct the production of a pilus that resembles conjugative pili (50), and VirB2 is the major subunit of this pilus (77). VirB7 may help to anchor this pilus, since it is an outer membrane lipoprotein that forms disulfide bonds with the periplasmically localized VirB9 (6, 13, 130). VirD4 is considered to be closely associated with the VirB protein complex. VirD4 is absolutely required for transfer and pilus formation (83, 112). The N-terminal one-third of VirD4 is secreted into the periplasmic space, while the C terminus is cytoplasmic (104). VirB1 possesses sequence motifs found in bacterial transglycosylases and eukaryotic lysozymes, suggesting a role in the assembly of the transport apparatus by localized digestion of the peptidoglycan (100).

The VirB apparatus delivers the T-strand to the host cytoplasm, and additional steps are required to transport this DNA to the nucleoplasm and to integrate it into host DNA. VirD2 appears to play central roles in both processes. The carboxyl terminus of this protein contains a bipartite nuclear localization signal (NLS) that is thought to guide nuclear targeting by interacting with members of the karyopherin alpha family (11, 61). This NLS is also sufficient for nuclear localization of VirD2 in mammalian cells (58, 115). A different region of VirD2 was reported to bind cyclophilins of *Arabidopsis* (41). A site directly adjacent to the NLS, designated omega, has also been implicated in DNA integration (101).

The VirE2 protein is also transferred to host cells, and genetic evidence suggests that this protein is transferred separately from T-DNA. Mutations in *virE2* can be complemented extracellularly (31). The complementing strain must express *virE1, virE2,* the *virB* operon, and *virD4* but does not require the *virC* operon or T-DNA (90, 135). Conversely, the T-DNA donor must express the *virB* operon, the *virD* operon, and the *virC* operon but does not need to express the *virE* operon. The observations that VirE1 is needed only to export VirE2 and that VirC proteins are needed solely to export T-DNA are reminiscent of

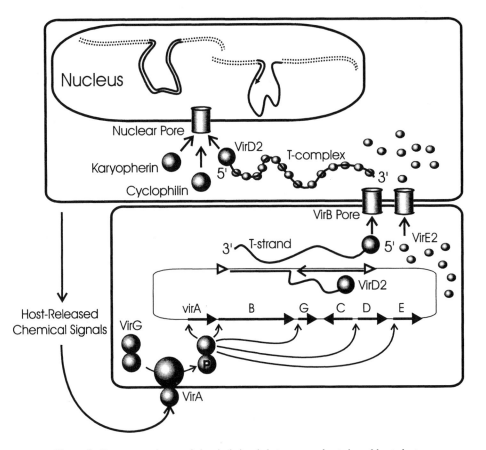

Figure 2. Two-way exchange of chemical signals between agrobacteria and host plants. Host-released chemical signals (including phenolic compounds, monosaccharides, and acidity) are perceived by the VirA to VirG proteins, which transcribe *vir* promoters. T-DNA is nicked by VirD2, and single-stranded, linear T-strands are formed by strand displacement. T-strands and VirE2 separately exit the bacteria via a conjugal pore encoded by the *virB* operon, and they form a T-complex within the plant cytoplasm. T-complexes are transported into the nucleoplasm via two classes of host transport proteins, and the T-DNA is integrated into genomic DNA. For the sake of clarity, the relative orientations of *vir* genes and T-DNA have been inverted.

observations that transport of toxins via type III translocation systems requires dedicated cytoplasmic chaperone proteins (26, 37). Supporting evidence that VirE2 is transferred separately from T-DNA comes from experiments studying the inhibition of tumorigenesis, which can be observed either by providing derivatives of plasmid RSF1010 to *A. tumefaciens* strains or by expressing the *osa* gene of plasmid pSa (26, 134). In extracellular complementation experiments, both forms of inhibition were more effective at blocking VirE2 transport than at blocking T-DNA transport.

VirE2 protein binds tightly and cooperatively to single-stranded nucleic acids (31, 33, 122) and is thought to bind to the T-DNA molecules within the host cytoplasm, forming a so-called T-complex (Fig. 2) (32, 34). Mutational analysis of VirE2 indicates that the carboxyl-terminal half of the protein is responsible for DNA binding while the amino-terminal half mediates cooperative interactions (44). Imaging VirE2-DNA complexes by scanning transmission electron microscopy showed that VirE2 packages DNA into hollow, coiled, cylindrical filaments (32).

A considerable body of evidence indicates that VirE2 functions solely in the plant cells. The best evidence for this is that transgenic plants expressing VirE2 can be transformed at high efficiency by *virE2* mutants of *A. tumefaciens* (34). Like VirD2, VirE2 contains NLSs that mediate the transport of T-DNA from the cytoplasm to the nucleoplasm (102, 118). Two such sites have been identified, each of which acts independently. Microinjection of single-stranded DNA coated with wild-type VirE2 resulted in localization of the DNA in the nucleus, while microinjection of DNA coated with mutant VirE2 lacking its NLSs abolished nuclear import (159). The NLSs of wild-type VirE2 did not function in *Xenopus* nuclei, but alteration of one amino acid residue restored nuclear import (58).

VirF also appears to be exported to the plant host by the *vir*-encoded transport apparatus, since (i) a *virF* mutant can be complemented extracellularly by an avirulent strain that expresses *virF* and the *vir* transfer apparatus and (ii) plants that are engineered to express *virF* can be efficiently transformed by *virF* mutant strains (114).

CONJUGATION MODEL FOR T-DNA TRANSFER

Many aspects of T-DNA transfer resemble interbacterial conjugal transfer of plasmid DNA (82). In both processes, transfer is initiated by single-stranded scissions (at border sites for T-DNA transfer and at *oriT* sites for conjugal plasmids), with the endonuclease remaining bound to the 5′ end of the cleaved strand. In both cases, DNA is transferred in a single-stranded form. Furthermore, proteins required for conjugation interact with Vir proteins, resulting in the transfer of a conjugal plasmid to other agrobacteria, plant cells, yeast, or filamentous fungi (15, 40, 81, 145). Perhaps the most direct evidence that T-DNA transfer resembles conjugation is the extensive sequence similarities between Vir proteins and certain Tra proteins. Each of the 11 proteins encoded by the *virB* region resembles a Tra protein encoded by the IncN plasmid pKM101, while 10 VirB proteins have homologs encoded by the IncW plasmid R388 (69, 111). These proteins also show a lower degree of similarity to the Tra proteins encoded by the IncP and IncF plasmids (81). The VirD1, VirD2, and VirD4 proteins also resemble proteins required for conjugation. In fact, the VirB and VirD operons together would constitute a complete set of conjugation proteins. Furthermore, the T-DNA border resembles the *oriT* sites of certain plasmids, and endonucleolytic cleavage occurs at identical positions (145). The gene family of Vir and Tra proteins also includes the Ptl proteins of *Bordetella pertussis,* which direct the export of pertussis toxin, and certain Cag proteins of *Helicobacter pylori* (3, 146). VirB, Tra, Ptl, and Cag proteins have been designated type IV export systems (119).

REGULATED EXPRESSION OF THE *vir* REGULON

The Vir proteins described above are expressed as a regulon and are coordinately induced in response to host-released chemical signals. This was first shown by cocultivating the bacteria with cultured roots or cultured mesophyll cells and later demonstrated by using synthetic inducing compounds (131). Two stimulatory molecules were purified from spent plant cell culture medium and identified as the phenolic compounds acetosyringone and α-hydroxyacetosyringone. Since then, a large number of inducing compounds have been identified, many of which are synthesized by plants (93, 129). Particular monosaccharides play a synergistic role in *vir* gene induction. Of these, the acidic sugars glucuronic acid and galacturonic acid were effective at extremely low concentrations, while higher concentrations of neutral sugars were required (7). This enhancement in *vir* gene expression was most evident when acetosyringone was provided in limiting amounts (22, 125). A third stimulus essential for *vir* gene induction is environmental acidity in the range of 5.0 to 5.5 (105, 131, 141). Phenolic compounds, monosaccharides, and acidity are thought to be ubiquitous exudates of roots and wound sites (70). The extremely broad host range of this organism is due in part to its ability to recognize ubiquitous plant-released compounds.

All *vir* promoters are positively regulated by the response regulator VirG, which is phosphorylated by the transmembrane two-component kinase VirA (Fig. 2) (123, 149). VirA is dimeric in both the presence and absence of inducing stimuli (107), and it contains four functional domains, denoted the periplasmic, linker, kinase, and receiver domains (24, 92, 148). Truncated VirA protein, lacking its periplasmic domain and transmembrane regions, can still respond to acetosyringone, indicating that any receptor for phenolics must lie in a cytoplasmic portion of the protein (24, 92). This truncation abolished the ability of the protein to detect sugars (22, 24, 125). The linker domain is essential for detection of phenolics and may contain a binding site for these compounds (24). There is still some controversy about whether phenolic compounds bind directly to VirA or whether they bind to some other receptor. A radiolabeled analog of acetosyringone failed to bind VirA but bound instead to two small soluble proteins (60, 78). However, convincing genetic evidence was obtained that VirA binds phenolics directly. This was shown by comparing the specificity of a variety of different VirA proteins for phenolics (79).

VirA contains a histidine kinase domain that resembles other two-component kinases, and VirA can undergo autophosphorylation in vitro, probably at His474 (64, 68, 97). At the carboxyl terminus of VirA is a domain that weakly resembles the receiver domain of VirG. This domain plays a purely inhibitory role, since removing it dramatically increases the activity of the kinase in vivo (24, 57). Several other two-component kinases have receiver domains at their carboxyl termini, and in many cases these domains are thought to be part of a phosphorelay, in which the kinase phosphorylates the receiver, which phosphorylates another intermediate, which finally kinases the response regulator (10, 62, 67, 91). However, since removal of the receiver domain of VirA increases kinase activity, this receiver cannot be part of an obligate phosphorelay. VirA transfers its phosphoryl group to the conserved and essential Asp52 residue of VirG (68, 117). The carboxyl-terminal domain of VirG, designated the output domain, has a helix-turn-helix motif characteristic of DNA-binding proteins and binds to 12-nucleotide sequences called *vir* boxes. One or two of these motifs are found directly upstream of all VirG-regulated promoters (9, 113, 117, 148).

A third protein, ChvE, is also required for efficient *vir* gene expression. ChvE is a periplasmic sugar-binding protein that is required for sugar utilization and for chemotaxis to particular sugars (63, 73). It is also required for detection of monosaccharides, since monosaccharides do not stimulate *vir* gene expression in a *chvE* mutant. Increased expression of ChvE potentiates *vir* gene expression and broadens the spectrum of inducers of phenolics (109). ChvE activity requires the periplasmic domain of VirA, since *virA* mutants lacking the periplasmic domain show the same phenotype as *chvE* null mutants do (22, 24). Different laboratories have isolated point mutations in the periplasmic domain of VirA that block the detection of monosaccharides (12, 45, 46, 124), and one such mutant was suppressed in an allele-specific fashion by a point mutation in *chvE* (124).

Some *vir* genes are subject to additional regulatory controls. *virG* is one example, in that it is expressed from two regulated promoters, only one of which (P1) is regulated by phospho-VirG. This promoter is also induced by phosphate starvation, probably via *Agrobacterium* equivalents of the PhoR and PhoB proteins (8). The other promoter (P2) is induced by environmental acidity, possibly through the ChvG-ChvI two-component system (25, 85). The *virC* and *virD* operons are subject to negative regulation by the chromosomally encoded Ros protein (35, 136). Both promoters are transcribed at elevated levels in *ros* mutants but are further induced by acetosyringone (35). Ros also represses the *ipt* gene, which is found on the T-DNA (28). This finding was quite surprising, since it indicates that *ipt* has a bacterial promoter as well as a plant promoter. Ros has a zinc finger motif and binds zinc (28). Ros has also been found in *Rhizobium* spp., where it positively regulates the synthesis of exopolysaccharides (18).

Some members of the *vir* regulon are not essential for tumorigenesis and may play other roles in pathogenesis. One example is the *virH* operon, which consists of two genes whose products are homologous to each other and to the family of P-450 monooxygenases (72), which oxidize their substrates by addition of one atom of molecular oxygen (99). In one study, *virH* mutants were slightly attenuated for virulence (72), suggesting that *virH* plays a direct but nonessential role in tumorigenesis. However, in another study, a deletion of both genes did not detectably affect tumorigenesis efficiency (71). Another example of a VirG-regulated gene not required for tumorigenesis is the *tzs* gene of nopaline-type Ti plasmids, which synthesizes cytokinin (1, 2, 98). We have recently identified additional members of the *vir* regulon (Fig. 1) that are not required for tumorigenesis, including *virM, virL,* and *virK* (71) and *virD5, virE3, virP,* and *virR* (unpublished data).

UPTAKE AND CATABOLISM OF OPINES

As described above, several T-DNA genes direct the synthesis of opines, which are exported from the plant cell and serve the bacteria as nutrient sources. Catabolism of opines provides the bacteria with sources of energy, carbon, and, in some cases, nitrogen or phosphorus. Each strain of *Agrobacterium* directs plants to synthesize more than one class of opine. Collectively, *Agrobacterium* strains synthesize an astonishing array of opines, and for all strains so characterized, a perfect match is found between transferred opine synthesis genes and nontransferred opine catabolism genes. The apparent rapid evolution of new opines is striking, since creating a novel opine should require the simultaneous evolution of a new opine synthase, a new opine uptake system, new catabolic genes, and new regulatory genes. This indicates that an extremely strong selective pressure must exist for opine diversification.

Opines activate the transcription of *Agrobacterium* genes whose products direct their uptake and catabolism (43). In the octopine-type Ti plasmid, more than 55 kb of DNA is devoted to opine uptake and degradation (including the *occ, mop, agr, aga, moa,* and possibly *oph* operons [Fig. 1]). This region contains no fewer than six ATP-binding cassette-type uptake systems, as well as a variety of cognate catabolic genes and regulatory genes. For example, the *occ* operon contains four genes that encode an octopine-specific uptake system and three genes that direct octopine catabolism. This operon is positively regulated by the product of the divergently transcribed *occR* gene (59, 144).

CELL DENSITY-DEPENDENT INTERBACTERIAL CONJUGATION OF Ti PLASMIDS

Ti plasmids contain complete sets of *tra* genes that are responsible for their interbacterial conjugal transfer (5, 48, 49, 150). Ti plasmid conjugation systems are fully independent of the T-DNA transfer systems described above, although the *tra* and *vir* systems do have a common ancestor (36). DNA sequence analysis indicates that both *vir* and *tra* systems have chimeric origins. Most components of the *tra* system resemble IncP-type *tra* genes, while one *tra* gene resembles an RSF1010 *mob* gene at its 5′ end and resembles an IncF *tra* gene at its 3′ end. Likewise, all 11 genes in the *virB* operon resemble IncN *tra* genes, while 2 genes in the *virD* operon resemble IncP-type *tra* genes (5, 49, 111). In all cases, sequence similarities between *tra* genes and *vir* genes are comparatively weak.

Transcription of the *tra* regulon is tightly regulated and requires host-released chemical signals, specifically opines (56, 74). Conjugation of octopine-type Ti plasmids requires octopine, while conjugation of nopaline-type Ti plasmids requires agrocinopine A or B. The mechanism by which opines regulate conjugation is more complex than was originally anticipated. In the case of octopine-type Ti plasmids, a gene designated *traR* is found at the distal end of the *occ* operon and is induced in response to octopine via the OccR regulatory protein (53). TraR, in turn, is a direct positive regulator of other *tra* genes (55). The *traR* gene of the nopaline-type Ti plasmid pTiC58 is repressed by a protein called AccR (14). In this case, agrocinopine neutralizes repression, allowing TraR synthesis.

TraR is a member of the LuxR family of quorum-sensing transcriptional regulators (52). Like other members of this family, its activity requires an *N*-acylhomoserine lactone. For TraR, the inducer was identified as *N*-3-oxooctanoyl-L-homoserine lactone (3-oxo-C_8-HSL) (66, 157). This compound is synthesized in the bacterial cytoplasm but diffuses across the cell envelope and acts as a bacterial pheromone, allowing the bacteria to estimate their population densities. This pheromone is synthesized by a protein encoded by the *traI* gene (55, 66). This protein utilizes 3-oxo-C_8-acyl carrier protein and *S*-adenosylmethionine as substrates (96).

Purified TraR binds one molecule of pheromone per protein monomer and binds to DNA sequences directly upstream of the divergent *traA* and *traC* promoters (158a). Bound TraR stimulates the transcription of these promoters in vitro on supercoiled templates but is largely inactive on linear templates. The in vivo activity of TraR is antagonized by a protein designated TraM. The mechanism of inhibition is not understood, and TraM does not resemble other known proteins (51, 65). Interestingly, the *traM* gene is positively regulated by TraR, thereby creating a negative autoregulatory loop (51, 65). In octopine-type Ti plasmids, TraR is also antagonized by the TrlR protein, which is extremely closely related to TraR but is truncated at its carboxyl terminus such that is contains a pheromone-binding domain but lacks a DNA-binding domain (103, 158). The mechanism by which TrlR antagonizes TraR probably involves the formation of inactive heterodimers. The *trlR* gene is positively regulated by mannopine (103, 158), possibly via the product of the *mocR* gene (Fig. 3). In wild-type strains, mannopine antagonizes octopine for *tra* gene expression and antagonism is abolished by a *trlR* mutation. Artificial overexpression of *trlR* also inhibits *tra* gene expression (103, 158). Expression of *trlR* was strongly inhibited by favored catabolites including succinate, glutamine, and tryptone, and these catabolites thereby restored *tra* gene expression (158).

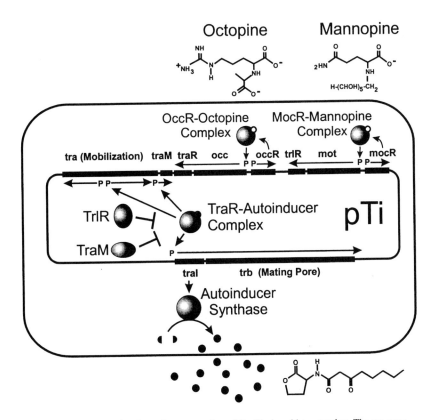

Figure 3. Cell density-dependent expression of the Ti plasmid *tra* regulon. The *tra* gene regulator TraR is synthesized in response to host-released opines. At high cell densities, TraR binds the pheromone 3-oxo-C_8-HSL and activates the transcription of other *tra* and *trb* promoters. TraR activity is antagonized by TraM and by TrlR. *traM* is part of the *tra* regulon, resulting in negative autoregulation, while *trlR* is induced in response to host-released mannopine. The role of MocR in the regulation of *mot* and *trlR* is speculative.

CONCLUSIONS

As described above, most of the genes of the Ti plasmid play direct or indirect roles in some aspect of tumorigenesis or tumor colonization. We understand the roles of most of the T-DNA genes, although the functions of a few of them remain mysterious. We have some insights into the processing and transfer of the T-DNA, although our understanding of the VirB-encoded pore is rudimentary, as is our understanding of the steps involved in nuclear transport and integration. VirA and VirG remain important paradigms for host detection, and the multidomain structure of VirA remains fertile ground for future work. Of the 34 known VirG-regulated genes, fully one-third are not required for tumorigenesis, strongly suggesting that plant-released *vir*-inducing signals elicit multiple bacterial responses.

It is striking that such a large portion of the Ti plasmid is devoted to opine catabolism, and few of these systems have been studied in any depth. Perhaps the most perplexing feature of Ti plasmids is their quorum-dependent regulation of conjugal transfer genes. Since Ti plasmids encode both TraI and TraR, each conjugal donor takes a census of other donors rather than of recipients. It is a challenge even to speculate about the adaptive value of such a system. The observation that two opines regulate conjugation in opposite ways is equally perplexing. Some genes regulated by TraR are not required for conjugation, suggesting that high cell densities may elicit multiple responses, and these remain to be described. We are left to conclude that the area of tumor colonization will be an especially fertile area for future studies.

Acknowledgments. We thank our many colleagues for their encouragement and their willingness to share unpublished data, insights, and ideas, which has helped to make this field so rewarding. Research in our laboratory is supported by NIH grant GM42893.

REFERENCES

1. **Akiyoshi, D. E., D. A. Regier, and M. P. Gordon.** 1987. Cytokinin production by *Agrobacterium* and *Pseudomonas* spp. *J. Bacteriol.* **169:**4242–4248.
2. **Akiyoshi, D. E., D. A. Regier, G. Jen, and M. P. Gordon.** 1985. Cloning and nucleotide sequence of the *tzs* gene from *Agrobacterium tumefaciens* strain T37. *Nucleic Acids Res.* **13:**2773–2788.
3. **Akopyants, N. S., S. W. Clifton, D. Kersulyte, J. E. Crabtree, B. E. Youree, C. A. Reece, N. O. Bukanov, E. S. Drazek, B. A. Roe, and D. E. Berg.** 1998. Analyses of the *cag* pathogenicity island of *Helicobacter pylori*. *Mol. Microbiol.* **28:**37–53.
4. **Albright, L. M., M. F. Yanofsky, B. Leroux, D. Q. Ma, and E. W. Nester.** 1987. Processing of the T-DNA of *Agrobacterium tumefaciens* generates border nicks and linear, single-stranded T-DNA. *J. Bacteriol.* **169:**1046–1055.
5. **Alt-Mörbe, J., J. L. Stryker, C. Fuqua, S. K. Farrand, and S. C. Winans.** 1996. The conjugal transfer system of *A. tumefaciens* octopine-type Ti plasmids is closely related to the transfer system of an IncP plasmid and distantly related to Ti plasmid *vir* genes. *J. Bacteriol.* **178:**4248–4257.
6. **Anderson, L. B., A. V. Hertzel, and A. Das.** 1996. *Agrobacterium tumefaciens* VirB7 and VirB9 form a disulfide-linked protein complex. *Proc. Natl. Acad. Sci. USA* **93:**8889–8894.
7. **Ankenbauer, R. G., and E. W. Nester.** 1990. Sugar-mediated induction of *Agrobacterium tumefaciens* virulence genes: structural specificity and activities of monosaccharides. *J. Bacteriol.* **172:**6442–6446.
8. **Aoyama, T., M. Takanami, K. Makino, and A. Oka.** 1991. Cross-talk between the virulence and phosphate regulons of *Agrobacterium tumefaciens* caused by an unusual interaction of the transcriptional activator with a regulatory DNA element. *Mol. Gen. Genet.* **227:**385–390.
9. **Aoyama, T., M. Takanami, and A. Oka.** 1989. Signal structure for transcriptional activation in the

upstream regions of virulence genes on the hairy-root-inducing plasmid A4. *Nucleic Acids Res.* **17:** 8711–8725.

10. **Arico, B., J. F. Miller, C. Roy, S. Stibitz, D. Monack, S. Falkow, R. Gross, and R. Rappuoli.** 1989. Sequences required for expression of *Bordetella pertussis* virulence factors share homology with prokaryotic signal transduction proteins. *Proc. Natl. Acad. Sci. USA* **86:**6671–6675.

11. **Ballas, N., and V. Citovsky.** 1997. Nuclear localization signal binding protein from *Arabidopsis* mediates nuclear import of *Agrobacterium* VirD2 protein. *Proc. Natl. Acad. Sci. USA* **94:**10723–10728.

12. **Banta, L. M., R. D. Joerger, V. R. Howitz, A. M. Campbell, and A. N. Binns.** 1994. Glu-255 outside the predicted ChvE binding site in VirA is crucial for sugar enhancement of acetsyringone perception by *Agrobacterium tumefaciens. J. Bacteriol.* **176:**3242–3249.

13. **Baron, C., Y. R. Thorstenson, and P. C. Zambryski.** 1997. The lipoprotein VirB7 interacts with VirB9 in the membranes of *Agrobacterium tumefaciens. J. Bacteriol.* **179:**1211–1218.

14. **Beck von Bodman, S., G. T. Hayman, and S. K. Farrand.** 1992. Opine catabolism and conjugal transfer of the nopaline Ti plasmid pTiC58 are coordinately regulated by a single repressor. *Proc. Natl. Acad. Sci. USA* **89:**643–647.

15. **Beijersbergen, A., A. Den Dulk-Ras, R. A. Shilperoort, and P. J. J. Hooykaas.** 1992. Conjugative transfer by the virulence system of *Agrobacterium tumefaciens. Science* **256:**1324–1327.

16. **Berger, B. R., and P. J. Christie.** 1994. Genetic complementation analysis of the *Agrobacterium tumefaciens virB* operon: *virB2* through *virB11* are essential virulence genes. *J. Bacteriol.* **176:**3646–3660.

17. **Bevan, M. W., and M.-D. Chilton.** 1982. T-DNA of the *Agrobacterium* Ti and Ri plasmids. *Annu. Rev. Genet.* **16:**357–384.

18. **Bittinger, M. A., J. L. Milner, B. J. Saville, and J. Handelsman.** 1997. *rosR*, a determinant of nodulation competitiveness in *Rhizobium etli. Mol. Plant-Microbe Interact.* **10:**180–186.

19. **Braun, A. C.** 1958. A physiological basis for autonomous growth of crown gall tumor cell. *Proc. Natl. Acad. Sci. USA* **44:**344–349.

20. **Bruce, W. B., and W. B. Gurley.** 1987. Functional domains of a T-DNA promoter active in crown gall tumors. *Mol. Cell. Biol.* **7:**59–67.

21. **Canaday, J., J. C. Gerad, P. Crouzet, and L. Otten.** 1992. Organization and functional analysis of three T-DNAs from the vitopine Ti plasmid pTiS4. *Mol. Gen. Genet.* **235:**292–303.

22. **Cangelosi, G. A., R. G. Ankenbauer, and E. W. Nester.** 1990. Sugars induce the *Agrobacterium* virulence genes through a periplasmic binding protein and a transmembrane signal protein. *Proc. Natl. Acad. Sci. USA* **87:**6708–6712.

23. **Cangelosi, G. A., L. Huang, V. Puvanesarajah, G. Stacey, D. A. Ozga, J. A. Leigh, and E. W. Nester.** 1987. Common loci for *Agrobacterium tumefaciens* and *Rhizobium meliloti* exopolysaccharide synthesis and their roles in plant interactions. *J. Bacteriol.* **169:**2086–2091.

24. **Chang, C. H., and S. C. Winans.** 1992. Functional roles assigned to the periplasmic, linker, and receiver domains of the *Agrobacterium tumefaciens* VirA protein. *J. Bacteriol.* **174:**7033–7039.

25. **Charles, T. C., and E. W. Nester.** 1993. A chromosomally encoded two-component sensory transduction system is required for virulence of *Agrobacterium tumefaciens. J. Bacteriol.* **175:**6614–6625.

26. **Chen, C. Y., and C. I. Kado.** 1994. Inhibition of *Agrobacterium tumefaciens* oncogenicity by the *osa* gene of pSa. *J. Bacteriol.* **176:**5697–5703.

27. **Chilton, M.-D., M. H. Drummond, D. J. Merlo, D. Sciaky, A. L. Montoya, M. P. Gordon, and E. W. Nester.** 1977. Stable incorporation of plasmid DNA into higher plant cells: the molecular basis of crown gall tumorigenesis. *Cell* **11:**263–271.

28. **Chou, A. Y., J. Archdeacon, and C. I. Kado.** 1998. *Agrobacterium* transcriptional regulator Ros is a prokaryotic zinc finger protein that regulates the plant oncogene *ipt. Proc. Natl. Acad. Sci. USA* **95:** 5293–5298.

29. **Christie, P. J.** 1997. *Agrobacterium tumefaciens* T-complex transport apparatus: a paradigm for a new family of multifunctional transporters in eubacteria. *J. Bacteriol.* **179:**3085–3094.

30. **Christie, P. J., J. E. Ward, Jr., M. P. Gordon, and E. W. Nester.** 1989. A gene required for transfer of T-DNA to plants encodes an ATPase with autophosphorylating activity. *Proc. Natl. Acad. Sci. USA* **86:** 9677–9681.

31. **Christie, P. J., W. E. Ward, S. C. Winans, and E. W. Nester.** 1988. The *Agrobacterium tumefaciens virE2* gene product is a single-stranded-DNA-binding protein that associates with T-DNA. *J. Bacteriol.* **170:**2659–2667.

32. **Citovsky, V., B. Guralnick, M. N. Simon, and J. S. Wall.** 1997. The molecular structure of agrobacterium VirE2-single stranded DNA complexes involved in nuclear import. *J. Mol. Biol.* **5:**718–727.

33. **Citovsky, V., M. L. Wong, and P. Zambryski.** 1989. Cooperative interaction of *Agrobacterium* VirE2 protein with single-stranded DNA: implications for the T-DNA transfer process. *Proc. Natl. Acad. Sci. USA* **86:**1193–1197.

34. **Citovsky, V., J. Zupan, D. Warnick, and P. Zambryski.** 1992. Nuclear localization of *Agrobacterium* VirE2 protein in plant cells. *Science* **256:**1802–1805.

35. **Close, T. J., P. M. Rogowsky, C. I. Kado, S. C. Winans, M. F. Yanofsky, and E. W. Nester.** 1987. Dual control of *Agrobacterium tumefaciens* Ti plasmid virulence genes. *J. Bacteriol.* **169:**5113–5118.

36. **Cook, D. M., P.-L. Li, F. Ruchaud, S. Padden, and S. K. Farrand.** 1997. Ti plasmid conjugation is independent of *vir:* reconstitution of the *tra* functions from pTiC58 as a binary system. *J. Bacteriol.* **179:** 1291–1297.

37. **Cornelis, G. R., and H. Wolf-Watz.** 1997. The *Yersinia* Yop virulon: a bacterial system for subverting eukaryotic cells. *Mol. Microbiol.* **23:**861–867.

38. **Costacurta, A., and J. Vanderleyden.** 1995. Synthesis of phytohormones by plant-associated bacteria. *Crit. Rev. Microbiol.* **21:**1–18.

39. **Dang, T. A., and P. J. Christie.** 1997. The VirB4 ATPase of *Agrobacterium tumefaciens* is a cytoplasmic membrane protein exposed at the periplasmic surface. *J. Bacteriol.* **179:**453–462.

40. **de Groot, M. J., P. Bundock, P. J. Hooykaas, and A. G. Beijersbergen.** 1998. *Agrobacterium tumefaciens*-mediated transformation of filamentous fungi. *Nat. Biotechnol.* **16:**839–842.

41. **Deng, W., L. Chen, D. W. Wood, T. Metcalfe, X. Liang, M. P. Gordon, L. Comai, and E. W. Nester.** 1998. Agrobacterium VirD2 protein interacts with plant host cyclophilins. *Proc. Natl. Acad. Sci. USA* **95:** 7040–7045.

42. **De Pater, B. S., M. P. Klinkhamer, P. A. Amesz, R. J. de Kam, J. Memelink, J. H. Hoge, and R. A. Schilperoort.** 1987. Plant expression signals of the *Agrobacterium* T-cyt gene. *Nucleic Acids Res.* **15:** 8267–8281.

43. **Dessaux, Y., A. Petit, and J. Tempe.** 1992. Opines in *Agrobacterium* biology, p. 109–136. *In* D. P. S. Verma (ed.), *Molecular Signals in Plant-Microbe Communications.* CRC Press, Inc., Ann Arbor, Mich.

44. **Dombek, P., and W. Ream.** 1997. Functional domains of *Agrobacterium tumefaciens* single-stranded DNA-binding protein VirE2. *J. Bacteriol.* **179:**1165–1173.

45. **Doty, S. L., M. Chang, and E. W. Nester.** 1993. The chromosomal virulence gene *chvE* of *Agrobacterium tumefaciens* is regulated by a LysR family member. *J. Bacteriol.* **175:**7880–7886.

46. **Doty, S. L., M. C. Yu, J. I. Lundin, J. D. Heath, and E. W. Nester.** 1996. Mutational analysis of the input domain of the VirA protein of *Agrobacterium tumefaciens. J. Bacteriol.* **178:**961–970.

47. **Douglas, C. J., R. J. Staneloni, R. A. Rubin, and E. W. Nester.** 1985. Identification and genetic analysis of an *Agrobacterium tumefaciens* chromosomal virulence region. *J. Bacteriol.* **161:**850–860.

48. **Farrand, S. K.** 1993. Conjugal transfer of *Agrobacterium* plasmids, p. 255–291. *In* D. B. Clewell (ed.), *Bacterial Conjugation.* Plenum Press, New York, N.Y.

49. **Farrand, S. K., I. Hwang, and D. M. Cook.** 1996. The *tra* region of the nopaline-type Ti plasmid is a chimera with elements related to the transfer systems of RSF1010, RP4, and F. *J. Bacteriol.* **178:**4233–4247.

50. **Fullner, K. J., J. C. Lara, and E. W. Nester.** 1996. Pilus assembly by *Agrobacterium* T-DNA transfer genes. *Science* **273:**1107–1109.

51. **Fuqua, C., M. Burbea, and S. C. Winans.** 1995. Activity of the *Agrobacterium* Ti plasmid conjugal transfer regulator TraR is inhibited by the product of the *traM* gene. *J. Bacteriol.* **177:**1367–1373.

52. **Fuqua, C., S. C. Winans, and E. P. Greenberg.** 1996. Census and consensus in bacterial ecosystems: the LuxR-LuxI family of quorum-sensing transcriptional regulators. *Annu. Rev. Microbiol.* **50:**727–751.

53. **Fuqua, C., and S. C. Winans.** 1996. Localization of OccR-activated and TraR-activated promoters that express two ABC-type permeases and the *traR* gene of Ti plasmid pTiR10. *Mol. Microbiol.* **20:**1199–1210.

54. **Fuqua, C., and S. C. Winans.** 1996. Conserved *cis*-acting promoter elements are required for density-dependent transcription of *Agrobacterium tumefaciens* conjugal transfer genes. *J. Bacteriol.* **178:**435–440.

55. **Fuqua, W. C., and S. C. Winans.** 1994. A LuxR-LuxI type regulatory system activates *Agrobacterium* Ti plasmid conjugal transfer in the presence of a plant tumor metabolite. *J. Bacteriol.* **176:**2796–2806.

56. **Genetello, C., N. van Larebeke, M. Holsters, A. De Picker, M. van Montagu, and J. Schell.** 1977. Ti plasmids of *Agrobacterium* as conjugative plasmids. *Nature* (London) **265:**561–563.

57. **Gubba, S., Y. H. Xie, and A. Das.** 1995. Regulation of *Agrobacterium tumefaciens* virulence gene expression: isolation of a mutation that restores virGD52E function. *Mol. Plant-Microbe Interact.* **8:**788–791.

58. **Guralnick, B., G. Thomsen, and V. Citovsky.** 1996. Transport of DNA into the nuclei of *Xenopus* oocytes by a modified VirE2 protein of *Agrobacterium. Plant Cell* **8:**363–373.

59. **Habeeb, L., L. Wang, and S. C. Winans.** 1991. Transcription of the octopine catabolism operon of the *Agrobacterium* tumor-inducing plasmid pTiA6 is activated by a LysR-type regulatory protein. *Mol. Plant-Microbe Interact.* **4:**379–385.

60. **Hess, K. M., M. W. Dudley, D. G. Lynn, R. D. Joerger, and A. N. Binns.** 1991. Mechanism of phenolic activation of *Agrobacterium* virulence genes: development of a specific inhibitor of bacterial sensor/response systems. *Proc. Natl. Acad. Sci. USA* **88:**7854–7858.

61. **Howard, E. A., J. R. Zupan, V. Citovsky, and P. C. Zambryski.** 1992. The VirD2 protein of *A. tumefaciens* contains a C-terminal bipartite nuclear localization signal: implications for nuclear uptake of DNA in plant cells. *Cell* **68:**109–118.

62. **Hrabak, E. M., and D. K. Willis.** 1992. The *lemA* gene required for pathogenicity of *Pseudomonas syringae* pv. *syringae* on bean is a member of a family of two-component regulators. *J. Bacteriol.* **174:**3011–3020.

63. **Huang, M. L., G. A. Cangelosi, W. Halperin, and E. W. Nester.** 1990. A chromosomal *Agrobacterium tumefaciens* gene required for effective plant signal transduction. *J. Bacteriol.* **172:**1814–1822.

64. **Huang, Y., P. Morel, B. Powell, and C. I. Kado.** 1990. VirA, a coregulator of Ti-specified virulence genes, is phosphorylated in vitro. *J. Bacteriol.* **172:**1142–1144.

65. **Hwang, I., D. M. Cook, and S. K. Farrand.** 1995. A new regulatory element modulates homoserine lactone-mediated autoinduction of Ti plasmid conjugal transfer. *J. Bacteriol.* **177:**449–458.

66. **Hwang, I., L. Pei-Li, L. Zhang, K. R. Piper, D. M. Cook, M. E. Tate, and S. K. Farrand.** 1994. TraI, a LuxI homolog, is responsible for production of conjugation factor, the Ti plasmid *N*-acylhomoserine lactone autoinducer. *Proc. Natl. Acad. Sci. USA* **91:**4639–4643.

67. **Iuchi, S., Z. Matsuda, T. Fujiwara, and E. C. Lin.** 1990. The *arcB* gene of *Escherichia coli* encodes a sensor-regulator protein for anaerobic repression of the *arc* modulon. *Mol. Microbiol.* **4:**715–727.

68. **Jin, S., T. Roitsch, R. G. Ankenbauer, M. P. Gordon, and E. W. Nester.** 1990. The VirA protein of *Agrobacterium tumefaciens* is autophosphorylated and is essential for *vir* gene regulation. *J. Bacteriol.* **172:**525–530.

69. **Kado, C. I.** 1994. Promiscuous DNA transfer system of *Agrobacterium tumefaciens:* role of the virB operon in sex pilus assembly and synthesis. *Mol. Microbiol.* **12:**17–22.

70. **Kahl, G.** 1982. Molecular biology of wound healing: the conditioning phenomenon, p. 211–268. *In* G. Kahl and J. S. Schell (ed.), *Molecular Biology of Plant Tumors.* Academic Press, Inc., New York, N.Y.

71. **Kalogeraki, V. S., and S. C. Winans.** 1998. Wound-released chemical signals may elicit multiple responses from an *Agrobacterium tumefaciens* strain containing an octopine-type Ti plasmid. *J. Bacteriol.* **180:**5660–5667.

72. **Kanemoto, R. H., A. T. Powell, D. E. Akiyoshi, D. A. Regier, R. A. Kerstetter, E. W. Nester, M. C. Hawes, and M. P. Gordon.** 1989. Nucleotide sequence and analysis of the plant-inducible locus *pinF* from *Agrobacterium tumefaciens. J. Bacteriol.* **171:**2506–2512.

73. **Kemner, J. M., X. Liang, and E. W. Nester.** 1997. The *Agrobacterium tumefaciens* virulence gene *chvE* is part of a putative ABC-type sugar transport operon. *J. Bacteriol.* **179:**2452–2458.

74. **Kerr, A., P. Manigault, and J. Tempe.** 1977. Transfer of virulence *in vivo* and *in vitro* in *Agrobacterium. Nature* (London) **265:**560–561.

75. **Kersters, K., and J. de Ley.** 1984. Genus III. *Agrobacterium* Conn 1942, 359[AL], p. 244–254. *In* N. R. Krieg and J. G. Holt (ed.), *Bergey's Manual of Systematic Bacteriology,* vol. 1. The Williams & Wilkins Co., Baltimore, Md.

76. **Korber, H., N. Strizhov, D. Staiger, J. Feldwisch, O. Olsson, G. Sandberg, K. Palme, J. Schell, and C. Koncz.** 1991. T-DNA gene 5 of *Agrobacterium* modulates auxin response by autoregulated synthesis of a growth hormone antagonist in plants. *EMBO J.* **10:**3983–3991.

77. **Lai, E. M., and C. I. Kado.** 1998. Processed VirB2 is the major subunit of the promiscuous pilus of *Agrobacterium tumefaciens. J. Bacteriol.* **180:**2711–2717.

78. **Lee, K., M. W. Dudley, K. M. Hess, D. G. Lynn, R. D. Joerger, and A. N. Binns.** 1992. Mechanism of activation of *Agrobacterium* virulence genes: identification of phenol-binding proteins. *Proc. Natl. Acad. Sci. USA* **89:**8666–8670.

79. **Lee, Y. W., U. H. Ha, W. S. Sim, and E. W. Nester.** 1998. Characterization of an unusual sensor gene (*virA*) of *Agrobacterium. Gene* **14:**307–314.

80. **Lee, Y.-W., S. Jin, W. S. Sim, and E. W. Nester.** 1996. The sensing of plant signal molecules by *Agrobacterium:* genetic evidence for direct recognition of phenolic inducers by the VirA protein. *Gene* **179:**83–88.

81. **Lessl, M., D. Balzer, W. Pansegrau, and E. Lanka.** 1992. Sequence similarities between the RP4 Tra2 and the Ti VirB region strongly support the conjugation model for T-DNA transfer. *J. Biol. Chem.* **267:** 20471–20480.

82. **Lessl, M., and E. Lanka.** 1994. Common mechanisms in bacterial conjugation and Ti-mediated T-DNA transfer to plant cells. *Cell* **77:**321–324.

83. **Lin, T. S., and C. I. Kado.** 1993. The *virD4* gene is required for virulence while *virD3* and *orf5* are not required for virulence of *Agrobacterium tumefaciens. Mol. Microbiol.* **9:**803–812.

84. **Magrelli, A., K. Langenkemper, C. Dehio, J. Schell, and A. Spena.** 1994. Splicing of the *rolA* transcript of *Agrobacterium rhizogenes* in *Arabidopsis. Science* **266:**1986–1988.

85. **Mantis, N. J., and S. C. Winans.** 1993. The chromosomal response regulatory gene *chvI* of *Agrobacterium tumefaciens* complements an *Escherichia coli phoB* mutation and is required for virulence. *J. Bacteriol.* **175:**6626–6636.

86. **Matthysse, A. G.** 1986. Initial interactions of *Agrobacterium tumefaciens* with plant host cells. *Crit. Rev. Microbiol.* **13:**281–397.

87. **Matthysse, A. G., and S. McMahan.** 1998. Root colonization by *Agrobacterium tumefaciens* is reduced in *cel, att, attD,* and *attR* mutants. *Appl. Environ. Microbiol.* **64:**2341–2345.

88. **Matthysse, A. G., D. L. Thomas, and A. R. White.** 1995. Mechanism of cellulose synthesis in *Agrobacterium tumefaciens. J. Bacteriol.* **177:**1076–1081.

89. **Mayerhofer, R., Z. Koncz-Kalman, C. Nawrath, G. Bakkeren, A. Crameri, K. Angelis, G. P. Redei, J. Schell, B. Hohn, and C. Koncz.** 1991. T-DNA integration: a mode of illegitimate recombination in plants. *EMBO J.* **10:**697–704.

90. **McBride, K. E., and V. C. Knauf.** 1988. Genetic analysis of the *virE* operon of the *Agrobacterium* Ti plasmid pTiA6. *J. Bacteriol.* **170:**1430–1437.

91. **McCleary, W. R., and D. R. Zusman.** 1990. FrzE of *Myxococcus xanthus* is homologous to both CheA and CheY of *Salmonella typhimurium. Proc. Natl. Acad. Sci. USA* **87:**5898–5902.

92. **Melchers, L. S., T. T. J. Regensburg, R. B. Bourret, N. J. Sedee, R. A. Schiperoort, and P. J. Hooykaas.** 1989. Membrane topology and functional analysis of the sensory protein VirA of *Agrobacterium tumefaciens. EMBO J.* **8:**1919–1925.

93. **Melchers, L. S., A. J. G. Regensburg-Tuink, R. A. Schiperoort, and P. J. Hooykaas.** 1989. Specificity of signal molecules in the activation of *Agrobacterium* virulence gene expression. *Mol. Microbiol.* **3:** 969–977.

94. **Messens, E., A. Lenaerts, M. VanMontagu, and R. W. Hedges.** 1985. Genetic basis for opine secretion from crown gall tumor cells. *Mol. Gen. Genet.* **199:**344–348.

95. **Miranda, A., G. Janssen, L. Hodges, E. G. Peralta, and W. Ream.** 1992. *Agrobacterium tumefaciens* transfers extremely long T-DNAs by a unidirectional mechanism. *J. Bacteriol.* **174:**2288–2297.

96. **Moré, M. I., L. D. Finger, J. L. Stryker, C. Fuqua, A. Eberhard, and S. C. Winans.** 1996. Enzymatic synthesis of a quorum-sensing autoinducer through use of defined substrates. *Science* **272:**1655–1658.

97. **Morel, P., B. S. Powell, and C. I. Kado.** 1990. Demonstration of 3 functional domains responsible for a kinase activity in VirA, a transmembrane sensory protein encoded by the Ti plasmid of *Agrobacterium tumefaciens. C. R. Acad. Sci. Ser. III* **310:**21–26.

98. **Morris, R. O.** 1990. Genes specifying auxin and cytokinin biosynthesis in prokaryotes, p. 636–655. *In* P. J. Davies (ed.), *Plant Hormones and Their Role in Plant Growth and Development.* Kluwer Academic Publishers, Dordrecht, The Netherlands.

99. **Munro, A. W., and J. G. Lindsay.** 1996. Bacterial cytochromes P-450. *Mol. Microbiol.* **20:**1115–1125.

100. **Mushegian, A. R., K. J. Fullner, E. V. Koonin, and E. W. Nester.** 1996. A family of lysozyme-like virulence factors in bacterial pathogens of plants and animals. *Proc. Natl. Acad. Sci. USA* **93:**7321–7326.

101. **Mysore, K. S., B. Bassuner, X. B. Deng, N. S. Darbinian, A. Motchoulski, W. Ream, and S. B. Gelvin.** 1998. Role of *Agrobacterium tumefaciens* VirD2 protein in T-DNA transfer and integration. *Mol. Plant-Microbe Interact.* **11:**668–683.

102. **Narasimhulu, S. B., X. B. Deng, R. Sarria, and S. B. Gelvin.** 1996. Early transcription of *Agrobacterium* T-DNA genes in tobacco and maize. *Plant Cell* **8:**873–886.

103. **Oger, P., K.-S. Kim, R. L. Sackett, K. R. Piper, and S. K. Farrand.** 1998. Octopine-type Ti plasmids code for a mannopine-inducible dominant-negative allele of *traR*, the quorum-sensing activator that regulates Ti plasmid conjugal transfer. *Mol. Microbiol.* **27:**277–288.

104. **Okamoto, S., A. Toyoda-Yamamoto, K. Ito, I. Takebe, and Y. Machida.** 1991. Localization and orientation of the VirD4 protein of *Agrobacterium tumefaciens* in the cell membrane. *Mol. Gen. Genet.* **228:**24–32.

105. **Olson, E. R.** 1993. Influence of pH on bacterial gene expression. *Mol. Microbiol.* **8:**5–14.

106. **Ophel, K., and A. Kerr.** 1990. *Agrobacterium vitis* sp. nov. for strains of *Agrobacterium* biovar 3 from grapevines. *Int. J. Syst. Bacteriol.* **40:**236–241.

107. **Pan, S. Q., T. Charles, S. Jin, Z. L. Wu, and E. W. Nester.** 1993. Preformed dimeric state of the sensor protein VirA is involved in plant-*Agrobacterium* signal transduction. *Proc. Natl. Acad. Sci. USA* **90:**9939–9943.

108. **Pansegrau, W., F. Schoumacher, B. Hohn, and E. Lanka.** 1993. Site-specific cleavage and joining of single-stranded DNA by VirD2 protein of *Agrobacterium tumefaciens* Ti plasmids: analogy to bacterial conjugation. *Proc. Natl. Acad. Sci. USA* **90:**11538–11542.

109. **Peng, W. T., Y. W. Lee, and E. W. Nester.** 1998. The phenolic recognition profiles of the *Agrobacterium tumefaciens* VirA protein are broadened by a high level of the sugar binding protein ChvE. *J. Bacteriol.* **180:**5632–5638.

110. **Peralta, E. G., and L. W. Ream.** 1985. T-DNA border sequences required for crown gall tumorigenesis. *Proc. Natl. Acad. Sci. USA* **82:**5112–5116.

111. **Pohlman, R. F., H. D. Genetti, and S. C. Winans.** 1994. Common ancestry between IncN conjugal transfer genes and macromolecular export systems of plant and animal pathogens. *Mol. Microbiol.* **14:**655–668.

112. **Porter, S. G., M. F. Yanofsky, and E. W. Nester.** 1987. Molecular characterization of the *virD* operon from *Agrobacterium tumefaciens*. *Nucleic Acids Res.* **15:**7503–7517.

113. **Powell, B. S., and C. I. Kado.** 1990. Specific binding of VirG to the *vir* box requires a C-terminal domain and exhibits a minimum concentration threshold. *Mol. Microbiol.* **4:**2159–2166.

114. **Regensburg-Tuink, A. J., and P. J. Hooykaas.** 1993. Transgenic *N. glauca* plants expressing bacterial virulence gene *virF* are converted into hosts for nopaline strains of *A. tumefaciens*. *Nature* (London) **363:**69–71.

115. **Relic, B., M. Andjelkovic, L. Rossi, Y. Nagamine, and B. Hohn.** 1998. Interaction of the DNA modifying proteins VirD1 and VirD2 of *Agrobacterium tumefaciens:* analysis by subcellular localization in mammalian cells. *Proc. Natl. Acad. Sci. USA* **95:**9105–9110.

116. **Rogowski, P. M., B. S. Powell, K. Shirasu, T.-S. Lin, P. Morel, E. M. Zyprian, T. R. Steck, and C. I. Kado.** 1990. Molecular characterization of the *vir* regulon of *Agrobacterium tumefaciens:* complete nucleotide sequence and gene organization of the 28.63 kbp regulon cloned as a single unit. *Plasmid* **23:**85–106.

117. **Roitsch, T., H. Wang, S. G. Jin, and E. W. Nester.** 1990. Mutational analysis of the VirG protein, a transcriptional activator of *Agrobacterium tumefaciens* virulence genes. *J. Bacteriol.* **172:**6054–6060.

118. **Rossi, L., B. Hohn, and B. Tinland.** 1996. Integration of complete transferred DNA units is dependent on the activity of virulence E2 protein of *Agrobacterium tumefaciens*. *Proc. Natl. Acad. Sci. USA* **9:**126–130.

119. **Salmond, G. P., and P. J. Reeves.** 1993. Membrane traffic wardens and protein secretion in gram-negative bacteria. *Trends Biochem. Sci.* **18:**7–12.

120. **Sawada, H., H. Ieki, H. Oyaizu, and S. Matsumoto.** 1993. Proposal for rejection of *Agrobacterium tumefaciens* and revised descriptions for the genus *Agrobacterium* and for *Agrobacterium radiobacter* and *Agrobacterium rhizogenes*. *Int. J. Syst. Bacteriol.* **43:**694–702.

121. **Scheiffele, P., W. Pansegrau, and E. Lanka.** 1995. Initiation of *Agrobacterium tumefaciens* T-DNA processing. Purified proteins VirD1 and VirD2 catalyze site- and strand-specific cleavage of superhelical T-border DNA *in vitro*. *J. Biol. Chem.* **270:**1269–1276.

122. **Sen, P., G. J. Pazour, D. Anderson, and A. Das.** 1989. Cooperative binding of *Agrobacterium tumefaciens* VirE2 protein to single-stranded DNA. *J. Bacteriol.* **171:**2573–2580.

123. **Sheng, J., and V. Citovsky.** 1996. *Agrobacterium*-plant cell DNA transport: have virulence proteins, will travel. *Plant Cell* **8:**1699–1710.

124. **Shimoda, N., A. Toyoda-Yamamoto, S. Aoki, and Y. Machida.** 1993. Genetic evidence for an interaction between the VirA sensor protein and the ChvE sugar-binding protein of *Agrobacterium*. *J. Biol. Chem.* **268:**26552–26558.

125. **Shimoda, N., A. Toyoda-Yamamoto, J. Nagamine, S. Usami, M. Katayama, Y. Sakagami, and Y. Machida.** 1990. Control of expression of *Agrobacterium vir* genes by synergistic actions of phenolic signal molecules and monosaccharides. *Proc. Natl. Acad. Sci. USA* **87:**6684–6688.

126. **Shirasu, K., Z. Koukolikova-Nicola, B. Hohn, and C. I. Kado.** 1994. An inner-membrane-associated virulence protein essential for T-DNA transfer from *Agrobacterium tumefaciens* to plants exhibits ATPase activity and similarities to conjugative transfer genes. *Mol. Microbiol.* **11:**581–588.

127. **Shurvington, C. E., and W. Ream.** 1991. Stimulation of *Agrobacterium tumefaciens* T-DNA transfer by overdrive depends on a flanking sequence but not on helical position with respect to the border repeat. *J. Bacteriol.* **173:**5558–5563.

128. **Smith, E. F., and C. O. Townsend.** 1907. A plant tumor of bacterial origin. *Science* **25:**671–673.

129. **Spencer, P. A., and G. H. N. Towers.** 1988. Specificity of signal compounds detected by *Agrobacterium tumefaciens*. *Phytochemistry* **27:**2781–2785.

130. **Spudich, G. M., D. Fernandez, X. R. Zhou, and P. J. Christie.** 1996. Intermolecular disulfide bonds stabilize VirB7 homodimers and VirB7/VirB9 heterodimers during biogenesis of the *Agrobacterium tumefaciens* T-complex transport apparatus. *Proc. Natl. Acad. Sci. USA* **93:**7512–7517.

131. **Stachel, S. E., E. Messens, M. Van Montagu, and P. C. Zambryski.** 1985. Identification of the signal molecules produced by wounded plant cells that activate T-DNA transfer in *Agrobacterium tumefaciens*. *Nature* (London) **318:**624–629.

132. **Stachel, S. E., B. Timmerman, and P. Zambryski.** 1986. Generation of single-stranded T-DNA molecules during the initial stages of T-DNA transfer from *Agrobacterium tumefaciens* to plant cells. *Nature* (London) **322:**706–712.

133. **Stachel, S. E., B. Timmerman, and P. Zambryski.** 1987. Activation of *Agrobacterium tumefaciens vir* gene expression generates multiple single-stranded T-strand molecules from the pTiA6 T-region: requirement for 5' *virD* gene products. *EMBO J.* **6:**857–863.

134. **Stahl, L. E., A. Jacobs, and A. N. Binns.** 1998. The conjugal intermediate of plasmid RSF1010 inhibits *Agrobacterium tumefaciens* virulence and VirB-dependent export of VirE2. *J. Bacteriol.* **180:**3933–3939.

135. **Sundberg, C., L. Meek, K. Carroll, A. Das, and W. Ream.** 1996. VirE1 protein mediates export of the single-stranded DNA-binding protein VirE2 from *Agrobacterium tumefaciens* into plant cells. *J. Bacteriol.* **178:**1207–1212.

136. **Tait, R. C., and C. I. Kado.** 1988. Regulation of the *virC* and *virD* promoters of pTiC58 by the *ros* chromosomal mutation of *Agrobacterium tumefaciens*. *Mol. Microbiol.* **2:**385–392.

137. **Thomashow, M. F., J. E. Karlinsey, J. R. Marks, and R. E. Hurlbert.** 1987. Identification of a new virulence locus in *Agrobacterium tumefaciens* that affects polysaccharide composition and plant cell attachment. *J. Bacteriol.* **169:**3209–3216.

138. **Thomashow, M. F., R. Nutter, A. L. Montoya, M. P. Gordon, and E. W. Nester.** 1980. Integration and organization of Ti plasmid sequences in crown gall tumors. *Cell* **19:**729–739.

139. **Tinland, B., and B. Hohn.** 1995. Recombination between prokaryotic and eukaryotic DNA: integration of *Agrobacterium tumefaciens* T-DNA into the plant genome. *Genet. Eng.* **17:**209–229.

140. **Tinland, B., P. Fournier, T. Heckel, and L. Otten.** 1992. Expression of a chimaeric heat-shock-inducible *Agrobacterium* 6b oncogene in *Nicotiana rustica*. *Plant Mol. Biol.* **18:**921–930.

141. **Turk, S. C., L. S. Melchers, H. den Dulk-Ras, T. A. J. Regensburg, and P. J. Hooykaas.** 1991. Environmental conditions differentially affect *vir* gene induction in different *Agrobacterium* strains. *Plant Mol. Biol.* **16:**1051–1059.

142. **van Larebeke, N., C. Genetello, J. Schell, R. A. Schilperoort, A. K. Hermans, J. P. Hernalsteens, and M. Van Montagu.** 1975. Acquisition of tumor inducing ability by non-oncogenic agrobacteria as a result of plasmid transfer. *Nature* **255:**742–743.

143. **Wagner, V. T., and A. G. Matthysse.** 1992. Involvement of a vitronectin-like protein in attachment of *Agrobacterium tumefaciens* to carrot suspension culture cells. *J. Bacteriol.* **174:**5999–6003.

144. **Wang, L., J. D. Helmann, and S. C. Winans.** 1992. The *A. tumefaciens* transcriptional activator OccR causes a bend at a target promoter, which is partially relaxed by a plant tumor metabolite. *Cell* **69:**659–667.

145. **Waters, V. L., K. H. Hirata, W. Pansegrau, E. Lanka, and D. G. Guiney.** 1991. Sequence identity in the nick regions of IncP plasmid transfer origins and T-DNA borders of *Agrobacterium* Ti plasmids. *Proc. Natl. Acad. Sci. USA* **88:**1456–1460.

146. **Weiss, A. A., F. D. Johnson, and D. L. Burns.** 1993. Molecular characterization of an operon required for pertussis toxin secretion. *Proc. Natl. Acad. Sci. USA* **90:**2970–2974.

147. **Willems, A., and M. D. Collins.** 1993. Phylogenetic analysis of rhizobia and agrobacteria based on 16S rRNA gene sequences. *Int. J. Syst. Bacteriol.* **43:**305–313.

148. **Winans, S. C., S. Jin, T. Komari, K. M. Johnson, and E. W. Nester.** 1987. The role of virulence regulatory loci in determining *Agrobacterium* host range, p. 573–582. *In* D. von Wettstein and N.-H. Chua (ed.), *Plant Molecular Biology.* Plenum Press, New York, N.Y.

149. **Winans, S. C.** 1992. Two-way chemical signaling in *Agrobacterium*-plant interactions. *Microbiol. Rev.* **56:**12–31.

150. **Winans, S. C., J. Zhu, and M. I. Moré.** 1999. Cell density-dependent gene expression by *Agrobacterium tumefaciens* during colonization of crown gall tumors, p. 117–128. *In* G. M. Dunny and S. C. Winans (ed.), *Cell-Cell Signaling in Bacteria.* ASM Press, Washington, D.C.

151. **Yadav, N. S., J. Vanderlayden, D. R. Bennett, W. M. Barnes, and M.-D. Chilton.** 1982. Short direct repeats flank the T-DNA on a nopaline Ti plasmid. *Proc. Natl. Acad. Sci. USA* **79:**6322–6326.

152. **Yamada, T., C. J. Palm, B. Brooks, and T. Kosuge.** 1985. Nucleotide sequence of the *Pseudomonas sevastanoi* indoleacetic acid genes show homology with *Agrobacterium tumefaciens* T-DNA. *Proc. Natl. Acad. Sci. USA* **82:**6522–6526.

153. **Yanofsky, M. F., S. G. Porter, C. Young, L. M. Albright, M. P. Gordon, and E. W. Nester.** 1986. The *virD* operon of *Agrobacterium tumefaciens* encodes a site-specific endonuclease. *Cell* **7:**471–477.

154. **Young, C., and E. W. Nester.** 1988. Association of the VirD2 protein with the 5′ end of T strands in *Agrobacterium tumefaciens.* *J. Bacteriol.* **170:**3367–3374.

155. **Zaenen, I., N. Van Larebeke, H. Teuchy, M. Van Montagu, and J. Shell.** 1974. Supercoiled circular DNA in crown-gall inducing *Agrobacterium* strains. *J. Mol. Biol.* **86:**109–127.

156. **Zambryski, P., J. Tempe, and J. Schell.** 1989. Transfer and function of T-DNA genes from *Agrobacterium* Ti and Ri plasmids in plants. *Cell* **27:**193–201.

157. **Zhang, L., P. J. Murphy, A. Kerr, and M. E. Tate.** 1993. *Agrobacterium* conjugation and gene regulation by *N*-acyl-ʟ-homoserine lactones. *Nature* (London) **362:**446–448.

158. **Zhu, J., and S. C. Winans.** 1998. Activity of the quorum-sensing regulator TraR of *Agrobacterium tumefaciens* is inhibited by a truncated, dominant defective TraR-like protein. *Mol. Microbiol.* **27:**289–297.

158a. **Zhu, J., and S. C. Winans.** 1999. Autoinducer binding by the quorum-sensing regulator TraR increases affinity for target promoters *in vitro* and decreases TraR turnover rates in whole cells. *Proc. Natl. Acad. Sci. USA* **96:**4832–4837.

159. **Zupan, J. R., V. Citovsky, and P. Zambryski.** 1996. *Agrobacterium* VirE2 protein mediates nuclear uptake of single-stranded DNA in plant cells. *Proc. Natl. Acad. Sci. USA* **93:**2392–2397.

Pathogenicity Islands and Other Mobile Virulence Elements
Edited by J. B. Kaper and J. Hacker
© 1999 American Society for Microbiology, Washington, D.C.

Chapter 16

The *hrp* Cluster of *Pseudomonas syringae*: a Pathogenicity Island Encoding a Type III Protein Translocation Complex?

Steven W. Hutcheson

Bacteria are associated with a number of economically important diseases of plants. Proteobacteria (gram-negative bacteria) of the genera *Agrobacterium, Pseudomonas, Erwinia, Ralstonia, Xanthomonas,* and *Xylella* include plant-pathogenic strains (1). Among the Firmicutes (gram-positive bacteria), strains of *Clavibacter, Mycoplasma, Rhodococcus, Streptomyces,* and *Spiroplasma* can cause plant diseases. Localized necrotic lesions of leaves, stems, and fruits, called spots, blights (larger-scale necrotic lesions affecting whole plant organs), or cankers (large necrotic lesions of woody tissue), are common manifestations of infection by some of the above bacteria. Other strains can cause massive tissue maceration known as bacterial soft rot, a common postharvest disease of plants. Still other strains colonize the vascular system of plants, causing wilts (systemic tissue dehydration), stunts (reduced growth rates), or various developmental aberrations (atypical structure of newly developed organs). Bacteria such as *Agrobacterium* strains induce neoplastic tumors in plants by causing genetic transformation of the host (see chapter 15).

It is not possible or desirable to review what is known of the molecular mechanisms of pathogenesis for all of these bacteria in this chapter. Instead, this chapter focuses on the pathogenicity determinants of *Pseudomonas syringae* as a paradigm for microbial pathogenesis in plants. It focuses specifically upon genetic determinants of *P. syringae* strains necessary for colonization of plant tissue. What is emerging from these studies is the remarkable similarity in the genetic mechanisms involved in pathogenesis by bacteria, irrespective of the host. As in mammalian pathogens, essential pathogenicity determinants of several plant-pathogenic bacteria are localized in apparent pathogenicity islands (PAIs). The reader is also directed to several other recent reviews related to this subject (4, 46, 48, 49, 65, 74).

PATHOGENESIS BY *P. SYRINGAE* STRAINS

P. syringae van Hall 1902 is a fluorescent pseudomonad, now included in the gamma subgroup of the *Proteobacteria* (purple nonsulfur bacteria [77]), that was originally isolated

---

Steven W. Hutcheson • Department of Cell Biology and Molecular Genetics, Microbiology Building, University of Maryland, College Park, MD 20742.

from diseased lilac tissue (78). The species is now known to include a large number of plant-pathogenic strains. Pathogenic strains are facultative pathogens of plants, causing spots, blights, or cankers in susceptible hosts. Most agronomically important plant species are susceptible to at least one strain of *P. syringae*. This includes species from divergent taxonomic groups of Angiosperms, including both monocotyledonous (grasses) and dicotyledonous (broad-leafed) plants. Although biochemically indistinguishable from one another in most cases, individual strains of *P. syringae* usually have very limited host ranges. A strain may cause disease in only one plant species, and in some cases only a few genetic variants of that plant species (known as cultivars, varieties, or ecotypes) are susceptible to a specific strain. The taxonomic designations of most pathogenic *P. syringae* strains therefore normally include a pathovar designation to indicate the host range of the strain at the plant species level (25). For example, strains of *P. syringae* that specifically cause a characteristic blight in *Phaseolus vulgaris* L. (bean) are designated *P. syringae* pv. phaseolicola strains. At present, more than 50 unique pathovars of *P. syringae,* which cause characteristic diseases in specific host plant species, have been defined. In some cases, a race designation is also included in a strain designation to indicate a subspecific limitation of host range.

The primary habitat of *P. syringae* strains appears to be the asymptomatic epiphytic growth on the external surfaces of plant organs, such as leaves (41). Both host and nonhost plant species can support epiphytic populations of a *P. syringae* strain, but larger epiphytic populations have been detected on susceptible host plants. Only ephemeral populations are present in the soil. When a virulent strain of the bacterium invades plant tissue, usually assisted by wetting (heavy dew, spray irrigation, or rain) or wounding, *P. syringae* cells adsorb to nearby cells of parenchymatous tissue (70). Such tissue consists of loosely packed thin-walled cells separated by gaseous spaces. It is not known whether specific adhesins are involved in this process or whether the association is simply the result of water absorption by plant cells or evaporation bringing the bacterial cells into close proximity to the plant cells (40, 80). *P. syringae* strains have been reported to produce a type IV pilus that could be involved in adhesion (85, 88). Although the motility of *P. syringae* strains is important for population dispersal and invasion of wetted tissue (presumably due to chemotactic attraction of the bacteria to infection sites), motility does not appear to be essential for colonization of tissue. Nonmotile mutants retained virulence when infiltrated into susceptible plant tissue (79).

Colonization of the tissue begins with growth in the intercellular spaces of the tissue. *P. syringae* strains are noninvasive and remain external to the cell wall of living plant cells during pathogenesis (70). The cell wall prevents direct contact of the bacteria with the plasma membrane of the host cells. Few if any strains of *P. syringae* have the ability to enzymatically degrade plant cell walls. Furthermore, the turgor pressure of plant cells impedes the direct uptake of bacterial cells into plant cells. Only modest changes in morphology of parasitized host cells are observed during early stages of *P. syringae* pathogenesis. Convolution of the cell membrane and deposition of new cell wall components (papillae) have been found at sites adjacent to colonizing *P. syringae* cells (18). Altered K^+ fluxes and sucrose efflux have also been detected at these tissues (8). During later stages of pathogenesis, macroscopic symptoms, such as water soaking (accumulation of water in the intercellular spaces of the tissue) and tissue necrosis, are commonly observed.

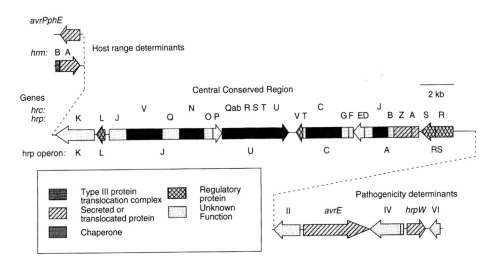

Figure 1. Organization of the *P. syringae hrp* cluster. Shaded polygons or boxes represent genes. The arrowhead indicates the deduced direction of transcription for the operon. Operon designations are indicated below the figure, and gene designations are given above their respective component. Gene designations are segregated into *hrp* and *hrc* according to the terminology of Bogdanove et al. (13). *hrc* genes are indicated by medium gray shading. The dashed lines connect the variable-host-range and semiconserved pathogenicity regions to the central conserved region. In the host range region, the *hrmBA* operon of *P. syringae* Pss61 (5, 39) and the *avrPphE* locus of *P. syringae* pv. phaseolicola 1302A (71) are shown to indicate the variability of the region. HrmA and AvrPphE do not show homology to each other. *P. syringae* pv. tomato DC3000 lacks either locus. A key to the deduced functions of the gene products is included. See Table 1 for references.

Translocated proteins (see below), derivatized peptide toxins (11, 35), extracellular polysaccharides (61, 90), and plant hormones (31) produced by the bacterium contribute to symptom development. A hydroscopic capsule, formed of the extracellular polysaccharides alginate and levan, is produced by many *P. syringae* strains early in pathogenesis (61, 91). The bacterium then spreads in the tissue as an expanding colony growing on surfaces of cells until a physical barrier, such as a vascular bundle, is reached or until the plant's cellular defense mechanisms prevent further spread of the bacterium.

Bacterial disease occurs in plants when a bacterium is able to colonize new cells in the tissue before the cellular defense responses of the initially colonized host cells become active (48). The failure of the plant cells to rapidly detect the presence of a pathogen or suppression of cellular defense responses by toxins or other virulence factors results in successful colonization of the tissue and disease development. Pathogenesis of *P. syringae* strains and the plant's ability to recognize and respond to these invaders are now known to involve a common mechanism. Proteins translocated by a type III protein translocation complex (PTC) similar to that of its mammalian counterparts mediate both the pathogenicity and host range of *P. syringae* strains. It is the recognition of one or more of these translocated proteins by surveillance systems of resistant plants that leads to the initiation of cellular defense responses and disease resistance.

Table 1. Properties of known gene products of the *P. syringae hrp* cluster

Gene product[a]	Size[b]		Selected homologs[c]		Probable cell location[d]	Deduced function	Reference(s)[e]
	aa	kDa	Other PAI(s)	Flagellar			
HrmB	96	10.9	P.a. ExcC, Y.p. orf 7	ND	Cyto.	Chaperone for HrmA	5
HrmA	375	41.5	ND	ND	Trans.	Pathogenicity or host range determinant	39
HrpK (HrpY)	767	80.2	ND	ND	Cyto.	Unknown	71, 107
HrpL	184	21.2	P.a. AlgU	FliA	Cyto.	Sigma factor for *hrp* regulon	107
HrpJ	346	37.7	ND	ND	Cyto.	Unknown	45
HrcV	695	76.5	LcrD	FlhA	IM	Type III PTC	45
HrpQ	324	35.3	R.s. HrpW	ND	Cyto.	Unknown	63
HrcN	449	48.9	YscN family	FliI	Peri. IM	ATPase for type III PTC	63
HrpO	148	17.3	ND	ND	Cyto.	Unknown	63
HrpP	192	20.7	ND	ND	Cyto.	Unknown	63
HrcQab	238, 212	26, 23.6	YscQ family	ND	Cyto.	Type III PTC	43, 63
HrcR	208	23.2	YscR family	FliP	IM	Type III PTC	43
HrcS	88	9.4	YscS family	FliQ	IM	Type III PTC	43
HrcT	264	28.5	YscT family	FliR	IM	Type III PTC	43
HrcU	359	39.9	YscU family	FlhB	IM	Type III PTC	43
HrpV	115	13.4	ND	ND	Cyto.	Negative-acting regulator	24, 82
HrpT	67	7.4	ND	ND	OM	Putative lipoprotein	24
HrcC	701	76.6	YscC family	ND	OM	Outer membrane pore for type III PTC	24
HrpG	149	16.1	ND	ND	OM?	Unknown	24
HrpF	74	8.0	ND	ND	OM?	Unknown	24
HrpE	193	21.5	YscL	ND	OM	Unknown	83

Table 1. *Continued*

Gene product[a]	Size[b]		Selected homologs[c]		Probable cell location[d]	Deduced function	Reference(s)[e]
	aa	kDa	Other PAI(s)	Flagellar			
HrpD	176	20.3	YscK	ND	OM	Unknown	83
HrcJ	268	29.1	YscJ family	ND	OM	Lipoprotein	83
HrpB	124	12.7	YscI	ND	OM	Unknown	83
HrpZ	341	34.7	ND	ND	Secr.	Unknown	38, 83
HrpA	108	11.0	ND	ND	Secr.	Structural protein of PTC pilus	83, 87
HrpS	302	33.3	DctD family of response regulators	ND	Cyto.	Regulator of *hrpL*	34, 107
HrpR	314	34.7	DctD family of response regulators	ND	Cyto.	Regulator of *hrpL*	24, 33, 107
Orf II			ND	ND		Probable pathogenicity factor	67
AvrE	494	54.0	ND	ND	Trans.	Pathogenicity factor	67
Orf IVab			ND	ND		Unknown; sigma 54 dependent	19, 67
HrpW	425	42.9	Several Pel genes	FliC?	Secr.	Pathogenicity factor	19
Orf VI			ND	ND		Probable pathogenicity factor	19

[a] See reference 13 for former genetic designations.
[b] Deduced properties of the indicated gene product derived from sequence data. aa, amino acids.
[c] Representative homologs in other bacteria. *Yersinia* Ysc homologs are used as the primary reference homolog. The following abbreviations were used for other bacteria: P.a., *P. aeruginosa*; R.s., *R. solanacearum*; Y.p., *Y. pestis*. ND, none detected or not reported.
[d] Probable location deduced from structural features of the deduced protein, properties of the protein family, biochemical localization, and/or gene fusion localization. Abbreviations: Cyto., cytoplasm; Peri., peripheral; IM, inner membrane; OM, outer membrane; Secr., secreted protein found in culture filtrates; Trans., putative translocated protein.
[e] Reference for gene sequence and characterization.

TYPE III PROTEIN TRANSLOCATION COMPLEX
OF *P. SYRINGAE* STRAINS

The early genetic characterization of *P. syringae* pathogenicity determinants identified a clustered set of chromosomal transposon mutations that affected pathogenicity in the normally susceptible plant species (see reference 106 for references). These mutants also failed to elicit the hypersensitive response when infiltrated into leaves of resistant plants. The hypersensitive response is a manifestation of a cascade of induced cellular defense responses that culminates in a form of programmed cell death (23, 48). This cluster of genes was designated *hrp* (66). A clone carrying a nearly complete *hrp* gene cluster was phenotypically active when expressed in heterologous bacteria, such as *Escherichia coli* K-12 strains, enabling transconjugants to elicit cellular defense responses but not disease (44). Sequence analysis of the region has revealed 35 open reading frames clustered in a 35-kb region of the *P. syringae* genome (Fig. 1). Contiguously arranged genes transcribed from a HrpL-dependent promoter (see below) were deduced to represent transcriptional units (43, 108).

An indication of the biochemical function of this cluster came from the similarity of products of 12 of the genes of the *P. syringae hrp* gene cluster to pathogenicity determinants of several mammalian pathogens (Table 1). As described elsewhere in this book, these conserved gene products form key components of a type III PTC. Like other type III PTCs, the inner membrane components also have similarity to components of the flagellar biosynthesis apparatus, whereas an outer membrane component is related to a pore-forming protein involved in filamentous-phage assembly (4, 46, 49). Among the mammalian pathogens, the *Yersinia* Ysc products are usually the closest homologs to the corresponding *P. syringae* Hrp products. In an effort to simplify the nomenclature of these genes in plant-pathogenic bacteria in general, *hrp* genes whose products are conserved in type III PTCs of other plant pathogens as well as in those of mammalian pathogens have been redesignated *hrc* genes (13). For easy comparison to other type III PTCs, the letter designation given to an *hrc* gene represents the corresponding *Yersinia* Ysc homolog in most cases.

The *hrp* cluster of *P. syringae* strains can be divided into three regions. On the left-hand side as drawn is a variable region that contains host range determinants in some strains (see below). In strain Pss61, this region consists of the *hrmBA* operon (5, 39, 42). In other strains, host range determinants called *avr* genes can be located in this region (see below). For example, *avrPphE* is located at this site of the *P. syringae* pv. phaseolicola *hrp* cluster (71). In at least one other strain (DC3000), this region is missing (27). The conserved central region of the cluster includes the *hrpK*, *hrpL*, *hrpJ*, *hrpU*, *hrpC*, *hrpA*, and *hrpRS* operons encoding structural and regulatory components of the type III PTC. The region adjacent to *hrpRS* is a semiconserved region that encodes at least two translocated proteins involved in pathogenicity (19, 56).

TRANSLOCATED PATHOGENICITY AND HOST RANGE DETERMINANTS
OF *P. SYRINGAE* STRAINS

The extensive similarity of Hrp products to components of type III PTCs of mammalian pathogens led to the prediction that one or more translocated proteins are involved in *P. syringae* pathogenicity. Consistent with this hypothesis, several proteins have been shown by biochemical or genetic methods to be secreted by the *hrp*-encoded PTC of *P. syringae* strains (110). Additional proteins, originally identified genetically as host range determinants, appear to be specifically translocated by the *hrp*-encoded PTC into plant cells (4, 49). Genetic evidence also suggests that presently cryptic pathogenicity determinants may also be translocated into plant cells by this mechanism as well.

HrpZ was the first protein shown to be secreted by the *hrp*-encoded PTC of *P. syringae* strains and can be detected as a 34.5-kDa protein in heat-treated culture filtrates of *P. syringae* strains (38). HrpZ is a member of the harpin family of proteins (3). These proteins are glycine-rich, cysteine-deficient, heat-stable proteins that can induce cellular defense responses when infiltrated at high concentrations into the tissue of an indicator plant (2, 20). Like other proteins secreted by type III PTCs, this protein lacks any obvious signal sequence or other structural features associated with secretion. Although HrpZ was originally proposed to be the primary effector molecule of the *hrp* cluster, later studies showed the locus to be dispensable for this activity. Δ*hrpZ* mutants retained pathogenicity in susceptible plants and were only slightly affected, if at all, in their ability to elicit cellular defense responses in resistant plants (2, 81). This locus appears to be moderately conserved among *P. syringae* strains and retains >75% similarity in the amino acid sequence among tested *P. syringae* strains (24, 83).

HrpA is the structural protein of a *hrp*-encoded pilus (86, 87). This 8-nm-diameter pilus is formed concurrently with induced expression of *hrp* genes in *P. syringae* pv. tomato DC3000 and presumably other *P. syringae* strains as well. Consistent with an important role of HrpA in the translocation process, Δ*hrpA* mutants lack most *hrp*-associated phenotypes and fail to secrete HrpZ (64, 87). This would suggest that HrpA functions in the translocation process in a manner similar to that proposed for enteropathogenic *E. coli* EspA (see chapter 3). Interestingly, both *hrpA* and *hrpZ* are transcribed as part of a large operon that also includes genes encoding homologs to *Yersinia* YscIJKL, which are constituents of the *Yersinia* PTC (83). HrpA is among the most variable proteins produced by the *hrp* gene cluster. For example, the *P. syringae* pv. tomato DC3000 HrpA retains only 28% amino acid sequence identity and 45% similarity to its counterpart in several other *P. syringae* strains (83).

HrpW is a recently identified secreted 43-kDa protein that has two distinct domains: the N-terminal region is a glycine-rich, cysteine-deficient, harpin-like domain, whereas the C-terminal region exhibits sequence similarity to several pectate lyases (19). Pectate lyases usually function in the degradation of the pectate polymer of plant cell walls, but HrpW did not exhibit typical pectate lyase activities when tested. Instead, HrpW bound to pectate molecules without cleaving the polymer. HrpW did exhibit the harpin-like ability to elicit a form of cellular defense responses in plants when infiltrated into tissue at high concentrations. A Δ*hrpW* mutant exhibited a diminished ability to elicit cellular defense responses in an indicator plant but only when *hrpZ* was also inactivated. This suggests the presence of proteins with redundant function in this bacterial strain or an accessory role in the translocation process. Hybridization analysis indicates that all *P. syringae* strains carry a homolog to HrpW and that a homolog is present in the closely related *Erwinia hrp* cluster (56). The pectate lyase-like domain was the most highly conserved region of the protein from two *P. syringae* strains.

Indirect evidence indicates that the products of *avr* genes are also secreted by the *hrp*-encoded PTC of *P. syringae* strains and appear to be specifically translocated into plant cells. *avr* genes are important host range determinants for many plant pathogens, including *P. syringae* strains, but their phenotype is distinct from known host range factors of mammalian pathogens. *avr* genes were originally identified in *P. syringae* by the altered host range of transconjugants carrying a genomic library of another *P. syringae* strain (96). Expression of an *avr* gene in a *P. syringae* strain restricted the host range of that *P. syringae* strain to cultivars of the susceptible plant species that lacked a corresponding resistance gene. Resistance gene products have been postulated to act as receptors for Avr products (48). For disease to occur, genetic evidence indicates that either a pathogenic strain does not express an *avr* gene or the host lacks a corresponding resistance gene and thus fails to recognize and respond to the invading pathogen. Nineteen distinct *avr* genes have been identified in a variety of *P. syringae* strains, and their products vary in size from 18 to 100 kDa (60, 101); however, their mechanism of action was not obvious. Infiltration of tissue with purified Avr products failed to elicit a response in most cases, and the phenotype encoded by *avr* genes was produced only by pathogenic strains. The products of most resistance genes characterized thus far that mediate responses to *P. syringae* Avr products appear to be cytoplasmic proteins (36). Since the products of these resistance genes appear not to have extracellular domains, a mechanism to translocate bacterial Avr products into plant cells would be required for the predicted protein-protein interactions to occur.

The potential interaction of Avr products with the products of *hrp* genes was first indicated by the coordinated regulation of *hrp* and *avr* transcription (53). Expression of these genes is controlled by the same mechanism (see below). In addition, several *avr* genes were found to be associated with the *P. syringae hrp* cluster. *avrPphE, hrmA,* and *avrE* are located in the regions flanking the core *hrc* genes of the *hrp* cluster (Fig. 1), suggesting that they are components of the *hrp* gene cluster (however, others are dispersed elsewhere in the genome). Furthermore, the phenotype encoded by several *avr* genes was lost in *P. syringae hrp*::Tn mutants (65), but it was unclear whether the phenotype was due to an interaction between gene products or an indirect effect attributable to the inability of the mutant to multiply in the tissue. A pivotal observation linking the activity of Avr products with that of the *hrp* cluster was the demonstration that the phenotypic expression of seven distinct *avr* genes in heterologous nonpathogenic bacteria was dependent upon secretion activities of a cloned *hrp*-encoded PTC (32, 81).

The above observations strongly suggested that Avr products are translocated by the *hrp*-encoded PTC into plant cells. Attempts to identify translocated Avr proteins in culture filtrates of strains expressing *hrp* and *avr* genes or in lysates of inoculated plant cells by biochemical, immunological, or radiographic techniques, however, have been unsuccessful (32, 64). Experiments involving gene fusions have been equally frustrating. Although epitope-tagged Avr products are phenotypically active when expressed in bacteria carrying a functional *hrp* cluster, various fusions with the above reporter domains have been unde-tectable in lysates of inoculated plant cells. Fusions of Avr products to reporter enzymes, such as adenylate cyclase, β-glucuronidase, or green fluorescent protein, either lost pheno-typic activity or failed to accumulate to detectable levels in plant tissue. The inability to detect these apparently translocated Avr products in plant cells by the above methods could be due to (i) translocation of the Avr product at levels below the sensitivity of the assay, (ii) processing of the protein prior to translocation, (iii) steric hindrance blocking translocation of the chimeric protein, or (iv) rapid degradation of Avr products once translocated into plant cells. Consistent with the hypothesis that Avr products are translocated into plant cells by the *hrp*-encoded PTC are the observations that *avr* genes produce a phenotype when transiently expressed in the plant cells (32, 62, 93, 97, 99). An apparent programmed cell death response is induced when a genetic construct expressing an *avr* gene is introduced into plant cells but only when those cells express the corresponding resistance gene.

Taken together, the aforementioned results provide a compelling argument that Avr products must be translocated by the *hrp*-encoded PTC into plant cells. Resistant plants have acquired the ability to recognize and respond to these translocated proteins to initiate cellular defense responses. Consistent with this model, the interaction of an Avr product with the product of the corresponding resistance gene has been detected by using the yeast two-hybrid assay (93, 97). Recently, eukaryotic myristylation sites have been identified in the amino termini of several Avr products (reference 22 and see below). If functional, this observation would suggest that Avr products are likely to be peripheral plasma membrane proteins. The resistance gene product mediating responses to one of these potentially myristylated Avr products has been shown to be a peripheral plasma membrane protein (16).

If Avr products are the stimuli that initiate a host defense response, why carry them? Several studies have reported that several Avr products also play a role in pathogenicity (see, e.g., references 55 and 68). *P. syringae* Δ*avr* mutants can exhibit reduced virulence in their normally susceptible host. There is some evidence to suggest that *P. syringae* strains may translocate additional proteins that function as pathogenicity determinants. *E. coli* transformants expressing *hrp* and *avr* genes do not become pathogens. *P. syringae* Δ*hrpW* Δ*hrpZ* mutants retained virulence when inoculated into susceptible tissue. Since inactivation of the *hrp*-encoded PTC causes a complete loss in virulence, one or more additional translocated proteins must be involved in *P. syringae* pathogenesis.

Relatively little is known about the mechanisms by which any of the above proteins are translocated out of the *P. syringae* cells. Presumably these *P. syringae* proteins are secreted by a mechanism similar to that used by *Yersinia* strains to secrete Yops (see chapter 6). This would predict that translocated proteins could require chaperones to maintain conformation prior to translocation, as observed in most mammalian pathogens. Putative chaperones have been identified for only two of the proteins translocated by *P. syringae* strains. HrmB is a weak homolog of the *P. aeruginosa* ExsC chaperone (5) and is proposed to function as a chaperone for HrmA, a protein with an Avr-like phenotype that is produced by some *P. syringae* strains (5, 39). Both genes are transcribed as part of a single operon. A second candidate chaperone may be associated with the *avrE* locus. The phenotype of *avrE* is dependent upon a second open reading frame (orf IV), whose function has not been established (67; see also reference 14). In contrast, most other proteins translocated by *P. syringae* strains do not appear to require dedicated chaperones. There is no obvious chaperone for HrpA, HrpZ, or HrpW in the *hrp* cluster, and genetic evidence suggests that translocation of most other Avr products does not involve dedicated chaperones. The phenotypic activity of seven distinct Avr products expressed by an *E. coli* K-12 strain carrying a cloned *P. syringae hrp* cluster (presumably due to translocation of the proteins) required only minimal clones of the tested *avr* genes (81). Either these *P. syringae* proteins do not require a chaperone for translocation or a presently cryptic chaperone encoded by the *hrp* cluster functions in the translocation of these proteins.

ENVIRONMENTAL REGULATION OF THE *P. SYRINGAE* TYPE III PROTEIN TRANSLOCATION COMPLEX

Like many other type III PTCs, the *hrp*-encoded PTC of *P. syringae* strains is environmentally regulated at the transcriptional level (for a review, see reference 51). The *hrp* regulon is presently known to consist of the *hrp* operons encoding components of the PTC, the *hrmBA* operon, pathogenicity region orf II, *avrE*, *hrpW*, orf VI, and all known *avr* genes of *P. syringae* strains. Expression of the *hrp* regulon is strongly repressed during growth in any rich medium containing broad-spectrum amino acid sources (84, 109). Enhanced expression can be detected during pathogenesis in either susceptible or resistant plants beginning 1 to 2 h after inoculation of plant tissue. It is not yet clear whether this enhanced expression is due to contact-dependent regulation as seen in several mammalian pathogens or is simply the result of the change in growth conditions. Enhanced expression can also be induced by transferring strains to defined media that mimic in planta growth conditions. Minimal-salt media activate the expression of *P. syringae hrp* and *avr* genes. The carbon source, medium pH, and temperature all influence the magnitude of *hrp* gene expression once induced (52). The role of plant cell contact in the regulation of *P. syringae hrp* genes is under investigation. Higher expression has been observed in planta than could be detected in culture (84), which could be indicative of contact-mediated regulation of the *hrp* regulon.

Four products of the *hrp* cluster appear to mediate the environmental regulation of the *hrp* regulon. HrpR and HrpS are positive transcriptional factors for the *hrpL* promoter (33, 107). HrpR and HrpS are 35- and 33-kDa proteins, respectively, that both exhibit similarity to the response regulator family of two-component regulatory proteins that includes *Rhizobium* DctD. Both proteins differ, however, from other members of this protein family by the absence of the N-terminal "receiver" domain that functions in related proteins to modulate regulatory activity through kinase-mediated phosphorylation. This suggests that HrpR and HrpS are not part of typical two-component regulatory systems. Consistent with this concept, both proteins are fully active as transcriptional factors when expressed from minimal clones in *E. coli* K-12 strains (107). The *hrpL* promoter is a typical σ^{54}-dependent promoter that is distinguished from other promoters in the regulon by the presence of a 90-bp region with a low G+C content (20%) that probably represents a region of bendable DNA. An area of dyad symmetry upstream of the low-G+C region has been proposed to function as the recognition motif for HrpR and HrpS (51).

HrpL, in turn, is an alternative sigma factor related to the extracellular factor (ECF) family of sigma factors (51, 107). HrpL is a 21-kDa protein that is among the smallest sigma factors identified to date. This protein consists primarily of domains 2 and 4 found in the sigma 70 family of sigma factors; these domains recognize the −10 and −35 regions of a promoter motif. Insertional inactivation of *hrpL* in *P. syringae* strains abolishes the transcription of all regulon genes except *hrpL* and *hrpRS*. Expression of *hrpL* in heterologous bacteria is sufficient to direct the transcription of the operons encoding components of the PTC as well as the genes for secreted effector proteins. A conserved bipartite sequence motif has been identified in the promoter region of the *hrpK, hrpJ, hrpU, hrpC,* and *hrpA* operons, as well as *hrmBA,* orf II, orf VI, *hrpW* and all known *P. syringae avr* genes, and this motif functions as a HrpL-dependent promoter (19, 108). Transcription initiates 6 to 8 bp downstream of this promoter sequence (54, 92, 94).

The fourth regulatory determinant, HrpV, is a negative-acting regulatory factor that was identified by its effect on production of several Hrp products (24, 82). HrpV is a 13.4- to 13.9-kDa protein that lacks homology to other proteins with known biochemical functions in the current databases. *hrpV*::Kan mutants overproduce several constituent proteins of the *hrp*-encoded PTC. Attempts to complement the mutation strongly suppressed the expression of secreted proteins. The *hrpV* gene is located at the 3′ end of the *hrpC* operon, which includes several putative outer membrane components of the *hrp*-encoded PTC (24). HrpV could function to coordinate the assembly of inner and outer membrane components of the *hrp*-encoded PTC, but it does not appear to be an anti-sigma factor. The activity of HrpL was independent of *hrpV* expression levels. Instead, HrpV has been proposed to regulate the *hrpRS* operon by an unspecified mechanism, but other interpretations of this data are possible. Interestingly, *hrpV*::Kan mutants retained the wild-type ability to elicit a cellular defense response in resistant plants but exhibited reduced pathogenicity in susceptible plants. Thus, negative regulation of the *hrp* regulon mediated by HrpV must be important for pathogenesis.

The mechanism by which environmental signals are transduced through HrpR, HrpS, HrpL, and HrpV to control the transcription of *hrp, hrc, hrm,* and *avr* genes has not been elucidated. However, it is apparent that regulation of the *P. syringae* type III secretion system is distinct from that of other pathogenic bacteria. In most other pathogenic bacteria, homologs of AraC frequently are key regulatory factors controlling the expression of type III PTCs (46). The *P. syringae hrp* regulatory system appears to lack this component. Instead, regulation of the *P. syringae hrp* regulon shares features with that of flagellar biosynthesis (69). The principal regulatory factor controlling the expression of the *hrp* regulon is an alternative sigma factor, similar to σ^{28}, that controls the expression of late genes of flagellar biosynthesis. Intriguing questions remain about whether the regulation of the *hrp* cluster involves an anti-sigma factor analogous to FlgM to coordinate the assembly of the *hrp*-encoded PTC (47) and about the role of plant cell contact in the environmental regulation of these genes.

THE *hrp-avr* GENE CLUSTER AS A PAI

From the discussion above, it is apparent that *P. syringae* strains carry a clustered set of genes that are essential for pathogenicity. Both the gene products and genetic organization of the cluster are conserved in all pathogenic strains of *P. syringae* examined thus far, except for the left-hand host range determinant region. This cluster encodes (i) a type III PTC that in mammalian pathogens is found as part of a PAI, (ii) translocated effector proteins that mediate host responses to the bacterium, and (iii) a dedicated and unique regulatory system controlling the transcription of cluster genes. The cloned cluster enables heterologous bacteria, such as *E. coli,* to translocate effector proteins into plant cells. Thus, the *hrp* cluster can function as an independent unit in several bacteria to perform pathogenesis-related activities. As such, the *P. syringae hrp* cluster probably forms a PAI that has undergone horizontal transfer between *P. syringae* strains as well as other bacteria (see below). Unfortunately, too little is known about *P. syringae* chromosomal genetics to be able to define borders for this apparent PAI. DNA sequence information for regions flanking the *P. syringae hrp* cluster is just beginning to be investigated. There is no direct evidence as yet to indicate the mobility of the cluster, but, as discussed below, taxonomically distinct bacteria carry very similar *hrp* clusters that most probably arose through horizontal transfer of a progenitor PAI. The G+C content of the cluster (58%) is within the normal range for *P. syringae* chromosomal DNA. In contrast, 14 of the 19 known *avr* genes of *P. syringae* strains are associated with mobile genetic elements, such as insertion sequences or transposons, or bacteriophage-mediated events (57).

EVOLUTIONARY RELATIONSHIP AMONG APPARENT PAIs OF PLANT-PATHOGENIC BACTERIA

Putative PAIs similar to those of *P. syringae* strains have been identified in the plant-pathogenic enteric bacteria *Erwinia amylovora* (12), *E. carotovora* (75), *E. chrysanthemi* (10), *E. herbicola* pv. gypsophilae (76), and *E. stewartii* (21). *E. amylovora* causes severe blights in rosaceous plants, such as apples and pears. *E. chrysanthemi* and *E. carotovora*, in contrast, are causal agents of bacterial soft rot. *E. herbicola* pv. gypsophilae is a tumorigenic pathogen, whereas *E. stewartii* is a vascular pathogen of corn and causes a wilt disease. Although these bacteria cause diseases with very distinct symptoms, a *hrp*-encoded PTC is essential to the pathogenicity of each species (4).

The *hrp* clusters of these *Erwinia* spp. appear to be nearly identical to the *P. syringae hrp* cluster (4, 12, 58, 59). At present, the *E. amylovora hrp* cluster is the best characterized. With the exception of HrpR and HrpK, homologs of all *P. syringae hrp* and *hrc* genes are present in the *E. amylovora hrp* cluster (13) (Fig. 2). The genes of the *P. syringae hrpJ, hrpU, hrpC,* and *hrpA* operons are colinear with their *E. amylovora* counterparts, except for *hrpZ* (4). The *hrpZ* homolog in *E. amylovora, hrpN,* is located in the virulence region of the cluster (56). While constituent operons are conserved between these bacteria, the organization of operons is different. In the *Erwinia hrp* clusters, the *hrpS, hrpA,* and *hrpC* operons are located to the left of *hrpL* (4) (Fig. 2). Some differences in organization are also apparent in the virulence region that includes *avrE* and *hrpW* (19, 56). Another similarity between these *hrp* clusters is the mechanism of environmental regulation. The regulatory components HrpL, HrpS, and HrpV have been detected in *Erwinia hrp* clusters (24, 82, 103). A homolog to *hrpR,* however, is absent from *Erwinia hrp* clusters. Unique to the *Erwinia hrp* cluster are *hrpXY,* which encode components of a typical two-component regulatory system (104). HrpN (the HrpZ homolog) (102), DspEF (the AvrE homolog) (14), and HrpW (56) are known translocated effector proteins of *E. amylovora* that have homologs in the *P. syringae hrp* cluster. Because of the similarity in components, organization, and regulation of the *hrp* clusters of *P. syringae* and *Erwinia* spp., these *hrp* clusters have been designated group I *hrp* clusters (4, 49). The strong similarities in operon structure and regulation strongly suggest that these *hrp* clusters arose through horizontal transfer by either conjugal transfer or transfection. The differences in operon organization can be explained by a single transposition event. In *E. herbicola,* the *hrp* cluster has been localized to a plasmid that carries several pathogenicity determinants (76) and could be transferred to other bacteria by conjugation.

Hrp clusters that are part of potential PAIs have also been identified in *Xanthomonas campestris* (references in reference 26) and *Ralstonia solanacearum* (references in refer-

Group I Hrp Clusters

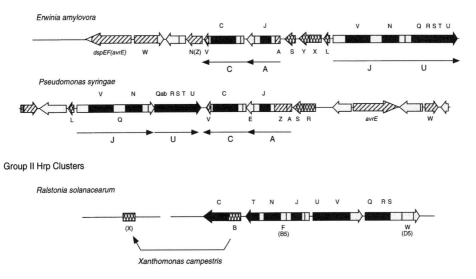

Figure 2. Comparison of group I and group II *hrp* clusters. The *hrp* clusters of *P. syringae*, *E. amylovora, R. solanacearum,* and *X. campestris* are represented. Conserved *hrc* genes are indicated by the medium gray boxes as in Fig. 1 and are labeled above the corresponding gene. Selected *hrp* genes referred to in the text are labeled below the corresponding gene. The labeled black arrows in the group I *hrp* clusters represent conserved operons. For group I *hrp* clusters, note similarities in the organization of genes within individual operons. In *E. amylovora,* the *hrpJ* and *hrpU* operons are merged into a single operon. The designations for homologs, when different, are indicated in parentheses. Only the central region of group II *hrp* clusters encoding apparent components of the PTC is shown. The *hrp* clusters of *X. campestris* and *R. solanacearum* are colinear except for the difference in the position of HrpX. *X. campestris* designations for selected *hrp* genes are shown in parentheses. Note the difference in the organization of *hrc* genes between the two groups of *hrp* clusters. See the text for references and Fig. 1 for fill pattern codes.

ence 100). *X. campestris,* a gamma subgroup proteobacterium, causes blights and spots in susceptible hosts, and over 140 pathovars of unique host range are known to exist (78). *R. solanacearum* (also known as *P. solanacearum* and *Burkholderia solanacearum*) is a member of the beta subgroup of the *Proteobacteria* (77). This bacterium is able to actively penetrate plant tissue and colonize the vascular system of the infected plants to cause wilts in over 100 taxonomic families of plants. Like the bacteria utilizing group I *hrp* clusters in pathogenesis, clustered mutations could be detected in *X. campestris* and *R. solanacearum* transposon mutants that lose pathogenicity and the ability to elicit cellular defense responses in resistant plants (references in reference 65). Because of the similarity in phenotype, these genes were also called *hrp* genes in these bacteria. However, because of prominent differences, the *hrp* clusters of *X. campestris* and *R. solanacearum* have been classified as group II *hrp* clusters (4, 49). These group II *hrp* clusters are nearly identical to each other, differing primarily in the position of a regulatory gene (Fig. 2). The components conserved among all type III PTCs are also present in group II *hrp* clusters (100), and these conserved elements have also been designated *hrc* genes, as described above for group I *hrp* clusters (13). As such, the group II *hrp* cluster must also encode type III PTCs that function in protein translocation. PopA is a harpin-like protein secreted by the group II *hrp*-encoded PTC of *R. solanacearum* (7), and several Avr products are translocated into plant cells from *X. campestris* strains by a *hrp*-dependent mechanism (99). In *R. solanacearum* strains, the *hrp* cluster resides on a large megaplasmid (15).

Although similarly named, group I and group II *hrp* clusters do not appear to be closely related. The levels of similarity detected for Hrc products of group II *hrp* clusters to their counterparts of group I *hrp* clusters are usually lower than those to their homologs of *Yersinia, Salmonella,* and enteropathogenic *E. coli* strains (6, 59, 100). The other gene products of the group II *hrp* clusters showed little if any similarity to Hrp products of group I *hrp* clusters. The only homologies detected are weak similarities between *P. syringae* HrpQ and *R. solanacearum* HrpW (*X. campestris* HrpD5) and between *P. syringae* HrpE and *R. solanacearum* HrpF (*X. campestris* HrpB5). The genetic organization of clusters and regulatory mechanisms controlling environmental regulation are clearly distinct between the two groups of *hrp* clusters. For example, the primary regulatory factor for the *X. campestris* and *R. solanacearum hrp* clusters is an AraC homolog (HrpX and HrpB, respectively [30, 105]). A homolog to this protein has not been detected in group I *hrp* clusters. In apparent contrast to *P. syringae* strains, *R. solanacearum hrp* gene expression is strongly induced by plant cell contact by a mechanism transduced through HrpB (17, 72). The differences in composition, organization, and regulation and the low levels of similarity to group I Hrc components argue that the *hrp* clusters of *R. solanacearum* and *X. campestris* arose by a different mechanism from the group I *hrp* clusters.

EMERGING CONCEPTS OF BACTERIAL PATHOGENESIS IN PLANTS

What develops from the preceding discussion is that pathogenesis by several plant-pathogenic bacteria has some similarities to that reported for enteric bacteria that cause gastroenteritis in mammals. By analogy to mammalian pathogens, pathogenesis by plant-pathogenic bacteria, such as *P. syringae,* probably involves (i) adhesion of the bacteria to plant cells, (ii) activation of a type III PTC, (iii) translocation of pathogenicity determinants into plant cells, (iv) physiological changes in the host cells to stimulate the release of nutrients, (v) production of virulence factors to facilitate the growth of the bacteria, and (vi) growth and spread of the bacteria to surrounding cells in the tissue.

There are intriguing hints to molecular events occurring during each stage of pathogenesis. Bacterial cells, such as *P. syringae,* adhere nonspecifically to plant cells. Both pili and lipopolysaccharides have been implicated in the process of adhesion to plant cells (88). Early studies on the hypersensitive response suggested that bacterial adhesion to plant cells may be important to pathogenesis (9). Contact between bacterial and plant cells is required for initiation of the cellular defense responses that are now known to result from host recognition of proteins translocated into the cytoplasm (50, 95, 98). Close association of bacterial cells with host cells would be required for translocation of effector proteins into host cells. Plant cells usually do not take up proteins by endocytosis, and Avr proteins lack activity when simply infiltrated into tissue.

The aforementioned plant-pathogenic bacteria all utilize type III PTCs, encoded by apparent PAIs, that are regulated by environmental conditions, such as medium composition and host cell interactions. The type III PTCs of plant-pathogenic bacteria carrying group I *hrp* clusters secrete some proteins to the medium, whereas others appear to be specifically translocated into host cells since they are essentially undetectable in culture filtrates. Of the secreted proteins, only HrpA has a clearly demonstrated function as a structural protein of a pilus. HrpW is a candidate adhesin that could interact with the pectic polymers of plant cell walls, but this activity has not been examined experimentally. The function of HrpZ has yet to be established but must involve altering the membrane permeability (2).

The function of translocated proteins in pathogenesis is just beginning to be elucidated. The only known activity for translocated proteins is as a stimulus for cellular defense responses that usually culminate in programmed cell death. However, since several of these proteins also function in pathogenesis, they must also function to facilitate the parasitism of plant cells. Presumably, the translocated proteins affect the plasma membrane function of the host cells of susceptible plants to enhance the release of nutrients to the invading bacterium. The identification of myristylation sites in several *avr* genes and the association of a resistance gene product mediating the responses to one of these potentially myristylated Avr products with the plasma membrane (16) are intriguing. This suggests that Avr products may be processed after translocation into plant cells to anchor the products to the plant cell membranes. These gene products would then be strategically located to influence membrane function. Some of the translocated Avr products of *X. campestris* strains have functional eukaryotic nuclear localization signals (28, 99), suggesting that the site of action for these proteins is in the nucleus.

As mentioned above, some remarkable parallels are emerging between the plant defense responses and selected cellular defenses of mammals. Pathogen-induced programmed cell death has been observed in some responding mammalian cells (73, 89). Presumably this programmed cell death is a response to cytotoxins, but some of the proteins translocated by the PTCs of the mammalian pathogen are similar to known avirulence determinants secreted by the plant-pathogenic bacteria. For example, *Salmonella* AvrA and *Yersinia* YopJ show significant amino acid sequence similarity to the *Xanthomonas* AvrRxv (29, 37, 60). Mammalian cells have recently been shown to carry counterparts of plant defense genes that are involved in the initiation of programmed cell death. The human apoptotic protease-activating factor, Apaf-1, is similar to the products of several plant defense genes (111). These interesting observations suggest that mammalian cells may carry surveillance systems similar to those used by plant cells to initiate some cellular defense responses. The aforementioned similarities indicate that the lessons learned from cellular defense mechanisms of plants may not be as specific as previously thought. Current efforts are being directed to elucidate the regulation and function of the proteins translocated into plant cells.

Acknowledgments. I express my appreciation to colleagues who sent reprints and prepublication materials to assist in the preparation of this chapter. My research mentioned in the text has been supported by grants from the National Science Foundation, the USDA National Research Initiative Competitive Grants Program and the Center for Agricultural Biotechnology of the University of Maryland Biotechnology Institute. I thank Kyong Pak for his assistance in the preparation of this chapter and Jamie Bretz and Tom Sussan for their comments on the manuscript.

REFERENCES

1. **Agrios, G. N.** 1988. *Plant Pathology,* 3rd ed. Academic Press, Inc., New York, N.Y.
2. **Alfano, J. R., D. W. Bauer, T. M. Milos, and A. Collmer.** 1996. Analysis of the role of the *Pseudomonas*

syringae pv. *syringae* HrpZ harpin in elicitation of the hypersensitive response in tobacco using functionally nonpolar deletion mutations, truncated HrpZ fragments and *hrmA* mutations. *Mol. Microbiol.* **19:**715–728.

3. **Alfano, J. R., and A. Collmer.** 1996. Bacterial pathogens in plants: life up against the wall. *Plant Cell* **8:**1683–1698.

4. **Alfano, J. R., and A. Collmer.** 1997. The type III (Hrp) secretion pathway of plant pathogenic bacteria: trafficking harpins, Avr proteins, and death. *J. Bacteriol.* **179:**5655–5662.

5. **Alfano, J. R., H.-S. Kim, T. P. Delaney, and A. Collmer.** 1997. Evidence that the *Pseudomonas syringae* pv. *syringae hrp*-linked *hrmA* gene encodes an Avr-like protein that acts in a *hrp*-dependent manner within tobacco cells. *Mol. Plant-Microbe Interact.* **10:**580–588.

6. **Arlat, M., C. L. Gough, C. Boucher, and M. J. Daniels.** 1991. *Xanthomonas campestris* contains a cluster of *hrp* genes related to the larger *hrp* cluster of *Pseudomonas solanacearum. Mol. Plant-Microbe Interact.* **4:**593–601.

7. **Arlat, M., F. Van Gijsegem, J. C. Huet, J. C. Pernollet, and C. A. Bouncher.** 1994. PopA1, a protein which induces a hypersensitivity-like response on specific *Petunia* genotypes, is secreted via the Hrp pathway of *Pseudomonas solanacearum. EMBO J.* **13:**543–553.

8. **Atkinson, M. M., and C. J. Baker.** 1987. Alteration of plasmalemma sucrose transport in bean leaves by *Pseudomonas syringae* pv. syringae and its association with K^+/H^+ exchange. *Phytopathology* **77:**1573–1578.

9. **Atkinson, M. M., J.-S. Huang, and C. G. Van Dyke.** 1981. Adsorption of pseudomonads to tobacco cell walls and its significance to bacterium-host interactions. *Physiol. Plant Pathol.* **18:**1–5.

10. **Bauer, D. W., A. J. Bogdanove, S. V. Beer, and A. Collmer.** 1994. *Erwinia chrysanthemi hrp* genes and their involvement in soft rot pathogenesis and elicitation of the hypersensitive response. *Mol. Plant-Microbe Interact.* **7:**573–581.

11. **Bender, C. L.** 1997. Phytotoxin production in *Pseudomonas syringae*, p. 124–144. *In* G. Stacey and N. T. Keen (ed.), *Plant-Microbe Interactions*, vol. 3. Chapman & Hall, New York, N.Y.

12. **Bogdanove, A., Z.-M. Wei, L. Zhao, and S. V. Beer.** 1996. *Erwinia amylovora* secretes harpin via a type III pathway and contains a homolog of *yopN* of *Yersinia* spp. *J. Bacteriol.* **178:**1720–1730.

13. **Bogdanove, A. J., S. V. Beer, U. Bonas, C. A. Boucher, A. Collmer, D. L. Coplin, G. R. Cornelis, H. C. Huang, S. W. Hutcheson, N. J. Panopoulos, and F. VanGijsegem.** 1996. Unified nomenclature for broadly conserved *hrp* genes of phytopathogenic bacteria. *Mol. Microbiol.* **20:**681–683.

14. **Bogdanove, A. J., J. F. Kim, Z.-M. Wei, P. Kolchinsky, A. O. Charkowski, A. K. Conlin, A. Collmer, and S. V. Beer.** 1998. Homology and functional similarity of an *hrp*-linked pathogenicity locus, *dspEF*, of *Erwinia amylovora* and the avirulence locus *avrE* of *Pseudomonas syringae* pathovar tomato. *Proc. Natl. Acad. Sci. USA* **95:**1325–1330.

15. **Boucher, C., A. Martinel, P. Barberis, G. Alloing, and C. Zischek.** 1986. Virulence genes are carried by a megaplasmid of the plant pathogen *Pseudomonas solanacearum. Mol. Gen. Genet.* **205:**270–275.

16. **Boyes, D. C., J. Nam, and J. L. Dangl.** 1998. The *Arabidopsis thaliana RPM1* disease resistance gene product is a peripheral plasma membrane protein that is degraded coincident with the hypersensitive response. *Proc. Natl. Acad. Sci. USA* **95:**15849–15854.

17. **Brito, B., M. Marenda, P. Barberis, C. Boucher, and S. Genin.** 1999. *prhJ* and *hrpG*, two new components of the plant signal-dependent regulatory cascade controlled by PrhA in *Ralstonia solanacearum. Mol. Microbiol.* **31:**237–251.

18. **Brown, J. R., and J. W. Mansfield.** 1988. An ultrastructural study, including cytochemistry and quantitative analyses, of the interactions between pseudomonads and leaves of *Phaseolus vulgaris* L. *Physiol. Mol. Plant Pathol.* **33:**351–361.

19. **Charkowski, A. O., J. R. Alfano, G. Preston, J. Yuan, S. Y. He, and A. Collmer.** 1998. The *Pseudomonas syringae* pv. tomato HrpW protein has domains similar to harpins and pectate lyases and can elicit the plant hypersensitive response and bind to pectate. *J. Bacteriol.* **180:**5211–5217.

20. **Charkowski, A. O., H. C. Huang, and A. Collmer.** 1997. Altered localization of HrpZ in *Pseudomonas syringae* pv. syringae *hrp* mutants suggests that different components of the type III secretion pathway control protein translocation across the inner and outer membrane of gram-negative bacteria. *J. Bacteriol.* **179:**3866–3874.

21. **Coplin, D. L., R. D. Frederick, D. R. Majerczak, and L. D. Tuttle.** 1992. Characterization of a gene cluster that specifies pathogenicity in *Erwinia stewartii. Mol. Plant-Microbe Interact.* **5:**81–88.

22. **Dangl, J.** Personal communication.

23. **Dangl, J. L., R. A. Dietrich, and M. H. Richberg.** 1996. Death don't have no mercy: cell death programs in plant-microbe interactions. *Plant Cell* **8:**1793–1807.

24. **Deng, W. L., G. Preston, A. Collmer, C.-J. Chang, and H.-C. Huang.** 1998. Characterization of the *hrpC* and *hrpRS* operons of *Pseudomonas syringae* pathovars syringae, tomato and glycinea and analysis of the ability of *hrpF, hrpG, hrcC, hrpT,* and *hrpV* mutants to elicit the hypersensitive response and disease in plants. *J. Bacteriol.* **180:**4523–4531.

25. **Dye, D. W., J. F. Bradbury, M. Goto, A. C. Hayward, R. A. Lelliott, and M. N. Schroth.** 1980. International standards for naming pathovars of phytopathogenic bacteria and a list of pathovar names and pathotype strains. *Rev. Plant Pathol.* **59:**153–168.

26. **Fenselau, S., and U. Bonas.** 1995. Sequence and expression analysis of the *hrpB* pathogenicity operon of *Xanthomonas campestris* pv. *vesicatoria* which encodes eight proteins with similarity to components of the Hrp, Ysc, Spa and Fli secretion systems. *Mol. Plant-Microbe Interact.* **8:**845–859.

27. **Fouts, D. E., and A. Collmer.** Personal communication.

28. **Gabriel, D. W.** 1997. Targeting of protein signals from *Xanthomonas* to the plant nucleus. *Trends Plant Sci.* **2:**204–206.

29. **Galan, J.** 1998. "Avirulence genes" in animal pathogens? *Trends Microbiol.* **6:**3–6.

30. **Genin, S., C. L. Gough, C. Zischek, and C. A. Boucher.** 1992. Evidence that the *hrpB* gene encodes a positive regulator for pathogenicity genes of *Pseudomonas solanacearum. Mol. Microbiol.* **6:**3065–3076.

31. **Glickman, E., L. Gardan, S. Jacquet, S. Hussain, M. Elasi, A. Petit, and Y. Dessaux.** 1998. Auxin production is a common feature of most pathovars of *Pseudomonas syringae. Mol. Plant-Microbe Interact.* **11:**156–162.

32. **Gopalan, S., D. W. Bauer, J. R. Alfano, A. O. Loniello, S. Y. He, and A. Collmer.** 1996. Expression of the *Pseudomonas syringae* avirulence protein AvrB in plant cells alleviates its dependence on the hypersensitive response and pathogenicity (Hrp) secretion system in eliciting genotype-specific hypersensitive cell death. *Plant Cell* **8:**1095–1105.

33. **Grimm, C., W. Aufsatz, and N. J. Panopoulos.** 1995. The *hrpRS* locus of *Pseudomonas syringae* pv. phaseolicola constitutes a complex regulatory unit. *Mol. Microbiol.* **15:**155–165.

34. **Grimm, C., and N. J. Panopoulos.** 1989. The predicted protein product of a pathogenicity locus from *Pseudomonas syringae* pv. phaseolicola is homologous to a highly conserved domain of several prokaryotic regulatory proteins. *J. Bacteriol.* **171:**5031–5038.

35. **Gross, D. C.** 1991. Molecular and genetic analysis of toxin production by pathovars of *Pseudomonas syringae. Annu. Rev. Phytopathol.* **29:**247–278.

36. **Hammond-Kosack, K. E., and J. D. G. Jones.** 1997. Plant disease resistance genes. *Annu. Rev. Plant Physiol. Plant Mol. Biol.* **48:**575–607.

37. **Hardt, W.-D., and J. E. Galan.** 1997. A secreted *Salmonella* protein with homology to an avirulence determinant of plant pathogenic bacteria. *Proc. Natl. Acad. Sci. USA* **94:**9887–9892.

38. **He, S. Y., H. C. Huang, and A. Collmer.** 1993. *Pseudomonas syringae* pv. syringae Harpin$_{Pss}$: a protein that is secreted via the Hrp pathway and elicits the hypersensitive response in plants. *Cell* **73:**1255–1266.

39. **Heu, S., and S. W. Hutcheson.** 1993. Nucleotide sequence and properties of the *hrmA* locus associated with the *P. syringae* pv. syringae 61 *hrp* gene cluster. *Mol. Plant-Microbe Interact.* **6:**553–564.

40. **Hildebrand, D. C., M. C. Alosi, and M. N. Schroth.** 1980. Physical entrapment of pseudomonads in bean leaves by films formed at air-water interfaces. *Phytopathology* **70:**98–109.

41. **Hirano, S. S., and C. D. Upper.** 1990. Population biology and epidemiology of *Pseudomonas syringae. Annu. Rev. Phytopathol.* **28:**155–177.

42. **Huang, H. C., S. W. Hutcheson, and A. Collmer.** 1991. Characterization of the *hrp* cluster from *Pseudomonas syringae* pv. syringae 61 and Tn*phoA* tagging of exported or membrane-spanning Hrp proteins. *Mol. Plant-Microbe Interact.* **4:**469–476.

43. **Huang, H. C., R. H. Lin, C. J. Chang, A. Collmer, and W. L. Deng.** 1995. The complete *hrp* gene cluster of *Pseudomonas syringae* pv. syringae 61 includes two blocks of genes required for harpin$_{Pss}$ secretion that are arranged colinearly with *Yersinia ysc* homologs. *Mol. Plant-Microbe Interact.* **8:**733–746.

44. **Huang, H. C., R. Schuurink, T. P. Denny, M. M. Atkinson, C. J. Baker, I. Yucel, S. W. Hutcheson, and A. Collmer.** 1988. Molecular cloning of a *Pseudomonas syringae* pv. *syringae* gene cluster that enables *Pseudomonas fluorescens* to elicit the hypersensitive response in tobacco. *J. Bacteriol.* **170:**4748–4756.

45. **Huang, H. C., Y. Xiao, R.-H. Lin, Y. Lu, S. W. Hutcheson, and A. Collmer.** 1993. Characterization

of the *Pseudomonas syringae* pv. syringae 61 *hrpJ* and *hrpI* genes: homology of HrpI to a superfamily of proteins associated with protein translocation. *Mol. Plant-Microbe Interact.* **6:**515–520.

46. **Hueck, C. J.** 1998. Type III protein secretion systems in bacterial pathogens of animals and plants. *Microbiol. Mol. Biol. Rev.* **62:**379–433.

47. **Hughes, K. T., K. L. Gillen, M. J. Semon, and J. E. Karlinsky.** 1993. Sensing structural intermediates in bacterial flagellar assembly by export of a negative regulator. *Science* **262:**1277–1280.

48. **Hutcheson, S. W.** 1998. Current concepts of active defense in plants. *Annu. Rev. Phytopathol.* **36:**59–90.

49. **Hutcheson, S. W.** 1997. The *hrp*-encoded protein export systems of *Pseudomonas syringae* and other plant pathogenic bacteria and their role in pathogenicity, p. 145–179. *In* G. Stacey and N. Keen (ed.), *Plant-Microbe Interactions,* vol. 3. Chapman & Hall, New York, N.Y.

50. **Hutcheson, S. W., A. Collmer, and C. J. Baker.** 1989. Elicitation of the hypersensitive response by *Pseudomonas syringae. Physiol. Plant.* **76:**155–163.

51. **Hutcheson, S. W., S. Heu, S. Jin, M. C. Lidell, M. U. Pirhonen, and D. L. Rowley.** 1996. Function and regulation of *Pseudomonas syringae hrp* genes, p. 512–521. *In* T. Nakazawa, K. Furukawa, D. Haas, and S. Silver (ed.), *Molecular Biology of Pseudomonads.* American Society for Microbiology, Washington, D.C.

52. **Hutcheson, S. W., S. Jin, M. C. Lidell, and X. Fu.** 1996. *Pseudomonas syringae hrp* genes: regulation and role in avirulence phenotypes, p. 153–158. *In* G. Stacey, B. Mullin, and P. M. Gresshoff (ed.), *Biology of Plant-Microbe Interactions.* International Society for Molecular Plant-Microbe Interactions, St. Paul, Minn.

53. **Huynh, T., D. Dahlbeck, and B. J. Staskawicz.** 1989. Bacterial blight of soybean: regulation of a pathogen gene determining host cultivar specificity. *Science* **245:**1374–1377.

54. **Innes, R. W., A. F. Bent, B. N. Kunkel, S. R. Bisgrove, and B. J. Staskawicz.** 1993. Molecular analysis of avirulence gene *avr*Rpt2 and identification of a putative regulatory sequence common to all known *Pseudomonas syringae* avirulence genes. *J. Bacteriol.* **175:**4859–4869.

55. **Kearney, B., and B. J. Staskawicz.** 1990. Widespread distribution and fitness contribution of *Xanthomonas campestris* avirulence gene *avrBs2. Nature (London)* **346:**385–386.

56. **Kim, J. F., and S. V. Beer.** 1998. HrpW of *Erwinia amylovora,* a new harpin that contains a domain homologous to pectate lyases of a distinct class. *J. Bacteriol.* **180:**5203–5210.

57. **Kim, J. F., A. O. Charkowski, J. R. Alfano, A. Collmer, and S. V. Beer.** 1998. Sequences related to transposable elements and bacteriophages flank avirulence genes of *Pseudomonas syringae. Mol. Plant-Microbe Interact.* **11:**1247–1252.

58. **Kim, J. F., J. H. Ham, D. W. Bauer, A. Collmer, and S. V. Beer.** 1998. The *hrcC* and *hrpN* operons of *Erwinia chrysanthemi* EC16 are flanked by *plcA* and homologs of hemolysin/adhesion genes and accompanying activator/transporter genes. *Mol. Plant-Microbe Interact.* **11:**563–567.

59. **Laby, R. J., and S. V. Beer.** 1992. Hybridization and functional complementation of the *hrp* gene cluster from *Erwinia amylovora* strain Ea321 with DNA of other bacteria. *Mol. Plant-Microbe Interact.* **5:**412–419.

60. **Leach, J. E., and F. F. White.** 1996. Bacterial avirulence genes. *Annu. Rev. Phytopathol.* **34:**153–179.

61. **Leigh, J. A., and D. L. Coplin.** 1992. Exopolysaccharides in plant-bacterial interactions. *Annu. Rev. Microbiol.* **46:**307–346.

62. **Leister, R. T., F. M. Ausubel, and F. Katagiri.** 1996. Molecular recognition of pathogen attack occurs inside of plant cells in plant disease resistance specified by the *Arabidopsis* genes *RPS2* and *RPM1. Proc. Natl. Acad. Sci. USA* **93:**3459–3464.

63. **Lidell, M., and S. W. Hutcheson.** 1994. Characterization of the *hrpJ* and *U* operons of *Pseudomonas syringae* pv. syringae Pss61: similarity with components of enteric bacteria involved in flagellar biogenesis and demonstration of their role in harpin$_{Pss}$ translocation. *Mol. Plant-Microbe Interact.* **7:**488–497.

64. **Lidell, M. C.** 1998. Ph.D. thesis. University of Maryland, College Park.

65. **Lindgren, P. B.** 1997. The role of *hrp* genes during plant-bacterial interactions. *Annu. Rev. Phytopathol.* **35:**129–152.

66. **Lindgren, P. B., R. C. Peet, and N. J. Panopoulos.** 1986. Gene cluster of *Pseudomonas syringae* pv. phaseolicola controls pathogenicity on bean plants and hypersensitivity on nonhost plants. *J. Bacteriol.* **168:**512–522.

67. **Lorang, J. M., and N. T. Keen.** 1995. Characterization of *avrE* from *Pseudomonas syringae* pv. tomato: a *hrp*-linked avirulence locus consisting of at least two transcriptional units. *Mol. Plant-Microbe Interact.* **8:**49–57.

68. **Lorang, J. M., H. Shen, D. Kobayashi, D. Cooksey, and N. T. Keen.** 1994. *avrA* and *avrE* in *Pseudomonas syringae* pv. tomato PT23 play a role in virulence on tomato plants. *Mol. Plant-Microbe Interact.* **7:** 508–515.

69. **Macnab, R. M.** 1996. Flagella and motility, p. 123–145. *In* F. C. Neidhardt, R. Curtiss III, J. L. Ingraham, E. C. C. Lin, K. B. Low, B. Magasanik, W. S. Reznikoff, M. Riley, M. Schaechter, and H. E. Umbarger (ed.), *Escherichia coli* and *Salmonella: Cellular and Molecular Biology,* 2nd ed., vol. 1. ASM Press, Washington, D.C.

70. **Mansfield, J., I. Brown, and A. Maroofi.** 1994. Bacterial pathogenicity and the plant's response: ultrastructure, biochemical and physiological perspectives, p. 85–106. *In* D. D. Bills and S. D. Kung (ed.), *Biotechnology and Plant Protection: Bacterial Pathogenesis and Disease Resistance.* World Scientific Publishing, Singapore.

71. **Mansfield, J., C. Jenner, R. Hockenhull, M. A. Bennett, and R. Stewart.** 1994. Characterization of *avrPphE*, a gene for cultivar-specific avirulence from *Pseudomonas syringae* pv. *phaseolicola* which is physically linked to *hrpY*, a new *hrp* gene identified in the halo-blight bacterium. *Mol. Plant-Microbe Interact.* **7:**726–739.

72. **Marenda, M., B. Brito, D. Callard, S. Genin, P. Barberis, C. A. Boucher, and M. Arlat.** 1998. PrhA controls a novel regulatory pathway required for the specific induction of *Ralstonia solanacearum hrp* genes in the presence of plant cells. *Mol. Microbiol.* **27:**437–454.

73. **Mills, S. D., A. Boland, M.-P. Sory, P. Van Der Smissen, C. Kerbourch, B. B. Finlay, and G. R. Cornelis.** 1997. *Yersinia enterocolitica* induces apoptosis in macrophages by a process requiring functional type III secretion and translocation mechanisms and involving YopP, presumably acting as an effector protein. *Proc. Natl. Acad. Sci. USA* **94:**12638–12643.

74. **Mudgett, M. B., and B. J. Staskawicz.** 1997. Protein signaling via type II secretion pathways in phytopathogenic bacteria. *Curr. Opin. Microbiol.* **1:**109–114.

75. **Mukherjee, A., Y. Cui, Y. Liu, C. K. Dumenyo, and A. K. Chatterjee.** 1997. Molecular characterization and expression of the *Erwinia carotovora hrpN$_{Ecc}$* gene, which encodes an elicitor of the hypersensitive response. *Mol. Plant-Microbe Interact.* **10:**462–471.

76. **Nizan, R., I. Barash, L. Valinsky, A. Lichter, and S. Manulis.** 1997. The presence of *hrp* genes on the pathogenicity-associated plasmid of the tumorigenic bacterium *Erwinia herbicola* pv. *gypsophilae. Mol. Plant-Microbe Interact.* **11:**763–771.

77. **Olsen, G. J., C. R. Woese, and R. Overbeek.** 1994. The winds of (evolutionary) change: breathing new life into microbiology. *J. Bacteriol.* **176:**1–6.

78. **Pallaroni, N. I.** 1984. *Pseudomonaceae,* p. 141–210. *In* N. R. Krieg and J. G. Holt (ed.), *Bergey's Manual of Systematic Bacteriology,* vol. 1. The Williams & Wilkins Co., Baltimore, Md.

79. **Panopoulos, N. J., and M. N. Schroth.** 1974. Role of flagellar motility in the invasion of bean leaves by *Pseudomonas phaseolicola. Phytopathology* **64:**1389–1397.

80. **Peuppke, S. G., and D. A. Kluepfel.** 1985. Responses of plant cells to absorbed bacteria, p. 404–435. *In* D. C. Savage and M. Fletcher (ed.), *Bacterial Adhesion. Mechanisms and Physiological Significance.* Plenum Press, New York, N.Y.

81. **Pirhonen, M. U., M. C. Lidell, D. Rowley, S. W. Lee, S. Silverstone, Y. Liang, N. T. Keen, and S. W. Hutcheson.** 1996. Phenotypic expression of *Pseudomonas syringae avr* genes in *E. coli* is linked to the activities of the *hrp*-encoded secretion system. *Mol. Plant-Microbe Interact.* **9:**252–260.

82. **Preston, G., W.-L. Deng, H.-C. Huang, and A. Collmer.** 1998. Negative regulation of *hrp* genes in *Pseudomonas syringae* by Hrp V. *J. Bacteriol.* **180:**4532–4537.

83. **Preston, G., H. C. Huang, S. Y. He, and A. Collmer.** 1995. The HrpZ proteins of *Pseudomonas syringae* pvs. syringae, glycinea, and tomato are encoded by an operon containing *Yersinia ysc* homologs and elicit the hypersensitive response in tomato but not soybean. *Mol. Plant-Microbe Interact.* **8:**717–732.

84. **Rahme, L. G., M. N. Mindronos, and N. J. Panopoulos.** 1992. Plant and environmental sensory signals control the expression of *hrp* genes in *Pseudomonas syringae* pv. phaseolicola. *J. Bacteriol.* **174:**3499–3507.

85. **Roine, E., D. M. Raineri, M. Romantschuk, M. Wilson, and D. N. Nunn.** 1998. Characterization of type IV pilus genes in *Pseudomonas syringae* pv. *tomato* DC3000. *Mol. Plant-Microbe Interact.* **11:** 1048–1056.

86. **Roine, E., J. Saarinen, N. Kalkkinen, and M. Romantshuk.** 1997. Purified HrpA of *Pseudomonas syringae* pv. *tomato* DC3000 reassembles into pili. *FEBS Lett.* **417:**168–172.

87. **Roine, E., W. Wei, J. Yuan, E.-L. Nurmiaho-Lassila, N. Kalkkinen, M. Romantschuk, and S.-Y. He.**

1997. Hrp pilus: an *hrp*-dependent bacterial surface appendage produced by *Pseudomonas syringae* pv. *tomato* DC3000. *Proc. Natl. Acad. Sci. USA* **94**:3459–3464.

88. **Romantschuk, M., E. Roine, and K. Bjorklof.** 1997. Attachment of *Pseudomonas syringae* to plant surfaces, p. 3–10. *In* K. Rudolph, T. J. Burr, J. W. Mansfield, D. Stead, A. Vivian, and J. von Kietzell (ed.), Pseudomonas syringae *Pathovars and Related Pathogens.* Kluwer Academic Publishers, Dordrecht, The Netherlands.

89. **Ruckdeschel, K., A. Roggenkamp, V. Lafont, P. Mangeat, J. Heeseman, and B. Rouot.** 1997. Interaction of *Yersinia enterocolitica* with macrophages leads to macrophage cell death through apoptosis. *Infect. Immun.* **65**:4813–4821.

90. **Rudolph, K., and B. Sonnenberg.** 1997. Role of polysaccharides from *Pseudomonas syringae* pathovars in pathogenesis, p. 265–270. *In* K. Rudolph, T. J. Burr, J. W. Mansfield, D. Stead, A. Vivian, and J. von Kietzell (ed.), Pseudomonas syringae *Pathovars and Related Pathogens.* Kluwer Academic Publishers, Dordrecht, The Netherlands.

91. **Rudolph, K. W. E., M. Gross, F. Ebrahim-Nesbat, M. Nollenburg, A. Zomorodian, K. Wydra, M. Neugebauer, U. Hettwer, W. El-Shouny, B. Sonnenberg, and Z. Klement.** 1994. Role of extracellular polysaccharides as virulence factors for phytopathogenic pseudomonads and xanthomonads, p. 357–378. *In* C. I. Kado and J. H. Crosa (ed.), *Molecular Mechanisms of Bacterial Virulence.* Kluwer Academic Publishers, Dordrecht, The Netherlands.

92. **Salmeron, J. M., and B. J. Staskawicz.** 1993. Molecular characterization and *hrp*-dependence of the avirulence gene *avrPto* from *Pseudomonas syringae* pv. tomato. *Mol. Gen. Genet.* **239**:6–10.

93. **Scofield, S. R., C. M. Tobias, J. P. Rathjen, J. H. Chang, D. T. Lavelle, R. W. Michelmore, and B. J. Staskawicz.** 1996. Molecular basis of gene-for-gene specificity in bacterial speck disease of tomato. *Science* **274**:2063–2065.

94. **Shen, H., and N. T. Keen.** 1993. Characterization of the promoter of avirulence gene D from *Pseudomonas syringae* pv. tomato. *J. Bacteriol.* **175**:5916–5924.

95. **Stall, R. E., and A. A. Cook.** 1979. Evidence that bacterial contact with the plant cell is necessary for the hypersensitive reaction but not the susceptible reaction. *Physiol. Plant Pathol.* **14**:77–84.

96. **Staskawicz, B. J., D. Dahlbeck, and N. T. Keen.** 1984. Cloned avirulence gene of *Pseudomonas syringae* pv. *glycinea* determines race-specific incompatibility on *Glycine max* (L.) Merr. *Proc. Natl. Acad. Sci. USA* **81**:6024–6028.

97. **Tang, X., R. D. Frederick, J. Zhou, D. A. Halterman, Y. Jia, and G. B. Martin.** 1996. Initiation of plant disease resistance by physical interaction of AvrPto and Pto kinase. *Science* **274**:2060–2063.

98. **Turner, J. G., and A. Novacky.** 1974. The quantitative relation between plant and bacterial cells involved in the hypersensitive reaction. *Phytopathology* **64**:885–890.

99. **Van den Ackerveken, G., E. Marois, and U. Bonas.** 1996. Recognition of the bacterial avirulence protein AvrBs3 occurs inside the host plant cell. *Cell* **87**:1307–1316.

100. **VanGijsegem, F., C. Gough, C. Zischek, E. Niqueux, M. Ariat, S. Genin, P. Barberis, S. German, P. Castello, and C. Boucher.** 1995. The *hrp* gene locus of *Pseudomonas solanacearum,* which controls the production of a type III secretion system, encodes eight proteins related to components of the bacterial flagellar biogenesis complex. *Mol. Microbiol.* **15**:1095–1114.

101. **Vivian, A., and M. J. Gibbon.** 1997. Avirulence genes in plant-pathogenic bacteria: signals or weapons. *Microbiology* **143**:693–704.

102. **Wei, Z.-M., R. J. Laby, C. H. Zumoff, D. W. Bauer, S. H. He, A. Collmer, and S. V. Beer.** 1992. Harpin, elicitor of the hypersensitive response produced by the plant pathogen *Erwinia amylovora. Science* **257**:85–88.

103. **Wei, Z. M., and S. V. Beer.** 1995. *hrpL* activates *Erwinia amylovora hrp* gene transcription and is a member of the ECF subfamily of sigma factors. *J. Bacteriol.* **177**:6201–6210.

104. **Wei, Z. M., and S. V. Beer.** Personal communication.

105. **Wengelnik, K., and U. Bonas.** 1996. HrpXv, an AraC-type regulator, activates expression of five of six loci in the *hrp* cluster of *Xanthomonas campestris* pv. vesicatoria. *J. Bacteriol.* **178**:3462–3469.

106. **Willis, D. K., J. J. Rich, and E. M. Hrabak.** 1991. The *hrp* genes of phytopathogenic bacteria. *Mol. Plant-Microbe Interact.* **4**:132–138.

107. **Xiao, Y., S. Heu, J. Yi, Y. Lu, and S. W. Hutcheson.** 1994. Identification of a putative alternate sigma factor and characterization of a multicomponent regulatory cascade controlling the expression of *Pseudomonas syringae* pv. *syringae* Pss61 *hrp* and *hrmA* genes. *J. Bacteriol.* **176**:1025–1036.

108. **Xiao, Y., and S. W. Hutcheson.** 1994. A single promoter sequence recognized by a newly identified alternate sigma factor directs expression of pathogenicity and host range determinants in *Pseudomonas syringae. J. Bacteriol.* **176:**3089–3091.

109. **Xiao, Y., Y. Lu, S. Heu, and S. W. Hutcheson.** 1992. Organization and environmental regulation of the *Pseudomonas syringae* pv. syringae 61 *hrp* cluster. *J. Bacteriol.* **174:**1734–1741.

110. **Yuan, J., and S. Y. He.** 1996. The *Pseudomonas syringae* Hrp regulation and secretion system controls the production and secretion of multiple extracellular proteins. *J. Bacteriol.* **178:**6399–6402.

111. **Zou, H., W. J. Henzel, X. Liu, A. Lutschg, and X. Wang.** 1997. Apaf-1, a human protein homologous to *C. elegans* CED-4, participates in cytochrome c-dependent activation of caspase-3. *Cell* **90:**405–413.

Pathogenicity Islands and Other Mobile Virulence Elements
Edited by J. B. Kaper and J. Hacker
© 1999 American Society for Microbiology, Washington, D.C.

Chapter 17

Conjugative Transposons: Transmissible Resistance Islands

Abigail Salyers, Nadja Shoemaker, George Bonheyo, and Jorge Frias

CONJUGATIVE TRANSPOSONS AND PATHOGENICITY ISLANDS

Conjugative transposons are integrated DNA segments that excise from the chromosome to form a circular intermediate. The circular intermediate transfers itself to a recipient, where it integrates once again in the chromosome (Fig. 1) (32–34). Conjugative transposons vary considerably in size, from 18 to over 150 kbp. They also vary in their target site specificity. Some integrate site specifically, whereas others integrate almost randomly (33, 34). Another type of integrated transmissible element that excises and transfers itself similarly to the conjugative transposons is a type of integrated plasmid found in streptomycetes (3, 5, 22, 46). Integrated plasmids differ from conjugative transposons in that they are capable of replication in some strains of streptomycetes whereas conjugative transposons have so far not been shown to replicate in any host.

The features of conjugative transposons are similar enough to those of pathogenicity islands (PAIs) to raise the question whether some PAIs are actually conjugative transposons. PAIs have been loosely defined as clusters of chromosomal virulence genes that appear to be transmissible. The transmissibility of the island can be inferred from the presence of the same island in different bacteria or from the fact that the G+C content of the region is different from that of the rest of the chromosome. Often, it is difficult to demonstrate the transmissibility of a suspected transmissible element. For one thing, excision and transfer may be tightly regulated, so that no transfer is seen unless the appropriate inducing conditions are found. This was the case for a group of *Bacteroides* conjugative transposons. Only the accidental discovery that tetracycline induced their transfer made it possible to detect transfer at all (33). Alternatively, a transmissible integrating element may have ends that are unstable in a particular host, resulting in deletions at the ends that render the element incapable of excision. This appears to have happened to the conjugative transposon CTn*916* in *Neisseria* spp. (43). For these reasons, it is helpful to have some way of deciding on the basis of sequence information whether there is sufficient reason to suspect that a PAI belongs to a particular class of integrating transmissible elements to justify more intensive attempts to demonstrate transmissibility. One purpose of this

Abigail Salyers, Nadja Shoemaker, George Bonheyo, and Jorge Frias • Department of Microbiology, University of Illinois, Urbana, IL 61801.

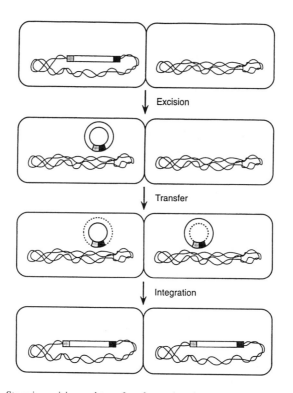

Figure 1. Steps in excision and transfer of a conjugative transposon. The conjugative transposon (shown as an open bar with differently hatched ends to indicate a lack of identity between the ends) is normally integrated into the chromosome. To transfer, it first excises to form a covalently closed circle, resealing the chromosomal site in the process, and then transfers by conjugation to a recipient. The single-stranded form of the donor and recipient circular forms is then copied (dashed line) to regenerate the double-stranded circular intermediate. The circular intermediate then integrates once again into the chromosome.

chapter is to review the features associated with conjugative transposons and other transmissible integrated elements. Another purpose is to alert scientists interested in PAIs to the existence of conjugative transposons.

Since most of the work on conjugative transposons has focused on elements that carry antibiotic resistance genes, scientists interested in PAIs may not think that conjugative transposons are relevant to their studies. However, at one time, plasmids were associated almost exclusively with the transmission of antibiotic resistance genes. We know that plasmids can serve equally well as vehicles of virulence gene transmission (see, for example, chapters 6 and 8); therefore, conjugative transposons and integrated plasmids might also play such a role.

Recently, a 70-kb plasmid of *Shigella dysenteriae* has been shown to carry genes for lipopolysaccharide synthesis and HeLa cell adherence as well as genes for resistance to antibiotics (10). This report raises an interesting question: how often does linkage between virulence genes and antibiotic resistance genes occur? There have been few examples so far of resistance genes and virulence genes occupying the same conjugal element, but the lack of such examples may not reflect a true lack of resistance gene-virulence gene linkage as much as the fact that scientists interested in resistance genes rarely look for virulence genes on the transmissible elements they study and vice versa. As more PAIs are completely sequenced, it will be interesting to see whether any of them contain antibiotic resistance genes as well as virulence genes. Similarly, conjugative transposons may prove to carry virulence genes as well as antibiotic resistance genes.

CONJUGATIVE TRANSPOSONS TRANSCEND CONVENTIONAL CATEGORIES OF GENE TRANSFER ELEMENTS

Conjugative transposons do not fit neatly into any of the traditional categories of mobile elements such as transposons, bacteriophages, and plasmids; instead, they combine features of all of them (32–34). Conjugative transposons resemble conventional transposons in that they integrate into DNA, but the mechanism of integration used by conjugative transposons is completely different from that used by transposons. Conjugative transposons, unlike transposons, regenerate the DNA segment from which they are excising and form a circular transfer intermediate that is self-transmissible by conjugation. Conjugative transposons resemble self-transmissible plasmids in that they are transferred by conjugation and have a circular transfer intermediate, but the circular intermediate does not replicate.

Conjugative transposons differ from the Hfr type of integrated plasmid in that the conjugative transposons excise and circularize prior to transferring and thus transfer as an intact element, whereas only a portion of an Hfr enters the recipient. Conjugative transposons that have moved into a recipient are still fully capable of self transfer to another bacterial cell. Conjugative transposons and the integrating actinomycete plasmids turn out to be most like lysogenic bacteriophages, except that they are transferred by conjugation rather than by phage transduction. They have similar integrases, and many of them integrate into the 3′ ends of tRNA genes (1, 13, 22, 33, 46), a common feature of lambdoid phages (6).

NOMENCLATURE

The name ''conjugative transposon'' has caused considerable confusion because it suggests that conjugative transposons are just a variety of transposon that can transfer themselves by conjugation. However, conjugative transposons are different from conventional transposons in a number of ways. The mistaken idea that conjugative transposons are just like conventional transposons except for their transmissibility is reinforced by the fact that many conjugative transposons have been given transposon designations. To distinguish between conjugative and conventional transposons, we have suggested the use of ''CTn'' instead of ''Tn'' to denote a conjugative transposon. We use the CTn designation in this chapter to identify elements that have been called conjugative transposons. It is perhaps premature, however, to become too deeply obsessed with nomenclature at this point. The elements that have been called conjugative transposons are an extremely heterogeneous group. In future years, as we learn more about their properties and activities, we may come to consider ourselves naive for having initially placed them all in a single group.

DISTRIBUTION AND SIGNIFICANCE OF CONJUGATIVE TRANSPOSONS

First found in streptococci and enterococci (1, 7), conjugative transposons have now been detected in a number of other gram-positive bacteria (2, 7, 12, 28, 29). In the gram-positive bacteria, conjugative transposons have been associated with the transfer of resistance to tetracycline, erythromycin, chloramphenicol, and aminoglycosides (Fig. 2). Recently, a conjugative transposon carrying vancomycin resistance genes has been identified (12). Conjugative transposons have also been found in gram-negative genera such as *Neisseria, Butyrivibrio,* and *Bacteroides* (17, 24, 31, 34, 35, 43). In *Neisseria* and *Butyrivibrio,* conjugative transposons frequently carry the ribosome protection-type resistance gene *tetM*. In *Bacteroides* and related genera, conjugative transposons are generally associated with a different ribosome protection-type tetracycline resistance gene, *tetQ* (Fig. 3). *Bacteroides* conjugative transposons can also carry genes that confer resistance to clindamycin (*ermF* and *ermG*) (9, 33). Recently, a conjugative transposon carrying resistance to sulfamethoxazole and trimethoprim has been found in the pandemic *Vibrio cholerae* O139 (STX element) (47) and a conjugative transposon carrying sucrose catabolism genes has been found in a strain of *Salmonella senftenberg* (CTncr94) (13). These are

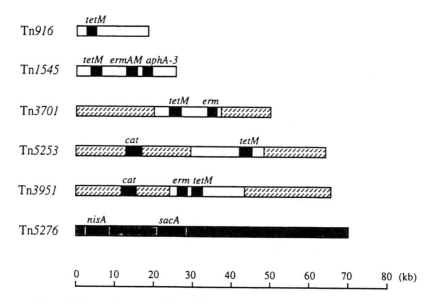

Figure 2. Schematic representation of the structures of some of the better-studied gram-positive bacterial conjugative transposons. Areas with the same fill cross-hybridize with each other. The designations are the old names. Currently, we designate them CTn*916*, CTn*1545*, CTn*3701*, CTn*5253*, CTn*3951*, and CTn*5276* (top to bottom). CTn*916* and CTn*1545* are nearly identical except for the extra antibiotic resistance genes (solid boxes) in CTn*1545*. CTn*3701*, CTn*5253*, and CTn*3951* cross-hybridize in the indicated regions but may not be as similar as CTn*916* and CTn*1545*. Each of these three larger elements contains an insertion of a CTn916-related element. CTn*5276*, from *Lactococcus lactis*, is completely unrelated to the others and carries a nisin gene and a gene for sucrose metabolism rather than the resistance genes seen on the other conjugative transposons.

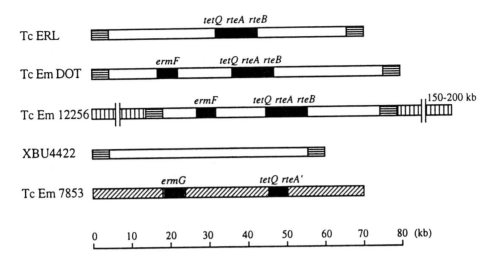

Figure 3. Schematic representation of the known *Bacteroides* conjugative transposons. The names in the figure are those under which information about the element was first published. Currently, we designate these elements CTn*ERL*, CTn*DOT*, CTn*12256*, CTn*XBU4422*, and CTn*7853*, (24, 32) (top to bottom). CTn*ERL* and CTn*DOT* are very similar to each other in the unfilled regions and are virtually identical in the area that contains *tetQ*, *rteA*, and *rteB*. CTn*DOT* has a 6- to 8-kbp insertion that contains *ermF*. CTn*12256* is a hybrid element with a CTn*DOT*-type element embedded in another similarly sized element. CTn*XBU4422* is a cryptic element that cross-hybridizes with CTn*ERL* but is more distantly related to it than is CTn*DOT*. CTn*7853* is unrelated to the other elements except that it contains *tetQ* (9).

the first sightings of conjugative transposons in bacterial species closely related to *Escherichia coli*. Clearly, conjugative transposons are widely distributed in the bacterial world.

Conjugative transposons usually have a very broad host range. In the laboratory, conjugative transposons such as CTn*916* can move between gram-positive and *Escherichia coli*-group gram-negative bacteria (7, 33). The *Bacteroides* conjugative transposons can transfer DNA from *Bacteroides* species to *E. coli* (32, 33), although they do not integrate in *E. coli* (27). *Bacteroides* conjugative transposons can transfer to other members of the *Bacteroides* phylogenetic group, such as the oral anaerobe *Porphyromonas* and the rumen anaerobe *Prevotella* (11, 31). Evidence that such transfers occur frequently in nature is beginning to accumulate. *tetM* and *tetQ* have been found in natural isolates from many different genera of bacteria, indicating that horizontal transfer has occurred under natural conditions (16, 17, 23, 31). Unlike phages and some plasmids, most conjugative transposons do not exclude closely related elements unless they have a single site that is no longer available once it is filled. This allows a bacterial strain to acquire more than one conjugative transposon. There is some evidence that related conjugative transposons increase each other's transposition frequencies when they are present in the same strain (7). Thus, having multiple conjugative transposons may not only expand the repertoire of resistance genes of a bacterium but also increase the potential of the bacterium to donate the genes to other bacteria. Moreover, conjugative transposons, with some exceptions (see, e.g., reference

43), are very stable in most hosts (33). Thus, once a conjugative transposon enters a strain, it is likely to stay there for a long time, even without selection for the genes it carries.

Most conjugative transposons were found by accident. Attempts to search in a more direct manner for new conjugative transposons have been hindered by the fact that there is no systematic way to screen natural isolates for them. There are probes related to the well-studied conjugative transposons, such as CTn*916* (Fig. 2) or the *Bacteroides* CTn*DOT* (Fig. 3), but as more conjugative transposons have been identified, it is becoming evident that this group of elements is quite diverse. As already mentioned, the ribosome protection-type resistance genes *tetM* and *tetQ* seem to be carried on many conjugative transposons and could thus be considered markers indicating the presence of a conjugative transposon, but these resistance genes are not found on all conjugative transposons. They are not part of the conjugative transposons of *V. cholerae* and *Salmonella senftenberg*. In *Neisseria* species, *tetM* is found on conjugal plasmids, which would seem to contradict the observation that *tetM* is almost always associated with a conjugative transposon; however, results of a recent study of *tetM*-carrying *N. gonorrhoeae* strains suggest that the *tetM* plasmid may actually have been created by integration of a *tetM*-containing conjugative transposon followed by deletion of the ends of the conjugative transposon (44). Therefore, although *tetM* and *tetQ* can be used as guides to where a conjugative transposon might be lurking, they are not infallible indicator genes.

Conjugative transposons do not always carry antibiotic resistance genes. Since people who stumble across conjugative transposons are usually looking for the force behind the movement of resistance genes or interesting metabolic genes rather than any conjugative element, the incidence of "cryptic" conjugative transposons has undoubtedly been under-estimated. Oggioni et al. (26) have suggested on the basis of analysis of DNA sequences of *tetM* alleles that the introduction of *tetM* onto conjugative transposons may have been a relatively recent evolutionary event. If so, CTn*916* started out as a cryptic conjugative transposon, and some copies of that form of the element should still be present in natural isolates. We found a cryptic member of the *Bacteroides* conjugative transposon family, CTn*XBU4422* (Fig. 3). This cryptic element was detected when it integrated into a nonmobilizable plasmid, allowing conjugal transfer of that plasmid to a recipient (33). Using a mating-out strategy is one way to look for conjugative transposons. However, it would not work for all conjugative transposons. CTn*916,* for example, excises from the plasmid it occupies during transfer and does not comobilize plasmid markers (33, 34).

STRUCTURES AND RELATEDNESS OF CONJUGATIVE TRANSPOSONS

Conjugative transposons vary considerably at the DNA sequence level and, as already mentioned, also vary in size and site specificity. The diversity of the conjugative transposons and related elements can be seen from Fig. 2 and 3, which illustrate the best-studied gram-positive bacterial and *Bacteroides* conjugative transposons, respectively. The gram-positive bacterial conjugative transposons shown in Fig. 2 are related to each other, but even in cases where two elements exhibit some cross-hybridization on Southern blots, they are clearly not identical because the hybridization is not uniform and there are restriction polymorphisms (Fig. 2). Just as a number of the gram-positive bacterial conjugative transposons are related to CTn*916,* many of the *Bacteroides* conjugative transposons are related to CTn*DOT*. Another *Bacteroides* conjugative transposon, CTn*7853,* however, is completely different from the CTn*DOT*-type elements except in the region around *tetQ* (9, 24). Furthermore, although CTn*XBU4422* cross-hybridizes with CTn*DOT,* the hybridization is weak, there are restriction polymorphisms, and some genes of CTn*DOT* are clearly missing from CTn*XBU4422* (33). The conjugative transposons from *V. cholerae* and *Salmonella senftenberg* are completely distinct from each other and from the conjugative transposons depicted in Fig. 2 and 3.

Hybrid conjugative transposons are common. For example, some of the large transposons in gram-positive bacteria carry a copy of a CTn*916*-like conjugative transposon (Fig. 2). The *Bacteroides* conjugative transposon CTn*12256* contains an element related to CTn*DOT* (Fig. 3). The fact that these hybrids are stably maintained through numerous transfers indicates that their ability to excise might be repressed. In fact, the copy of CTn*916* in CTn*5253* can excise if part of the larger element is deleted (1). Thus, there appears to be a repressor of excision encoded somewhere on the larger element. Whether this is true of the *Bacteroides* conjugative transposon CTn*12256* remains to be seen. PAIs may also prove to have been cobbled together from disparate integrating elements. Therefore, it is important to analyze sequences interior to the island for indications of this type of hybrid structure. Another type of hybrid is also seen in conjugative transposons. Some conjugative transposons contain insertion sequences (4, 28). These insertions do not occur at the end of the conjugative transposon, although they may occur near the end, and they appear to have nothing to do with excision or integration of the element. Thus, finding an insertion sequence adjacent to a PAI does not rule out the possibility that the island is a conjugative transposon. Conjugative transposons might be described as shopping-cart elements that travel around accumulating new DNA accessories. This strategy for adaptation to new conditions has been very successful.

STEPS IN TRANSPOSITION

Excision and Integration

Despite their structural differences, all conjugative transposons so far identified have a common pathway of excision, transfer, and integration (Fig. 1). The first step is excision to form a covalently closed circular double-stranded DNA molecule. Usually, the abundance of the circular intermediate is too low to allow it to be seen by ethidium bromide staining or Southern blotting of a plasmid preparation. One exception to this rule has been found, CTn*5381,* a CTn*916*-like element from *Enterococcus faecalis* (29). Another exception is CTn*916* cloned in a high-copy-number plasmid in *E. coli,* where the excision rate is high enough that added to the high copy number of the element, circular forms of the element can be visualized on stained gels. In cases where the circular form cannot be visualized on stained gels of plasmid preparations, the joined ends of the circular form can be detected by PCR. The fact that the site from which the transposon excised can also be detected by PCR amplification confirms that the process of excision leaves an intact donor molecule behind. A model for integration and excision of CTn*916* has been proposed (Fig. 4). An integrase protein, encoded near one end of the conjugative transposon, makes staggered cuts 6 bp from each end of the conjugative transposon (21, 30). A ligation reaction occurs that produces a covalently closed circle and a resealed site. Since the 6-bp segments at the two ends of the element (coupling sequences) are not homologous to

338   Salyers et al.

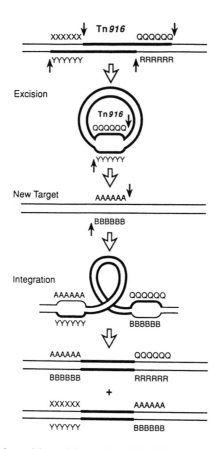

Figure 4. Model for excision and integration of CTn*916* (34). The coupling sequences are marked with X(Y)s and Q(R)s to show that the coupling sequences do not base pair with each other. Thus, when the element excises, a 6-bp region of heterology is created that is resolved to copy one coupling sequence of the other (21, 30). Integration occurs by a similar process. Because of the mode of excision and integration, a conjugative transposon can bring along to its new site bases that were adjacent to one end in its former location (XXXXXX/YYYYYY in this case). This type of integration mechanism usually does not duplicate the target site, although it can appear to do so if a region near one end is identical to a region near the target site, as was the case with CTn*XBU4422* (33).

each other, a small region of heterology is produced (Fig. 4). Evidence for such regions of heterology comes from experiments in which PCR amplification is done first with a single primer that recognizes one or the other of the strands of the excised circle and then with addition of the second primer to create many copies of the products. The amplicons are then sequenced. When this was done with CTn*916* in *E. coli,* both of the heterologous sequences were detected, in a ratio of about 1:1 (34). In *Enterococcus,* the heterology was not seen when this approach was used (21). This latter result indicates that the heterology is resolved more rapidly in some hosts than in others. How the heterologous regions are resolved remains to be determined. It is not done by the homologous recombination system, because excision and integration are independent of RecA function (8, 34).

Because of the way in which CTn916 excises, it takes 6 bp of adjacent chromosomal DNA with it and can either restore the donor molecule to its original sequence or leave a new 6-bp sequence behind. These "footprints" of the conjugative transposon aid in monitoring the transfer of the conjugative transposon from strain to strain. Also, their existence is further evidence to support the hypothesis that the excising conjugative transposon does in fact repair the donor molecule. Integration into the recipient genome probably occurs by a process that is the reverse of excision (Fig. 4). Once again, small regions of heterology are introduced, this time at both ends of the integrated element. The resolution of these regions to give base-paired regions leaves the 6-bp sequence that was brought in by the conjugative transposon at one end of the element. As the model predicts, CTn916 places this new sequence at one end or the other, with approximately equal frequency, when it integrates. This type of integration mechanism usually does not generate target site duplications. It can appear to do so, however, if a sequence within one end of the conjugative transposon matches a sequence in or near the target site. Two examples of this apparent target site duplication have been seen so far with the *Lactococcus lactis* conjugative transposon CTn5276 (28) and the *Bacteroides* conjugative transposon CTnXBU4422 (33).

Evidence that the integrating form is a double-stranded circle comes from transformation experiments. The excision frequency of CTn916 is so high in *E. coli* that the circular form can actually be seen in plasmid preparations. When isolated circles from *E. coli* were used to used to transform protoplasts of *Bacillus subtilis,* integration occurred (34). Presumably, the circular form that integrates after conjugation would have a homologous coupling-sequence region, because any heterology would be resolved during the conjugation process, which replicates the complementary strand of the incoming single-stranded copy of the circle.

The mechanisms of integration and excision are less well established for *Bacteroides* conjugative transposons. Initially, we thought that insertion occurred by a blunt-ended ligation mechanism, but more recent work suggests that the *Bacteroides* conjugative transposons integrate and excise similarly to CTn916 except that the coupling sequences are only 4 bp long (27).

CTn916 integrates in many different sites in most hosts, and there are no immediately obvious target sites for this class of conjugative transposons. However, transposition of CTn916 is not completely random. Jaworski and Clewell (14) compared regions around a number of CTn916 integration sites and noted that all of these sites were flanked by a T-rich region on one side and an A-rich region on the other and that these regions were separated by 6 bp, the exact size of the coupling sequences. Possibly, CTn916 is targeting bends in the DNA rather than specific sequences. Although the integration of CTn916 appears to be relatively random, indicating that integration occurs readily at many sites, the site into which CTn916 integrates has a major effect on excision of the element. Excision frequencies differ by several log units from one site to another, with no clear sequence pattern to explain the difference in excision frequencies (14, 20). Other gram-positive bacterial conjugative transposons are quite site specific (1), and the integrating *Streptomyces* plasmids are very site specific in their integration because they recognize a target site that can be as large as 50 kbp (5). Integration of the *Streptomyces* plasmids, in contrast to most conjugative transposons, creates a large target site duplication.

Bacteroides conjugative transposons also appear to be more site selective than CTn916, and excision from different sites appears to be equally efficient. The site selectivity of the *Bacteroides* conjugative transposons may be mediated by a 13-bp sequence located about 4 bp from one end that is identical to a 13-bp sequence that lies 4 bp from the site of integration into the chromosome (33). Possibly, proteins binding to the 13-bp site align the circular form with the preferred entry site before the actual integration event occurs.

CTn916 and other gram-positive bacterial conjugative transposons carry a single integrase gene located near the end of the element. The protein encoded by this gene is a member of the lambda family of integrases (33, 34). Although there is relatively little amino acid sequence identity between the integrases of CTn916 and lambda outside the catalytic region of the protein, all of the residues in the catalytic region of lambda integrase that are known to be essential for lambda excision are found in the CTn916 integrase sequence. Downstream of the *int* gene on CTn916 is a small gene that encodes a small basic protein similar to lambda Xis. Whether this gene plays a role analogous to that encoding lambda Xis remains to be established. The fact that the integrase of CTn916 appeared to be more similar to lambda integrase than to transposases or restriction enzymes was very perplexing at first, because the model proposed for CTn916 excision—a model that has so far been supported by all available evidence—seemed so different from the model proposed for lambda integration. In particular, there was no region of identity between the chromosomal *att* site and the joined ends of the circular intermediate. Thus, strand migration, a staple of the model for lambda integration, could not occur. Nonetheless, lambda does integrate in secondary sites where there is little or no identity between the *att* site on the phage and the target site. Recently, Nunes-Duby et al. (25) have proposed a strand-swapping model for phage lambda integration in which branch migration does not occur. If this model is correct, it brings the mechanism of lambda integration much closer to that proposed for integration of CTn916.

An important advance in testing the model proposed for CTn916 was the overproduction and purification of the CTn916 integrase by Lu and Churchward (20). Using the purified integrase, they showed that the integrase binds to sequences that overlap the joint between the ends of CTn916 and adjacent chromosomal DNA. More recently, Taylor and Churchward (44) have shown that the purified integrase makes staggered cuts in the expected places and forms a covalent bond with the integrase, as expected on the basis of similarities to lambda integrase. The finding that CTn916 integrase binds to sequences in adjacent chromosomal DNA as well as to sequences at the end of CTn916 helps to explain the previous observation of Jaworski and Clewell (14) that the frequency of excision of CTn916 could vary as much as 1,000-fold depending on the sequences adjacent to the ends of the integrated copy of CTn916. Taylor and Churchward (44) found that binding of integrase to sites associated with high excision frequencies was stronger than binding to sites associated with low excision frequencies.

Not much is known about the integrase genes of *Bacteroides* conjugative transposons, but since their integration and excision seem to resemble those of CTn916, it seems likely that their integrases are members of the lambda integrase family. The integrating *Streptomyces* plasmids also have a lambda-type integrase (3). Since lambda-type integrases seem to be a common theme among conjugative transposons and related elements, the presence of a lambda-type integrase gene may be a good indicator of the presence of a conjugative transposon. A word of caution is in order, however. The types of lambdoid integrase genes found so far on most conjugative transposons are not easy to spot in Blast searches and must be checked at the amino acid level for the conserved amino acid signature.

Transfer Step

Most of the coding capacity of CTn*916*—the smallest known conjugative transposon—is devoted to the genes encoding proteins that comprise the mating machinery and proteins that nick at the transfer origin to begin the transfer process. Not much can be said about the mechanism of CTn*916* at this point because no biochemical studies of the mating bridge proteins have been done. The location of the transfer origin (*oriT*) has recently been determined (15). Two noteworthy aspects of the transfer region of CTn*916* are its small size (about 12 kbp) and the lack of homologies to known transfer gene sequences. The small size may be because this is a pilin-independent type of conjugal system. A large portion of the much larger transfer regions of conjugal plasmids is taken up by the pilin export and assembly genes. The transfer regions of conjugative transposons appear to be stripped-down versions of the transfer regions of conjugative plasmids. We are finding the same thing in the *Bacteroides* conjugative transposons: the transfer region is less than 16 kbp, and there are few homologs to known plasmid transfer genes (4). Similarly, the transfer origin (*oriT*) regions of CTn*916* and CTn*DOT* (from *Bacteroides*) have virtually no similarity to each other or to the *oriT* sequences from *E. coli-Pseudomonas* group plasmids (19). Thus, the failure to find homologs of known transfer genes does not rule out the transmissibility of a PAI. Sequence gazing is a notoriously unreliable way to find *oriT* regions. There is a simple way to test directly for *oriT* function: clone the proposed *oriT* region in a nonmobilizable plasmid and examine whether it is mobilized in *trans* by the PAI (18, 42). A note of caution is in order here too: a positive result is interpretable as a ''yes'' answer, but a negative result may simply mean that the mobilization proteins do not work in *trans* well enough for their activities to be detectable.

REGULATION OF TRANSFER AND OTHER ACTIVITIES

Excision and transfer of at least some of the conjugative transposons are stimulated by the antibiotic tetracycline (29, 33, 39). This stimulation is seen only with tetracycline and its derivatives, not with other protein synthesis-inhibiting antibiotics. For CTn*916,* the increase in transfer frequency produced by exposure to tetracycline was only about 20- to 50-fold (39) but Rice et al. (29) detected what appeared to be a higher fold enhancement of excision of a CTn*916*-related element, CTn*5381,* in *Enterococcus faecalis.* Therefore, the host in which the element is located, as well as features of the element itself, may dictate to what extent tetracycline controls conjugative transposon activities. For *Bacteroides* conjugative transposons of the CTn*DOT* type, tetracycline is required to see any excision and transfer at all, and the increase in transfer frequency when tetracycline is present is at least 1,000-fold (33). This is not true of all *Bacteroides* conjugative transposons. CTn*7853* and CTn*12256* transfer constitutively (33).

The elements whose excision and transfer are regulated by tetracycline illustrate how antibiotic use may be stimulating the spread of resistance genes as well as selecting for strains that acquire them. There is an important lesson in the tetracycline induction story for people interested in learning whether PAIs are transmissible: it may be necessary to have the right inducing conditions to detect transmission. If someone had not stumbled, quite by accident, across the tetracycline effect, the transmissibility of the *Bacteroides* conjugative transposons would have been missed completely.

The mechanism for regulation of the excision and transfer of gram-positive bacterial conjugative transposons has not been determined. At least part of the regulatory machinery of the *Bacteroides* conjugative transposons of the CTn*DOT* type has been identified. There are three genes located near *tetQ* on the element, i.e., *rteA, rteB,* and *rteC,* which are essential for transfer of the element and appear to be part of the regulatory apparatus that responds to tetracycline stimulation (33). RteA and RteB look like a classical two-component regulatory system at the amino acid sequence level, but the way in which they work is still under study. RteC has an apparent DNA binding motif, but here, too, there is no direct proof that this is in fact a regulatory protein.

INTERACTION WITH OTHER CONJUGAL ELEMENTS

Coresident Plasmids

Conjugative transposons are very interactive elements. Like self-transmissible plasmids, they can mobilize coresident plasmids in *trans,* by providing the mating apparatus, or in *cis,* by integrating into the plasmid to form a self-transmissible chimera. One sign that a conjugative transposon is in a bacterial strain is the transfer of a plasmid too small to be capable of self-transfer. The mobilization region of a mobilizable *Bacteroides* plasmid has been analyzed in some detail, and it bears little relationship to mobilization regions of plasmids of the *E. coli* phylogenetic group (41). This is somewhat surprising because *Bacteroides* plasmids that are mobilized by *Bacteroides* conjugative transposons are also mobilized by the IncP plasmids RK2 and R751 (33).

The *Bacteroides* conjugative transposons can also act in *trans* to trigger excision and circularization of unlinked and apparently unrelated integrated elements called nonreplicating *Bacteroides* units (NBUs) (36–38). The circular form of the NBU is then mobilized in *trans* by the conjugative transposon to the recipient, where the NBU integrates into the chromosome. NBUs and NBU-type elements are described in more detail in the next section. Less is known about the ability of gram-positive bacterial conjugative transposons to mobilize coresident plasmids, and so the extent to which these conjugative transposons play a role in plasmid transfer is still unknown. Nothing analogous to the NBUs has yet been found in the gram-positive bacteria.

Tn*4555* and the NBUs

NBU1, NBU2, and Tn*4555* are integrated elements of 10 to 12 kbp that are excised and transferred in *trans* by *Bacteroides* conjugative transposons (33). At first they appeared to be very closely related to each other, because the sequences of the mobilization regions of these three elements were very similar (18, 40, 41). The mobilization region is located near the middle of all three elements and consists of an *oriT* and a single *mob* protein. This small region is all that is needed to allow the circular form to be mobilized by the conjugative transposon. This is somewhat unusual, because mobilizable plasmids have at least two mobilization genes, one that encodes the protein that binds and nicks at the *oriT* and one that encodes a helicase that aids in strand separation. Apparently, the single *mob* gene on NBU1, NBU2, and Tn*4555* carries out both of these functions.

A surprising finding was that NBU1 and NBU2, and presumably Tn*4555* as well, are not only mobilized out of *Bacteroides* by the conjugative transposons but can also be mobilized out of *E. coli* by IncP plasmids, RK2 and R751 (18). Since the IncP plasmids have so far proven to have no sequence similarities to the conjugative transposons and the transfer origin of NBU1 bears no resemblance to the transfer origins of plasmids mobilized by R751 and RK2, this finding was unexpected. It demonstrates, however, that mobilization regions can be promiscuous. On the other side of the NBU1 *oriT* from the *mob* gene is a gene that encodes a protein with high amino acid similarity to the N-terminal half of chromosomally encoded primases (18). The function of this gene is still unknown, but it is part of the region shared by NBU1 and NBU2. Outside this region, however, the sequence similarity between NBU1 and NBU2 drops off abruptly, and the remaining part of these three elements is quite dissimilar.

NBU1, NBU2, and Tn*4555* may have different integration mechanisms. Tribble et al. (45) have shown that Tn*4555* integrates and excises similarly to CTn*916*. Like CTn*916*, Tn*4555* integrates into many different sites, although it has a preferred site in *Bacteroides fragilis* that is not found in other *Bacteroides* species. By contrast, NBU1 integrates site specifically in *Bacteroides* into a site that is identical to a 13-bp sequence formed by the joined ends of the circular form, thus creating a 13-bp duplication at its ends (38). The integration site is in the 3′ end of a leucine-tRNA gene, a type of target favored by lambdoid phages (6, 36). The integrase of NBU1 is a member of the lambda integrase family, as is the integrase of Tn*4555* (38). In *E. coli*, NBU1 integrates more randomly than in *Bacteroides*, but when a primary site was provided in *E. coli*, integration into this site occurred at more than a 10-fold-higher frequency than into sites with less homology to the joined ends of NBU1 (37). Thus, NBU1 seems more lambda-like, whereas Tn*4555* seems more like CTn*916*. The integration mechanism of NBU2 has not been established. The integrase gene is in the lambda integrase family, but NBU2 integrase is actually less closely related to NBU1 integrase than the NBU1 integrase is to lambda integrase (48). The picture that is beginning to emerge from all this is of a mobile DNA segment containing an *oriT*, a *mob* gene, and in some cases a primase homolog, a segment that has been inserted in a variety of different elements, including some plasmids as well as integrated elements (41). There is no room on the conserved segment for transposase genes; therefore, presumably the segment was integrated by functions encoded elsewhere. DNA that hybridizes to this mobilization segment is widespread in *Bacteroides* isolates, and it remains to be seen how many different elements this mobilization segment has invaded.

ARE CONJUGATIVE TRANSPOSONS A COHERENT GROUP?

As the diversity of elements called conjugative transposons increases, the question arises of the rules for inclusion in this group. CTn*916* should obviously be considered the prototype. One criterion could be that all elements in the group must integrate and excise by the same mechanism as CTn*916*. However, if we accept the argument that phage lambda may integrate by a very similar process, even though it looks different at the DNA sequence level and is more site specific, this criterion is clearly not sufficient unless we are willing to call bacteriophages conjugative transposons. The ability to transfer by conjugation is another obvious criterion. Then, is Tn*4555,* which integrates and excises like CTn*916* and can be transferred by conjugation, a conjugative transposon even though it must be mobilized by other elements whereas CTn*916* carries all of the genes needed to transfer itself? Target site specificity is another possible criterion, but this is also problematic if the element is more site specific in one host than in another. For the time being, the best strategy is to await further developments and hope that a better understanding of various integrated, transmissible elements will reveal shared features that make it more obvious how these elements should be grouped. What is likely to happen, however, is that more detailed information about conjugative transposons will confirm that there are no discrete groups but, rather, a continuum of element types that includes the lambdoid phages and the integrating actinomycete plasmids.

REFERENCES

1. **Alarcon-Chaidez, F., J. Sampath, P. Srinivas, and M. N. Vijayakumar.** 1997. Tn*5252*: a model for complex streptococcal conjugative transposons. *Adv. Exp. Med. Biol.* **418:**1029–1032.
2. **Bannam, T. L., P. K. Crellin, and J. I. Rood.** 1995. Molecular genetics of the chloramphenicol-resistance transposon Tn*4551* from *Clostridium perfringens:* the TnpX site-specific recombinase excises a circular transposon intermediate. *Mol. Microbiol.* **16:**535–551.
3. **Boccard, F., T. Smokvina, J.-L. Pernodet, A. Friedmann, and M. Guerineau.** 1989. The integrated conjugative plasmid pSAM2 of *Streptomyces ambofaciens* is related to temperate bacteriophages. *EMBO J.* **8:**973–980.
4. **Bonheyo, G., and A. A. Salyers.** Unpublished data.
5. **Brown, D. P., K. B. Idler, and L. Katz.** 1990. Characterization of the genetic elements required for site-specific integration of plasmid pSE211 in *Saccharopolyspora erythraea. J. Bacteriol.* **172:**1877–1888.
6. **Campbell, A.** 1992. Chromosomal insertion sites for phages and plasmids. *J. Bacteriol.* **174:**7495–7499.
7. **Clewell, D. B., S. E. Flannagan, and D. D. Jaworski.** 1995. Unconstrained bacterial promiscuity: the Tn*916*-Tn*1545* family of conjugative transposons. *Trends Microbiol.* **3:**229–236.
8. **Cooper, A. J., A. P. Kalinowski, N. B. Shoemaker, and A. A. Salyers.** 1997. Construction and characterization of a *Bacteroides thetaiotaomicron recA* mutant: transfer of *Bacteroides* integrated conjugative elements is RecA independent. *J. Bacteriol.* **179:**6221–6227.
9. **Cooper, A. J., N. B. Shoemaker, and A. A. Salyers.** 1996. The erythromycin resistance gene from the *Bacteroides* conjugative transposon Tc^{r}Em^{r}7853 is nearly identical to *ermG* from *Bacillus sphaericus. Antimicrob. Agents Chemother.* **40:**506–508.
10. **Datta, S., A. Pal, S. Basu, and P. C. Banergee.** 1997. Involvement of a 70 bp plasmid of the epidemic *Shigella dysenteriae* type 1 (Dt66) strain in drug-resistance, lipopolysaccharide synthesis and virulence. *Microb. Drug Resist.* **3:**351–357.
11. **Gardner, R. G., J. B. Russell, D. B. Wilson, G.-R. Wang, and N. B. Shoemaker.** 1996. Use of a modified *Bacteroides-Prevotella* shuttle vector to transfer a reconstructed β-1,4-D-endoglycanase gene into *Bacteroides uniformis* and *Prevotella ruminicola* B$_1$4. *Appl. Environ. Microbiol.* **62:**196–202.
12. **Handwerger, S., and J. Skoble.** 1995. Identification of chromosomal mobile element conferring high-level vancomycin resistance in *Enterococcus faecium. Antimicrob. Agents Chemother.* **39:**2446–2453.
13. **Hochhut, B., K. Jahreis, J. W. Lengeler, and K. Schmid.** 1997. CTn*scr94*, a conjugative transposon found in enterobacteria. *J. Bacteriol.* **179:**2097–2102.
14. **Jaworski, D. D., and D. B. Clewell.** 1994. Evidence that coupling sequences play a frequency-determining role in conjugative transposition of Tn*916. J. Bacteriol.* **176:**3328–3335.
15. **Jaworski, D. D., S. E. Flannagan, and D. B. Clewell.** 1996. Analyses of *traA, int-Tn,* and *xis-Tn* mutations in the conjugative transposon Tn*916* in *Enterococcus faecalis. Plasmid* **36:**201–208.
16. **Lacroix, J.-M., and C. B. Walker.** 1995. Detection and incidence of the tetracycline resistance determinant *tet(M)* in the microflora associated with adult periodontitis. *J. Periodontol.* **66:**102–108.
17. **Leng, Z., D. E. Riley, R. E. Berge, J. N. Krieger, and M. C. Roberts.** 1997. Distribution and mobility of the tetracycline resistance determinant *tetQ. J. Antimicrob. Chemother.* **40:**551–559.

18. **Li, L.-Y., N. B. Shoemaker, G.-R. Wang, S. P. Cole, M. Hashimoto, J. Wang, and A. A. Salyers.** 1995. The mobilization regions of two integrated *Bacteroides* elements, NBU1 and NBU2, have only a single mobilization protein and may be on a cassette. *J. Bacteriol.* **177:**3940–3945.

19. **Li, L.-Y., N. B. Shoemaker, and A. A. Salyers.** 1995. Localization and characterization of the transfer origin of a *Bacteroides* conjugative transposon. *J. Bacteriol.* **177:**4992–4999.

20. **Lu, F., and G. Churchward.** 1995. Tn*916* sequences bind the C-terminal domain of integrase protein with different affinities that correlate with transposon insertion frequency. *J. Bacteriol.* **177:**1938–1946.

21. **Manganelli, R., S. Ricci, and G. Pozzi.** 1997. The joint of Tn*916* circular intermediates is a homoduplex in *Enterococcus faecalis*. *Plasmid* **38:**71–78.

22. **Mazodier, P., C. Thompson, and F. Boccard.** 1990. The chromosomal integration site of the *Streptomyces* element pSAM2 overlaps a putative tRNA gene conserved among actinomycetes. *Mol. Gen. Genet.* **222:** 431–434.

23. **Nikolich, M., G. Hong, N. Shoemaker, and A. A. Salyers.** 1994. Evidence that conjugal transfer of a tetracycline resistance gene (*tetQ*) has occurred very recently in nature between the normal microflora of animals and the normal microflora of humans. *Appl. Environ. Microbiol.* **60:**3255–3260.

24. **Nikolich, M. P., N. B. Shoemaker, and A. A. Salyers.** 1994. Characterization of a new type of *Bacteroides* conjugative transposon, Tc^rEm^r7853. *J. Bacteriol.* **176:**6606–6612.

25. **Nunes-Duby, S. E., M. A. Azaro, and A. Landy.** 1995. Swapping DNA strands and sensing homology without branch migration in lambda site-specific recombination. *Curr. Biol.* **5:**139–148.

26. **Oggioni, M. R., C. G. Dowson, J. M. Smith, R. Provvedi, and G. Pozzi.** 1996. The tetracycline resistance gene *tet(M)* exhibits mosaic structure. *Plasmid* **35:**156–163.

27. **Paszkhiet, B., and A. A. Salyers.** Unpublished data.

28. **Rauch, P. J., and W. M. de Vos.** 1994. Identification and characterization of genes involved in excision of the *Lactococcus lactis* conjugative transposon Tn*5276*. *J. Bacteriol.* **176:**2165–2171.

29. **Rice, L. B., S. H. Marshall, and L. L. Carias.** 1992. Tn*5381*, a conjugative transposon identifiable as a circular form in *Enterococcus faecalis*. *J. Bacteriol.* **174:**7308–7315.

30. **Rudy, C. K., and J. R. Scott.** 1994. Length of the coupling sequence of Tn*916*. *J. Bacteriol.* **176:**3386–3388.

31. **Salyers, A. A., and N. B. Shoemaker.** 1996. Resistance gene transfer in anaerobes: new insights, new problems. *Clin. Infect. Dis.* **23**(Suppl.):S36–S43.

32. **Salyers, A. A., and N. B. Shoemaker.** 1997. Conjugative transposons. *Genet. Eng.* **19:**89–99.

33. **Salyers, A. A., N. B. Shoemaker, L. Y. Li, and A. M. Stevens.** 1995. Conjugative transposons: an unusual and diverse set of integrated gene transfer elements. *Microbiol. Rev.* **59:**579–590.

34. **Scott, J. R., and G. C. Churchward.** 1995. Conjugative transposition. *Annu. Rev. Microbiol.* **49:**367–397.

35. **Scott, K. P., T. M. Barbosa, K. J. Forbes, and H. J. Flint.** 1997. High-frequency transfer of a naturally occurring chromosomal tetracycline resistance element in the ruminal anaerobe *Butyrivibrio fibrisolvens*. *Appl. Environ. Microbiol.* **63:**3405–3411.

36. **Shoemaker, N. B., G. R. Wang, and A. A. Salyers.** 1996. The *Bacteroides* mobilizable insertion element, NBU1, integrates into the 3′ end of a tRNA gene and has an integrase that is a member of the lambda integrase family. *J. Bacteriol.* **178:**3594–3600.

37. **Shoemaker, N. B., G. R. Wang, and A. A. Salyers.** 1996. NBU1, a mobilizable site-specific integrated element from *Bacteroides* spp., can integrate nonspecifically in *Escherichia coli*. *J. Bacteriol.* **178:** 3601–3607.

38. **Shoemaker, N. B., G.-R. Wang. A. M. Stevens, and A. A. Salyers.** 1993. Excision, transfer and integration of NBU1, a mobilizable site-selective insertion element. *J. Bacteriol.* **175:**6578–6586.

39. **Showsh, S. A., and R. E. Andrews.** 1992. Tetracycline enhances Tn*916*-mediated conjugal transfer. *Plasmid* **28:**213–224.

40. **Smith, C. J., and A. C. Parker.** 1993. Identification of a circular intermediate in the transfer and transposition of Tn*4555*, a mobilizable transposon from *Bacteroides* spp. *J. Bacteriol.* **175:**2682–2691.

41. **Smith, C. J., and A. C. Parker.** 1996. A gene product related to TraI is required for the mobilization of *Bacteroides* mobilizable transposons and plasmids. *Mol. Microbiol.* **20:**741–750.

42. **Srinivas, P., A. O. Kilic, and M. N. Vijayakumar.** 1997. Site-specific nicking *in vitro* at *oriT* by the DNA relaxase of Tn*5252*. *Plasmid* **37:**42–50.

43. **Swartley, J. S., C. F. McAlister, R. A. Hajjeh, D. W. Heinrich, and D. S. Stephens.** 1993. Deletions of Tn*916*-like transposons are implicated in *tetM*-mediated resistance in pathogenic *Neisseria*. *Mol. Microbiol.* **10:**299–310.

44. **Taylor, K. L., and G. Churchward.** 1997. Specific DNA cleavage mediated by the integrase of conjugative transposon Tn*916*. *J. Bacteriol.* **179:**1117–1125.

45. **Tribble, G. D., A. C. Parker, and C. J. Smith.** 1997. The *Bacteroides* mobilizable transposon Tn*4555* integrates by a site-specific recombination mechanism similar to that of the gram-positive bacterial element Tn*916*. *J. Bacteriol.* **179:**2731–2739.

46. **Vogli, M., and S. N. Cohen.** 1992. The chromosomal integration site for the *Streptomyces* plasmid SLP1 is a functional tRNA[Tyr] gene essential for cell viability. *Mol. Microbiol.* **6:**3041–3050.

47. **Waldor, M. K., H. Tschape, and J. J. Mekalanos.** 1996. A new type of conjugative transposon encodes resistance to sulfamethoxazole, trimethoprim, and streptomycin in *Vibrio cholerae* O139. *J. Bacteriol.* **178:** 4157–4165.

48. **Wang, J., and A. A. Salyers.** Unpublished data.

INDEX